Maimonides *Commentary on Hippocrates'* Aphorisms

Volume 1

The Medical Works
of Moses Maimonides

Series Editor

Gerrit Bos (*Cologne*)

VOLUME 14/1

The titles published in this series are listed at *brill.com/mwmm*

This series, now published by Brill, used to be part of the

Middle Eastern Texts Initiative

Founding Editor

Daniel C. Peterson

Director

D. Morgan Davis

∴

The Medical Works of Moses Maimonides

Academic Board

Gerrit Bos (*University of Cologne*), *general editor*
Lawrence I. Conrad (*University of Hamburg*)
Alfred I. Ivry (*New York University*)
Y. Tzvi Langermann (*Bar Ilan University, Israel*)
Michael R. McVaugh (*University of North Carolina, Chapel Hill*)

∴

NEAL A. MAXWELL INSTITUTE
FOR RELIGIOUS SCHOLARSHIP
BRIGHAM YOUNG UNIVERSITY

Maimonides
Commentary on Hippocrates' Aphorisms

*A New Parallel Arabic-English Edition and Translation,
with Critical Editions of the Medieval
Hebrew Translations*

VOLUME 1

By

Gerrit Bos

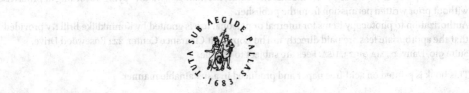

BRILL

LEIDEN | BOSTON

Cover illustration: MS Paris, BN, héb. 1103, fol. 45ᵛ, the beginning of Maimonides' *Talkhīṣ K. Ḥīlat al-burʾ* (*Summary of Galen's "De Methodo Medendi"*). The illumination hails from the workshop of Ferrer and Arnau Bassa in Barcelona. Cf. M. Garel, *D'une main forte: Manuscrits hébreux des collections françaises*, Paris 1991, no. 48. The cover design is a copy of the original design by Brigham Young University Press.

Library of Congress Cataloging-in-Publication Data

Names: Maimonides, Moses, 1135–1204, author. | Maimonides, Moses, 1135–1204.
  Sharḥ fuṣūl Abuqrāṭ. Arabic. | Maimonides, Moses, 1135–1204. Sharḥ fuṣūl
  Abuqrāṭ. English. | Maimonides, Moses, 1135–1204. Sharḥ fuṣūl Abuqrāṭ.
  Hebrew. | Bos, Gerrit, 1948- translator, editor. | Maimonides, Moses, 1135–1204.
  Medical works of Moses Maimonides.
Title: Maimonides, Commentary on Hippocrates' Aphorisms : a new parallel
  Arabic-English edition and translation, with critical editions of the medieval
  Hebrew translations / by Gerrit Bos.
Other titles: Commentary on Hippocrates' Aphorisms
Description: Leiden ; Boston : Brill, 2020. | Series: The medical works of Moses
  Maimonides, 2589-6946 ; volume 14 | Includes bibliographical references and
  index. | Introduction in English; text in Arabic and parallel English translation,
  Hebrew.
Identifiers: LCCN 2019048195 (print) | LCCN 2019048196 (ebook) |
  ISBN 9789004412873 (hardback) | ISBN 9789004412880 (ebook)
Subjects: LCSH: Hippocrates. Aphorisms. | Medicine–Aphorisms–Early works to
  1800.
Classification: LCC R126.H6 A859 2020 (print) | LCC R126.H6 (ebook) |
  DDC 610–dc23
LC record available at https://lccn.loc.gov/2019048195
LC ebook record available at https://lccn.loc.gov/2019048196

Typeface for the Latin, Greek, and Cyrillic scripts: "Brill". See and download: brill.com/brill-typeface.

ISSN 2589-6946
ISBN 978-90-04-42566-8 (hardback, set)
ISBN 978-90-04-41287-3 (hardback, vol. 1)   ISBN 978-90-04-41288-0 (e-book, vol. 1)
ISBN 978-90-04-42552-1 (hardback, vol. 2)   ISBN 978-90-04-42553-8 (e-book, vol. 2)

Copyright 2020 by Koninklijke Brill NV, Leiden, The Netherlands.
Koninklijke Brill NV incorporates the imprints Brill, Brill Hes & De Graaf, Brill Nijhoff, Brill Rodopi, Brill Sense, Hotei Publishing, mentis Verlag, Verlag Ferdinand Schöningh and Wilhelm Fink Verlag.

Contents

Preface

Hippocrates' *Aphorisms* enjoyed great popularity in the ancient and medieval world. According to Maimonides, it was Hippocrates' most useful work as it contains aphorisms, which every physician should know by heart. He adds that he even saw how non-physicians have schoolchildren memorize them in school, so that subsequently people who are not physicians know many of these aphorisms by heart from learning them in school. The *Aphorisms* were very popular in Jewish circles as well. They were translated into Hebrew several times, the earliest dated translation written on the basis of an unknown Latin *Vorlage* between 1197 and 1199 by an anonymous author who—after his conversion to Christianity—called himself Doeg ha-Edomi. Other translations based on the Latin version by Constantine the African are by Hillel ben Samuel of Verona (ca. 1220–1295) and possibly by Judah (Astruc) ben Samuel Shalom (ca. 1450). Ḥunayn ibn Isḥāq's Arabic version of Hippocrates' *Aphorisms*—i.e., of the lemmata in Galen's commentary—was the basis for the translation by Nathan ha-Me'ati and the otherwise unknown Jacob bar Joseph ibn Zabara. However, it was Maimonides' commentary on Hippocrates' *Aphorisms* that was primarily responsible for the profound influence that the work had in Jewish circles. Maimonides' Arabic commentary was translated into Hebrew in the year 1260 by Moses ibn Tibbon (fl. 1244–1283). Other translations of Maimonides' commentary are that by R. Zeraḥyah ben Isaac ben She'altiel Ḥen (end of the thirteenth century) and by an anonymous author. An indication of the esteem in which Hippocrates' *Aphorisms* were held by generations of Jewish scholars is the fact that it was twice parodied, namely by the Provençal writer Maimón Gallipapa (fourteenth–fifteenth century?) and by the Haskalah satirist Isaac Erter (1791–1851) under the title *Pirkei ha-Zahav*.

The edition of Maimonides' Arabic commentary and its Hebrew translations is part of a project to critically edit Maimonides' medical works that have not been edited at all or have been edited in unreliable editions. The project started in 1995 at the University College London with the support of the Wellcome Trust and was continued at the University of Cologne with the support of the Deutsche Forschungsgemeinschaft. So far it resulted in the publication of critical editions of Maimonides' *On Asthma* (2 vols.), *Medical Aphorisms* (5 vols.), *On Poisons and the Protection against Lethal Drugs*, *On Hemorrhoids*, *On Rules Regarding the Practical Part of the Medical Art*, *On Coitus*, *On the Regimen of Health*, and *On the Elucidation of Some Symptoms and the Response to Them*.

The first ten volumes in the series were published by the Middle Eastern Texts Initiative at Brigham Young's Neal A. Maxwell Institute for Religious

Scholarship. From *On Coitus* on, the series is continued by E.J. Brill, Leiden. I thank Jessica Kley for her assistance, Felix Hedderich for compiling the Hebrew indexes and copy editing and proofreading the text, and also Fabian Käs for checking the proofs.

Introduction

1 Biography

Moses Maimonides, known by his Arab name, Abū 'Imrān Mūsā ibn 'Ubayd Allāh ibn Maymūn, and his Jewish name, Moshe ben Maimon, was not only one of the greatest Jewish philosophers and experts in Jewish law (*halakhah*),[1] but an eminent physician as well. Born in Córdoba in 1138,[2] he was forced to leave his native city at age thirteen because of persecutions by the fanatical Muslim regime known as the Almohads and the policy of religious intolerance adopted by them.[3] After a sojourn of about twelve years in southern Spain, the family moved to Fez in the Maghreb. Some years later, probably around 1165, they moved again because of the persecutions of the Jews in the Maghreb, this time going to Palestine. After staying there for some months, the family moved on to Egypt and settled in Fusṭāṭ, the ancient part of Cairo.

It was in Cairo that Maimonides started to practice and teach medicine, as well as pursue his commercial activities in the India trade.[4] He became physician to al-Qāḍī al-Fāḍil, the famous counsellor and secretary to Saladin.[5] Later,

---

1 For Maimonides' biographical data, see art. "Ibn Maymūn," in E.I.[2], vol. 3, pp. 876–878 (Vajda); art. "Maimonides, Moses," in *Encyclopaedia Judaica*, vol. 11, cols. 754–764 (Rabinowitz); Lewis, "Maimonides, Lionheart and Saladin," pp. 70–75; Goitein, "Ḥayyei ha-Rambam," pp. 29–42; idem, "Moses Maimonides, Man of Action," pp. 155–167; ed. Shailat, in Maimonides, *Iggerot ha-Rambam*, vol. 1, pp. 19–21; Cohen, "Maimonides' Egypt," pp. 21–34; Ben-Sasson, "Maimonides in Egypt," pp. 3–30; Levinger, "Was Maimonides 'Rais al-Yahud' in Egypt?," pp. 83–93; Davidson, "Maimonides' Putative Position," pp. 115–128; Kraemer, "Life of Moses ben Maimon," pp. 413–428; idem, "Maimonides' Intellectual Milieu in Cairo," pp. 1–37; for a fundamental discussion of all the available data concerning Maimonides' biography, see now: Davidson, *Moses Maimonides*, pp. 3–74, and Kraemer, *Maimonides*. For Maimonides' training and activity as a physician, see ed. Bos, introduction to Maimonides, *On Asthma*, vol. 1, pp. xxv–xxx, and idem, "Maimonides' Medical Works."

2 While traditionally, his date of birth is set at 1135, Maimonides himself wrote in 1168, in the colophon to his *Commentary on the Mishnah*, that he was then in Egypt and thirty years old; Goitein, "Moses Maimonides, Man of Action," p. 155, argued on the basis of this that the actual year of his birth should be put at 1138; see also Leibowitz, "Maimonides," pp. 75–76.

3 Following Graetz, *Geschichte der Juden*, vol. 7, p. 265, it is generally assumed that the family left Córdoba in the year 1148, when the city was conquered by the Almohads. Accordingly, Maimonides was ten.

4 Goitein, "Moses Maimonides, Man of Action," p. 163, has shown that Maimonides was already involved in this trade before his younger brother David perished in a shipwreck in 1169, and that he still had a hand in it in 1191 when he was practising as a physician.

5 See art. "al-Ḳāḍī al-Fāḍil," in E.I.[2], vol. 4, pp. 376–377 (Brockelmann/Cahen).

© KONINKLIJKE BRILL NV, LEIDEN, 2020 | DOI:10.1163/9789004412880_002

he became court physician of al-Malik al-Afḍal, after the latter's ascension to the throne in the winter of 1198/1199. It is generally assumed that Maimonides died in 1204. The theory, that for some years he served as *ra'īs*, or head of the Jewish community, is disputed. While Davidson argues against it,[6] Friedman argues in favour of it;[7] and according to Kraemer, Maimonides did serve as *ra'īs* for the Jews from September 1171 until 1173, to secure for the Jewish communities a favorable position with the Ayyubids who had replaced the Fatimids as the ruling dynasty.[8] After that, he performed many of the functions of *ra'īs* without holding the title, as his opponents held the office.[9] According to some sources, he served a second time in the 1190s, possibly between 1198 and 1199.[10]

2   Medical Works

Maimonides was a prolific author in the field of medicine, composing ten works considered as authentic.[11] These ten works consist of the following major compositions: 1. *Sharḥ fuṣūl Abuqrāṭ* (*Commentary on Hippocrates' Aphorisms*); 2. *K. al-sumūm wa-l-taḥarruz min al-adwiya al-qattāla* (*On Poisons and the Protection against Lethal Drugs*); 3. *Fuṣūl Mūsā fī l-ṭibb* (*Medical Aphorisms*); 4. *Mukhtaṣarāt li-kutub Jālīnūs* (*Epitomes from the Works of Galen*). The following treatises are considered minor works: 1. *K. fī l-jimāʿ* (*On Coitus*) probably written in 1190 or 1191 at the request of an anonymous high ranking client; 2. *Fī tadbīr al-ṣiḥḥa* (*On the Regimen of Health*), written at the request of al-Malik al-Afḍal; 3. *Maqāla fī bayān baʿḍ al-aʿrāḍ wa-l-jawāb ʿanhā* (*On the Elucidation of Some Symptoms and the Response to Them*), written for the same al-Malik al-Afḍal, when his condition did not improve; 4. *Sharḥ asmāʾ al-ʿuqqār* (*Commentary*

---

6   See Davidson, "Maimonides' Putative Position."

7   See Friedman, "Ha-Rambam 'Ra'īs al-Yahūd' be-Miẓrayim."

8   See Kraemer, *Maimonides*, pp. 191–192, 222–226.

9   I thank Yoel Kraemer for this personal information.

10   See Kraemer, *Maimonides*, p. 227.

11   For his medical works, see Meyerhof, "Medical Work of Maimonides," pp. 265–299; Friedenwald, *Jews and Medicine*, vol. 1, pp. 200–216; Baron, *Social and Religious History of the Jews*, vol. 8, pp. 259–262; Ullmann, *Medizin im Islam*, pp. 167–169; art. "Maimonides, Moses," in *Encyclopaedia Judaica*, vol. 11, cols. 777–779 (Muntner); ed. Avishur, in Maimonides, *Shivḥei ha-Rambam*, pp. 33–36; Ackermann, "Moses Maimonides;" ed. Bos, introduction to Maimonides, *On Asthma*, vol. 1, pp. xxxi–xxxii; Davidson, *Moses Maimonides*, pp. 429–483; Langermann, "Œuvre médicale de Maïmonide," pp. 275–302. For a survey of editors and translators of Maimonides' medical works, see Dienstag, "Translators and Editors," pp. 95–135; for Muntner's activity, see esp. pp. 116–121.

on the Names of Drugs); 5. *Risāla fī l-bawāsīr* (*On Hemorrhoids*); 6. *Maqāla fī l-rabw* (*On Asthma*). In addition to these ten works featuring in the current bio-bibliographical literature, Maimonides is the author of the *K. Qawānīn al-juz' al-'amalī min ṣinā'a al-ṭibb* (*On Rules Regarding the Practical Part of the Medical Art*).

3   Maimonides' *Commentary on Hippocrates'* Aphorisms[12]

Maimonides composed the *Commentary* at an unknown date, after the *Epitomes from the Works of Galen*[13] and after the *Medical Aphorisms*, which he quotes in aphorism 2.33 (85). At the same time, however, the *Commentary* seems to have been composed before his treatise *On Asthma*, as the *Commentary* is quoted there in section 13.19.[14] Maimonides gives the following explanation for his decision to compose a commentary on the *Aphorisms* and not upon one of the other Hippocratic works:

> And since I consider Hippocrates' *Aphorisms* to be the most useful of the books [he composed], I decided to explain them; for these are aphorisms, which every physician should know by heart. I have even seen how non-physicians have schoolchildren memorize them, so that [subsequently] people who are not physicians know many of these aphorisms by heart from learning them as young children at school.[15]

For the composition of his commentary, Maimonides consulted the *Aphorisms* as they were transmitted through the commentary composed by Galen of Pergamum, and translated by Ḥunayn ibn Isḥāq al-'Ibādī (809–873). In his *Risāla ilā 'Alī b. Yaḥyā* ... (*Missive to 'Alī b. Yaḥyā*),[16] a detailed survey of the various translations of Galen's works as available at his time, Ḥunayn remarks that

---

12   For an adapted version of the introduction, cf. NM 3, pp. 11–13.

13   Cf. preface (13): "Every explanation that I will mention anonymously is that of Galen, according to its sense (figuratively), for I do not envisage (intend) to be precise in [quoting] his words as I did in the *Epitomes* [from Galen's writings]." For the *Epitomes*, see Bos, "Maimonides on Medicinal Measures and Weights."

14   Maimonides, *On Asthma* 13.19, trans. Bos, vol. 1, p. 91: "Consequently, a lifetime is too short to attain perfection in even one part of it, as I explained in my commentary to Hippocrates' *Aphorisms*."

15   Cf. preface (12).

16   Ḥunayn, *Syrische und arabische Galen-Übersetzungen*, ed. and trans. Bergsträsser. See also Bergsträsser, *Neue Materialien*; Käs, "Neue Handschrift."

he first corrected the poor Syriac translation of Galen's commentary by Ayyūb[17] and the even poorer one by Jibrīl ibn Bakhtīshūʿ through collating these versions with the Greek.[18] Ḥunayn remarks, if I understand his words correctly, that he first translated Galen's commentary and then added this translation to that of the Hippocratic *Aphorisms* themselves.[19] Following the revised Syriac version, he prepared an Arabic translation in two phases, a first part at the request of Abū l-Ḥassan Aḥmad ibn al-Mudabbir (d. 883 or 884), who was a high official, courtier, and man of letters in Bagdad, Damascus, and Fusṭāṭ.[20] As for Arabic translations of the *Aphorisms* themselves, we know about at least two translations, one from the hand of Ḥunayn and another earlier one from an anonymous source.[21]

On occasion, Ḥunayn's translation of the *Aphorisms* deviates from the Greek text as it has come down to us.[22] Since Maimonides consulted the Arabic translation of the *Aphorisms* by Ḥunayn, such deviations recur in his commentary. For instance in aphorism 4.36 (173), the twenty-fourth day is missing in the Greek Hippocrates and in the Greek Galen[23] but features in the Arabic Hippocrates and Arabic Galen. And in aphorism 7.32 (384), Maimonides' statement هذا بيّن ويريد بقوله رقيقا أنْ يكون أعلى الثفل رقيق فيكون شكله صنوبري) This is clear. With

---

17   I.e., Ayyūb al-Ruḥāwī al-Abrash (d. 835). For this translator into Syriac, cf. Baumstark, *Geschichte der syrischen Literatur*, p. 230; Meyerhof, "New Light on Ḥunayn Ibn Isḥāq," pp. 703–704.; Ullmann, *Medizin im Islam*, p. 101; Strohmaier, "Syrischer und arabischer Galen," p. 2001. See also Barry, *Syriac Medicine*, p. xviii. Unfortunately, this study was only published after the completion of the manuscript of my edition. Therefore, it could only be used cursorily.

18   Cf. Ḥunayn, *Syrische und arabische Galen-Übersetzungen* §8, ed. and trans. Bergsträsser, p. 40: وقد كان ترجمه أيوب ترجمة رديئة ورام جبريل بن بختيشوع إصلاحه فزاده فسادا فقابلت به اليوناني وأصلحتُه إصلاحا شبيها بالترجمة. For Jibrīl ibn Bakhtīshūʿ, cf. Baumstark, ibid., p. 227; Meyerhof, ibid., p. 705; Ullmann, ibid., p. 109; art. "Bukhtīshūʿ," in E.I.², vol. 1, p. 1298 (Sourdel).

19   Cf. Ḥunayn, ibid.: وأضفتُ اليه فصّ كلام بقراط على حدّته. Pormann/Joosse, "Commentaries on Hippocratic *Aphorisms*," p. 217, translate the Arabic فصّ كلام بقراط as: "the essence of Hippocrates' text."

20   For Abū l-Ḥassan Aḥmad ibn al-Mudabbir, cf. art. "Ibn al-Mudabbir," in E.I.², vol. 3, pp. 879–880 (Gottschalk).

21   Cf. Klamroth, "Ueber Auszüge aus griechischen Schriftstellern," pp. 196–198; Bergsträsser, *Ḥunain b. Isḥāḳ und seine Schule*, p. 51; Ullmann, *Medizin im Islam*, p. 28. The Arabic translation by Ḥunayn has been edited by John Tytler.

22   For the Greek text, I consulted the following editions: Hippocrates, *Aphorisms*, ed. and trans. Littré, vol. 4, pp. 458–609; ed. and trans. Jones, pp. 97–221.

23   For Galen's commentary, cf. Galen, *In Hippocratis Aphorismos commentarius*, ed. Kühn, vol. 17b, pp. 345–887; and vol. 18a, pp. 1–195.

"thin" he means that the upper part of the sediment is thin and that its shape is like that of pine nuts) does not feature in Galen's commentary, but is derived from Ḥunayn's additional statement to his translation (S, fols. 145ᵇ–146ᵃ), that it is shaped like a cone (مخرط).[24] Instead of Ḥunayn's مخرط (shaped like a cone), which is a mathematical term, Maimonides uses the botanical term صنوبري (like a pine nut). In addition to these textual differences, aphorisms 7.63–87 are missing both in Ḥunayn's translation of the *Aphorisms* and in Maimonides' commentary.[25]

And in cases where Ḥunayn's Arabic translation of Hippocrates' *Aphorisms* themselves deviates from his translation of the *Aphorisms* in Galen's commentary, Maimonides' version usually agrees with that of the Galenic text. For instance, in aphorism 5.25 (245), Maimonides states وسكّن الوجع بإحداثه الخدر (the pain is relieved because it causes numbness) which conforms to the Arabic Galen, whereas the Arabic Hippocrates has: وسكّن الوجع بما يحدث من الخدر. And in aphorism 5.45 (265), Maimonides' version تقعير الرحم (lit., the fundus of the uterus; Greek αἱ κοτυληδόνες; i.e., cotyledons) is a variant of the Arabic Galen قعر الرحم, whereas the Arabic Hippocrates has نقر الرحم. In a few cases, however, Maimonides' version agrees with that of the Arabic Hippocrates and deviates from that of the Arabic Galen, as, for instance, in aphorism 4.32 (169), where Maimonides has من انتشل من مرض (if someone is recovering from an illness) for the Greek Ὁκόσοισι δὲ ἀνισταμένοισιν ἐκ τῶν νούσων,[26] whereas the Arabic Galen has من انتعش من مرض.[27]

In addition to the reason for composing his commentary on Hippocrates' *Aphorisms* quoted above, Maimonides gives four reasons for composing a commentary to a certain work in general:

1. The brevity of the text; its meaning may be clear to the author himself, but not to the reader, especially not in later generations.

---

24 Cf. S, fols. 145ᵇ–146ᵃ: إنّ اللفظة التي يسمّي بها أبقراط الرقيق في هذا الفصل يحتمل أن يكون معناها الرقيق في القوام ويحتمل أن يكون معناها الرقيق في الشكل فقد يجوز على هذا القياس عندي أن يكون أبقراط أراد بقوله أعلاه رقيق أيّ مخرط أعلاه ويميل إلى الدقّة لأنّ الثفل الراسب في البول إذا كان غليظا ثقيلا نيّا كان سطحه الأعلى شبيها بالمسطح وإذا كان رقيقا خفيفا نضيجا كان أعلاه مخرط. For other examples where Ḥunayn adds a commentary of his own, which is mostly of a linguistic nature, see aphorisms 1.12 (E, fol. 91ᵃ); 1.13 (E, fol. 92ᵇ); 1.14 (E, fol. 96ᵃ); 1.15 (E, fol. 100ᵇ); 2.5 (only in V, fol. 27ᵃ); 6.32 (E, fols. 59ᵃ–60ᵃ); 7.32 (E, fol. 76ᵇ).

25 Note however that the Hebrew translation by Zeraḥyah has preserved three more aphorisms: 7.68, 70, and 81.

26 Cf. Hippocrates, *Aphorisms*, ed. Tytler, p. 33.

27 Cf. E, fol. 11ᵃ; V, fol. 61ᵇ.

2. The author has omitted the premises, because he falsely assumed that the reader has preliminary knowledge of them.

3. Certain statements by the author are ambiguous, allowing for different interpretations.

4. The work contains different errors, repetitions, or useless matters.

Regarding the commentaries on Hippocrates' works, Maimonides states that most of them are composed for the first, third, and fourth reason, and some for the second reason. At the same time, Maimonides criticizes Galen for denying that Hippocrates' works contain errors, by manipulating and interpreting them in a way that they seem to be correct:

> And all the commentaries written on the books by Hippocrates, are mostly composed for the first, third, and fourth reason, while some of its statements are commented upon for the second reason. However, Galen denies this and does not think in any way that the works of Hippocrates contain errors. But he (i.e., Galen) offers explanations which cannot be supported by the text and provides commentaries to [certain] statements that are not alluded to by those statements.[28]

He remarks that, contrary to Galen, he will give a fair, honest verdict of those aphorisms that are problematic, self-evident, repetitive, useless, or completely mistaken. For the other aphorisms, his commentary will be an abbreviated version of that by Galen, insofar that the latter is correct.

A close look at Maimonides' commentary itself indeed shows that he criticizes Hippocrates for the reasons mentioned above. For instance, in aphorism 2.20 (72), he comments upon Hippocrates' statement that "who has loose bowels when he is young will have constipated ones when he grows old, and he who has constipated bowels when he is young will have loose bowels when he grows old," that it is a faulty generalization (logical conclusion) based upon the observation of only one or two cases, and adds that Galen gave it a semblance of truth by attaching certain conditions and prerequisites to it. And in aphorisms 5.53 (273), Maimonides remarks:

> In general, all these indications are neither correct nor do they occur most frequently. In my opinion, all these aphorisms and their like follow from his observation of what happened [only] once or twice, for Hippocrates was [merely] a beginner in the [medical] art.[29]

---

28   Cf. preface (6–7).
29   See also aphorisms 5.40 (260), 5.65 (285), 6.40 (332), 6.49 (341), 7.62 (414).

In addition to criticizing Galen for trying to justify Hippocrates' faulty aphorisms, Maimonides attacks Galen for his own interpretation of certain aphorisms. For instance, in aphorism 5.48 (268), he exclaims "I wish I knew whether
he received this [knowledge] by divine revelation or by analogical reasoning. If
he has defined and formulated this argument through analogical reasoning, it
is an astonishing and strange logical conclusion," as a reaction to Galen's statement that "the semen that comes from the woman from the right side, from one
of her ovaries, is thick and warm, while that which comes from the left side is
thin and watery and colder than the other."[30] In a few cases, Maimonides' critique of Galen is unjustified and wrong, as for instance in aphorism 1.25 (52),
where Hippocrates states: "If the body is purged from the kind [of matter] it
should be purged from, it is beneficial and easily borne [by the patient]; but
if the opposite is the case, it is [borne] with difficulty," and Maimonides comments:

> In my opinion, this aphorism is not a repetition of the contents of the sec-
> ond aphorism, because that aphorism deals with that which is evacuated
> spontaneously, whereas this aphorism deals with that which we evacuate
> by means of drugs. Since Galen thought that the second aphorism deals
> with both matters, he sought to give a reason for the repetition of this
> aphorism.

Maimonides' statement that aphorism 1.2 (29) deals with spontaneous evacuation and aphorism 1.25 (52) with artificial evacuation is wrong, since both
forms of evacuation are explicitly discussed in aphorism 1.2. Thus, Galen is
right to consider this aphorism a repetition of the second and that it therefore needs a different sort of explanation. And sometimes Maimonides' critique or affirmation of Galen is based on his own observation, thus provid-
ing us a glimpse into his own medical experience.[31] For instance, in aphorism
7.29 (381), Maimonides remarks that he has seen twice how someone who
suffers from dropsy of the flesh is cured when he is attacked by violent diarrhea.

    In his critique of Galen as a medical doctor, Maimonides stands in a long tra-
dition of Galenic criticism, going back to Byzantine physicians like Alexander
of Tralles (ca. 525–ca. 605),[32] and continuing with Arab physicians, above all

---

30   See also aphorism 5.48 (268).
31   For Maimonides' own medical experience, see Bos, "Maimonides' Medical Works,"
      pp. 255–257.
32   For Maimonides' critique of Galen, see ibid., pp. 261–265.

al-Rāzī (865–932), who devoted a special monograph to the subject entitled
K. al-shukūk ʿalā Jālīnūs (Doubts Concerning Galen).[33] Maimonides criticizes
Galen above all in treatise twenty-five of his *Medical Aphorisms*. The first part,
i.e., aphorisms 1–58, contains Maimonides' critique of the medical inconsisten-
cies found in Galen's works, and the second part, covering aphorisms 59–68,
contains Maimonides' refutation of Galen's denial of the Mosaic doctrines of
God's omnipotence and creation of the world. In addition to treatise twenty-
five, we find Maimonides criticizing Galen in the other treatises of his *Medical
Aphorisms* as well, as I showed in my editions of these treatises.[34]

4   Popularity of Hippocrates' *Aphorisms*[35]

The didactic features of Hippocrates' *Aphorisms* mentioned above were an
important factor in making them extremely popular, as is borne out by numerous quotations and commentaries. Already in early antiquity, the work was
commented upon, for instance, by Rufus of Ephesus, whose commentary has
been lost. In late antiquity, Stephen of Alexandria and Palladius[36] composed
commentaries that are still extant today. Subsequently, numerous Arab physicians commented upon the *Aphorisms*, generally consulting the translation by
Ḥunayn ibn Isḥāq of the lemmata featuring in the commentary by Galen of
Pergamum.[37]

The *Aphorisms* occupied a prominent position in the Hebrew medical tradition as well. On the evidence of the extant manuscript material, the work was
translated into Hebrew no less than eleven times, whether as an independent
text or as part of a later commentary.[38] The earliest dated Hebrew translation

---

33   See al-Rāzī, *Doutes sur Galien*, ed. and trans. Koetschet.
34   Cf. ed. Bos, introductions to Maimonides, *Medical Aphorisms*, vol. 1, p. xxv; vol. 2, pp. xxii–
      xxiii; vol. 3, pp. xix–xx.
35   I thank my friend Eric Pellow for proofreading and correcting this section of the introduc-
      tion.
36   His commentary is no longer extant in Greek, but it has recently been rediscovered by
      Hinrich Biesterfeldt and Y. Tzvi Langermann, who hope to publish a preliminary study of
      Palladius' commentary in the near future, to be followed by a full edition and analysis.
37   For a detailed discussion of the extant commentaries, cf. Pormann/Joosse, "Commentaries
      on Hippocratic *Aphorisms*."
38   In a forthcoming article, Katelyn Mesler discusses several more translations, which she
      discovered during her research at the Institute of Microfilmed Hebrew Manuscripts
      (IMHM) at the Jewish National and University Library in Jerusalem. For a detailed discus-
      sion of Hippocrates' *Aphorisms* and their medieval Hebrew translations and terminology,
      see NM 3, pp. 1–20.

of Hippocrates' *Aphorisms* was written by an anonymous author living in the Midi who, after his conversion to Christianity, called himself Doeg ha-Edomi.[39] Between 1197 and 1199, he completed his translation of a corpus of twenty-four medical texts, both practical and theoretical, from Latin into Hebrew. These texts were the first complete Hebrew translations of works by non-Jewish authors on secular subjects. Doeg's translation of Hippocrates' *Aphorisms* under the title *Sefer Agur* was highly esteemed and widely distributed in Jewish circles; it survives in eleven manuscripts, nine of which were copied in the fifteenth century.

Another translation of Hippocrates' *Aphorisms*, based on Constantine the African's Latin version, is that by Hillel ben Samuel of Verona (ca. 1220–1295), a talmudic scholar, philosopher, physician, and translator of medical works.[40] In a letter to his friend Isaac—the pope's physician, more widely known as Master Gaio—Hillel remarks that although he already possessed the Latin translation by Constantine and the commentary by Burgundius of Pisa, he still wanted the commentary by Maimonides in addition to Maimonides' *Medical Aphorisms* in order to solve the 'hundred' queries he had, so he entreats Gaio: "Do not care about the cost, and make a scribe copy them, and I shall immediately send you the scribe's salary and [the price] of the paper and the corrections, as much as demanded. Even if it turns out to be a substantial expenditure it will become smaller [in my mind] when considering how much I love them [the books]."[41]

Another translation, perhaps based on Constantine's Latin version, is incorporated in the commentary on the *Aphorisms* written by Judah (Astruc) ben Samuel Shalom (ca. 1450) for his student, the physician Raphael ben David ha-Kohen from Lunel. Judah developed a distinctive terminology, which precludes the ascription of his translations to others.

Ḥunayn ibn Isḥāq's Arabic version of Hippocrates' *Aphorisms*—i.e., of the lemmata in Galen's commentary—was the basis for the translation by Nathan ha-Me'ati (of Cento), a translator of scientific texts, and especially of medical works, from Arabic into Hebrew in the city of Rome in the final decades of the

---

39   See Steinschneider, *Hebräische Übersetzungen des Mittelalters*, pp. 659–660, 713; Barkai, *History of Jewish Gynaecological Texts*, pp. 20–29; Freudenthal, "Aim and Structure of Steinschneider," pp. 201–204; Zonta, "Hebrew Translations of Philosophical and Scientific Texts," pp. 22–23 (nos. 29–46); Freudenthal, "Father of Latin-into-Hebrew Translations," pp. 105–120; idem, "Avi ha-Metargemim min ha-Latinit le-Ivrit," pp. 23–53.

40   On Hillel as a translator, cf. NM 1, pp. 9–15.

41   Cf. the Hebrew text in Richler, "Another Letter from Hillel;" trans. Shatzmiller, *Jews, Medicine, and Medieval Society*, p. 46; NM 1, p. 9.

thirteenth century.[42] Another translation based on the Arabic was prepared by the otherwise unknown Jacob bar Joseph ibn Zabara. However, as Alexander Marx remarks, Ibn Zabara extensively used Moses ibn Tibbon's Hebrew translation of Maimonides' commentary on the *Aphorisms* for his translation of the Hippocratic lemmata.[43]

Despite the availability of various translations, it was Maimonides' commentary on Hippocrates' *Aphorisms* that was primarily responsible for the profound influence that the work had in Jewish circles. Maimonides' Arabic commentary was translated into Hebrew in 1260 by the well-known translator Moses ibn Tibbon (fl. 1244–1283), a member of the famous dynasty of translators known as the "Tibbonides," who was active as a physician, merchant, and translator in Lunel.[44] The enduring popularity of this translation among Jewish scholars is amply demonstrated by the fact that thirteen of the fourteen extant MSS were copied in the fifteenth century or later.

Another translation of Maimonides' commentary is that by R. Zerahyah ben Isaac ben She'altiel Ḥen (also known as Zerahyah Gracian), who, in the years 1277–1291, was active in Rome as a teacher of philosophy, commentator on the Bible, and translator.[45] While Steinschneider was unaware of the translation by Zerahyah, he pointed to the existence of an anonymous translation in three manuscripts, two of which were located in the Bodleian Library.[46] However, upon closer examination, it is evident that the translation extant in the two Oxford manuscripts is the work of Zerahyah, as the following comparison of aphorisms 1.7 (34) and 2.54 (106) demonstrates:

---

42   On Nathan, see NM 2, pp. 21–27, 95–108. The translation of the *Aphorisms* is missing in Zonta, "Hebrew Translations of Philosophical and Scientific Texts," pp. 17–73.

43   Marx, "Targum ha-Aphorismim," p. 208.

44   On Moses ibn Tibbon as a translator, see NM 1, pp. 47–51. For this translation, cf. Steinschneider, *Hebräische Übersetzungen des Mittelalters*, p. 769; Zonta, "Hebrew Translations of Philosophical and Scientific Texts," p. 31, no. 143.

45   The identification of the translator is based upon the colophon of MS Udine, Biblioteca Arcescovile, 246 ebr. 12: העתקת זרחיה בן יצחק חן מעיר ווירדזילונא זצ״ל. Cf. Tamani, "Codici ebraici Pico Grimani," p. 18; Zonta, "Hebrew Translations of Philosophical and Scientific Texts," p. 35, no. 181. On Zerahyah as a translator, see NM 1, pp. 121–127; ed. Bos, introduction to Maimonides, *Medical Aphorisms: Hebrew Translation by R. Zerahyah ben Isaac ben She'altiel Ḥen* (forthcoming).

46   The MSS containing the 'anonymous' translation, as identified by Steinschneider, are: (1) Oxford, Bodleian Library, Opp. 685, fols. 1ª–122ᵇ; (2) Oxford, Bodleian Library, Reggio 7, fols. 39ᵇ–102ᵇ; (3) Leiden, Universiteitsbibliotheek, Cod. Warneriani 30 (= Or. 4768). Note that ed. Schliwski, introduction to Maimonides, *Šarḥ fuṣūl Abuqrāṭ*, p. XXXIX, tentatively attributed the two Oxford manuscripts to Nathan ha-Me'ati: "vielleicht Nathan ha-Meathi."

'Anonymous' translation, MSS Oxford, Bodleian Library, Reggio 7 and Opp. 685	Zeraḥyah's translation, MS Udine, Biblioteca Arcescovile, 246 ebr. 12
ובהיות החולי חד מאד והכאבים בתכלית האחרון הקצוי יבואו בו תחלה, ראוי בהכרח בתכלית האחרון שיעשה בו הנהגה אשר מן הדקות. ואם לא יהיה כן, ויהיה הענין הפך אבל יהיה סובל מן ההנהגה מה שהיא יותר עב מזה, יהיה ראוי שתהיה ההנהגה (הירידה MS²) לפי רפיון החולי וחסרונו על התכלית הקצוי וכשהפליג החולי לבוא החולי עד תכונתו, הוא ראוי בהכרח שיעשה ההנהגה אשר היא בתכלית הקצוי מן הדקות.	ובהיות החולי חם מאד והכאבים אשר בתכלית האחרון הקצוי יבוא (יבואו MS¹) בו תחלה, וראוי בהכרח שיעשה בו הנהגה אשר בתכלית האחרון מן הדקות. ואם מה לא יהיה כן, ויהיה הענין הפך אבל יהיה סובל מן ההנהגה מה שהיא יותר עב מזה יהיה ראוי שתהיה הירידה לפי רפיון החולי וחסרונו על התכלית הקצוי, וכשהפליג החולי לבוא עד תכונתו (עמידתו MS¹), הוא ראוי בהכרח שיעשה ההנהגה אשר היא בתכלית הקצוי מן הדקות.
גודל הגוף בזמן המ' שנה אינו רחוק אבל הוא נאהב, אבל בזמן הזקנה יכבד ויקשה לשאת אותו, ויהיה יותר רע מהקטן אשר הוא יותר חסר ממנו.	גודל הגוף בזמן הארבעים שנה אינו רחוק אבל הוא נאהב, אבל בזמן הזקנה יכבד ויקשה לשאת אותו, ויהיה יותר רע מהבטן (*מהקטן) אשר הוא יותר חסר ממנו.

This comparison of the 'anonymous' translation to Zeraḥyah's text is sufficient to establish their identity. Note, however, that even if the manuscripts were fragmentary, recent research on the techniques and terminologies of medieval translators of medical works from Arabic and Latin into Hebrew would allow identification of this text as Zeraḥyah's work. His distinctive translation of e.g., Arab. منتهى (climax) as Hebrew עמידה;[47] Arab. تطيل (fomentation) as Hebrew טיבולים;[48] and Arab. معدن (mineral) as Hebrew מקור,[49] is sufficient to differentiate his efforts from those of other translators, such as Nathan ha-Me'ati and Moses ibn Tibbon.

In addition to these translations by both Moses ibn Tibbon and Zeraḥyah Ḥen, Maimonides' commentary on Hippocrates' *Aphorisms* was also translated by an anonymous author. Steinscheider found this translation in MS Leiden,

---

47   Cf. preface (9); the term is also found in his translation of Maimonides' *Medical Aphorisms* 9.18; cf. NM 1, p. 176.

48   Cf. aphorism 1.2 (29); the term also appears in his translation of Maimonides, ibid. 8.2, cf. NM 1, p. 153, where Nathan ha-Me'ati uses the term יציקה; cf. NM 2, p. 38.

49   Cf. aphorism 1.2 (29); the same term appears in his translation of Maimonides, ibid. 7.72; cf. NM 1, p. 166.

Universiteitsbibliotheek, Cod. Warneriana 30; another copy is extant in MS Paris, Bibliothèque Mazarine, 4478.

Next to the comprehensive translations of—and commentaries on—the *Aphorisms*, there is a commentary on the first two aphorisms in Joseph Solomon Delmedigo's *Sefer Elim* (*Book of Palms*), an encyclopedic work covering mathematics, astronomy, the natural sciences, and metaphysics.[50] However, as Isaac Barzilay notes, "a comparison of the commentaries of Yashar (i.e., Joseph Solomon Delmedigo) and Galen on the first two aphorisms ... leaves no doubt as to the total reliance of Yashar on Galen."[51]

The first aphorism—"Life is short, and the art is long, and time is limited, and experience is dangerous, and judgment is difficult"—was particularly popular in the Jewish tradition.[52] The opening phrase of the aphorism is resonant with—and consequently cited in the context of—the well-known saying in *Mishnah Avot* 2.15: רבי טרפון אומר: היום קצר והמלאכה מרובה והפועלים עצלים והשכר הרבה ובעל הבית דוחק ("R. Tarfon said: The day is short and the task is great and the labourers are idle and the wage is abundant and the master of the house is urgent").[53] For example, the Spanish philosopher, linguist, and poet Moses ibn Ezra (ca. 1055–after 1035) remarks in his treatise on rhetoric and poetry, *K. al-Muḥāḍara wa-l-Mudhākara:* קאל בקראט: אלעמר קציר ואלצנאעה טוילה. ומתלה קאל אואילנא: היום קצר והמלאכה מרבה ("Hippocrates says: Life is short and the art is long. Likewise, our forefathers said: The day is short and the task is great").[54] Another parallel between this aphorism and the saying in *Avot* can be found in the *Ṭibb al-nufūs*, written by the Spanish philosopher and poet Joseph ibn Aknin (ca. 1160–1226).[55] Isaac Israeli, the Jewish physician and philosopher (ca. 855–ca. 955), quotes the opening phrase of this aphorism in his *Book on the Elements*.[56] In his testament, the translator Judah ibn Tibbon (ca. 1120–1190) exhorts his son "to be prompt, but to apply a sure remedy, avoiding doubtful treatment," in accord with Hippocrates' statement: "Time is short, and experiment dangerous."[57] The first aphorism also reverberates in Maimonides' letter to his student Joseph ben Judah ibn Shim'on, which was written in 1187 or 1190:

---

50   Cf. Barzilay, *Yoseph Shlomo Delmedigo*, pp. 128–130.

51   Ibid., p. 129 n. 1.

52   On the popularity of this aphorism in the Arabic tradition, see Rosenthal, "Life is Short, Art is Long."

53   Trans. Danby, *Mishnah*, p. 449.

54   Ibn Ezra, *K. al-Muḥāḍara wa-l-Mudhākara*, ed. and trans. Halkin, p. 142.

55   Cf. Güdemann, *Jüdisches Unterrichtswesen*, p. 128; Rosenthal, "Life is Short, Art is Long," pp. 229–230.

56   Trans. Altmann, *Isaac Israeli*, p. 134.

57   Trans. Abrahams, *Hebrew Ethical Wills*, p. 80.

"For you know how long and difficult this art is for someone who is conscientious and fastidious."[58] Again, in his treatise *On the Regimen of Health* 4.11, Maimonides writes: "Concerning the matter discussed by al-Rāzī in this aphorism, Galen has remarked many times in his books that the crafty find this art easy and insignificant, while Hippocrates finds it difficult and time-consuming."[59]

Indeed, the phrase "life is short, and the art is long"—without explicit attribution to Hippocrates—joined the stock of phrases upon which medieval and later Jewish scholars drew. The Spanish poet and philosopher Judah ha-Levi (ca. 1075–1141) uses the phrase incidentally in his *Kuzari* 5.2, and the Provençal polemicist Abba Mari ben Moses ben Joseph Astruc (late thirteenth–early fourteenth century) employs it in his correspondence with Solomon ben Abraham Adret.[60] Judah ibn Tibbon, apparently influenced by the familiar formulation in *Avot*, rendered the phrase as החיים קצרים והמלאכה מרובה (life is short, and the task is great) in his translation of the *Kuzari*, despite the resultant loss of verbal symmetry (short/long vs. short/great); and in that form it was cited by later Jewish scholars, such as Moses ben Barukh Almosnino (ca. 1515–ca. 1580).[61]

An indication of the esteem in which Hippocrates' *Aphorisms* was held by generations of Jewish scholars is the fact that it was twice parodied. In the first of these satires, apparently the work of the otherwise unknown Provençal writer Maimón Gallipapa (fourteenth–fifteenth century?), the aphorisms open with "the enemy said," rather than "Hippocrates said."[62] The following quotation, in which physicians are ridiculed for their pomposity as well as their incompetence, conveys the tenor of Gallipapa's parody:

> The enemy said: When one has a spot or cloudiness covering the eye or is blind, and "Jericho was straightly shut up"[63] [i.e., the eye is tightly closed] and the doctor is consulted about the disease, he answers with pride and arrogance: "Who is wise and able to explain this, and who, like me, in past

---

58 Maimonides, *Iggerot*, trans. Kafih, pp. 134–135; idem, *Iggerot ha-Rambam*, ed. Baneth, pp. 69–70; see also Bos, "Maimonides' Medical Works," p. 252.

59 Cf. Maimonides, *On the Regimen of Health*, trans. Bos, p. 124; see also Davidson, *Moses Maimonides*, p. 440.

60 Astruc, *Sefer Minḥat Kenaʾot*, p. 134, letter no. 62. Note that Astruc inverted the phrase in accordance with the rhyme scheme of the letter.

61 Almosnino, *Pirqei Moshe*, ed. Baṣri, Jerusalem 1995, p. 234 (final Mishnah of *Avot* 5).

62 Ibn Zabara, *Shalosh halaẓot*, ed. Davidson, pp. 13–23. Although Davidson erred in his initial attribution of the parody to Ibn Zabara, he corrected the error in his later edition of Ibn Zabara's *Sepher Shaʿashuim*, pp. XCIX–CI.

63 Js 6:1.

or future, can interpret it? For those who suffer with their eyes, my knowledge reaches to the heavens, and for all humankind have I established my
covenant. My wisdom is greater than that of the angels; when the sight
becomes dim, I do wondrous works to clear it; I bring healing to the eye."
The patient's relatives honor him [i.e., the physician], they almost carry
him on their hands. He visits with words of flattery and sits in the entrance
of the house; he prepares in his hand the salt of Sodom[64] and the poison
of a serpent, thorns and thistles, makes a plaster of them and puts it on the
eye; but this is as a sword and spear, and the pain increases exceedingly
and the patient cries bitterly, for his eyes are blinded.[65]

The other parody of the *Aphorisms* was composed by the Haskalah satirist
Isaac Erter (1791–1851),[66] who had studied medicine in Budapest. The parody,
which bears the title *Pirkei ha-Zahav* (*The Golden Aphorisms*),[67] is part of his
humorous monograph *Ha-Ṣofeh le-Veit Yisrael*.[68] Characteristic of Erter's parody, which is less exuberant than that of his predecessor, is the following advice
to physicians:

When you visit the home of a patient, do not investigate his illness to
understand [the cause of] his pain, but consider his attendants, who
stand around his bed, so that you know what to say to them. And when
you leave, say: "I don't believe that he will live." If he dies, they will say:
"Did he [i.e., the physician] not tell us from the outset? He understood
[the seriousness of the illness]; he investigated and ascertained it." And
if he [i.e., the patient] recovers and walks, they will not say: "You are an
ass,"[69] because you did not understand [i.e., diagnose his illness correctly],
rather, they will call it a miracle, saying: "he restores soul to the dead."[70]

---

64   This 'salt' was allegedly so caustic that it could blind the eyes, when one would touch them
     with one's fingers to which it would adhere after the meal. The danger of Sodomite salt
     is one of the explanations given for the obligation to wash one's hands after meals (מים
     אחרונים). See Krauss, *Talmudische Archäologie*, vol. 1, p. 119, and p. 501 n. 660; Preuss, *Bib-
     lical and Talmudic Medicine*, ed. and trans. Rosner, p. 525.
65   Trans. Friedenwald, *Jews and Medicine*, vol. 1, p. 88.
66   On Isaac Erter, see Zinberg, *History of Jewish Literature*, ed. and trans. Martin, vol. 10,
     pp. 92–100, 108–110.
67   Note that the title refers not only to the *Aphorisms* of Hippocrates, but also to the *Golden
     Verses* of Pythagoras; see Erter, *Ha-Ṣofeh le-Veit Yisrael*, p. 55.
68   Ibid., pp. 55–57.
69   Here 'ass' is not only an expression of derision, but also a reference to the previous tale, in
     which the soul of the physician was incarnated into an ass.
70   Erter, *Ha-Ṣofeh le-Veit Yisrael*, pp. 55–56 (trans. Bos and Pellow). Note that the last phrase
     is a play on the text of one of the traditional morning benedictions, אלהי נשמה.

5   Editions and Translations of Maimonides' *Commentary on Hippocrates'* Aphorisms

So far, Maimonides' *Commentary* has been published in the following editions and translations.[71] The Arabic text has been edited recently, together with a translation into German, by Carsten Schliwski.[72] The introduction to the treatise has been edited by Moritz Steinschneider on the basis of MS Oxford, Bodleian Library, Hunt. 427, which was transcribed into Hebrew script and compared with two Hebrew manuscripts and translated into German.[73] The section from the introduction dealing with al-Fārābī's division of medicine into seven parts, the knowledge of which constitutes the art of medicine, has been edited by Martin Plessner.[74] Maimonides' commentary on the first aphorism was translated by Ariel Bar-Sela and Hebbel E. Hoff on the basis of the Arabic MS Oxford, Bodleian Library, Hunt. 427, and three Hebrew manuscripts.[75] A first edition of a medieval Hebrew translation was published in the years 1934/1935.[76] The Hebrew translation by Moses ibn Tibbon was edited by Suessmann Muntner on the basis of MS Munich, Bayerische Staatsbibliothek, 275, with variant readings from the anonymous translation as extant in MS Oxford, Bodleian Library, Reggio 7 (cat. Neubauer 1319).[77] This edition was the basis for the English translation by Fred Rosner[78] and the Spanish translation by Lola Ferre.[79] A new edition of the Arabic text was deemed necessary since the edition by Schliwski is based on a very small number of manuscripts, as he did not

---

71   For a complete list, cf. ed. Schliwski, introduction to Maimonides, *Šarḥ fuṣūl Abuqrāṭ*, p. XL; see also ed. Muntner, introduction to Maimonides, *Perush le-firqei Abuqraṭ*, pp. XXXIII–XXXIV; trans. Rosner in Maimonides, *Commentary on the Aphorisms of Hippocrates*, ch. "Bibliography: B. Printed Editions" (no pagination).

72   Maimonides, *Šarḥ fuṣūl Abuqrāṭ*, ed. and trans. Schliwski.

73   Idem, "Vorrede zu seinem Commentar über die Aphorismen des Hippokrates," ed. and trans. Steinschneider, pp. 218–234. This edition was corrected and translated into Hebrew in: idem, *Iggerot*, ed. and trans. Kafih, pp. 141–147.

74   Plessner, "Al-Fārābī's Introduction," pp. 310–312.

75   Bar-Sela/Hoff, "Maimonides' Interpretation."

76   Cf. Heilperin, "Perush pirqei Abuqraṭ;" Maimonides, "Perush le-firqei Abuqraṭ," ed. Hasida.

77   Maimonides, *Perush le-firqei Abuqraṭ*, ed. Muntner. For a critical evaluation of this edition, see eds. Bar-Sela/Hoff/Faris in Maimonides, "Two Treatises on the Regimen of Health," p. 10: "This text is profusely edited, but almost completely without any indication of the source or basis for the many additions, deletions, interpretations, and interpolations. We were therefore unable to utilize this text because it is impossible to distinguish textual variations from editorial interpolations without resort to the original manuscripts."

78   Maimonides, *Commentary on the Aphorisms of Hippocrates*, trans. Rosner.

79   Idem, *Comentario a los aforismos de Hipócrates*, ed. and trans. Ferre.

have access to the Tehran MSS mentioned below. For this reason, he was forced to consult the Hebrew translations for sections missing in the Arabic MSS available to him. The accompanying full English translation to this new edition is the first that is based on the Arabic text. In addition to the Arabic text, I have prepared critical editions of all the extant Hebrew translations, i.e., those by Moses ibn Tibbon, Zeraḥyah ben Isaac ben She'altiel Ḥen, and the anonymous Hebrew translation, since Muntner's edition only covers the Hebrew translation by Moses ibn Tibbon and is based on one manuscript only, namely MS Munich, Bayerische Staatsbibliothek, 275.

6 Manuscripts of the Arabic Text of Maimonides' *Commentary*

The Arabic text of Maimonides' Commentary is extant in the following MSS:

1. Tehran, Millī, 1142/1 (**A**); pp. 1–54; the text was copied in an Arabic script in the seventh/thirteenth century.[80]
2. Tehran, Majlis, 6405/2 (**B**); fols. 9ᵇ–70ᵇ; the text was copied in an Arabic script in the eighth/fourteenth century.[81] This MS abbreviates the Hippocratic text from aphorism 1.15 (42) onwards.
3. Oxford, Bodlein Library, Hunt. 427/1 (**C**); fols. 1ᵃ–51ᵃ; the text was copied in an Arabic script in the eighth/fourteenth century.[82] The preface until معان مختلفة is missing. As Savage-Smith has noted, fols. 16ᵇ–18ᵃ have extracts from a commentary on the *Aphorisms* specified as the *'Umdah*, which was composed by al-Sīwāsī. According to the colophon on fol. 51ᵃ, the MS was collated against the author's original.
4. Paris, BN, héb. 412 (cat. Zotenberg 1202) (**P**); the text was copied in a Hebrew script in 1465 and bears the title: כתאב אלתכוין לגאלינוס ואבוקר. The MS begins at aphorism 3.25 (131): لا سيّما; missing is aphorism 4.34 (171): المرض الذي هو من نوع واحد (177) until aphorism 4.40 (177): الا ختناق.[83]
5. St. Petersburg, Russian National Library, Evr. Arab. I 2170 (**D**); the text was copied in a Hebrew script; the outer and sometimes also the inner margins contain Moses ibn Tibbon's Hebrew translation of Hippocrates' *Aphorisms* in addition to a part of Moses ibn Tibbon's Hebrew transla-

80 Cf. Sezgin, *Geschichte des arabischen Schrifttums*, vol. 3, p. 30.
81 Cf. ibid.
82 Cf. Savage-Smith, *New Catalogue of Arabic Manuscripts*, pp. 16–18.
83 Cf. ed. Zotenberg, *Catalogues des manuscrits hébreux*; and the online catalogue of the Institute of Microfilmed Hebrew Manuscripts (IMHM) at the Jewish National and University Library, Jerusalem.

tion of Maimonides' *Commentary*; the inner margins also contain many explanatory notes. The MS is fragmentary, in poor condition, and suffers from many mistakes by the copyist.[84]

In addition to these MSS, small fragments can be found in the Cambridge Genizah Collection, namely T-S Ar. 39.72 (cat. Isaacs no. 150); Arabic script, containing parts from aphorisms 1.12–13 (39–40); and T-S Ar. 43.328 (cat. Isaacs no. 564); Hebrew script, containing parts from aphorisms 1.23–2.5 (50–57).[85]

The following critical edition is based on C, as it was collated against the author's original, and its readings are more correct than those of the other MSS. Sections missing from C have been supplemented from other MSS. Neither D nor the Genizah fragments have been used, since D is very defective and has many faulty readings and mistakes, and the fragments do not offer any significant variant readings. Since Maimonides' commentary is primarily based on the Hippocratic lemmata as they feature in Galen's commentary, I refer to that commentary as edited by Kühn for textual comparisons and references. My English translations of the original Greek terms featuring in this commentary are derived from the translations of the Hippocratic *Aphorisms* by Littré and Jones, as far as these terms are identical with those featuring in the Galenic commentary.

7 Manuscripts of the Hebrew Translations of Maimonides' *Commentary*

As mentioned above, the Hebrew tradition of Maimonides' commentary is extant in three translations, namely by Moses ibn Tibbon, by Zeraḥyah ben Isaac ben She'altiel Ḥen, and by an anonymous author.

(a) Moses ibn Tibbon: This translation is extant in the following MSS:

1. Munich, Bayerische Staatsbibliothek, 275; fols. 30ᵃ–61ᵃ; no title (א). The MS was copied in 1483 by Samuel ha-Ṣaʿir Elʿazar Parnas.[86] It has several, sometimes very lengthy learned marginal expositions; it also has short additional supralinear annotations, sometimes derived from other

---

84 Cf. the IMHM online catalogue.
85 Cf. Isaacs/Baker, *Medical and Para-Medical Manuscripts*.
86 Cf. colophon fol. 61ᵃ: בעזר האל נשלם יום שני י״ד לחדש אייר שנת הרמ״ג ליצירה מכתב שמאל הצעיר אלעזר פרנס; cf. Steinschneider, *Hebräische Handschriften München*; see also the IMHM online catalogue (also for all the following Hebrew MSS).

manuscript versions.[87] The text of the MS is very unequivocal, giving the impression of being compiled from a variety of versions. In many cases, the text seems to be contaminated by versions hailing from other translations, such as the anonymous translation and that by Zeraḥyah.[88] Likewise, it shares with Zeraḥyah's translation an additional number of aphorisms at the end of bk. 7, that do not feature in the other translations, but do feature in the Greek Hippocrates[89] and in the Arabic Galenic commentary.[90] Sometimes the MS has preserved early, faulty versions that have been revised at a later stage, presumably by Moses ibn Tibbon, and feature in the MS tradition represented by ד.[91] And in a few cases, the MS has preserved unique correct readings, presumably hailing from Ibn Tibbon's revised version.[92] These correct readings have been adopted as basic readings for the edition. In other cases it seems as if an original literal correct version has been replaced by a free translation.[93] In yet other cases it seems as if an original faulty translation featuring in the other MSS has been replaced by a non-standard correct one.[94]

2. Oxford, Bodleian Library, Poc. 405, Uri 420 (cat. Neubauer 2116); fols. 202ª–240ª (ב).[95] The MS, bearing the title ספר מן פצול אבוקרט, was copied in the fifteenth century in a Sephardic script; it suffers from mistakes

---

87 Cf. aphorism 1.19 (46): נ״א קודם; and aphorism 2.25 (77): ויתקשו שם (cf. trans. Anonymous: יתקשו); and aphorism 3.2 (108): בזמן הקור (= trans. Anonymous); and aphorism 4.68 (205): יעצרנו שום דבר במעבריו (= trans. Anonymous).

88 Cf. appendix 1 below.

89 Aphorisms 7.68, 70 and 81; cf. Hippocrates, *Aphorisms*, ed. and trans. Jones, pp. 210–215.

90 Cf. appendix 2 below.

91 Cf. preface (3): האנשים for Arab. الأشخاص instead of האישים featuring in ד; and aphorism 2.20 (72): מוחלט for Arab. مهمل, where ד has סתום; and ibid.: כולל for Arab. حكّ على, where דבקים instead of لازمة لنظامها for Arab. נוהגין כסדרן and aphorism 3.8 (114): ד has דין על; and aphorism 3.8 (114): בסדורם in ד.

92 Cf. aphorism 2.31 (83): לוקח מן המזון for Arab. ويحظا من الطعام; and aphorism 3.5 (111): ועכירות בראות for Arab. وغشاوة في البصر; and ibid.: והפלצות for Arab. والاقشعرار; and ibid.: ראוי שתפחד מהתחדש בחולים for Arab. ينبغي أن يتوقع في الأمراض; and aphorism 3.8 (114): רע הנקיון for Arab. سمج البحران; and aphorism 4.27 (164): כאשר יחלישהו ישוב ברכות הטבע for Arab. عندما ينقه فيغذا يلين بطنه; and aphorism 6.35 (327): עד שיגיע בקנה הריאה for Arabic إلى أن تبلغ قصبة الرئة.

93 Cf. aphorism 2.54 (106), where Arab. ليس يكره بل يستحبّ has been rendered as יותר טוב while א has: לא יגונה אבל ישובח ויותר נאה.

94 Cf. aphorism 5.22 (242), where it has כלי התשמיש לזכר ולנקבה for Arab. فرج (genitals), where the other MSS have: קיבה (stomach).

95 Cf. Neubauer, *Catalogue of Hebrew Manuscripts in Oxford*; and *Supplement*, comp. Beit-Arié and ed. May.

and omissions; part of the text is out of order; aphorisms 2.7–13 (59–65) feature on fols. 232ᵇ–233ᵃ in-between aphorisms 5.70 (290) and 6.16 (308), and aphorisms 7.56–62 (408–414) have been written in a different hand.

3. London, British Library, Or. 10526, fols. 1ᵃ–57ᵇ (ד). The MS has no title and was copied in the fifteenth century in a Sephardic script; the section from aphorism 6.38 (330) טוב until aphorism 6.60 (352) הליחה ההיא is missing. The MS suffers from occasional staining and fading of the ink, and from the occasional intervention of a learned scribe, as in aphorism 2.18 (70), where it has (together with ה): ועניין מהר שיבשל הטבע מה שיאכל ראשון, while the other MSS read: ועניין מהר אחר שיקח אותו בזמן ראשון קודם שיתקבץ, for Arabic: ‏ومعنى سريعا بعد تناولها بزمان يسير‎. The MS also seems to have preserved early, sometimes faulty versions by Ibn Tibbon, that have been revised at a later stage and feature in the MS tradition represented by א.[96]

4. Hamburg, Staats- und Universitätsbibliothek, Levy 128, fols. 2ᵃ–27ᵇ (ה).[97] The MS with the title פרקי אבוקראט written in a different hand, was copied in Baghdad in 1821. It misses the introduction and starts at aphorism 1.1 (14): אמר אבוקרט: החיים קצרים. The copyist also had access to and consulted other versions (translations).[98]

5. Berlin, Staatsbibliothek Preußischer Kulturbesitz, Or. Qu. 809 (cat. Steinschneider 237); fols. 4ᵃ–42ᵇ (ה). The MS was copied in a Sephardic script in the fifteenth century[99] and is entitled: ספר מן פצל אבקרט. The text of the MS closely resembles that of ב, sharing the same corruptions, mistakes, and peculiarities.

The following MSS have been looked into as well, but have not been consulted for the edition since they suffer from many corruptions and omissions:

---

96 Cf. aphorism 2.31 (83): יחטא מרוב האכילה for Arab. ‏ويحظا من الطعام‎; and aphorism 3.5 (111): ראוי for Arab. ‏والاقشعرار‎; and ibid.: וסמור for Arab. ‏وغشاوة في البصر‎; and ibid.: וסנויר בראות for Arab. ‏ينبغي أن يتوقّع في الأمراض حدوث‎; and aphorism 3.8 (114): שיפול בחליים התחדשות for Arab. ‏سمج البحران‎; and aphorism 4.27 (164): כאשר יחלישהו ישוב ברכות for Arab. ‏عندما ينقه فيغذّا يلين بطنه‎; and aphorism 6.35 (327): עד שיתעלוג בקנה הריאה for Arab. ‏إلى أن تبلغ قصبة الرئة‎ for Arab. והנקיון משונה for Arab.

97 Cf. Steinschneider, *Katalog der hebräischen Handschriften in Hamburg*.

98 Cf. aphorism 1.12 (39): הרקיקה (נ״א רקיקת הדם) הצד (נ״א בחולי) בבעלי; and ibid.: and ibid.: והאיברים (נ״א והאיברים שראוי שיורקו); and aphorism 1.21 (48): והשגעון ממרה שחורה; and aphorism 2.18 (70): פתאום (נ״א המזונות אשר יגדלו(?) =) זונו) מהר פתאום תהיה (מהם; and aphorism 7.36 (388): ואם יהיה הכאב מבפנים תפול היציאה מבפנים (יציאתם מהר). One of these versions is the commentary by Palladius; cf. aphorism 3.5 (111).

99 Cf. Steinschneider, *Verzeichniss der hebräischen Handschriften in Berlin*.

1.   Parma, Biblioteca Palatina, Cod. Parm. 2279 (cat. De Rossi 312; Richler
      1559).[100]

2.   Berlin, Staatsbibliothek Preußischer Kulturbesitz, Or. Qu. 836 (cat. Stein-
      schneider 232).

The MSS that are listed above, which form the basis for the edition, can be
divided into the families בח and אדה, whereby each of the MSS in the last family forms a subfamily on its own. The critical edition is based on ר since its
readings are generally better than those of the other MSS and since it suffers
from contamination to a lesser degree than the other MSS. In the case of scribal
corruptions, mistakes, and hiatuses, one of the other MSS has been consulted.
From the description of the MSS it may be clear that the reconstruction of a
version that can truly be ascribed to Moses ibn Tibbon, be it original or revised,
is in several cases one that could only be achieved tentatively.

(b)   Zeraḥyah ben Isaac ben She'altiel Ḥen: This translation is extant in the
      following MSS:

1.   Oxford, Bodleian Library, Opp. 685 (cat. Neubauer 2084), fols. 1ᵃ–122ᵇ; no
      title (ט); the MS was copied in an Italian script in the fourteenth century
      and contains in the margin a version of the *Sefer Agur*.[101] It has marginal
      and supralineal variant readings derived from the ל tradition, and derived
      from the translation by Moses ibn Tibbon. It also has an unknown com-
      mentary on several aphorisms as on aphorism 4.13 (150) on fol. 61ᵇ, intro-
      duced by the letter ג'.[102]

2.   Oxford, Bodleian Library, Reggio 7 (cat. Neubauer 1319), fols. 39ᵇ–102ᵇ, no
      title (ז). The MS was copied in the year 1375 in an Italian script and con-
      tains in the margin a version of the *Sefer Agur*.[103] In addition, the MS has
      marginal and supralineal variant readings derived from the ל tradition,
      and the same unknown commentary as the previous manuscript. It is thus
      a close copy of the previous manuscript.

---

100   See Richler, *Hebrew Manuscripts in the Biblioteca Palatina*.

101   Cf. Neubauer, *Catalogue of Hebrew Manuscripts in Oxford*; and *Supplement*, comp. Beit-
      Arié and ed. May.

102   The commentary on aphorism 4.13 (150) states: ג': בעבור ששתיית האליבורו הוא סכנה
      כשלא תשלים פעולתו על כן אומר שצריך לנו לדעת שהגוף יהיה מוכן לעשות פעולת הקיא
      ואם איננו מוכן בטבע לזה צריך להכינו בשני דרכים בהרבות מזון לח ובמנוחת הגוף המלחלחת
      הדרכים והאליבורו הלבן יעשה פעולתו מלמעלה בעבור קלותו בערך לשחור שעושה פעולתו
      מלמטה לכבידותו.

103   Cf. Neubauer, *Catalogue of Hebrew Manuscripts in Oxford*; and *Supplement*, comp. Beit-
      Arié and ed. May.

3.   Udine, Biblioteca Arcescovile, 246 ebr. 12, fols. 1ᵃ–29ᵇ; no title (ל). The MS
     was copied in an Italian script in the city of Tivoli in 1342. According to
     the colophon on fol. 29ᵇ, the translation hails from the hand of Zeraḥyah
     ben Isaac Ḥen.[104] The MS has marginal variant readings derived from the
     MS tradition preserved in זט.

These MSS can be divided into two families: זט and ל. The critical edition is
based on ל. Significant variants from זט feature in the critical apparatus.

(c)   Anonymous translation: This translation is extant in the following MSS:

1.   Leiden, Universiteitsbibliotheek, Cod. Warneriani 30, Or. 4768 (cat. Stein-
     schneider);[105] fols. 266ᵃ–314ᵃ; no title (צ); copied in a Karaite script in 1623.
     The MS suffers from many corruptions and mistakes caused by the copy-
     ist(s). On fol. 314ᵃ it has the following colophon: נשלמו פרקי אבוקרט על ידי
     יוסף ביו׳ ב׳ ט״ו לאייר השפ״ג ול׳ למספר.
2.   Paris, Bibliothèque Mazarine, 4478; pp. 1–120; no title (ק); copied in a
     Sephardic script in the fifteenth century. The readings of this MS are by
     far better than those in צ, however it suffers from increased staining, so
     that parts of the text cannot be read.

This translation is at times poor and impossible to understand without the
original, as the translator lacks knowledge of the standard Hebrew general and
technical terminology developed by the Tibbonids and other major translators
like Nathan and Zeraḥyah.[106] Several mistakes result from an incorrect reading
of the Arabic, as in aphorism 1.14 (41), where he translates Arabic أما أن يصف
אמנם שיספר לבד מה שצריך לעשותו ברוח פיו as פקט מא ינבغي أن يفعل ويروح, resulting
from misreading the Arabic ويروح as ويروح (and [only] with the breath [of his
mouth], i.e., by words only, not by action). Sometimes he uses a correct term
in one aphorism, as עונות for Arabic نوائب in aphorisms 2.30 (82), but a faulty
term in another aphorism, such as in aphorisms 4.30 (167), where he translates
the same Arabic term as וסת; cf. ibid.: וסתות הקדחת for Arabic نوائب الحمى. And
sometimes he does not give one standard translation for the same Arabic term

---

104   Cf. Tamani, "Codici ebraici Pico Grimani," p. 35 (no. 181).
105   Cf. Steinschneider, *Catalogus Codicum Hebraeorum*.
106   Cf. aphorism 1.1 (28): עצירת תשומת כלי for Arab. والحقّن; ibid.: כריתת הברזל for Arab. بط;
      and aphorism 1.2 (29): גרישת הבטן for Arab. اسطلاق البطن; and aphorism 1.3 (30): טרחנים
      for Arab. مصارعين (wrestlers); and aphorism 1.7 (34): תחת זמן for Arab. نوائب; and apho-
      rism 1.8 (35): התערובות for Arab. الأخلاط; and aphorism 1.12 (39): חולי הדאגה for Arab.
      في أكثر الأمر. Cf. also the use of the particle ודאי to
      render Arab. فإنه throughout his translation.

but different terms.[107] In other cases he uses the Hebrew term for different Arabic terms.[108] In several cases, the translation is not a faithful reflection of the original, but an adaptation of the original text, through extension, omission, interpretation, or explanation.[109]

The critical edition is based on ק, as its readings are more reliable and correct than those in ע. Copyists' mistakes have been emended as far as possible.[110]

---

107 Cf. Arab. فضاء, which he translates as חדרים in aphorisms 5.15 (235) and 5.60 (280), as חדרי הבטן in aphorism 6.20 (312), and as רוחב החדר in aphorism 6.27 (319), and Arabic حران, which he translates in aphorism 7.4 (356) both as גבול and as נקיון.

108 Cf. Hebrew חלל for Arab. الموضع الخالي in aphorism 7.24 (376), but also for غضروف in aphorism 7.28 (380), and Arab. اضطراب is translated as התפעמות הפעמות in aphorisms 7.9 (361) and 7.33 (385), and as בלבול in aphorisms 6.26 (318) and 6.31 (323), and as הצטערות in aphorism 2.13 (65).

109 Cf. Steinschneider, *Catalogus Codicum Hebraeorum*, p. 134: "locis nonnullis textus magis paraphrasticus videtur." For an addition, cf. aphorism 1.7 (34): וכאשר הגיע החולי בתכליתו ועם זה צריך שיהיה ההנהגה אשר היא בקצה האחרון מן הדקות; see also the aphorism and explanation in 3.3 (109), that is missing in both the Greek and Arabic traditions. For an explanation, cf. also aphorism 6.59 (351): רטיבות רירי דומה לליחה היוצאת מהנחירים.

110 For instance, in aphorism 3.17 (123), both MSS read ורחיצת בשר for Arab. والمنتنة, which I emended as: ומסרחת בשר; cf. preface (26): מסריח for Arab. منتن.

Sigla and Abbreviations

Arabic Text

Manuscripts

A	Tehran, Millī, 1142/1, pp. 1–54
B	Tehran, Majlis, 6405/2., fols. 9^b–70^b
B^1	marginal note in B
C	Oxford, Bodleian Library, Hunt. 427/1, fols. 1^a–51^a
C^1	marginal note in C
C^2	supralinear note in C
D	St. Petersburg, Russian National Library, Evr. Arab. I 2170
P	Paris, BN, héb. 412 (cat. Zotenberg 1202)
P^1	marginal note in P
P^2	supralinear note in P

Galen, Commentary on Hippocrates' *Aphorisms* (*Arabic Trans. Ḥunayn*)

E	Escorial 789
F	Paris 2837
S	Escorial 791
V	Vatican 426

Editions

b	Maimonides, *Medical Aphorisms*, vol. 2 (*Treatises 6–9*), ed. Bos
d	Pseudo-Galen, *Pseudogaleni in Hippocratis de Septimanis Commentarium ab Hunaino*, ed. Bergsträsser
s	Maimonides, "Vorrede des Maimonides zu seinem Commentar über die Aphorismen des Hippokrates," ed. Steinschneider
t	Hippocrates, *Aphorisms*, Arabic trans. Ḥunayn, ed. Tytler

© KONINKLIJKE BRILL NV, LEIDEN, 2020 | DOI:10.1163/9789004412880_003

Hebrew Translations

Manuscripts
Moses Ibn Tibbon

א	Munich, Bayerische Staatsbibliothek, 275, fols. 30ᵃ–61ᵃ
¹א	marginal note in א
²א	supralinear note in א
ב	Oxford, Bodleian Library, Poc. 405, Uri 420 (cat. Neubauer 2116), fols. 202ᵃ–240ᵃ
²ב	supralinear note in ב
ד	London, British Library, Or. 10526, fols. 1ᵃ–57ᵇ
²ד	supralinear note in ד
ה	Hamburg, Staats- und Universitätsbibliothek, Levy 128, fols. 2ᵃ–27ᵇ
ח	Berlin, Staatsbibliothek Preußischer Kulturbesitz, Or. Qu. 809 (cat. Steinschneider 237), fols. 4ᵃ–42ᵇ
¹ח	marginal note in ח

Zeraḥyah ben Isaac ben She'altiel Ḥen

ז	Oxford, Bodleian Library, Reggio 7 (cat. Neubauer 1319), fols. 39ᵇ–102ᵇ
¹ז	marginal note in ז
²ז	supralinear note in ז
ט	Oxford, Bodleian Library, Opp. 685 (cat. Neubauer 2084), fols. 1ᵃ–122ᵇ
¹ט	marginal note in ט
²ט	supralinear note in ט
ל	Udine, Biblioteca Arcescovile, 246 ebr. 12, fols. 1ᵃ–29ᵇ
¹ל	marginal note in ל

Anonymous

צ	Leiden, Universiteitsbibliotheek, Cod. Warneriani 30, Or. 4768 (cat. Steinschneider), fols. 266ᵃ–314ᵃ
ק	Paris, Bibliothèque Mazarine, 4478, pp. 1–120

Editions

a	Arabic edition of Maimonides' *Commentary on Hippocrates'* Aphorisms

Abbreviations and Symbols

add.	added in
corr.	corrected in
del.	deleted in
inv.	inverted in
om.	omitted in
O.Occ.	Old Occitan
⟩ ⟨	to be deleted in Arabic and Hebrew text
⟨ ⟩	supplied by editor in Arabic and Hebrew text
[ ]	supplied by translator in English text
(!)	corrupt reading
(?)	doubtful reading

PART 1

Arabic Text and Translation

∴

Commentary on Hippocrates' Aphorisms: Arabic Text with English Translation

In the name of God, the Merciful, the Compassionate

[1] Says the master, the erudite, the eminent, the leader, Mūsā ibn ʿUbayd Allāh, the Israelite from Cordova, may God bless his soul: I do not think that any scholar who composes books would write a book in any kind of science with the intention that the contents of his book cannot be understood, unless they are explained. If any author would have such an intention, he would thwart the purpose of his composition, because an author does not write a book so that he alone will understand its contents. However, he writes a book so that others will understand it. And if a book he wrote can only be understood by another book he has thwarted the purpose of its composition.

[2] In my view, there are four reasons why later [authors] were prompted to explain the books of earlier [authors] and to comment upon them:

The first reason is the perfection of the degree [of knowledge] of the author. Because of his excellent intellect, he speaks briefly about things that are obscure, hidden, and difficult to understand [for others], but which are clear to him [so that] he does not need to use more words. If someone in a later generation wants to understand those matters that were [written down] in such a concise way, it is very difficult for him. A commentator must add an explanation to his words so that the meaning of the matters, which the first author had in mind, can be understood.

[3] The second reason is the omission of premisses in a book. For the author sometimes composes a book assuming that the reader will have preliminary knowledge of certain premisses. But if someone who does not know those premisses wants to understand that book, he is unable to do so. Then the commentator has to supply and explain those premisses, or to refer [the reader] to books in which those premisses are explained and to direct [him] to them. For the same reason the commentator has to explain the causes of things that were not mentioned by the author.

© KONINKLIJKE BRILL NV, LEIDEN, 2020 | DOI:10.1163/9789004412880_004

بسم الله الرحمن الرحيم وبه نستعين

[١] قال السيّد العالم الفاضل الإمام موسى بن عبيد الله القرطبي الإسرائيلي قدّس الله نفسه: ما أظنّ
أحدا من العلماء الذين ألّفوا الكتب ألّف كتابا في نوع من أنواع العلوم وهو يقصد أن لا يفهم ما
تضمّنه كتابه حتّى يشرح ولو قصد هذا أحد من واضعي الكتب لكان قد أبطل غاية تأليف كتابه لأنّ
المؤلّف ما يؤلّف تأليفه ليفهم نفسه ما يضمّنه ذلك التأليف وإنّما يؤلّف ما ألّف ليفهم ذلك غيره وإذا
كان ما ألّفه لا يفهم إلّا بتأليف آخر فقد أبطل غاية كتابه.

[٢] وإنّما الأسباب الداعية للمتأخّرين إلى شرح كتب المتقدّمين وتفسيرها عندي أحد أربعة أسباب:
الأوّل منها كمال فضيلة المؤلّف فإنّه لجودة ذهنه يتكلّم في أمور غامضة خفيّة بعيدة الإدراك بكلام
وجيز ويكون ذلك بيّنا عنده لا يحتاج إلى زيادة. فإذا رام المتأخّر بعده فهم تلك المعاني من ذلك
الكلام الوجيز عسر ذلك عليه جدّا فيحتاج الشارح إلى بسط زائد في القول حتّى يفهم المعاني الذي
قصده المؤلّف الأوّل.

[٣] والسبب الثاني حذف مقدّمات الكتاب وذلك أنّ المؤلّف قد يؤلّف كتابه متّكلا على أن يكون
الناظر قد تقدّم له علم المقدّمات الفلانيّة. فإذا رام فهم ذلك الكتاب من لا علم له بتلك المقدّمات لم
ينفهم له شيء فيحتاج الشارح إلى إحضار تلك المقدّمات وتبيينها أو ينبّه على الكتب التي تبيّنت فيها
تلك المقدّمات ويرشد إليها وبحسب هذا السبب أيضا يبيّن الشارح علل ما لم يذكر المؤلّف علّته.

١–٣١.٢ بسم ... معان: .om.C ١ نستعين: شرح فصول أبقرﻂ للرئيس للأفضل العالم الأوحد المتفنّن الفيلسوف الأكمل أبي عمرن موسى عبيد الله القرطبي رضي الله عنه .add. B ٢ السيّد العالم الفاضل الإمام: .om B || قدّس الله نفسه .om. B ١٢ متّكلا: معتمدا B ١٤ وتبيينها أو ينبّه: ويبيّنها وينبّه A

[4] The third reason is the [correct interpretation] of a statement. For most statements in any language can be interpreted [in various ways]. They can have meanings that are different and sometimes even opposite or contradictory. Consequently, disagreement arises between those who look at that statement. One person gives it a certain interpretation and says that the author only meant this and another person gives it another interpretation. The commentator of that statement must declare one interpretation for correct and adduce proof for its correctness and declare the other interpretations for false.

[5] The fourth reason is the errors that befall the author, or words that are repetitive or [even] utterly useless. The commentator must draw [the reader's] attention to these words and prove that they are futile, useless, or repetitive. This should not really be called a commentary, but a refutation or annotation. However, when people study a book and most of its contents is correct, they usually consider the annotations to the few [erroneous] places to be part of the commentary, [in which] it is said: "the error of the author is such and such and the truth is such and such," or: "this should not have been mentioned," or: "this is repetitious," all this is explained. However, if the contents of that book are mostly mistaken, then the later work, which exposes those mistakes is called a refutation, not a commentary. When the work with the refutation cites a correct statement, it will say: "such and such statement is correct."

[6] It seems to me that all the commentaries on the books of Aristotle were composed for the first and the third reason. All the commentaries on the books on the mathematical sciences were composed for the second reason, although it is also possible that some mathematical statements have been commented upon because of the fourth reason. For the book [called] *Almagest*,[1] in spite of the eminence of its author, has errors that were pointed out by a group of Andalusian authors in the books they composed regarding that matter.[2]

---

1 For the *Almagest*, the famous astronomical handbook composed by Claudius Ptolemaeus from Alexandria and its medieval translations, see art. "Baṭlamiyūs," in E.I.[2], vol. 1, pp. 1100–1102 (Plessner).

2 The conflict over Ptolemaic astronomy and Aristotelean cosmology that arose in twelfth century Spain was about the fact that Ptolemaic astronomy posits epicycles and eccentrics that enable the astronomer to make precise predictions of planetary motions, while Aristotelian cosmology requires all heavenly motion to be uniform, circular, and about the center of the earth. Some of Maimonides' near-contemporaries rejected Ptolemaic astronomy and some tried to construct alternative theories. Maimonides himself exploited, as Stern, "Maimonides'

[٤] والسبب الثالث ترجّح القول وذلك أنّ أكثر الأقاويل في كلّ لغة تحتمل التأويل ويمكن أن
ينفهم من ذلك القول معان مختلفة بل بعضها متضادّة بل متناقضة فيقع الاختلاف بين النظّارين
في ذلك القول ويتأوّله شخص تأويلا ما ويقول ما أراد به المؤلّف إلّا هذا المعنى ويتأوّله شخص آخر
تأويلا آخر فيحتاج الشارح لذلك القول إلى ترجيح أحد التأويلات والاستدلال على صحّته وتزييف
٥ ما سواه.

[٥] والسبب الرابع الأوهام الواقعة للمؤلّف أو الكلام المكرّر أو لا فائدة فيه أصلا فيحتاج الشارح
أن ينبّه عليها ويستدلّ على بطلانها أو على كون ذلك القول غير مفيد أو مكرّر. وهذا لا يسمّى شرحا
بالحقيقة بل ردّا وتنبيها. لكن قد جرت العادة عند الناس أن ينظر الكتاب فإن كان ما قيل فيه
أكثره صواب فينعدّ التنبيه على تلك المواضع القليلة من جملة الشرح ويقال: وهم المؤلّف في قوله كذا
١٠ والحقّ هو كذا وهذا لا يحتاج إلى ذكره أو هذا تكرّر القول فيه وتبيّن ذلك كلّه. فأمّا إن كان ما قيل
في ذلك الكتاب أكثره خطاء فيسمّى التأليف الأخير الذي يكشف تلك الأغلاط ردّا لا شرحا.
وإذا ذكر في كتاب الردّ شيء من الأقاويل الصحيحة التي ذكرت في التأليف الأوّل قيل أمّا قوله كذا
فصحيح.

[٦] وكلّ ما شرح أو يشرح من كتب أرسطو إنّما شرح بحسب السبب الأوّل والثالث فيما ظهر
١٥ لنا وكلّ ما شرح من كتب التعاليم إنّما شرح بحسب السبب الثاني. وقد يشرح بعض أقاويل تعليميّة
بحسب السبب الرابع أيضا لأنّ هذا كتاب المجسطي مع جلالة مؤلّفه قد وقعت له في كتابه أوهام نبّه

٢ متضادّة: متضاددة B ‖ النظّارين: الناظرين C ٧ أن ينبّه: إلى التنبيه B ‖ يسمّى: يستمى C ٨ قد: om.
A ‖ كان: om. A ١٠ لا: B om. ١١ الأخير: الأخر A ‖ الأغلاط: الأغاليط A ١٢ في التأليف: C¹
١٤ أرسطوا: أرسطو B ١٦ مع: بحسب C

Epistemology," p. 119, remarks, "the conflict in order to motivate 'the true perplexity' of Aristotelean cosmology, that is, the irresolvable disagreement that is symptomatic of the lack of demonstrative knowledge and hence the limitations of the intellect." See also Maimonides, *Dalālat al-ḥāʾirīn*, trans. Pines: *Guide of the Perplexed* 1.31, 2.24, pp. 65–67, 322–327; and Sabra, "Andalusian Revolt against Ptolemaic Astronomy."

And all the commentaries written on the books by Hippocrates are mostly composed for the first, third, and fourth reason, while some of its statements are commented upon for the second reason.

[7] However, Galen denies this and does not think in any way that the works of Hippocrates contain errors.[3] But he (i.e., Galen) offers explanations, which cannot be supported by the text and provides commentaries to [certain] statements that are not alluded to by those statements. We can see how he did so in his commentary on the book *On Humors*,[4] even though he was doubtful whether this book was written by Hippocrates or by someone else. He was prompted to do so because of the confusion in matters [discussed by him] and because it resembles the works of the alchemists or is [even] worse than these.[5] In my opinion, it would be more correct to call it "The Book of [Mental] Confusion."[6] However, because of the fame of Hippocrates and the ascription of the book to him, he (i.e., Galen) composed this strange commentary. Everything that Galen said in that commentary is correct from a medical viewpoint; however, the text that he commented upon does not indicate (relate to) anything of the commentary that he wrote. [His commentary] should not really be called a commentary, because a commentary brings to actuality that which can potentially be understood from a text, so that, if you look once again at that commented text, once you have understood the commentary, you will see that that text indicates (relates to) what you have understood from the commen-

---

3   Cf. Galen's statement in *De usu partium* 1.8, ed. Helmreich, vol. 1, p. 15, ll. 13–16; trans. May: *On the Usefulness of the Parts of the Body*, p. 77: "Nor are the writings of Hippocrates adequate, since he treats some subjects obscurely and omits others altogether, though in my estimation, at any rate, he has written nothing that is incorrect." For Galen's admiration of Hippocrates, see Jouanna, *Hippocrates*, pp. 353–357. For Maimonides' critical attitude towards Galen, see Bos, "Maimonides' Medical Works," pp. 261–265.

4   This commentary, *Hippocratis de humoribus liber et Galeni in eum commentarii tres*, ed. Kühn, vol. 16, pp. 1–488, is according to Deichgräber, *Hippokrates'* De humoribus, a forgery dating from the Renaissance, probably from the hand of Rasarius. Deichgräber pointed out that Maimonides' quotations—in the form of the old Latin translation—were used by Rasarius for reconstructing part of the text. By comparing these quotations with parallels from Oribasius, Deichgräber also showed how problematic it is to distinguish between the Maimonidean and the genuine Galenic elements.

5   Although Maimonides' does not provide a rationale for his rejection of alchemy, one may suppose that it is for the same epistemological reasons for which he rejected astrology; cf. Langermann, "Maimonides' Repudiation of Astrology."

6   The term *ikhtilāṭ* or *ikhtilāṭ al-'aql* is common in Maimonides' *Medical Aphorisms* for "mental confusion" or "delirium." Note the wordplay between Arabic *ikhtilāṭ* (confusion) and *akhlāṭ* (humors), i.e., the Arabic title of Hippocrates' *On Humors*.

عليها جماعة من الأندلسيين وقد ألّفوا في ذلك. وكلّ ما شرح أو يشرح من كتب أبقراط فهو بحسب
السبب الأوّل والثالث والرابع أكثرها وبعض أقواله يشرح بحسب السبب الثاني.

[٧] إلّا أنّ جالينوس يأبى ذلك ولا يرى بوجه أنّ في كلام أبقراط وهم بل يتأوّل ما لا يحتمل التأويل
ويجعل شرح القول ما لا يدلّ ذلك القول على شيء منه كما نراه منه كا نزاه فعل كما في شرحه لكتّاب الأخلاط وإن
٥ كان قد شكّ جالينوس في كتّاب الأخلاط هل هو لأبقراط أو لغيره ودعاه لذلك ما هو عليه ذلك
الكتّاب من اختلاط المعاني وكونها شبه تواليف أصحاب الكيمياء أو أنزل منها. وأحقّ التسميات به
عندي أن يسمّى كتّاب الإختلاط لكنّه لشهرة اسمه ونسبته لأبقراط شرحه ذلك الشرح العجيب.
وكلّ ما قاله جالينوس في ذلك الشرح هو كلّه كلام صحيح بحسب صناعة الطبّ لكن لا يدلّ ذلك
الكلام المشروح على شيء من الشرح وما يسمّى هذا شرحا على التحقيق لأنّ الشرح هو إخراج ما
١٠ هو في ذلك الكلام بالقوة عند الفهم إلى الفعل حتّى أنّك إذا رجعت وتأمّلت الكلام المشروح بعد
ما فهمته من الشرح رأيت ذلك الكلام دالّا على ما فهمته من الشرح. هذا هو الذي يسمّى شرحا

١ كتب: om. A ٢ السبب: om. B ٥ هو: (...) C ٧ اسمه ونسبته: نسخته B نسبته C ٨ يدلّ: شيء
من add. B ١٠ هو: om. C ١١ هذا: عندي add. B

tary. This is what should be called a real commentary, but [this is not the case] if someone makes true statements and maintains that they are a commentary to the words of the author, as Galen did with regard to some of the statements by Hippocrates. The same holds good for those who draw conclusions from the words of a certain person and call it a commentary. In my opinion, it is not a commentary but another work, like most of the commentary by al-Nayrīzī[7] on Euclid.[8] I do not call that whole work a commentary.

[8] Similarly, we find that Galen in his commentaries on the works by Hippocrates, explains [certain] statements contrary to their meaning so that he turns that statement into a correct one. He does so in the book *De septimanis*,[9] where Hippocrates says that the earth surrounds the water. Galen explains this statement by saying that it is possible that he meant with this statement that the water surrounds the earth.[10] [He says] all this so that he would not have to say that Hippocrates made a mistake or committed an error in this statement. And when the matter baffled him [because] he found a statement that was clearly mistaken and he did not find any [other] way out, he would say that this [statement] is [falsely] ascribed to Hippocrates and interpolated into his words, or that these are the words of a certain Hippocrates but not the well-known Hippocrates. He did so in his commentary on *De natura hominis*.[11] [He did] all this to defend Hippocrates; although Hippocrates is without any doubt one of the most eminent physicians, [such] a defense is not a virtue, even in the case of an eminent [man].

[9] It is well known that not everything in a book that has been commented on or that will be commented on needs an explanation. There are inevitably statements in it, which are clear and do not need an explanation. However, the goal

---

7   For al-Nayrīzī (fl. 900 in Baghdad), well known in the history of mathematics because of his commentary on Euclid's *Elements*, see art. "al-Nayrīzī," in E.I.[2], vol. 7, p. 1050 (Hogendijk).

8   In his letter to Samuel ibn Tibbon, Maimonides characterizes the works of Euclid, in addition to those by Pythagoras, Hermes, and Porphyrius, as "ancient philosophy" and their study as "a waste of time;" cf. Marx, "Texts by and about Maimonides," p. 380.

9   The original Greek text of this pseudo-Hippocratic work has been lost; it is, however, extant in the Arabic translation of Pseudo-Galen, *In Hippocratis de Septimanis Commentarium ab Hunaino*, ed. and trans. Bergsträsser.

10   Cf. ibid., trans. Bergsträsser, p. 19: "Die Erde umfaßt das Wasser, das süße und salzige; oder vielleicht meint er mit diesen Worten, daß das Wasser die Erde umfaßt."

11   Cf. Galen, *In Hippocratis de natura hominis commentarius* 2.7, ed. Kühn, vol. 15, pp. 147–148; ed. Mewaldt, pp. 75–76.

بالحقيقة لا أن يأتي الإنسان بأقاويل صحيحة ويقول هذا شرح قول القائل كذا كما يفعل جالينوس في بعض أقاويل أبقراط. وكذلك أيضا هؤلاء الذين ينتجون نتائج من كلام شخص ويسمّون ذلك شرحا. ليس هذا عندي شرح بل تأليف آخر كأكثر شرح أقليدس للنيريزي فإنّي لا أسمّي ذلك كلّه شرحا.

٥ [٨] وكذلك نجد جالينوس أيضا في شروحه لكتب أبقراط قد يشرح القول بضدّ مفهومه حتّى يجعل ذلك القول صوابا كما فعل في كتاب الأسابيع حيث قال أبقراط إنّ الأرض تحيط بالماء. فسّر جالينوس هذا القول بأن قال: عسى أن يكون عنى بقوله هذا أنّ الماء يحيط بالأرض. كلّ هذا حتّى لا يقول إنّ أبقراط غلط أو وهم في هذا القول. وإذا غلب في الأمر ووجد قولا بيّن الخطاء ولا يتّسع له في حيلة قال: هذا منسوب لأبقراط ودخيل في كلامه أو هو كلام أبقراط الفلاني لا أبقراط المشهور كما فعل في شرحه لطبيعة الإنسان. وكلّ هذا تعصّب لأبقراط وإن كان أبقراط من أعظم

١٠ فضلاء الأطبّاء بلا شكّ فليس التعصّب فضيلة ولو كان ذلك في حقّ فاضل.

[٩] ومعلوم أنّ كلّ كتاب شرح أو يشرح كلّ ما فيه يحتاج إلى الشرح بل لا بدّ أن يكون فيه قول بيّن لا يحتاج إلى شرح. لكن أغراض الشارحين في شروحهم كطريقة المؤلّفين في تواليفهم

ـــــــــــــــــــــــ

١ أن: الشرح c ‖ هذا: هذه c add. c   ٣ أقليدس: أوقليدس c؟   ٥ شروحه: شرحه A   ٥-٦ حتّى يجعل ذلك القول صوابا: om. B   ٦-٧ إنّ ... بالأرض: إنّ الأرض تحيط بالماء العذب منه والمالح أو عسى أن يكون عنى بقوله هذا أنّ الماء يحيط بالأرض d   ٨ إنّ: om. A ‖ غلب: om. A   ٩ أبقراط: بقراط AC   ١٢ أن: أو AC   ١٣ إلى: إليه ولا إلى شرح A ‖ أغراض: أعراض c ‖ شروحهم: شرحهم A

of the commentators with their commentaries is comparable to the method of the authors in their compositions. Some authors strive for brevity, which does not affect the meaning so that if, for example, to fulfill the purpose of the composition in one hundred words they would not use one hundred and one words. Other [authors] aim at long-windedness and verbosity at composing a voluminous work of many parts, even though the total work does not have much content. The same applies to commentators: Some of them explain something that needs to be explained as briefly as possible, and omit the rest; others are long-winded and explain that which does not need to be explained or explain that which needs to be explained more verbosely than necessary.

[10] I thought that Galen is a very verbose commentator, as most of his [commentaries are very lengthy] until I noticed that he remarks in the beginning of his commentary on Plato's *Laws*,[12] and these are his words: "I have noticed that a commentator explained the following statement of Hippocrates on more than one hundred folios without any reason [to do so] and without [any actual] content: 'When the disease reaches its climax, then the regimen [of the patient] should be extremely thinning.'"[13]

[11] Says Mūsā: When I saw this statement of Galen, I excused him for his works and commentaries as I realized that he had been very brief therein in comparison with the works of his contemporaries. On the other hand, [these works] are [so] verbose that it can only be denied by someone who is biased. I am only speaking to those who are free of unfounded predilections and who seek the truth in everything.[14] Galen remarks in *De methodo medendi* 6 that his colleagues discussed these statements (i.e., by Hippocrates) lengthily.[15]

---

12   This compendium has been lost in the original Greek, but has been partly preserved in the Arabic tradition and translated into Latin: Galen, *Compendium Timaei Platonis aliorumque dialogorum synopsis quae extant fragmenta*, eds. and trans. Kraus/Walzer; see also Ullmann, *Medizin im Islam*, pp. 63–64. For Maimonides' quotation, see Galen, ibid., pp. 39 (Arabic text); 100–101 (Latin trans.).

13   Cf. Hippocrates, *Aphorisms* 1.8, trans. Jones, p. 103: "It is when the disease is at its height that it is necessary to use the most restricted regimen."

14   Cf. Maimonides, *Dalālat al-ḥāʾirīn* 2.23; eds. Munk/Joel, pp. 224–225; trans. Pines: *Guide of the Perplexed*, pp. 321–322.

15   Cf. Galen, *De methodo medendi* 6.1, ed. Kühn, vol. 10, p. 384: 'I know that to some it may seem that I speak too lengthily, as I am still explaining one kind of disease. However, it is appropriate that these people should not accuse me of lengthiness but rather those people who, as their understanding is deficient, attempt to attack the words correctly spoken by Hippocrates.'

لأنّ من المؤلّفين من يقصد الإيجاز الذي لا يحلّ بالمعنى حتّى لو أمكنه الكلام في ما قصد لتأليفه في مائة كلمة مثلا لمّا جعلها مائة كلمة وكلمة. وثمّ من قصده التطويل والتكثير وتكبير حجم الكتاب وتكثير عدّة أجزائه وإن كان بجموع ذلك كلّه قليل المعاني. كذلك الشارحون منهم من يشرح الشيء المحتاج للشرح بأوجز ما يمكن ويترك ما سوى ذلك ومنهم من يطوّل ويشرح ما لا يحتاج إلى شرح أو ما

٥   يحتاج إلى شرح بأكثر مما يحتاج.

[١٠] وقد كنت أظنّ أنّ جالينوس من المطوّلين في شروحه جدًّا كأكثر تواليفه حتّى رأيته أعني جالينوس يقول في أوّل شرحه لكتاب النواميس لأفلاطون كلاما هذا نصّه قال: قد رأيت بعض المفسّرين فسّر هذا القول من قول أبقراط وهو هذا: وإذا بلغ المرض منتهاه فعند ذلك ينبغي أن يكون التدبير في الغاية القصوى من اللطافة فإنّه فسّر هذا في أكثر من مائة جلد بلا معنى ولا سبب.

١٠   [١١] قال موسى: فلمّا رأيت هذا الكلام لجالينوس عذرته في تواليفه وشروحه وعلمت أنّه قد أوجز فيها كثيرا بالإضافة إلى تواليف أهل تلك الأعصار لكنّها على حال فيها تطويل لا يناكر في ذلك إلّا متعصّب. وأنا إنّما أخاطب من يتعرّى عن الأهواء ويقصد الحقّ في كلّ شيء. وقد ذكر جالينوس في المقالة السادسة من حيلة البرء أنّ أصحابه استطالوا كلامهم في تلك المقالات.

---

٢ مثلا: مثالا A ‖ التطويل: لتطويل A ‖ الكتاب: الكتب الذي تقصد إلى تصنيفها add. A   ٣ الشارحون: الشارحين AC   ٥ يحتاج: إلى شرح add. A   ٧ لأفلاطون: لأفلاطن A ‖ قد: om. B   ٨ وإذا: إذا B   ٩ جلد: مجلد B   ١١ الأعصار: الأعصيار s ‖ لكنّها: لكن B   ١٣ كلامهم: emendation editor كلامه ABC

[12] And since I consider Hippocrates' *Aphorisms* to be the most useful of the books [he composed], I decided to explain them; for these are aphorisms, which every physician should know by heart.[16] I have even seen how non-physicians have schoolchildren memorize them, so that [subsequently] people who are not physicians know many of these aphorisms by heart from learning them as young children at school.

[13] Among these aphorisms of Hippocrates are some that are problematic and require explanation, some that are self-evident, some that are repeated, some that are useless for the medical art, and some that are completely mistaken. However, Galen denies this and explains [such statements] as he wishes. But I will explain them in a fair (honest) way, that is, I will only explain that which needs an explanation, and will comply therein with Galen's goals (opinions), except for a few aphorisms, where I will give my opinion, in my name. Every explanation that I will mention anonymously is that of Galen, according to its sense (figuratively), for I do not envisage (intend) to be meticulous in [quoting] his words as I did in the *Epitomes* [from Galen's writings].[17] In this commentary, my only intention is to abbreviate so that it will be easy to memorize the meaning of those aphorisms that require explanation. [To achieve that] I try to use as few words as possible, except for the first aphorism, on which I will dwell a little longer. [I am not doing so in order to compose] a true commentary on that aphorism, but in order to [inform the reader about] some things in it that occurred to me as useful, [regardless] whether Hippocrates so intended them or not. Now it is time to start with the commentary.

---

16 The demand that every physician should know Hippocrates' *Aphorisms* by heart, already features in Ibn Riḍwān's *Fī l-taṭarruq bi-l-ṭibb ilā l-saʿāda*; cf. Ibn Riḍwān, *Über den Weg zur Glückseligkeit*, ed. and trans. Dietrich, pp. 19 l. 81 (Arabic text); 18 l. 114 (German trans.). On Alī ibn Riḍwān (991–1061/1068), active as a physician in Cairo, see art. "Ibn Riḍwān," in E.I.², vol. 3, pp. 906–906 (Schacht).

17 For Maimonides' *Epitomes from the Works of Galen*, see Bos, "Maimonides on Medicinal Measures and Weights."

[١٢] ولمّا رأيت كتاب الفصول لأبقراط أعظم كتبه فائدة رأيت أن أشرحها لأنّها فصول ينبغي أن يحفظها كلّ طبيب بل غير الأطبّاء رأيتهم يحفظونها للصبيان في المكتب حتّى أنّ فصولا كثيرة منها يحفظها من ليس بطبيب حفظ الصغر من المكتب.

[١٣] وهذه فصول أبقراط منها فصول مشكلة تحتاج إلى شرح ومنها بيّنة بنفسها ومنها مكرّرة ومنها ما

٥ لا تفيد في صناعة الطبّ ومنها وهم محض. لكنّ جالينوس كما علمت يأبى هذه الأشياء فيشرح كما يريد. أمّا أنا فأشرحها على طريق الإنصاف وذلك أنّي لا أشرح إلّا ما يحتاج إلى شرح وأتبع في ذلك أغراض جالينوس إلّا في بعض فصول فإنّي أذكر ما وقع لي فيها منسوبا إليّ. وأمّا كلّ ما شرح أذكره مطلقا فهو كلام جالينوس أعني معانيه لأنّي لم التفت إلى المشاحة على ألفاظه كما فعلت في المختصرات. وإنّما كان قصدي في هذا الشرح الإيجاز فقط ليسهل حفظ معاني هذه الفصول المحتاجة إلى شرح

١٠ وأروم تقليل الكلام في ذلك جهدي إلّا في الفصل الأوّل فإنّي أطول فيه قليلا ليس أنّ ذلك على طريق الشرح الحقيقي لذلك الفصل بل لأفيد بعض فوائد سنحت لي فيه كان أبقراط قصدها أو لم يقصدها.

وهذا حين أبتدئ بالشرح.

[The first part of the commentary on Hippocrates' *Aphorisms*]

(1.1)
[14] Says Hippocrates: Life is short, and the art is long,[18] and time is limited, and experience[19] is dangerous, and judgment is difficult. One (i.e., the physician) should not be content with the intention to do what is necessary without the patient and his attendants doing the same; and the external matters also.

[Says] the commentator: It is well known that short and long are[20] adjunctive attributes. If he wants, by saying "life is short," to refer to the art of medicine, then his statement "the art is long" is a repetition that is unnecessary, and there is no difference between this and saying "Zayd is shorter than 'Amr" and "'Amr is longer than Zayd." But if he meant to say that the life of an individual is short in comparison to perfection in any science and that the art of medicine is long in comparison to the other arts, then this reiteration is useful, as if he says how far man is from being perfect in this art—all this to urge persistence in it.

[15] As for the fact that the medical art is longer than the other theoretical and practical arts, this is obvious, because it [is an art] that cannot be comprehended nor perfection attained in it, except through its many parts. But the life of a single person is not sufficient to comprehend all those parts in a perfect and complete way.[21] Abū Naṣr al-Fārābī[22] has mentioned that there are seven

---

18   On the popularity of this aphorism, see the introduction above.
19   "experience is dangerous": Rosenthal, "Life is Short, Art is Long," p. 238, translates: "empiricism is a risk," cf. his excursus on the Arabic term *tajriba* (empiricism) on p. 233 n. 30, and section 19 below.
20   "are adjunctive attributes": Lit., "belong to the category of *iḍāfa* (genetive construction; annexation, attachment)."
21   About the difficulty of memorizing the different parts of the medical art, cf. Maimonides, *On Asthma* 13.19, trans. Bos, vol. 1, p. 91: "And if Galen—with his excellent intellect and long experience in the practice of medicine, his devotion to this art, and his strong aspirations [to excel] in it—casts doubts on his own practice and is tentative about it, how much more should this be the case in our generations, in which physicians have only very little experience, while [at the same time] much memorizing is needed, since the different parts of medicine have become so lengthy! Consequently, a lifetime is too short to attain perfection in even one part of it ...;" cf. ibid. 13.49, p. 109: "... rather, this art is difficult for most scholars not with respect to understanding it, but with respect to remembering it, because it requires [the command of] a very large amount of memorized material;" and Bos, "Maimonides' Medical Works," p. 253; and aphorism 1.4 (31) below.
22   For this statement by al-Fārābī (870?–950) from his *Treatise on Medicine*, see Plessner, "Al-Fārābī's Introduction," p. 312, and Stroumsa, "Al-Fārābī and Maimonides," p. 235; see also Maimonides, ibid. 13.6, p. 84.

(المقالة الأولى من شرح فصول أبقراط)

(1.1)

[١٤] قال أبقراط: العمر قصير والصناعة طويلة والوقت ضيّق والتجربة خطر والقضاء عسر. وقد ينبغي لك أن لا تقتصر على توخّي فعل ما ينبغي دون أن يكون ما يفعله المريض ومن يحضره كذلك والأشياء التي من خارج.

٥ المفسّر: معلوم أنّ القصير والطويل من مقولة الإضافة فإن كان يريد بقوله العمر قصير بإضافته إلى صناعة الطبّ فقوله والصناعة طويلة تكرار غير يحتاج إليه. ولا فرق بين هذا وبين قولك زيد أقصر من عمرو وعمرو أطول من زيد. وإن كان أراد أنّ عمر الشخص من الناس قصير بإضافته إلى استكمال أيّ علم كان من العلوم وصناعة الطبّ طويلة بإضافتها إلى سائر الصنائع هذا الترديد مفيد كأنّه يقول فما أبعد كمال الإنسان في هذه الصناعة. هذا كلّه ليحضّ على الدأب عليها.

١٠ [١٥] وأمّا كون صناعة الطبّ أطول من سائر الصنائع النظريّة والعمليّة فذلك بيّن لأنّها لا تلتئم وتحصل غايتها إلّا بأجزاء كثيرة لا يفي عمر شخص إنسان بالإحاطة بتلك الأجزاء كلّها على الكمال والتمام. وقد ذكر أبو نصر الفارابي أنّ الأجزاء التي تلتئم بمعرفتها صناعة الطبّ سبعة أجزاء. أوّلها ما

---

٥ المفسّر: الشرح BC   ٨ الترديد: التقرير B

parts, the knowledge of which constitutes the art of medicine. The first [part], pertaining to the physician, is the knowledge of the object of his art, namely, the human body, that is the science of anatomy, and the knowledge of the temperament of each of the organs in general, and the knowledge of its function and usefulness and the condition of its substance in firmness, softness, density and looseness, and the form of each of the organs, and the location of the organs (parts), both internal and external, and the connection of the organs to each other. Every[23] physician should have this degree [of knowledge] about everything of it or in it, although it may take a long time to acquire [this knowledge], as long as it does not concern things that are hidden.

[16] The second part related to our subject is the condition of the body, that is the knowledge of the [different] kinds of health of the whole body, in general, and the [different] kinds of health of every singular organ.

The third part consists of the knowledge of the [different] kinds of disease and its causes, and the pertinent symptoms in the whole body, in general, and in every singular part of the body.

The fourth part consists of the knowledge of the rules of deduction, that is, how to select from those afflictions affecting the subject, the indications from which one can draw conclusions about each and every kind of health and about each and every kind of disease, whether in the entire body or in any of its parts and how to distinguish between one disease and another when most of the indications are similar.

The fifth [part] consists of the rules of the regimen of the health of the body in general and the health of each of its organs for every age and for every season of the year and according to every place, so that every body and every organ will maintain the health specific to it.

The sixth [part] consists of the knowledge of the general rules according to which the illness should be treated so that the missing health is restored to the entire body or to the ailing organ.

The seventh [part] consists of the knowledge of the instruments, which the physician uses to preserve health when it is present or to restore it when it is lost, that is the knowledge of the different kinds of the foods of man and his medicines, both simple and compound; binding, bandaging, and douching are also part of this. Likewise, the instruments with which the flesh is lanced and

---

23   "Every physician ... are hidden": Bar-Sela/Hoff, "Maimonides' Interpretation," p. 349, translate: "The physician should not possibly be ignorant of anything, of it or in it, as long as it is not hidden."

يتعلّق بالطبيب من معرفة موضوع صناعته وهو بدن الإنسان وهذا هو علم التشريح ومعرفة مزاج كلّ عضو من الأعضاء على العموم ومعرفة فعله ومنفعته وحال جوهره في الصلابة واللين والكثافة والتخلخل وصورة كلّ عضو منها ومواضع الأعضاء الباطنة والظاهرة واتّصال الأعضاء بعضها ببعض. وهذا القدر لا يمكن أنْ يجهل الطبيب شيئا منه وفيه من الطول ما لا خفاء به.

[١٦] والجزء الثاني معرفة ما يلحق الموضوع من حال الصحّة وهو معرفة أنواع الصحّة على العموم لجملة ٥ البدن وأنواع صحّة عضو عضو.

والجزء الثالث معرفة أنواع الأمراض وأسبابها والأعراض التابعة لها في البدن كلّه على العموم أو في عضو عضو من أعضاء البدن.

والجزء الرابع معرفة قوانين الاستدلال وهو كيف يتّخذ من تلك الأعراض اللاحقة للموضوع دلائل يستدلّ بها على نوع نوع من أنواع الصحّة وعلى نوع نوع من أنواع المرض كان ذلك في البدن كلّه أو ١٠ في أيّ عضو من أعضائه وكيف يفرّق بين مرض ومرض آخر إذ قد يتشابه أكثر الدلائل.

والخامس قوانين تدبير صحّة البدن على العموم وصحّة كلّ عضو من أعضائه في كلّ سنّ من الأسنان وفي كلّ فصل من فصول السنة وبحسب بلد بلد حتّى يستدام كلّ بدن وكلّ عضو على صحّة التي تخصّه.

والسادس معرفة القوانين الكلّية التي يدبّر بها المرض حتّى يستردّ الصحّة المفقودة إلى البدن كلّه أو إلى ١٥ ذلك العضو الذي إعتلّ.

والسابع معرفة الآلات التي بها يعمل الطبيب حتّى يستديم الصحّة الموجودة أو يستردّ الصحّة المفقودة وهي معرفة أغذية الإنسان وأدويته على اختلاف أنواعها بسائطها ومركّباتها والشدّ والتقميط والتنطيل من هذا القبيل. وكذلك الآلات التي يبطّ بها ويقطع اللحم والصنّارات التي يعلق بها وسائر الآلات

---

٣ والتخلخل: والتخلل A   ٤ خفاء: خفي C   ٥ وهو معرفة: ومعرفة C   ١٢ صحّة البدن: الصحّة للبدن A
١٣ صحّة: صحّته A   ١٥ بها: كلّ .add B ‖ المرض: المرضي C

cut, the hooks that are used for suspension, and the other instruments that are used for wounds and for eye illnesses, all these belong to this category. Included in this part of the art of medicine is the knowledge of the form of every plant and mineral used in it, because, if you know only their name, you cannot gain their end. Likewise, you also need to know their various names in various places so that you know in each place with which name to ask for it.[24]

[17] It is well known that by knowing all these seven parts and by memorizing them from the books composed for each part, the physician will not attain the goal of his action, nor will [the physician] who has this knowledge acquire perfection in the art, until he attends to individual persons, both when they are healthy and sick, and [until] he acquires the skill to recognize the symptoms from which he can draw whatever conclusions and knows readily the condition of the temperament of that person and the condition of the temperament of each of his organs in what kind of health or illness it is, and, similarly, the state of function of each organ of that person and the condition of the substance of his organs. Likewise, through prolonged observation of a person and through those forms impressed in his mind,[25] he will readily know how to use those instruments, that is, foods, medicines, and the other instruments. This requires an extremely long time.

[18] It will be clear to you that the knowledge of these parts in general and the memorization of these rules, until nothing is lacking therefrom, needs a very long time. Likewise, attending to individual persons until one is trained in regimenting the health of one individual after another, in managing the cure of the diseases of one individual after another, in applying those instruments in individual cases, that is, one time [using them] alone and another time combining some of them with others, and in selecting a particular medicine or food over another of its kind, all this requires a very long time. It was rightly said that this

---

24   Maimonides' concern about the practical application of remedies in various places is actually his major motive for composing his *Sharḥ asmāʾ al-ʿuqqār* (*Glossary of Drug Names*), in which he explains the Arabic names of the remedies by means of the corresponding term in Romance and the term under which it is known amongst the people in the Maghreb and in Egypt; cf. Bos, "Maimonides' Medical Works," pp. 246–248.

25   The forms mentioned here are those that are abstracted from the sensible images by the intellect. For an extensive discussion of Maimonides' epistemology, see Stern, "Maimonides' Epistemology."

التي تستعمل في الجراحات وفي أمراض العين كلّها من هذا القبيل. وفي ضمن هذا الجزء من الصناعة معرفة صورة كلّ نبات وكلّ معدن يستعمل في صناعة الطبّ لأنّك إن لم تعلم منه غير اسمه فما حصلت على غاية. وكذلك أيضا تحتاج لمعرفة أسمائه المختلفة باختلاف المواضع حتّى تعلم في كلّ بلد أيّ اسم تطلب.

٥ [١٧] ومعلوم أنّ معرفة هذه الأجزاء السبعة كلّها وحفظها من الكتب الموضوعة لكلّ جزء منها لا تحصل به غاية فعل الطبيب ولا يحصل لذلك العارف كمال الصناعة حتّى يباشر الأشخاص في حال صحّتهم وحال مرضهم ويحصل له ملكة في تمييز الدلائل التي يستدلّ بها كيف يستدلّ ويعلم بسهولة حال مزاج هذا الشخص وحال مزاج كلّ عضو من أعضائه في أيّ نوع هو من أنواع الصحّة أو أنواع المرض وكذلك حال فعل كلّ عضو من أعضاء هذا الشخص وحال جوهر أعضائه. وكذلك

١٠ يعلم بسهولة بطول مباشرة الأشخاص وبتلك الصور المرتسمة في ذهنه كيف يصرّف تلك الآلات أعني الأغذية والأدوية وسائر الآلات. وهذا يحتاج إلى زمان طويل جدًّا.

[١٨] فقد بان لك أنّ معرفة تلك الأجزاء على العموم وحفظ تلك القوانين حتّى لا يشذّ عنه منها شيء يحتاج إلى زمان طويل جدًّا وكذلك مباشرة الأشخاص حتّى يرتاض في تدبير صحة شخص بعد شخص وفي تدبير شفاء مرض شخص بعد شخص وفي تصريف تلك الآلات تصريفا شخصيًّا أعني إفرادها

١٥ مرّة وتركيب بعضها مع بعض مرّة أخرى وتخيّر شخص هذا الدواء أو الغذاء على شخص آخر من نوعه كلّ هذا يحتاج إلى زمان طويل جدًّا. فبالحقّ قيل إنّ هذه الصناعة أطول من كلّ صناعة لمن يقصد

---

٦ حال: مزاج كلّ عضو من A add. ‏ ٨–٩ في ... أعضاء: C‏¹ ‏‖ أو أنواع: وأنواع B‏ ‏ ٩–١٠ وكذلك ... الأشخاص: A om.‏ ‏ ١٥ شخص: من C add.‏ ‏ ١٦ زمان: زمن C آخر BC add.

art is longer than every [other] art for him, who aims at perfection therein.[26] Galen has said in his commentary on the book *Timaeus*: No one can master the art of medicine completely.[27]

[19] Says the author: To be honest, you should know that every [physician] who is not perfect in [the art] does more harm than good because whether a person is healthy or sick, it is better not to be treated by a physician at all than to be treated according to the opinion of a physician who makes a mistake; his mistakes will be in proportion to his inadequacy, and if he happens to do something right, then it is by accident.[28] For this reason that eminent [physician] (i.e., Hippocrates) began his book with the exhortation to be perfect in this art by saying: "Life is short, and the art is long, and time is limited, and experience is dangerous, and judgment is difficult." As to experience being dangerous, that is clear, but I will add an explanation.

[20] As to his statement "time is limited," it seems to me that he means with this that the time for [treating] the disease is far too limited to experiment. If you do not know all matters already verified by experience,[29] but begin now to

---

26   On perfection in the medical art, see Kottek, "Maimonides on the Perfect Physician."

27   This quotation has not been preserved in Galen's commentary on the medical contents of Plato's work as published by eds. Schroeder/Kahle in Galen, *In Platonis Timaeum commentarii fragmenta*, as already noted by Rosenthal, "Life is Short, Art is Long," p. 236.

28   Cf. Maimonides, *On Asthma* 13.22, trans. Bos, vol. 1, p. 93: "On the other hand, the incompetent physician never stops rendering medical treatment and is always actively [involved], although he is ignorant of all these subjects. Sometimes he is successful [in his treatment], and sometimes he fails; but his failures are more frequent, while his successes are accidental and rare."

29   For Maimonides' concept of *tajriba*, i.e., experience or experiment, cf. ibid. 13.29, p. 96: "The greatest mistake is the belief that the experience which is mentioned and referred to in medicine is the experience of the [individual] physician in his own era. But this is not so. Rather, [medical] experience is the sum of the experience acquired over the course of past generations [even] before the time of Galen—namely, those things which have been written down in the medical books. Some of the drugs and compound remedies were tested for hundreds of years and were [then] written in books. But the individual practitioner of this art can in no way be qualified as experienced, since the right conditions for [acquiring] experience are missing; for not even an eminent physician carries out experiments because Hippocrates said: 'Experiment is dangerous.' But in our times experience is claimed only by pseudo-physicians, who make people believe in something which has not been proven in order to cover up their lack [of experience];" cf. Langermann, "Ibn Kammuna," p. 296: "*Tajriba* denotes conclusions drawn from repeated observation ...;" see also Rosenthal, "Life is Short, Art is Long," p. 233 n. 30.

الكمال فيها. وقال جالينوس في شرحه لكتاب طيماوس قال: لا يمكن الإنسان أن يكون عالما بصناعة الطبّ بأسرها.

[١٩] قال المؤلّف: وعند الإنصاف تعلم أنّ كلّ غير كامل فيها فإنّه يضرّ أكثر ممّا ينفع لأنّ كون الشخص صحيحا كان أو مريضا لا يتدبّر برأي طبيب أصلا أولى به من أن يتدبّر برأي طبيب يغلط
٥ عليه. وعلى قدر تقصير كلّ شخص يكون غلطه وإن وقعت منه إصابة فبالعرض. فمن أجل هذا استفتح هذا الفاضل كتابه بالحضّ على الكمال في هذه الصناعة بقوله العمر قصير والصناعة طويلة والوقت ضيّق التجربة خطر والقضاء عسر.

أمّا كون التجربة خطر بيّن لكنّي سأزيده بيانا.

[٢٠] وقوله الوقت ضيّق يبدو لي أنّه أراد به وقت المرض يضيق جدّا عن التجربة. فإنّك إذا لم تعلم
١٠ الأمور كلّها التي قد صحّت بالتجربة بل تستأنف الآن أن تجرّب أمورا في هذا المريض فالوقت يضيق

---

experiment with [certain] matters on this patient, time is too short for that and there is danger in beginning to experiment on this patient. All these words are in exhortation to be perfect in the art, so that all that has been tried throughout the years is present in your memory.

[21] As to his statement "judgment is difficult," it seems to me that he means by this the judgment whether the disease tends towards [the patient] being saved or perishing or to [another kind] of change. In general, prognosis is very diffi-cult in the art of medicine because the elements [of the body] are in a state of constant change and rarely remain in the same condition. You already know that most of the natural matters are not constant. How many times are the indications extremely bad, yet the patient is saved, and how many times one takes the favorable indications as a good omen, yet what they indicated does not come true. Therefore, lengthy training is needed in the observation of indi-vidual symptoms, for then you will be able to judge what will occur with a good intuition[30] that approaches the truth. This saying also urges to apply oneself with persistence and perseverance to this art.

[22] The meaning of "danger in experience" is as I will describe [now]. Know that in every natural body there are two kinds of accidents: accidents that adhere to it with respect to its matter and accidents that adhere to it with respect to its form. Man is an example of this: Health and illness, sleep and wakefulness adhere to him with respect to his matter, that is, with respect to his being a living being, and it adheres to him that he thinks, reflects, wonders, and laughs with respect to his form. Those accidents that adhere to his body with respect to its form are those that are called "specific properties," because they are specific to this species alone. Likewise, every plant, every mineral, and every organ of a living being has these two kinds of accidents.

[23] To each of these accidents belongs a certain action in our body. The actions performed by a drug in our body with respect to its matter is that it heats or cools or moistens or dries. These are the actions, which the physicians call "the primary powers" and say that this drug heats or cools by its nature. They also say that it does so by its quality. Similarly, the actions, which result from these

---

30   "intuition (حدس)": For this concept, cf. Langermann, ibid., pp. 286–302. Note however
      that in a medical context, the term is used in the Arabic translations of Galen for Greek
      στοχασμόν, i.e., conjecture; cf. Maimonides, *Medical Aphorisms* 11.1, ed. and trans. Bos,
      vol. 3, p. 20.

عن ذلك مع ما في استئناف التجربة في هذا المريض من الخطر ويكون الكلام كلّه في الحضّ على الكمال في الصناعة حتّى يكون كلّ ما جرّب على مرور السنين حاضرا في ذكرك.

[٢١] وأمّا قوله والقضاء عسر فيبدو لي أنّه يريد به القضاء على ميل المرض للخلاص أو للعطب أو لحدوث تغيّر من التغيّرات وبالجملة تقدمة المعرفة بما سيكون فإنّ ذلك عسر في صناعة الطبّ جدّا

٥ لسيلان العنصر وقلّة ثباته على حالة واحدة. وقد علمت أنّ الأمور الطبيعيّة كلّها أكثر لا دائمة فكم مرّة تكون الدلائل في غاية الرداءة وينجو المريض وكم مرّة يستبشر بجودة الدلائل ولا يصحّ ما دلّت عليه. فلذلك يحتاج إلى رياضة طويلة في مباشرة الدلائل الشخصيّة وحينئذ تقدر أن تقضي على ما يحدث بحدس جيّد يقرب من الحقّ. فيكون هذا القول أيضا في الحضّ على الدؤوب في ملازمة هذه الصناعة.

[٢٢] وأمّا وجه الخطر في التجربة فعل ما أصف. اعلم أنّ كلّ جسم طبيعي فيوجد فيه نوعين من ١٠ الأعراض: أعراض تلحقه من جهة مادّته وأعراض تلحقه من جهة صورته. مثال ذلك الإنسان: فإنّه تلحقه الصحّة والمرض والنوم واليقظة من جهة مادّته أعني من جهة ما هو حيوان ويلحقه أنّ يفكّر ويروي ويتعجّب ويضحك من جهة صورته. وهذه الأعراض التي تلحق الجسم من جهة صورته هي التي تسمّى الخواصّ لأنّها خاصّة بذلك النوع وحده. كلّ نبات وكلّ معدن وكلّ عضو من أعضاء ١٥ الحيوان يوجد له هذين النوعين من الأعراض.

[٢٣] ويتبع لكلّ عرض منها فعل ما في أبداننا. فالأفعال التي يفعلها الدواء في أبداننا من جهة مادّته هو أن يسخّن أو يبرّد أو يرطّب أو يجفّف. وهذه هي التي يسمّيها الأطبّاء القوى الأوّل ويقولون إنّ هذا الدواء يسخّن بطبيعته أو يبرّد وكذلك يقولون أيضا يفعل بكيفيّته وكذلك الأفعال التابعة لهذه

---

٣ وأمّا: أمّا BC ‖ فيبدو: فيبد A ‖ ميل: emendation editor مال ABC   ٥ حالة: حال A   ٨ الدؤوب: الدروب A ‖ ملازمة: مداومة A   ١٠ نوعين: نوعان C   ١٧ هي: om. B   ١٨ يفعل: C¹

primary powers, those which the physicians call "the secondary powers," such as when a drug hardens or softens or loosens or thickens, and the other [actions], which they enumerated, all of them are effected by the drug with respect to its matter.[31]

[24] The actions, which a drug performs in our body with regard to its specific form, are those, which the physicians call "specific properties."[32] Galen expounds this kind of action by saying that it acts by the whole of its essence,[33] that is to say, it performs its action with respect to its specific form through which that body is constituted[34] as a substance. This present action does not result from its quality. They also call these "tertiary powers," and these are, for example, the purgative effect of purgatives, the emetic effect of emetics, the lethal effect of poisons, or the life-saving effect [of drugs] for the ingestion of a poisonous substance or for the bite of a poisonous animal. All these actions result from the form [of the remedy], not its matter.

[25] Nutrients are also of this kind, that is to say, the fact that certain species of plants serve as nourishment for certain species of animals is not only attributable to the first qualities and also not to the hardness, softness, thickness, or looseness that follow from them. Rather, it is an action of the entire substance, as Galen says. Consider how we are nourished by things, which are close to the nature of wood and which our stomach acts upon and changes, such as dried chestnuts, dried acorns, and dried carobs. But our stomach does not at all change the peel and pits of grapes, nor the peel of apples and their like. As these enter the body so they leave, for it is not in their essence to be influenced (affected) by the stomach in any way.

---

31   For the theory of the primary, secondary, and tertiary powers of drugs, based on Galen's medical system, cf. Harig, *Bestimmung der Intensität*, pp. 111–114.

32   In his *Medical Aphorisms* 22, ed. and trans. Bos, vol. 5, pp. 1–22, Maimonides gives a long list of remedies effective through their specific properties, mostly consisting of all sorts of animals, their parts, excrements, and urine. See also idem, *On the Elucidation of Some Symptoms and the Response to Them* 3, ed. and trans. Bos, pp. 28–29; *On Hemorrhoids* 2.3, ed. and trans. Bos, pp. 9–11; *On Poisons and the Protection Against Lethal Drugs* 15, ed. and trans. Bos, p. 16. The subject is discussed in Schwartz, "Magiyah," pp. 35–38; Pseudo-Ibn Ezra, *Sefer Hanisyonot*, eds. and trans. Leibowitz/Marcus, pp. 17–20; Langermann, "Gersonides on the Magnet," pp. 273–274; Freudenthal, "Maimonides' Philosophy of Science," pp. 151–156; and ed. Bos, introduction to Maimonides, *Medical Aphorisms*, vol. 5, pp. xix–xxii.

33   Cf. Harig, *Bestimmung der Intensität*, pp. 107–110.

34   "constituted as a substance" (جوهر): Cf. Maimonides, *Dalālat al-ḥāʾirīn* 1.1, trans. Pines: *Guide of the Perplexed*, p. 22; cf. Friedländer, *Arabisch-deutsches Lexikon*, p. 21.

القوى الأوّل وهي التي يسمّيها الأطبّاء القوى الثواني مثل أن يكون الدواء يصلّب أو يلين أو يخلخل أو يكثّف وسائر ما عدّوا كلّها يفعلها الدواء من جهة مادّته.

[٢٤] والأفعال التي يفعلها الدواء في أبداننا من جهة صورته النوعية هي التي يسمّيها الأطبّاء الخاصّية. وجالينوس يعبّر عن هذا النوع من الأفعال بأن يقول: يفعل بجملة جوهره المعنى أنّه فعل يفعله من

٥   جهة صورته النوعية التي بها تجوهر ذلك الجسم وصار هذا لا أنّه فعل تابع لكيفيته ويسمّونها أيضا القوى الثوالث وهي مثل إسهال الأدوية المسهلة أو تقييئها أو كونها سمّ قاتل ومخلّصة من شرب السمّ أو من نهش أحد ذوات السموم. كلّ هذه الأفعال تابعة للصورة لا للمادّة.

[٢٥] والأغذية أيضا هي من هذا النوع أعني كون هذا النوع من النبات يغذو النوع الفلاني من الحيوان ليس هذا راجع لمجرّد الكيفيّات الأوّل ولا أيضا لما يلزم عنها من الصلابة واللين أو الكثافة

١٠ والتخلخل بل فعل بجملة الجوهر كما يقول جالينوس. تأمّل كيف نغتذي بأشياء هي قريبة من طبيعة الخشب وتفعل فيها معدنا وتحيلها كالقسطل اليابس والبلّوط اليابس والخرّوب اليابس ولا تحيل معدنا بوجه قشر حبّ العنب ولا قشر التفّاح ونحوها إلّا كما يردّ الجسم كما تخرج لأنّ ليس في جوهرها أن تقبل من معدنا أثرا بوجه.

٣-٢ من جهة مادّته والأفعال التي يفعلها الدواء: om. A   ٣ الخاصّية: الخاصّة C   ٤ فعل: ما add. A

٩ ليس: وليس B   ٩-١٤.53 أو الكثافة ... صارت أدوية: om. B   ١٢ قشر: C²   ١٣ أثرا: أثر C

[26] In his famous book *De simplicium medicamentorum* [*temperamentis ac facultatibus*], Galen has explained how to deduce from its taste the nature and action of a drug resulting from its quality.[35] As to the knowledge of what the drug does with respect to its specific form, and this is what is said [above] that it performs this action with its entire substance, we have no indication whatsoever, nor any other way by which to draw conclusions about this action, except by experience (*tajriba*).[36] How many drugs are bitter and extremely foul-smelling, and yet are beneficial drugs. But one may also find a plant that tastes and smells like the other nutrients, yet is a lethal poison, or a plant of which one thinks that it is one of the [different] kinds of nutrients, except that it is wild and not cultivated, yet it is a lethal poison. The danger of [applying a certain medication based on] experience should be clear to you, there is nothing more dangerous than it. Yet there is a great need for it, for the nutritional power of all the nutrients was not learned except by experience. Likewise, the actions of most drugs were not learned except by experience. Therefore, you should not give precedence to experimentation, but [first] seek help by remembering all that others have tried.

[27] Know that there are drugs whose action in our bodies, which occurs as a result of their matter, is clear and manifest, while their action, which results from their form, is very much hidden so that it is not perceived, like most drugs to which no specific property is ascribed and to which no specific action is attributed. But there are also drugs whose action in our body, which occurs as a result of their form, is very clear, like purgatives, poisons, and antidotes. These affect our bodies with respect to heating and cooling only very little, either because of the small quantity taken of them, even though they are warming or cooling, or because they do not have a predominant manifest quality. [In any case] it is absolutely necessary that these two actions are present, namely that which results from the matter and that which results from the form. Because of the action, which results from the form, there are drugs that are specific for the stomach, drugs that are specific for the liver, drugs that are specific for the spleen, drugs that are specific for the heart, and drugs that are specific for the brain. And because of the specific form the actions of the drugs are diverse,

---

35   Cf. Galen, *De simplicium medicamentorum temperamentis ac facultatibus* 4.26, ed. Kühn, vol. 11, pp. 784–786; Harig, *Bestimmung der Intensität*, pp. 107–110.

36   For *tajriba*, cf. section 20 above.

[٢٦] وقد بيّن جالينوس كيف يستدلّ على طبائع الأدوية وأفعالها التابعة لكيفيّاتها من طعومها في كتابه المشهور في الأدوية المفردة. أمّا معرفة ما يفعله الدواء من جهة صورته النوعية وهي التي يقال إنّه يفعلها بجملة جوهره فليس عندنا دليل بوجه يستدلّ به على ذلك الفعل ولا لمعرفة ذلك طريق آخر بوجه غير التجربة. وكم دواء مرّ منتن غاية النتن وهو دواء نافع وقد يوجد النبات الذي يكون طعمه

٥ ورائحته كسائر طعوم الأغذية وروائحها وهو سمّ قاتل بل قد يوجد نبات يظنّ أنّه من أنواع الأغذية إلّا أنّه بريّ فقط لا بستاني وهو سمّ قاتل. فقد تبيّن لك خطر التجربة ما أعظمه وشدّة الحاجة إليها مع ذلك لأنّ كلّ الأغذية ما علمت قواها من حيث هي غذاء إلّا بالتجربة وكذلك معظم الأدوية ما علمت أفعالها إلّا بالتجربة فينبغي لك أن لا تقدم بالتجربة وأن تستظهر بحفظ كلّ ما جرّبه كلّ ما جرّبه الغير.

[٢٧] واعلم أنّ ثمّ أدوية يكون فعلها في أبداننا التابع لمادّتها هو الظاهر البيّن وفعلها التابع لصورتها خفي

١٠ جدّا حتّى لا يشعر به كأكثر الأدوية التي لا توصف لها خاصّية ولا تخصّص بفعل. وثمّ أدوية يكون فعلها في أبداننا التابع لصورتها ظاهر عظيم كالأدوية المسهلة والسموم والمخلّصات ولا تؤثّر في أبداننا من جهة التسخين والتبريد إلّا أثر يسير جدّا إمّا من قبل نزارة ما يتناول منها وإن كانت حارّة أو باردة أو من قبل أن ليس لها كيفيّة غالب ظاهرة. ولا بدّ من وجود الفعلين ضرورة أعني التابع للمادّة والتابع للصورة. ومن أجل الفعل التابع للصورة صارت أدوية مخصوصة بالمعدة وأدوية مخصوصة

١٥ بالكبد وأدوية مخصوصة بالطحال وأدوية مخصوصة بالقلب وأدوية مخصوصة بالدماغ. ومن أجل الصورة النوعية أيضا تختلف أفعال الأدوية وإن كانت طبيعتها واحدة. أنت تتأمّل فتجد أدوية عدّة

---

٤ يوجد: يجود A ٨ أفعالها: فعالها A ١٢ نزارة: نزادة A ١٣ غالب ظاهرة: غالبة A ١٤ للصورة: لصورتها A

even though their nature is the same. If you look well, you will find numerous drugs that have exactly the same degree of heat and dryness, for instance, and each of these drugs has actions other than those of the other drug. All this was indeed brought out by experience in the course of time.

[28] Because of his great moral virtues, Hippocrates ordered in this aphorism, with which he began, that the physician should not be content with doing what is necessary only, and stop there, because that is not sufficient for the attainment of health for the patient. For the goal will only be achieved and [the patient] healed, if also the patient and all those around him will do what is necessary, and remove all external impediments that prevent the cure of the illness. It is as though he is commanding in this aphorism that the physician should apply his abilities to manage his patients, and make their treatment easy with, for instance, the ingestion of bitter medicines, clysters, lancing, cautery, and the like. He should admonish and warn the patient and those around him, against making mistakes, and make those around him take care of the treatment [of the patient], as is proper when the physician is absent. Similarly, he should remove the external impediments as well as he can, according to each individual case. For instance, if the patient is poor and he is in a place that increases his illness but he cannot afford another place, he (i.e., the physician) should move him from [that] place to another one. Likewise, he should provide him with nourishment and medication if he (the patient) does not have that. These and their like are the things, which exceed a physician's duty with respect to his art, yet are necessary for the attainment of the goal, which the physician wants to attain for this patient. Only to prescribe what is necessary to do [with regard to the medical art] and to leave it at that, he (i.e., the physician) should not do so, because then the goal intended will not be attained.[37]

---

37   The awareness of the special needs of poor patients can already be found in Galen's pharmacological writings. A prominent theme is his diatribe against the greed of the physicians, who deserve more to be called "sellers of drugs" than "physicans." In his treatise "The Best Doctor is Also a Philosopher," trans. Singer, Galen portrays Hippocrates, the ideal physician, as a physician who despises money and champions the poor. The medieval deontological treatises, clearly influenced by Hippocratic and Galenic writings, enjoin the treatment of the sick and poor for free. As for Maimonides and his great-great grandson, David II, we know for a fact that they gave medical advice and help to poor persons with whom they had dealings in their capacity as heads of their Jewish communities (cf. Goitein, *Mediterranean Society*, vol. 2, p. 133). For an extensive treatment of this subject, see Bos, "Ibn al-Jazzār on Medicine," esp. pp. 366–368.

في درجة واحدة بعينها من الحرارة واليبس مثلا ولكلّ دواء منها أفعال غير أفعال الدواء الآخر. وهذا كلّه إنّما أخرجته التجربة على مرور الأزمنة.

[٢٨] ولعظم فضيلة أخلاق أبقراط أمر في هذا الفصل الذي أفتح به أن لا يقتصر الطبيب على أن يفعل ما ينبغي فقط ويكفّ لأنّ ذلك غير كاف في حصول الصحّة للمريض. وإنّما تتمّ الغاية ويبرأ

٥ بأن يكون المريض أيضا وكلّ من حوله يفعل بالمريض ما ينبغي فعله ويرفع العوائق كلّها التي من خارج المانعة عن شفاء المرض. فكأنّه يأمر في هذا الفصل أنّ للطبيب قدرة على سياسة المرضى وتسهيل أعمال الطبّ عليهم كشرب الأدوية المرّة والحقن والبطّ والكيّ ونحوها وأن يخطب المريض ومن حوله ويحذّره من أن يخطئ على نفسه. ويجعل من حوله يقومون بتدبيره كما ينبغي في حال غيبة الطبيب. وكذلك يزيل العوائق التي من خارج ما أمكنه بحسب شخص شخص. مثاله إن يكون

١٠ المريض فقيرا وهو في موضع يزيد في مرضه ولا قدرة له على موضع آخر فينقله هو من موضع إلى موضع. وكذلك يهيّئ له الغذاء والدواء إذا لم يكن ذلك عنده. فهذه وأشباهها هي الأشياء الخارجة عمّا يلزم الطبيب من حيث صناعته لكنّها ضرورية في حصول الغاية التي يروم الطبيب حصولها لهذا المريض. أمّا أن يصف فقط ما ينبغي أن يفعل ويروح فلا يفعل ذلك لأنّه قد لا تحصل من ذلك الغاية المقصودة.

---

٣ ولعظم: ولعظيم AC ‖ به: على add. B ٥ المريض أيضا و-: om. B ‖ حوله: C¹ ٦ عن: من B

٨ يقومون: له add. B ١٠ فقيرا: فقير BC ١٢ لكنّها: ولكنّها A

(1.2)

[29] Says Hippocrates: If the [material] that is evacuated from the body during diarrhea or during vomiting, which happen spontaneously, is from the kind that should be purged from the body, it is beneficial and easy to bear. But if this is not the case, the contrary holds good. The same applies to the [artificial] emptying of the vessels. If they are emptied from the [material] they should be free from, it is beneficial and easy to bear. But if this is not the case, the contrary holds good. One should also consider the current time of the year, the place [where one lives], the age and the diseases as to whether the intended evacuation should be carried out or not.

Says the commentator: The statement "the same applies to the emptying of the vessels" means through micturiction or perspiration or through flow of blood (i.e., nosebleed or menses) or the opening of the orifices of the blood vessels. All these are things that occur spontaneously.[38] As for Galen, he says that with the "emptying of the vessels" he means the evacuation by means of a drug. In his opinion, the last part of his (i.e., Hippocrates') statement[39] is repetitious, so that it needs an explanation.[40] Then he states that if you intend an evacuation of [a humor, which is] of the kind [that should be evacuated] when the signs of its domination are clear to you, you should also take into consideration the [current] time of the year, the place [where one lives], the age, and the nature of that disease and deal with the matter accordingly. For the evacuation of yellow bile in winter or in cold places or in old age or in diseases [caused by cold] is difficult and cannot be tolerated [by the patient]. Likewise, the evacuation of phlegm in summer or in hot places or in the case of young people or of diseases [caused by heat] is difficult and cannot be tolerated [by the patient].[41]

---

38   Maimonides clearly interprets the Arabic خلاء العروق (lit., "state of emptiness of the ves-
      sels") (= V, fol. 9^b) contrary to the original meaning of the Hippocratic text, as the Greek
      κενεαγγείη (Galen, *In Hippocratis Aphorismos commentarius* 1.2, ed. Kühn, vol. 17b, p. 357),
      does not refer to a spontaneous evacuation but to an artificial one; cf. Liddell/Scott, *Greek-
      English Lexicon*, p. 937: "lowering or evacuant treatment;" Hippocrates, *Aphorisms*, trans.
      Jones, p. 99: "artificial evacuations."

39   I.e., "If they are emptied from the [material] they should be free from, it is beneficial and
      easy to bear. But if this is not the case, the contrary holds good."

40   Cf. Galen, *In Hippocratis Aphorismos commentarius* 1.2, ed. Kühn, vol. 17b, pp. 357–358.

41   Cf. ibid., pp. 359–360.

(1.2)

[٢٩] قال أبقراط: إن كان ما يستفرغ من البدن عند استطلاق البطن والقيء الذين يكونان طوعا

من النوع الذي ينبغي أن ينقّى منه البدن نفع ذلك وسهل احتماله وإن لم يكن كذلك كان الأمر

على الضدّ. وكذلك خلاء العروق فإنّها إن خلّت من النوع الذي ينبغي أن تخلو منه نفع ذلك وسهل

احتماله وإن لم يكن كذلك كان الأمر على الضدّ. فينبغي أيضا أن ينظر في الوقت الحاضر من أوقات

٥   السنة وفي البلد وفي السن وفي الأمراض هل يوجب استفراغ ما هممت باستفراغه أم لا.

قال المفسّر: قوله وكذلك خلاء العروق يعني بإدرار البول أو العرق أو النزف أو انفتاح أفواه العروق

ويكون هذا الفصل كلّه فيما يأتي طوعا. أمّا جالينوس فقال: يريد بخلاء العروق الاستفراغ الذي

يكون بالدواء ولذلك يكون الفصل الأخير من هذه المقالة عنده مكرّرا حتّى احتاج له لتأويل. ثمّ

ذكر إنّه إذا هممت باستفراغ النوع الذي ينبغي إذا بانت لك علامات غلبته فينبغي أيضا أن يجعل

١٠   لأوقات السنة والبلد والسن وطبيعة ذلك المرض حظّ ويدبّر الأمر بحسبه. فإنّ استفراغ الصفراء

في الشتاء أو في المواضع الباردة أو في سنّ الشيخ أو في الأمراض الباردة يعسر ولا يحتمل. وكذلك

استفراغ البلغم في الصيف أو في المواضع الحارّة أو من الشباب أو في الأمراض الحارّة يعسر ولا

يحتمل.

---

٤ أيضا: C om.   ٦ العروق: عروق C   ٨ ثمّ: انه B add.   ١٠ والسن: وللسن C

(1.3)

[30] Says Hippocrates: In those who do physical exercise, extreme stoutness of the body is dangerous, if they have reached the very limit therein. For they cannot stay or remain in that condition, and since they cannot stay [in that condition] and cannot become healthier, their condition can only become worse. For this reason one should reduce the stoutness of the body without delay so that it can start again to[42] assimilate the food, but the [reduction][43] should not be extreme, for that is [also] dangerous. It should only be to the degree, which can be tolerated by the nature (constitution) of the body, which one wants to [reduce]. Similarly, any evacuation carried out to the extreme is dangerous, and any feeding[44] that is extreme is also dangerous.

Says the commentator: With "those who carry out physical exercise" he means wrestlers and the like, among those who choose hard physical exercise for their profession. When their [blood] vessels are filled more than necessary one cannot be sure that they will not burst or that the innate heat will not be strangled in them, so that it becomes extinguished and they die. For the [blood] vessels need a vacuum to receive the food that reaches them.[45]

(1.4)

[31] Says Hippocrates: A[46] strict regimen is undoubtedly dangerous in all chronic diseases, and in acute diseases when[47] it is not endured. A[48] regimen that is extremely strict is undoubtedly difficult and reprehensible.

---

42   "to assimilate the food" (قبول الغذاء): Cf. ibid. 1.3, p. 361: ἀναθρέψιος; Hippocrates, *Aphorisms*, trans. Littré, vol. 4, p. 461: "la réparation;" trans. Jones, p. 101: "growth;" cf. Liddell/Scott, *Greek-English Lexicon*, p. 105, s.v. ἀναθρέψις: "renewal, restoration in physiological sense."

43   "[reduction]": Lit., "evacuation" (استفراغ); cf. Galen, ibid.: ξυμπτώσιας; Hippocrates, ibid., trans. Littré: "les atténuations;" trans. Jones: "reduction;" cf. Liddell/Scott, ibid., p. 1686, s.v. σύμπτωσις: "falling together, collapsing."

44   "feeding" (تغذية): Cf. Galen, ibid., p. 362: ἀναθρέψιες; Hippocrates, ibid., trans. Littré: "les réparations;" trans. Jones: "new growths."

45   Cf. Maimonides, *Medical Aphorisms* 18.9, trans. Bos, vol. 4, p. 41: "Strenuous physical exercise dries the body and makes it hard and slow of sensation and understanding. Therefore, wrestlers and those who carry heavy burdens and stones are ignorant and have little understanding. *De somno et vigilia*."

46   "A strict regimen": Cf. Galen, *In Hippocratis Aphorismos commentarius* 1.4, ed. Kühn, vol. 17b, p. 367: Ἀι λεπταὶ καὶ ἀκριβέες δίαιται; Hippocrates, *Aphorisms*, trans. Littré, vol. 4, p. 461: "Une diète tenue et stricte;" trans. Jones, p. 101: "A restricted and rigid regimen."

47   "when it is not endured": Cf. Galen, ibid.: οὗ μὴ ἐπιδέχεται; Hippocrates, ibid., trans. Littré, pp. 461, 463: "dans celles qui ne s'en accommodent pas;" trans. Jones: "where it is not called for."

48   "A regimen that is extremely strict is undoubtedly difficult and reprehensible": Cf. Galen,

(١.٣)

[٣٠] قال أبقراط: خصب البدن المفرط لأصحاب الرياضة خطر إذا كانوا قد بلغوا منه الغاية القصوى وذلك إنّه لا يمكن أن يثبتوا على حالتهم تلك ولا يستقرّوا ولما كانوا لا يستقرّون (و) لم يمكن أنْ يزدادوا صلاحا فبقي أن يميلوا إلى حالة أردأ فلذلك ينبغي أن ينقص خصب البدن بلا تأخير كيما يعود البدن فيبتدئ في قبول الغذاء ولا يبلغ من استفراغه الغاية القصوى فإنّ ذلك خطر لكن بمقدار احتمال طبيعة البدن الذي يقصد إلى استفراغه. وكذلك أيضا كلّ استفراغ يبلغ فيه الغاية القصوى فهو خطر ٥ وكلّ تغذية أيضا هي عند الغاية القصوى فهي خطر.

قال المفسّر: يريد بأصحاب الرياضة المصارعين ونحوهم ممن يتّخذ الرياضة العنيفة صناعة وذلك أنّ العروق إذا امتلأت أكثر ممّا ينبغي لم يؤمن أن تتصدع أو تختنق الحرارة الغريزية فيها فتطفأ فيموتوا فإنّه ينبغي أن يكون في العروق خلو لقبول ما يصل إليها من الغذاء.

(١.٤)

[٣١] قال أبقراط: التدبير البالغ في اللطافة في جميع الأمراض المزمنة لا محالة خطر وفي الأمراض ١٠ الحادّة إذا لم يحتمله والتدبير الذي يبلغ فيه الغاية القصوى من اللطافة فهو عسر مذموم لا محالة.

---

٢ حالتهم: حالهم C ‖ (و) لم: (و) لم t emendation editor following ٣ حالة: حال هي A ٥ كلّ: A om. A
٦ فهي: فهو C ٨ إذا: om. A ٩ ٦٥.٢ لقبول ... قال المفسّر: om. C ١٠ اللطافة: عسر مذموم add.
At ‖ لا محالة خطر: om. tV ١٠-١١ والتدبير الذي يبلغ فيه الغاية القصوى من اللطافة وفي ... لا محالة
في الأمراض الحادّة اذا لم يحتمله القوة عسر مذموم t والتدبير الذي يبلغ فيه الغاية القصوى من اللطافة في
الأمراض الحادّة اذا لم تحتمله فهو عسر مذموم V والتدبير الذي يبلغ في غاية القصوى من اللطافة في الأمراض
الحادّة لم تحتمل القوة فهو عسير مذموم D ١١ يحتمله: المريض add. B

---

ibid.: αἱ πληρώσιες αἱ ἐς το ἔσχατον ἀφιγμέναι χαλεπαί; Hippocrates, ibid., ed. and trans. Littré, pp. 462–463: αἱ πληρώσιες αἱ ἐν τῷ ἔσχατῳ ἐοῦσαι χαλεπαί ("car les réparations, à l'extrême limite, sont pénibles"); trans. Jones: "and in fact repletion too, carried to extremes, is perilous."

Says the commentator: A regimen that is extremely strict is that in which one absolutely abstains from taking any food, a regimen that is very strict but not extreme is the imbibition of honey water and the like. A regimen that is strict but not very [strict] consists of barley gruel and the like.

(1.5)
[32] Says Hippocrates: In a strict regimen, patients sometimes make mistakes, which cause severe harm to them. For all that happens [to them] as a result of [a strict regimen] is more serious than what happens [to them] as a result of [a regimen of] food that is slightly thickening (nourishing). For this reason, a strict regimen is also dangerous for healthy people, but they endure [the harm] resulting from a mistake in a thickening (nourishing) regimen more easily. Therefore, a strict regimen is in most cases more dangerous than a regimen that is slightly more thickening (nourishing).

Says the commentator: This is clear [and] evident.

(1.6)
[33] Says Hippocrates: In extreme diseases the[49] best regimen is that, which is extreme.

Says the commentator: Extreme diseases are those, which are extremely acute.

(1.7)
[34] Says Hippocrates: When the disease is very acute, extreme pains appear in the beginning and it is necessary to apply an extremely strict (lit., refining, thinning) regimen. If this is not the case, and a more thickening (nourishing) regimen is possible, the relaxation [of the extremely strict regimen] should be according to the mildness of the disease and its deviation from the extreme.

Says the commentator: Extreme pains are severe pains, such as [those occurring during] fever attacks and all [other] afflictions. [They happen during] the culmination of the disease, for the culmination is that [phase] of the disease that is most powerful in its (i.e., of the disease) symptoms. His statement "in the beginning" should be understood as [referring to] the first four days or a little bit later.

---

49   "the best regimen is that, which is extreme": Galen, ibid. 1.6, p. 372: αἱ ἔσχαται θεραπεῖαι ἐς
     ἀκριθείην, κράτισται; Hippocrates, ibid., trans. Littré, p. 463: "l' extrême exactitude du traite-
     ment est ce qu' il y a de plus puissant;" trans. Jones, p. 103: "extreme strictness of treatment
     is most efficacious."

قال المفسّر: التدبير الذي في غاية اللطافة هو ترك تناول الطعام البتّة والتدبير الذي هو في الغاية من اللطافة إلّا أنّه ليس في أقصاها هو تناول ماء العسل ونحوه والتدبير اللطيف الذي ليس في الغاية فماء كشك الشعير ونحوه.

(1.5)

[٣٢] قال أبقراط: في التدبير اللطيف قد يخطئ المرضى على أنفسهم خطأً يعظم ضرره عليهم وذلك

٥ أنّ جميع ما يكون منه أعظم ممّا يكون منه في الغذاء الذي له غلظ يسير ومن قبل هذه صار التدبير البالغ في اللطافة في الأصحّاء أيضا خطر إلّا أنّ احتمالهم لما يعرض من خطائهم في التدبير الغليظ أقلّ ولذلك صار التدبير البالغ في اللطافة في أكثر الحالات أعظم خطرا من التدبير الذي هو أغلظ قليلا.

قال المفسّر: هذا بيّن واضح.

(1.6)

[٣٣] قال أبقراط: أجود التدبير في الأمراض التي في الغاية القصوى التدبير التي في غاية القصوى.

١٠ قال المفسّر: الأمراض التي في الغاية القصوى هي الأمراض الحادّة جدًّا.

(1.7)

[٣٤] قال أبقراط: وإذا كان المرض حادًّا جدًّا فإنّ الأوجاع التي في الغاية القصوى تأتي فيه بدءا ويجب ضرورة أن يستعمل فيه التدبير الذي في الغاية القصوى من اللطافة. فإذا لم يكن كذلك لكن كان يحتمل من التدبير ما هو أغلظ من ذلك فينبغي أن يكون الانحطاط على حسب لين المرض ونقصانه عن الغاية القصوى.

١٥ قال المفسّر: الأوجاع التي في الغاية القصوى هي الأوجاع العظيمة يعني نوائب الحمّى وجميع الأعراض وهو منتهى المرض فإنّ ليس المنتهى شيء سوى أعظم أجزاء المرض في أعراضه وافهم قوله بدءا الأربعة الأيّام الأوّل أو بعدها قليلة.

---

٥ منه أعظم: منه من الخطاء أعظم ضررا t ‖ لأنّ a emendation editor: إلّا أنّ ٦ يعرض: لهم add. A

(1.8)

[35] Says Hippocrates: When the disease has reached its culmination one should apply a regimen that is extremely strict.

Says the commentator: This is because of the severity of the symptoms at that time, and so that the illness can be concocted. For nature should not be diverted through the concoction of new food that is delivered to it from the concoction of the humors that produced the disease. For at that time nature is wholeheartedly engaged in that with all its powers, and it only needs [to do] a little more until it has subdued them (i.e., the humors) completely.

(1.9)

[36] Says Hippocrates: One should also examine the strength of the patient and find out whether it can remain firm until the culmination of the disease, and investigate whether the strength of the patient will dwindle before the disease becomes extremely severe, and it (i.e., his strength) will not last on that diet, or whether the disease will decline first and lose its severity.

Says the commentator: This is evident.

(1.10)

[37] Says Hippocrates: The regimen of those whose illness reaches its climax [right] in the beginning should be strict (lit., fine, thin) straightaway. The[50] regimen of those whose illness culminates later on should be more thickening (nutritious) in the beginning, and then, when the culmination of the illness approaches, it (i.e., the regimen) should be restricted slowly in a way that the strength of the patient lasts. One should stop [the administration of] food during the culmination of the illness, for an increase[51] in [food] is harmful.

Says the commentator: This is evident.

---

50   "The regimen ... is harmful": Cf. Galen, ibid. 1.10, p. 379: ὁκόσοισι δὲ ἐς ὕστερον ἡ ἀκμὴ ἐς ἐκεῖνο καὶ πρὸ ἐκείνου σμικρὸν ἀφαιρετέον· ἔμπροσθεν δὲ πιωτέρως διαιτᾶν ὡς ἂν ἐξαρκέσῃ ὁ νοσέων; Hippocrates, ibid., trans. Littré, p. 465: "quand ce moment tarde davantage, il faut, à l'époque du *summum* et un peu avant cette époque, retrancher de la nourriture; auparavant, l'alimentation sera plus abondante, afin que le malade puisse résister;" trans. Jones: "When the height comes later, restrict regimen then and a little before then; before, however, use a fuller regimen, in order that the patient may hold out."

51   "increase": Cf. Galen, ibid. 1.11, pp. 379–380: τὸ προστιθέναι; Hippocrates, ibid., trans. Littré: "donner;" trans. Jones: "to give."

(1.8)

[٣٥] قال أبقراط: إذا بلغ المرض منتهاه فعند ذلك يجب ضرورة أن يستعمل التدبير الذي هو في الغاية القصوى من اللطافة.

قال المفسّر: وذلك لعظم الأعراض في ذلك الوقت ولكيما ينضج المرض وذلك أنّه لا ينبغي أن تشغل الطبيعة بإنضاج غذاء جديد تورده عليه عن إنضاج الأخلاط المولّدة للمرض إذ كانت في ذلك
٥ الوقت مكبّة عليها بقوّتها كلّها وإنّما بقي لها اليسير حتّى يستكمل الغلبة عليها.

(1.9)

[٣٦] قال أبقراط: وينبغي أن تزن أيضا قوّة المريض فتعلم إن كانت تثبت إلى وقت منتهى المرض وتنظر أقوّة المريض تخور قبل غاية المرض ولا تبقى على ذلك الغذاء أم المرض يخور قبل وتسكن عاديته.

قال المفسّر: هذا بيّن.

(1.10)

١٠ [٣٧] قال أبقراط: والذين يأتي منتهى مرضهم بدءا فينبغي أن يدبّروا بالتدبير اللطيف بدءا والذين يتأخّر منتهى مرضهم فينبغي أن يجعل تدبيرهم في ابتداء مرضهم أغلظ ثم ينقص من غلظه قليلا قليلا كلّما قرب منتهى المرض وفي وقت منتهاه بمقدار ما تبقى قوّة المريض عليه وينبغي أن يمنع من الغذاء في وقت منتهى المرض فإنّ الزيادة فيه مضرّة.

قال المفسّر: هذا بيّن.

---

١ هو: om. B ٦ أيضا: om. B ٩ قال المفسّر: om. B ‖ بيّن: ولا حاجة فيه إلى بيان add. A واضح add. D
١٠ والذين: والذي B ١١ غلظه: تغليظه B ١٢ كلّما قرب منتهى: وكلّما منتهى A

(1.11)

[38] Says Hippocrates: If the fever has cycles, one should stop [the administration of] food during its attacks, for an increase in it is harmful.

Says the commentator: This is evident.

(1.12)

[39] Says Hippocrates: The paroxysms and course[52] of a disease are indicated by the diseases themselves, the seasons of the year, the[53] increase in the cycles, [whether] they come every day or every two days or at a longer interval. [They are also indicated by] the [symptoms] that appear later; for example, in patients with pleuritis, if expectoration appears straightaway in the beginning of the disease, the disease will be a short one, but if it appears later, the disease will be prolonged. When urine, feces, and sweat appear later they may indicate whether the crisis of the disease will be benign or bad and whether the disease will be short or prolonged.

Says the commentator: From the nature of the illness itself one can know whether [the illness] ends quickly or slowly. Pleuritis, pneumonia, and phrenitis are acute diseases; angina, cholera, and spasms are very acute diseases; dropsy, delirium, internal suppuration, and phthisis, which is an [infection] of the lungs, are chronic diseases. Fever attacks mostly occur on alternate days in the case of pleuritis and phrenitis. They are mostly quotidian, especially during the night, in the case of those who have a purulent abscess in the stomach or liver or who suffer from phthisis. Fever attacks occur every three days in the case of those who suffer from an illness of the spleen or an illness resulting from black bile. The same holds good for the seasons of the year. Quartan fever is mostly short in the summer and long in autumn, especially when it is nearly winter.

An increase in attacks (cycles) indicates an increase [in the severity] of the disease and imminence of its culmination. The increase in the second attack can be distinguished from the first attack by three things: the first is the time of the attack of the fever, the second is the length of the attack, and the [third] is its strength, that is its severity.

---

52   "course of a disease" (نظام المرض) (مرتبة ونظام المرض) (cf. V, fol. 14ᵃ: مرتبة المرض): Cf. Galen, ibid. 1.12, ed. Kühn, p. 380: τὰς καταστάσιας; Hippocrates, ibid., trans. Littré: "les constitutions;" trans. Jones, p. 105: "constitutions." See also Barry, *Syriac Medicine*, pp. 155–157.

53   "the increase in the cycles": Cf. Galen, ibid. 1.12, pp. 380–381: αἱ τῶν περιόδων πρὸς ἀλλήλας ἀνταποδόσιες; Hippocrates, ibid., trans. Littré: "les correspondances réciproques des périodes;" trans. Jones: "the correspondence of periods to one another." For Arabic *ziyāda*

(1.11)

[٣٨] قال أبقراط: وإذا كان للحمّى أدوار فامنع من الغذاء في أوقات نوائبها فإنّ الزيادة فيه مضرّة.

قال المفسّر: هذا بيّن.

(1.12)

[٣٩] قال أبقراط: إنّه يدلّ على نوائب المرض ومرتبته ونظامه الأمراض أنفسها وأوقات السنة وتزيّد الأدوار بعضها على بعض نائبة كانت في كلّ يوم أو يوما ويوما لا أو في أكثر من ذلك الزمان. والأشياء أيضا التي تظهر بعد ومثال ذلك ما يظهر في أصحاب ذات الجنب فإنّه إن ظهر النفث بدئا منذ أوّل المرض كان المرض قصيرا وإن تأخّر ظهوره كان المرض طويلا. والبول والبراز والعرق إذا ظهرت بعد تدلّنا على جودة بحران المرض ورداءته وطول المرض وقصره.

قال المفسّر: من طبيعة المرض نفسه تعلم هل انقضاءه سريعا أو بطيئا. فإنّ ذات الجنب وذات الرئة والسرسام أمراض حادّة والذبحة والهيضة والتشنّج أمراض حادّة جدّا. والاستسقاء والوسواس ومدّة الجوف والسلّ وهي قرحة الرئة هي أمراض مزمنة. ونوائب الحمّى أكثر ما تكون في ذات الجنب والسرسام غبّا. وأكثر ما تكون من به خراج فيه مدّة في معدته أو في كبده أو في من به السلّ في كلّ يوم ولا سيّما الليل. وأكثر ما تكون نوائب الحمّى بمن علّته من طحاله وبالجملة من المرّة السوداء يوما ويومين لا. وكذلك أوقات السنة فإنّ حمّى الربع الصيفية قصيرة في أكثر الأمر والخريفية طويلة ولا سيّما إذا اتّصلت بالشتاء.

وتزيّد النوائب يدلّ على تزيّد المرض وقرب منتهاه. ويعرف تزيّد النوبة الثانية على النوبة الأولى من ثلاثة أشياء أحدها وقت نوبة الحمّى والآخر طول النوبة والآخر عظمها أعني شدّتها.

---

٣ يدلّ: يدلّك B ‖ ونظامه: om. C   ٤ يوما ويوما: يوم ويوم B   ٥ النفث: add. A فيهم   ٨ هل: المرض

١٠-١١ في ... تكون: ¹C   ١٢ نوائب: om. A   add. A

(increase), see the enlightening n. 24 by ed. Littré: "Galien (ibid., p. 387) a lu ἐπιδόσιες et a traduit par *augmentation*; il entend que cela signifie l'augmentation des accidents de période en période jusqu'au summum."

(1.13)

[40] Says Hippocrates: Old people bear fasting most easily; then adults. Young people bear fasting less well and least of all children, and especially those children who have a very strong appetite.

Says the commentator: The reason for what he said in this aphorism is mentioned by him in the next aphorism, namely, the stronger one's innate[54] heat, the more food one needs, since the dissolution in the bodies of young people is stronger because of their moisture. And regarding his statement that old people endure fasting [most easily], Galen said that this refers to old people who have not reached the stage of senility.[55] Extremely old people cannot endure fasting, but have to feed themselves with small quantities time and again, since their [innate] heat is close to extinction, and [consequently] have a constant need for that which reinforces it little by little.

(1.14)

[41] Says Hippocrates: Bodies that are growing have the greatest amount of innate heat. For fuel they need more food than the other bodies. If they do not take the [amount of] food they need, their body wastes away and becomes emaciated. Old people have little innate heat and for this reason they only require little fuel, because their [innate] heat would be extinguished by too much [fuel]. For this reason too, the fever of old people is less acute than that of young people, for their bodies are cold.

Says the commentator: Galen says that the substance that contains the [innate] heat in the case of children is very large in quantity and this is what he means in all those cases in which he says [about them] that their [innate] heat is greater in quantity, as he explains in De temperamentis.[56]

---

54   On the notion of "innate heat," the force sustaining life in living beings, see Galen, De usu
       partium, trans. May: Usefulness of the Parts of the Body, vol. 1, pp. 50–53.
55   Cf. idem, In Hippocratis Aphorismos commentarius 1.13, ed. Kühn, vol. 17b, p. 403.
56   Idem, De temperamentis 2.2, ed. Kühn, vol. 1, pp. 594, 598; cf. Bos/Fontaine, "Medico-
       philosophical Controversies," pp. 37–38.

(1.13)

[٤٠] قال أبقراط: المشائخ أحمل الناس للصوم ومن بعدهم الكهول والفتيان أقلّ احتمالا وأقلّ الناس احتمالا للصوم الصبيان. ومن كان من الصبيان أقوى شهوة فهو أقلّ احتمالا له.

قال المفسّر: الذي ذكره في هذا الفصل قد ذكر علّته في الفصل الذي بعده وذلك أنّ كلّ ما كان ٥ الحارّ الغريزي أكثر احتاج إلى غذاء أكثر. وتحلّل من أبدان الصبيان لرطوبتها أكثر. وهذا الذي ذكره من احتمال الشيوخ للصيام ذكر جالينوس أنّه الشيخ الذي لم يصل لحدّ الهرم. أمّا الشيوخ الذين في غاية الشيخوخة فلا يحتملوا الصبر عن الطعام بل يحتاجون إلى تناوله قليلا قليلا المرّة بعد المرّة لقرب حرارتهم من الانطفاء فتحتاج إلى متابعة ما يمدّها قليلا قليلا.

(1.14)

[٤١] قال أبقراط: ما كان من الأبدان في النشء فالحارّ الغريزي فيهم على غاية ما يكون من الكثرة ١٠ ويحتاج من الوقود إلى أكثر ممّا يحتاج إليه سائر الأبدان من الغذاء فإن لم يتناول من الغذاء ما يحتاج إليه ذبل بدنه وانتقص. وأمّا الشيوخ فالحارّ الغريزي فيهم قليل فمن قبل ذلك ليس يحتاجون من الوقود إلّا إلى اليسير لأنّ حرارتهم تطفأ من الكثير ومن قبل هذا أيضا ليس تكون الحمّى في المشائخ حادّة مثل ما تكون في النشء ذلك لأنّ أبدانهم باردة.

قال المفسّر: قال جالينوس: الجوهر الذي فيه الحرارة في الصبيان أكثر مقدارا وهذا المعنى هو الذي ١٥ يقول عنه جالينوس دائما إنّ الحرارة أزيد في الكمّيّة كما بيّن في المزاج.

---

١ ومن بعدهم: وبعدهم A ‖ الفتيان (= الفتيان F): الفتيان A ‖ الصبيان ABC الشبان t ٥ وتحلّل من أبدان الصبيان لرطوبتها أكثر: C¹ ٦ للصيام: للصبيان A ٧ قليلا: om. A ٨ متابعة ما: متابعة بما C ١٠ ممّا: ما BC ‖ سائر الأبدان: C¹ غيره A ‖ من الغذاء: om. A ١١ إليه: من الغذاء add. A ‖ ذبل: اذبل C ‖ وانتقص: ونقص A ‖ فيهم قليل: inv. C ١٢ المشائخ: المشيخة BC

(1.15)

[42] Says Hippocrates: During winter and spring, the[57] interior parts of the body are naturally the hottest and sleep is the longest. For this reason, one should take more food during these seasons, for [during that time] the body has much innate heat and thus needs more nourishment. This is proven by those who are young[58] men and wrestlers.[59]

Says the commentator: This is proven by [young men] and wrestlers. Galen says: For young men have more innate heat and therefore need more nourishment. Wrestlers can also take more nourishment, since their innate heat increases because of their intensive training.[60]

(1.16)

[43] Says Hippocrates: Moist foods are appropriate for all those who suffer from fever, especially in the case of children and others, [namely] those who are used to be nourished with moist foods.

Says the commentator: This is clear; it is an example [of a case] from which the general rule is deducted that every disease should be treated by opposite means.[61]

(1.17)

[44] Says Hippocrates: To some patients food should be given once, to others twice, in greater or smaller portions, while to [yet] others it should be given little by little. One should also consider the current time of the year (i.e., season), habit, and age.

Says the commentator: After first giving the rules regarding the [appropriate] quantity of the food, and then regarding the quality, he here begins with giving the rules regarding the [proper] way of its administration. The basic rule

---

57   "the interior parts" (الأجواف) (= V, fol. 19ᵇ): Cf. Galen, *In Hippocratis Aphorismos commentarius* 1.15, ed. Kühn, vol. 17b, p. 415: Αἱ κοιλίαι; Hippocrates, *Aphorisms*, trans. Littré, vol. 4, p. 467: "le ventre;" trans. Jones, p. 105: "Bowels."

58   "young men" (الأسنان): Cf. Galen, ibid.: αἱ ἡλικίαι; Hippocrates, ibid., trans. Littré: "les jeunes gens;" trans. Jones, p. 107: "the young." Greek ἡλικία in singular is regularly used to mean 'prime of life,' and to define 'young men.' It can also be used in both singular and plural to mean those of a certain age and then specifically those in the age group of the ἡλικία. I thank my colleague Vivian Nutton for this exposition.

59   "wrestlers": Cf. Galen, ibid.: ἀθληταί; Hippocrates, ibid., trans. Littré: "les athlètes;" trans. Jones: "athletes." See also Barry, *Syriac Medicine*, pp. 64–65.

60   Cf. Galen, ibid.

61   I.e., contraria contrariis curantur.

(1.15)

[٤٢] قال أبقراط: الأجواف في الشتاء والربيع أسخن ما تكون بالطبع والنوم أطول ما يكون. فينبغي في هذين الوقتين أن يكون ما يتناول من الأغذية أكثر وذلك أنّ الحارّ الغريزي في الأبدان في هذين الوقتين كثير ولذلك يحتاج إلى غذاء أكثر. والدليل على ذلك أمر الأسنان والصريعين.

قال المفسّر: ودليل على ذلك أمر الأسنان والصريعين. قال جالينوس: وذلك أنّ الصبيان لمّا الحارّ

٥ الغريزي أكثر ما فيهم احتاجوا من الأغذية إلى ما هو أكثر والصريعين أيضا لمّا كانت حرارتهم الغريزية تنمو بكثرة رياضتهم صاروا يقدرون أن يتناولوا من الأغذية أكثر.

(1.16)

[٤٣] قال أبقراط: الأغذية الرطبة توافق جميع المحمومين لا سيّما الصبيان وغيرهم ومن قد اعتاد أن يغتذي بالأغذية الرطبة.

قال المفسّر: هذا بيّن وهو مثال يؤخذ منه القانون العامّ وهو أنّ كلّ مرض يقابل بضدّه.

(1.17)

١٠ [٤٤] قال أبقراط: وينبغي أن يعطى بعض المرضى غذاءهم في مرّة واحدة وبعضهم في مرّتين ويجعل ما يعطونه منه أكثر أو أقلّ وبعضهم قليلا قليلا وينبغي أن يعطى الوقت الحاضر من أوقات السنة حظّه من هذا والعادة والسنّ.

قال المفسّر: لمّا أعطى القانون في كمّية الغذاء أوّلا ثمّ في كيفيّته أخذ أن يعطي هنا القانون في صورة تناوله. والأصل في ذلك اعتبار قوّة المريض واعتبار المرض ويعطى أيضا السنّ والعادة ومزاج الهواء

١-٤ والنوم ... ودليل على ذلك: إلى قوله B ٣ أكثر: كثير A ٤ om. B أمر: ٤ om. B ‖ قال جالينوس: om.

B ٧ جميع: سائر C ٨-٧ جميع ... أن يغتذي: إلى قوله B ٧ وغيرهم: om. E ١٢-١٠ في ... من هذا: إلى

قوله B ١٣ في: om. B ‖ يعطي هنا: يعطينا B يعطي هذا A

is that one should consider the strength of the patient and the power of the disease. One should also consider the age and habits [of the patient], and the climate. When the vigor [of the patient] is strong, his food intake should be all at one time, and when it is weak, it should be little by little.[62] When his body is lean and emaciated, one should give him much food, and when he is corpulent one should give him little food. It therefore follows that if his vigor is weak and his body lean, he should be nourished with small amounts of food at many times. But if his vigor his weak and his body is not lean, he should be nourished with little food only a few times. The same applies if his vigor is strong and his humors are plentiful. However, if the vigor [of the patient] is strong but his body is lean and its humors corrupt, he should be fed much food at many times because the condition of his body requires much food, and because his vigor is strong he is able to digest [the food]. But if fever attacks prevent him from eating frequently, one should feed him only a few times.

This is the reasoning regarding the vigor [of the patient] and the disease. As for the [current] time [of the year], the age and habits [of the patient] and similar factors, [the reasoning] is as follows: In summer one should eat more often but the amounts taken at each time should be smaller; in winter one should eat more food but less frequently. But [after] the middle of spring, when summer approaches, one should take little food at long intervals, because at this time the body tends to be full. This is because the humors, which were congealed during winter, melt and dissolve. But if someone suffers from fever during autumn, he needs an ample portion of healthy additional food because of the corruption of the humors at that time. The matter of the age and habits [of the patient] is clear.

(1.18)
[45] Says Hippocrates: In summer and autumn, bodies can [only] tolerate food with great difficulty, while in winter, and next in spring, it is very easy for them.

Says the commentator: Galen[63] remarks that [Hippocrates'] statement in this aphorism refers to sick people, while his earlier statement refers to healthy people.[64]

---

62   Cf. Maimonides, *Medical Aphorisms* 20.8, trans. Bos, vol. 4, p. 63: "Convalescents and weak people should be given stronger food in the evening. But since they cannot digest the food [properly], we should feed them little by little ..."

63   Cf. Galen, *In Hippocratis Aphorismos commentarius* 1.18, ed. Kühn, vol. 17b, pp. 433–434.

64   I.e., aphorism 1.15 (42) above.

حظّه. وذلك أنّ القوة القويّة توجب تناول الغذاء دفعة والضعيفة توجب تناوله قليلا قليلا. ونقصان البدن وهزاله يوجب أن يعطى غذاء كثيرا وامتلاؤه يوجب تقليل الغذاء. فيلزم من هذا أنّه إن كانت القوة ضعيفة والبدن في حال نقصان فيعطى طعامه قليلا مرارا كثيرة وإن كانت القوة ضعيفة والبدن ليس في حال نقصان فينبغي أن يعطى طعاما قليلا مرارا قليلة. وكذلك إذا كانت القوة قويّة

٥ والكيموسات كثيرة. أمّا إذا كانت القوة قويّة والبدن في حال نقصان أو حال فساد أخلاط فينبغي أن يطعم المريض طعاما كثيرا مرارا كثيرة لأنّ حال بدنه يحتاج إلى طعام كثير وقوّته قويّة تفي بإنضاجه. فإن عاقته نوائب الحمّى ولم يجد أوقاتا كثيرة للغذاء فاعطه في مرار قليلة.

فهكذا الاستدلال بحسب القوة والمرض. وأمّا الوقت والسنّ والعادة وما يجري مجراها فعل هذا المثال: الصيف يوجب تكثير المرّات وتقليل ما يتناول في كلّ مرّة والشتاء يوجب تكثير الطعام

١٠ وتقليل المرّات. وأمّا وسط الربيع وإذا قرب من الصيف فينبغي أن يغذوا بغذاء يسير فيما بين أوقات طويلة لأنّ هذا الوقت يكاد أن تكون الأبدان ممتلئة لأنّ الكيموسات التي كانت جامدة في الشتاء تذوب وتتحلّل. وأمّا الخريف فمن يحمّ فيه يحتاج إلى زيادة سابغة من غذاء محمود لفساد الكيموسات في ذلك الوقت وأمر الأسنان والعادات بيّن.

(1.18)

[٤٥] قال أبقراط: أصعب ما يكون احتمال الطعام على الأبدان في الصيف والخريف وأسهل ما

١٥ يكون احتماله عليها في الشتاء وبعده في الربيع.

قال المفسّر: قال جالينوس: كلامه في هذا الفصل في المرضى وكلامه المتقدّم في الأصحّاء.

---

١٣ وأمر: وأمّا B   ١٤-١٥ على ... الشتاء: إلى قوله B   ١٦ المتقدّم: في المتقدّم B

(1.19)

[46] Says Hippocrates: When fever attacks recur in cycles, one should not give the patient any [food] during [the attacks] nor force him to [take] anything; rather one should decrease the[65] food portions before the times[66] of separation (crises).

Says the commentator: Galen says: With his statement "before the times of separation," he means "before the times of the attacks." Since during this time one should decrease the [superfluous] matters so that the fever does not get worse, far be it from you to increase them in any way through nourishment.

(1.20)

[47] Says Hippocrates: When a body [suffers from a disease] that is attained by a crisis or when[67] the crisis has become full-blown, one should not disturb it, nor try any experiments, neither by purgatives nor other stimulants; rather it should be left alone.

Says the commentator: His words "that is attained" mean that the causes [of the crisis] are ready (to bring the crisis about) and that its symptoms are apparent and that it is immanent. His words "nor other stimulants" refer, for instance, to induce vomiting, perspiration, and micturiction or menstruation, and to massage. He stipulated that the crisis should be complete (full-blown). As to an incomplete crisis, one should complete what is missing and expel the remaining illness-producing humor in the easiest possible way. Galen says that

---

65   "the food portions" (زيادات) (= V, fol. 22ᵇ): An unattested semantic borrowing from the corresponding Greek πρόσθεσεις, which can mean both "administration of food, nourishment" and "addition, increase;" cf. Liddell/Scott, *Greek-English Lexicon*, p. 1514, s.v. προσθέ-σις; see also Hippocrates, *Aphorisms* 1.19, trans. Littré, vol. 4, p. 469: "la nourriture;" trans. Jones, p. 107: "nourishment."

66   "times of separation (crises)" (أوقات الانفصال): I.e., the times in which the different cycles are separated from each other.

67   "when the crisis has become full-blown": I have translated the Arabic على الكمال (= V, fol. 23ᵃ), lit., 'completely,' according to the sense in which it is interpreted by Maimonides. The term is actually a semantic borrowing from the corresponding Greek ἄρτιος, c.q. ἀρτίως; cf. Liddell/Scott, *Greek-English Lexicon*, p. 249, meaning "just." Thus, the meaning of the Hippocratic sentence is: "when the crisis has just passed;" cf. Hippocrates, *Aphorisms* 1.20, trans. Jones, p. 107: "just after a crisis." Note however that also Galen, *In Hippocratis Aphorismos commentarius*, ed. Kühn, vol. 17b, pp. 437–438, remarks that Greek ἀρτίως should be interpreted as meaning 'complete, perfect' in this context.

(1.19)

[٤٦] قال أبقراط: إذا كانت نوائب الحمّى لازمة لأدوار فلا ينبغي في أوقاتها أن يعطى المريض شيئا أو أن يضطرّ إلى شيء لكن ينبغي أن ينقص من الزيادات من قبل أوقات الانفصال.

قال المفسّر: قال جالينوس: يريد بقوله من قبل أوقات الانفصال من قبل أوقات النوائب وإذا كان هذا الوقت ينبغي فيه تنقيص المواد لئلّا تعظم الحمّى فناهيك أن تزيد فيها شيئا بالتغذية.

(1.20)

٥ [٤٧] قال أبقراط: الأبدان التي يأتيها أو قد أتاها البحران على الكمال لا ينبغي أن تحرّك ولا يحدث فيها حدث لا بدواء مسهل ولا بغيره من التهييج لكن يترك.

قال المفسّر: قوله يأتيها يعني أنّه تهيّأت أسبابه فظهرت علاماته وهو مزمع أن يكون. وقوله ولا بغيره من التهييج مثل التقيّء والتعريق وإدرار البول أو الطمث والدلك. واشترط أن يكون البحران كاملا. أمّا البحران الناقص فيلزم أن يكمل نقصه ويخرج ما بقي من الخلط الممرّض بالوجه الأسهل فيه. وقال

<hr>

٢-١ لازمة ... الزيادات: إلى قوله B ٢ أن يضطرّ (E =):emendation editor أن اضطرّ A أو اضطرّه C ٥ البحران: بحران C ٦-٥ على ... التهييج: إلى قوله B ٩-٤.٧٥ وقال ... البدن: يستدلّ على أنّ البحران تامّ كامل بستّة أشياء: أوّلها وهو أعظمها أن يتقدّمه النضج البيّن. الثاني أن يكون باستفراغ لا بخراج. الثالث أن يكون الشيء المستفرغ كيموسا رديئا. الرابع أن يكون الاستفراغ من جانب المرض. الخامس أن يكون في يوم بحران. السادس أن يتبعه الخفّ والراحة الكاملة. في شرحه لأولى الفصول b

a complete crisis is a combination of six things.[68] The first is that it is preceded by concoction. The second is that this occurs on one of the days of the crisis. The third is that [the crisis] occurs with plain matter that is evacuated from the body, but not with an abscess. The fourth is that the evacuated matter only consists of the harmful matter that causes the illness. The fifth is that the evacuation is done correctly, from the side of the illness. The sixth is that it is accompanied by relaxation and lightness of the body.[69]

Says Galen: If one or more of these [conditions] are missing, the crisis is neither perfect nor complete.

Says the commentator: At this point one should ask and say: How can the very illness-producing humor be evacuated, after its concoction on the day of the crisis, correctly, without being followed by lightness and relaxation [of the body]? Since Galen stipulates a sixth condition, namely, that it is accompanied by lightness and relaxation, it is proof that sometimes the five conditions can be fulfilled without occurring relaxation there. The answer is that this is possible if the evacuation is excessive. Although it is a kind of evacuation that comes with the other conditions [being fulfilled], yet, if it is excessive, it is not followed by lightness or relaxation, but by weakness and limpness of the body, and sometimes by a severe feebleness. You should know this.

(1.21)

[48] Says Hippocrates: The matters that should be evacuated, should be evacuated from the sites to which they tend mostly, through[70] those organs that are appropriate for their evacuation.

---

68   Cf. Galen, ibid., p. 438. Galen only enumerates five conditions, since he does not count the first condition separately, but combines it with the fifth condition as follows: 'The fifth that it (i.e., the evacuation) is done on a critical day when there is coction [of superfluous matter].'

69   Cf. Maimonides, *Medical Aphorisms* 11.30, trans. Bos, vol. 3, p. 27: "From six things, one can conclude that a crisis is complete and perfect. The first and the most important is that it is preceded by clear coction. The second is that it occurs through evacuation and not through an abscess. The third is that the evacuated matter consists of bad chyme. The fourth is that the evacuation is from the side of the illness. The fifth is that this is done on a critical day. The sixth is that it is followed by alleviation and total relaxation. *In Hippocratis Aphorismos commentarius* 4."

70   "through those organs that are appropriate for their evacuation": Cf. Galen, *In Hippocratis Aphorismos commentarius* 1.21, ed. Kühn, vol. 17b, p. 439: διὰ τῶν ξυμφερόντων χωρίων; Hippocrates, *Aphorisms*, trans. Littré, vol. 4, p. 469: "par les voies convenables;" trans. Jones, p. 107: "through the appropriate passages."

جالينوس إنّ البحران الكامل هو ما جمع ستّة أشياء: أوّلها أن يتقدّمه النضج. الثاني أن يكون في يوم
من أيّام البحران. الثالث أن يكون باستفراغ شيء بيّن يخرج عن البدن لا بخراج. الرابع أن يكون
الشيء المستفرغ هو الشيء المؤذي فقط الذي كان علّة المرض. الخامس أن يكون استفراغه على
استقامة من الجانب الذي فيه المرض. السادس أن يكون مع راحة وخفّة من البدن.

قال جالينوس: وإذا نقص واحد منها أو أكثر من واحد فليس البحران بصحيح ولا تامّ. ٥

قال المفسّر: ينبغي لك أن تسأل هنا وتقول: كيف يستفرغ الخلط الممرّض بعينه بعد النضج وفي يوم
بحران وعلى استقامة ولا يعقبه الخفّ والراحة لأنّ جالينوس يشترط شرطا سادسا وهو أن يكون
مع خفّ وراحة دليل أنّه قد تحصل الشرائط الخمسة ولا تكون راحة وجواب ذلك أنّه يمكن هذا
إذا أفرط الاستفراغ وعلى أنّه من نوع الذي ينبغي خروجه مع سائر الشروط فإنّه إذا أفرط لا يعقبه
خفّ ولا تكون معه راحة بل ضعف ورخاوة من البدن وقد ربّما غشي شديد فاعلم ذلك. ١٠

(1.21)

[٤٨] قال أبقراط: الأشياء التي ينبغي أن تستفرغ يجب أن تستفرغ من المواضع التي هي إليها أميل
بالأعضاء التي تصلح لاستفراغها.

---

١ الثاني: الثانية C ‖ يوم: أيّام B ٢ بيّن: C² ‖ يكون: C² ٤ من: om. A ٥ واحد: ذلك B ١١ يجب
أن تستفرغ: C¹ ‖ يجب ... التي: إلى قوله B

Says the commentator: Galen says that the matters that should be evacuated are the humors that produce those illnesses that have an incomplete crisis, and that the sites that are suitable for [their] evacuation are the intestines, stomach, urinary bladder, uterus, and skin. And also the palate[71] and the nostrils, if we want to cleanse the brain. The physician should seek [for an evacuation] that is based on his knowledge of the tendency of nature. If he finds that it tends in a direction that is appropriate to evacuate that, which [he wants to] evacuate, he should provide it with that, which she needs and help it. But if he sees that the opposite is the case and sees that [nature's] movement is harmful, he should prevent it and divert it and draw it in the direction that is opposite to the one [nature] tends to. I will give you an example of this: If there are humors in the liver that have produced an illness, it is good if they tend to [either one] of two sides (directions); one is that of the stomach. If they tend to that side their evacuation through purgation is better than that through emesis. The other side is that of the kidneys and urinary bladder. But it is not good if they tend to the side of the chest, lungs, or heart.

(1.22)

[49] Says Hippocrates: One should only administer drugs and move (disturb) [the body] once [the humors that cause] the illness are concocted. As long as they are crude and in the beginning of the illness one should not administer [drugs], unless the illness (i.e., the humors causing the disease) is stirred up, but in most cases it is not stirred up.

Says the commentator: With the word "drugs," he means purgatives,[72] and "the illness that is stirred up" is [an illness] in which the humors disturb the patient and harm him with their heat that is severe and [their] flow from organ to organ in the beginning of the illness. Consequently, they oppress the patient and disturb him and do not let him rest, as they move and stream from organ to organ. But this happens most rarely. In most cases the humors are motionless and stay in one organ, and in that organ their concoction takes place during the whole duration of the illness until they decrease.

---

71   "palate" (cf. Galen, ibid.: αἵ ὑπερῷαί): Arab. لهوة, Plur. لهوات (cf. E, fol. 107ᵃ), means "uvula" and is often used metonymically for: throat, gullet, mouth; cf. WKAS, vol. 2.3, p. 1594; cf. Blau, *Dictionary of Medieval Judaeo-Arabic Texts*, p. 641: "the innermost parts of the mouth."

72   Following the Greek φαρμακεύω (cf. Galen, ibid. 1.22, ed. Kühn, p. 441), Arabic استعمل الدواء can mean both 'to administer a drug' and 'to administer a purgative drug;' cf. Ullmann, *Wörterbuch*, pp. 723–724; Liddell/Scott, *Greek-English Lexicon*, p. 1917.

قال المفسّر: قال جالينوس: الأشياء التي ينبغي أن تستفرغ هي الأخلاط المولّدة للأمراض التي أتى فيها البحران غير تامّ. والمواضع التي تصلح للاستفراغ هي الأمعاء والمعدة والمثانة والرحم والجلد ومع هذا أيضا اللهوات والمنخرين إذا كّا نريد استفراغ الدماغ. فينبغي للطبيب أن يتفقّده بتعرّف ميل الطبيعة فإن وجد ميلها نحو ناحية تصلح لاستفراغ ما يستفرغه أعدّ لها ما يحتاج إليه وعاونها. وإن رأى

٥ الأمر على ضدّ ذلك ورأى حركتها حركة ضارّة منعها ونقلها وجذبها إلى ضدّ الناحية التي مالت نحوها. وأضرب لك في ذلك مثلا: إذا كانت في الكبد كيموسات قد أحدثت مرضا فالنواحي التي تصلح أن تميل إليها ناحيتان أحدهما ناحية المعدة وإذا كان الميل لتلك الناحية فالاستفراغ بالإسهال أجود من أن يكون بالقيء والناحية الأخرى ناحية الكلى والمثانة فأمّا ميل تلك الكيموسات إلى ناحية الصدر والرئة والقلب فليس بجيّد.

(1.22)

١٠ [٤٩] قال أبقراط: إنّما ينبغي لك أن تستعمل الدواء والتحريك بعد أن ينضج المرض فأمّا ما دام نيئا وفي أوّل المرض فلا ينبغي أن يستعمل ذلك إلّا أن يكون المرض مهتاجا وليس يكاد في أكثر الأمر أن يكون المرض مهتاجا.

قال المفسّر: قوله الدواء يريد به المسهل والمرض المهتاج هو الذي تكون الكيموسات أقلقت المريض وآذته بحرارة تكون لها قوّة وسيلان من عضو إلى عضو في ابتداء المرض فيكربه ويحدث له قلقا ولا

١٥ تدعه يستقرّ لكنها تتحرّك وتسيل من عضو إلى عضو وهذا أقلّ ما يكون. وأمّا في أكثر الأمر فتكون الكيموسات ساكنة ثابتة في عضو واحد وفي ذلك العضو يكون نضجها في مدّة زمان المرض كلّه إلى أن تنقص.

---

١ ينبغي أن: C¹ ‖ ١٠-١١ والتحريك ... إلّا: إلى قوله B ‖ ١١-١٢ وليس ... مهتاجا: om. AB ‖ ١٥ يستقرّ: يستفرغ A ‖ أقلّ: قلّ C

(1.23)

[50] Says Hippocrates: One should not conclude to the measure of that which should be evacuated from the body from its large quantity. But[73] one should take the opportunity to evacuate, as long as [only] that is [actually] evacuated that needs to be evacuated, and [as long as] the patient endures it easily and comfortably. When necessary, one should carry out the evacuation until the patient faints, but only if he can tolerate it.

Says the commentator: Galen says that if the prevailing [superfluous] matter is that which is being evacuated, then the body of the patient feels lighter than before.[74] But if together with the unnatural matter natural matter is evacuated, then the patient will necessarily lose strength, his vigor will weaken, he will feel heaviness and anxiety. The evacuation should be carried out to the point of fainting in the case of extremely large inflammations and extremely ardent fevers and extremely severe pains. But one should only resort to this amount of evacuation if the vigor [of the patient] is strong. I have tried this innumerable times and found it to be highly beneficial. I do not know any remedy that is stronger and more effective in the case of extremely severe pains than evacuation up to the point of fainting. [But one may only do so] once one has investigated and determined whether one should apply phlebotomy or purgation up to the point of fainting.[75]

(1.24)

[51] Says Hippocrates: In the beginning of acute diseases one should only rarely use purgatives and one should only do so after a proper examination [of the patient].

Says the commentator: He explained to us that we are not allowed to apply purgation in the beginning of diseases, except for some acute diseases and these are those that are stirred up, as he mentioned before.[76] Moreover, one should only do so very carefully and cautiously and after preparing the body as much as possible and after ascertaining the thinness (consistency) of the humors.

---

73   "But one should take the opportunity to evacuate, as long as [only] that is [actually] evacuated that needs to be evacuated": Cf. Galen, ibid. 1.23, p. 443: ἀλλ᾽ ὡς ἂν χωρέῃ οἷα δεῖ; Hippocrates, *Aphorisms*, trans. Littré, vol. 4, p. 471: "mais suivant qu'elles sortent telles qu'il convient;" trans. Jones, p. 109: "but by their conformity to what is proper."
74   I.e., the patient will feel relief.
75   Cf. Galen, *In Hippocratis Aphorismos commentarius* 1.23, ed. Kühn, vol. 17b, pp. 444–446.
76   Aphorism 1.22 (49) above.

(1.23)

[٥٠] قال أبقراط: ليس ينبغي أن يستدلّ على المقدار الذي يجب أن يستفرغ من البدن من كثرته لكنّه ينبغي أن يستغنم الاستفراغ ما دام الشيء الذي ينبغي أن يستفرغ هو الذي يستفرغ والمريض محتمل له بسهولة وخفّة وحيث ينبغي فليكن الاستفراغ حتّى يعرض الغشي. وإنّما ينبغي أن يفعل ذلك متى كان المريض محتملا له.

قال المفسّر: قال جالينوس: إن كان الشيء الغالب هو الذي استفرغ فإنّ بدن المريض يخفّ ضرورة عمّا كان فإن استفرغ مع الشيء الخارج عن الطبيعة شيء طبيعي فإنّ المريض يسترخي ضرورة وتضعف قوّته ويحسّ بثقل وقلق. وينبغي أن يكون الاستفراغ إلى حين يحدث عنه الغشي في الأورام الحارّة التي هي في غاية العظم وفي الحمّيات المحرقة جدّا والأوجاع الشديدة المفرطة. وتقدم على هذا المقدار من الاستفراغ إذا كانت القوة قويّة. وقد جرّبنا هذا مرارا كثيرة لا تحصى فوجدناه ينفع منفعة قويّة ولا نعلم في الأوجاع الشديدة المفرطة علاجا أقوى وأبلغ من الاستفراغ إلى أن يعرض الغشي بعد أن تحدّد وتعلم هل ينبغي أن يفصد عرق أو يستعمل الإسهال إلى أن يعرض الغشي.

(1.24)

[٥١] قال أبقراط: قد يحتاج في الأمراض الحادّة في الندرة إلى أن يستعمل الدواء المسهل في أوّلها. وينبغي أن يفعل ذلك بعد أن يتقدّم فيدبّر الأمر على ما ينبغي.

قال المفسّر: بيّن لنا أنّه لا يسوغ الإسهال في أوائل الأمراض إلّا في بعض الأمراض الحادّة وهي المهتاجة كما ذكر قبل. ومع ذلك ينبغي أن يفعل ذلك بحذر وتوقٍ كثير وبعد إعداد البدن ما أمكن وبعد معرفة رقّة الأخلاط.

١-٤ الذي ... ذلك: إلى قوله B   ٥ جالينوس: om. A   ٨ العظم: الغلظ B   ١٠-٩ وقد ... منفعة قويّة: .om

A   ١٣-١٢ في ... يتقدّم: إلى قوله B

Galen says that the danger (risk) of an improper use of purgatives in the case of acute diseases is very great [for the patient] because all purgatives are warming and drying and because fever in its capacity as fever does not need anything that heats and dries; rather it needs that which is the opposite, that is, something that cools and moistens. Purgatives are only used because of the presence of a humor that activates the fever. The benefit to be derived from the evacuation of the humor that produces the illness should be greater than the harm done to the body in that case as a result of [the application of] purgatives. And the benefit will only be greater if the harmful humor is evacuated completely without [causing] harm [to the body]. But one should first consider whether the body of the patient is prepared [and] ready for such a purgation. Those[77] whose illness starts from frequent indigestions or from viscous thick foods and those who suffer from stretching or swelling in the hypochondrium, or from an extremely severe heat [of[78] the urine], or from an [inflamed] tumor in one of the viscera, the body of none of these persons is ready to be purged. None of these [afflictions] should be present and the humors in the body of the patient should be as fluid as possible, that is to say, they should be thin and not at all thick. And the passages through which the evacuated matter has to pass should be widely open; there should not be any obstruction in it. We have to do these things and we have first to prepare the body by [bringing it into] this condition when we want to purge it.[79]

(1.25)
[52] Says Hippocrates: If the body is purged from the kind [of matter] it should be purged from, it is beneficial and easily borne [by the patient]; but if the opposite is the case, it is [borne] with difficulty.

---

77   "Those whose ... to be purged": Cf. Maimonides, *Medical Aphorisms* 8.50, trans. Bos, vol. 2, p. 52: "Those whose illness starts from many indigestions or from viscous thick foods and those who suffer from stretching or swelling in the hypochondrium, or from an extremely severe heat [of the urine], or from an inflamed tumor in one of the viscera are not ready to be purged. *In Hippocratis Aphorismos commentarius* 1."

78   "[of the urine]": Cf. Galen, *In Hippocratis Aphorismos commentarius* 1.24, ed. Kühn, vol. 17b, p. 448: τὰ οὖρα. Maimonides' version follows Ḥunayn's Arabic translation (E, fol. 110ᵇ), which also misses this term.

79   Cf. Galen, ibid., ed. Kühn, pp. 447–449.

قال جالينوس: الخطر في استعمال الدواء المسهل على غير ما ينبغي في الأمراض الحادّة عظيم لأنّ الأدوية المسهلة كلّها حارّة يابسة والحمّى من جهة ما هي حمّى ليس تحتاج إلى ما يسخّن ويجفّف لكنّها إنّما تحتاج إلى ضدّ ذلك أعني ما يبرّد ويرطب. وإنّما استعملت لمكان الكيموس الفاعل لها. فينبغي أن يكون الانتفاع باستفراغ الكيموس الذي عنه حدث المرض أكثر من الضرر الذي ينال

٥ الأبدان في تلك الحال بسبب الأدوية المسهلة. وإنّما يكون الانتفاع أكثر إذا استفرغ الكيموس الضارّ كلّه بلا أذى. فقد ينبغي أن ينظر أوّلا هل بدن المريض متهيّئ مستعدّ لذلك الإسهال. فإنّ الذين كان أوّل مرضهم من تخم كثيرة أو من أطعمة لزجة غليظة والذين بهم في ما دون الشراسيف تمدّد أو انتفاخ أو حرارة شديدة مفرطة أو هناك في بعض الأحشاء مع ذلك ورم ليس بدن أحد منهم متهيّئ للإسهال فينبغي أن لا يكون شيء من هذا موجودا وأن تكون الكيموسات في

١٠ بدن المريض على أفضل ما يمكن أن تكون من سهولة جريها أعني أن تكون رقيقة ولا يكون فيها شيء من اللزوجة وأن تكون المجاري التي تكون نفوذ ما يخرج بالإسهال فيها واسعة مفتوحة ليس فيها شيء من السدد. فقد نفعل نحن هذه الأشياء ونتقدّم ونهيّئ البدن بهذه الحال إذا أردنا أن نسهله.

(1.25)

[٥٢] قال أبقراط: إن استفرغ البدن من النوع الذي ينبغي أن ينقّى منه نفع ذلك واحتمل بسهولة

١٥ فإن كان الأمر على ضدّ ذلك كان عسرا.

---

٣ لكنّها: ولكنّها C ٦ بدن: الإنسان add. A ٦–٩ فإنّ ... للإسهال: الذين أوّل مرضهم من تخم كثيرة أو من أطعمة لزجة غليظة، والذين بهم فيما دون الشراسيف تمدّد أو انتفاخ أو حرارة شديدة مفرطة أو كان في بعض الأحشاء ورم فليس واحد من هؤلاء متهيّئ للإسهال. في شرحه للأولى من الفصول b ٧ أوّل: C¹ ٩ متهيّئ: بمتهيّئ C ١٠ أعني: يعني B ١١–١٢ ليس فيها شيء من السدد: C¹ ١٤ استفرغ: استفراغ ACE ١٤–١٥ من ... بسهولة فإن: إلى قوله B

Says the commentator: In my opinion, this aphorism is not a repetition of the contents of the second aphorism, because that aphorism deals with that which is evacuated spontaneously, whereas this aphorism deals with that which we evacuate by means of drugs. Since Galen thought that the second aphorism deals with both matters, he sought to give a reason for the repetition of this aphorism.[80]

This is the end of the first part. Praise be to God alone.

---

[80]   Maimonides is obviously wrong in stating that aphorism 1.2 (29) deals with spontaneous evacuation and aphorism 1.25 (52) with artificial evacuation, since both forms of evacuation are explicitly discussed in aphorism 1.2. Thus, Galen is right in considering this aphorism to be a repetition of the second and that it therefore needs a different sort of explanation.

قال المفسّر: هذا الفصل عندي ليس هو تكرار لما تضمّنه الفصل الثاني لأنّ ذلك الفصل فيما يستفرغ طوعا وهذا الفصل فيما نستفرغه نحن بأدوية. ولما جعل جالينوس الفصل الثاني يتضمّن المعنين جميعا التجأ ليعطي علّة في تكرار هذا الفصل.

كملت المقالة الأولى والحمد لله وحده.

---

١ لأنّ: أنّ B   ٤ والحمد لله: ولله الحمد B واهب العقل كما هو أهله add. A

In the name of God, the Merciful, the Compassionate
The second part of [the commentary on] Hippocrates' *Aphorisms*

(2.1)

[53] Says Hippocrates: If sleep causes pain in a certain disease, it is a fatal sign.
But if sleep is beneficial, it is not a fatal sign.

Says the commentator: With the term "pain," he means harm, because there
are illnesses and [cases] in which sleep is harmful. Therefore, the patient should
be ordered to stay awake during them, for if he sleeps, he will suffer harm.
On the other hand there are also [cases] in which sleep is beneficial, but if
the patient sleeps and suffers harm, it is a fatal sign; we hoped that it (i.e.,
sleep) would be beneficial, but it was harmful. This happens especially when
the humors of the body are very bad and suppress the innate heat. However, illnesses in which sleep is always harmful are when [one sleeps] in the beginning
of internal tumors and when [superfluous] matters stream into the stomach,
or in the beginning of a fever attack, especially when it is accompanied by cold
and shivering. The times during which sleep is beneficial are at the end of the
beginning of an attack or tumor, especially during the climax. Sleep is most
beneficial during the decline [of a disease]. If it is harmful at that time, it is a
fatal sign. If it is beneficial, according to what is known of its benefit during this
time, it does not tell us anything more [than that].

(2.2)

[54] Says Hippocrates: When sleep puts an end to mental confusion (delirium),
it is a good sign.

Says the commentator: This indicates that the innate heat has prevailed over
the humors and has subdued them.

(2.3)

[55] Says Hippocrates: If both sleep and sleeplessness exceed the measure of
moderateness (become immoderate), it is a bad sign.

Says the commentator: This is clear.

بسم الله الرحمن الرحيم
المقالة الثانية من (شرح) فصول أبقراط

(2.1)

[٥٣] قال أبقراط: إذا كان النوم في مرض من الأمراض يحدث وجعا فذلك من علامات الموت
وإذا كان النوم ينفع فليس ذلك من علامات الموت.

قال المفسّر: يريد بقوله وجعا ضررا وثمّ أمراض وأوقات من المرض يضرّ فيها النوم ولذلك ينبغي أن

٥   يؤمر المريض فيها بالانتباه وإن نام حينئذ استضرّ. وثمّ أوقات ينفع فيها النوم وإن نام فيها المريض
وحدث له الضرر فتلك علامة هلاك لأنّ حيث ترجّينا النفع جاء الضرر وهذا إنّما يجري إذا كانت
أخلاط البدن رديئة جدّا وقاهرة للحرارة الغريزية. وأمّا الأمراض التي يضرّ فيها النوم أبدا فهو عند
ابتداء أورام الأعضاء الباطنة أو عند سيلان الموادّ للمعدة أو في ابتداء نوبة الحمّى وبخاصّة إذا كان

١٠ معها برد واقشعرار. والأوقات التي ينفع فيها النوم فهو بعد انقضاء ابتداء النوبة أو الورم وبخاصّة في
وقت المنتهى. وأنفع ما يكون النوم وقت الانحطاط وإن ضرّ في هذا الوقت فهو علامة موت وإن
كان ينفع على ما قد علم من نفع النوم في هذا الوقت فليس يزيدنا في الدلالة شيئا.

(2.2)

[٥٤] قال أبقراط: متى سكّن النوم اختلاط الذهن فتلك علامة صالحة.

قال المفسّر: ذلك يدلّ على أنّ الحرارة الغريزية غلبت الكيموسات وقهرتها.

(2.3)

١٥ [٥٥] قال أبقراط: النوم والأرق إذا جاوز كلّ واحد منهما المقدار القصد فتلك علامة رديئة.

قال المفسّر: هذا بيّن.

---

١ بسم الله الرحمن الرحيم: om. ABP   ٣-٤ في ... فليس ذلك: إلى قوله B   ٤ من علامات: C¹   ١٠ التي:
الذي B   ١٣ الذهن: العقل B الذهن B¹   ١٥ القصد: القاصد B

(2.4)

[56] Says Hippocrates: Neither satiation nor hunger nor anything else is good when it exceeds the measure of nature.

Says the commentator: This is clear.

(2.5)

[57] Says Hippocrates: Spontaneous[81] fatigue indicates illness.

Says the commentator: This indicates that the humors move along channels that are not natural to them, and therefore cause pain to the organs, either because of their bad quality or because of their large quantity. For this reason they indicate illness.

(2.6)

[58] Says Hippocrates: If someone has a painful spot in his body, but does not feel the pain in most cases, he suffers from mental confusion.

Says the commentator: With "pain" overhere he means the cause of the pain. For instance, when the patient is affected by a hot tumor, erysipelas, wound, bruise,[82] crushing[83] [of a limb], and the like and does not feel it, then he suffers from mental confusion.

(2.7)

[59] Says Hippocrates: Bodies that become emaciated over a long period should be slowly restored with nutrition to [their normal] corpulence, while bodies that become emaciated over a short period [should be restored] quickly.

Says the commentator: For bodies that become emaciated in a short time are affected by that emaciation and leanness because of the evacuation of humors, and not because of a dissolution of the solid organs. But bodies that become emaciated and lean over a long period, their flesh is dissolved and the other organs in which digestion, distribution of the food in the body and production

---

81   "Spontaneous": Lit., "the cause of which is not known" (لا يعرف له سبب); cf. Galen, *In Hippocratis Aphorismos commentarius* 2.5, ed. Kühn, vol. 17b, p. 459: αὐτόματοι; cf. Liddell/Scott, *Greek-English Lexicon*, p. 281: "self-acting, spontaneous;" cf. Ullmann, *Wörterbuch*, p. 148: من تلقاء نفسه; من ذاته; من نفسه.

82   "bruise" (فسخ): Cf. Galen, ibid. 2.6, p. 460: θλάσμα; cf. Liddell/Scott, ibid., p. 802: "bruise;" see also Ullmann, ibid., p. 297, s.v. θλάσις: "Quetschung, Prellung" (bruise, contusion).

83   "crushing [of a limb]" (شدخ): Cf. Galen, ibid.: ῥῆγμα; Liddell/Scott, ibid., p. 1568: "breakage, fracture; lesion."

(2.4)

[٥٦] قال أبقراط: لا الشبع ولا الجوع ولا غيرهما من جميع الأشياء بمحمود إذا كان يجاوز المقدار الطبيعي.

قال المفسّر: هذا بيّن.

(2.5)

[٥٧] قال أبقراط: الإعياء الذي لا يعرف له سبب ينذر بمرض.

٥ قال المفسّر: ذلك يدلّ على أنّ الأخلاط قد تحرّكت على غير مجراها الطبيعي ولذلك تألّمت منها الأعضاء إمّا من رداءة كيفيّتها أو من كثرة كميّتها ولذلك تنذر بمرض.

(2.6)

[٥٨] قال أبقراط: من يوجعه شيء من بدنه ولا يحسّ بوجعه في أكثر حالاته فعقله مختلط.

قال المفسّر: يريد بالوجع هنا سبب الوجع مثل أن يكون بالمريض ورم حارّ أو حمرة والجرح والفسخ والشدخ وما أشبه ذلك وكان لا يحسّ به ففهمه مختلط.

(2.7)

[٥٩] قال أبقراط: الأبدان التي تضمر في زمان طويل فينبغي أن تكون إعادتها بالتغذية إلى الخصب ١٠ بتمهّل والأبدان التي ضمرت في زمان يسير ففي زمان يسير.

قال المفسّر: وذلك أنّ الأبدان التي تضمر في زمان يسير فإنّما حدث لها ذلك الضمور والقضف من استفراغ الرطوبات لا من ذوبان الأعضاء الجامدة. فأمّا الأبدان التي ضمرت وقضفت في زمان طويل فقد ذاب منها اللحم ودقّت منها ونهكت سائر الأعضاء التي بها يكون الهضم وانتشار الغذاء في

---

١ ولا ... يجاوز: إلى قوله B ‖ ١-٢ المقدار الطبيعي: المقادير الطبيعيّة C ٥ غير: om. B ٧ ولا: فلا C ‖ في أكثر حالاته: om. B ‖ فعقله: في أكثر أوقاته add. B ٩ وكان: كان C¹ ١٠-١١ في ... في زمان يسير: إلى قوله B ١١ ففي ... يسير: om. A ١٢ لها: من C add.

of blood take place become thin and emaciated, so that they cannot concoct
the amount of food, which the body needs. For that reason, their corpulence
should be restored over a long time.

(2.8)

[60] Says Hippocrates: If a convalescent takes food but does not become
stronger, it is a sign that he burdened his body (i.e., ate) more than it can tolerate. But if this happens while he takes none, it is a sign that evacuation is
required.[84]

Says the commentator: He explains the reason in the aphorism in which he
informs us that the more one feeds a body that is not clean, the more harm one
does.[85]

(2.9)

[61] Says Hippocrates: If one wants to purge a body, one should take care that
that, which one wants to be purged, should flow through it easily.

Says the commentator: This is done by opening all its passages widely and
by diluting, thinning, and dissolving its humors, if they have any [sort] of thickness and viscosity.

(2.10)

[62] Says Hippocrates: A body that is not clean, the more you nourish it the
more you harm it.[86]

Says the commentator: The reason for that is clear; this happens mostly if
the stomach is full with bad humors; for then that happens, which Hippocrates
has mentioned regarding a convalescent who cannot take any food.[87]

---

84   As ed. Jones in Hippocrates, *Aphorisms* 2.8, p. 111 n. 1, explains, "The commentators from
      Galen have been worried by this phrase and the apparent inconsequence of the second
      part of the proposition." According to Galen, ibid., p. 462, the sentence τροφὴν μὴ λαμβάνειν
      should be understood in the sense of "not to be hungry;" see also Hippocrates, ibid., ed.
      Littré, vol. 4, p. 472, and aphorism 4.41 (178) below. Note, that Ibn Tibbon interpreted the
      second part of the proposition as 'but if this happens while he does not take more than it
      can tolerate.'
85   Cf. aphorism 2.10 (62) below. According to Galen, ibid., pp. 463–464, the Hippocratic text
      should read: 'If a convalescent takes food but does not become stronger, it is a sign that
      he burdened his body (i.e., ate) more than it can tolerate. But if this happens while one
      does not take food, it is a sign that it needs evacuation. For the more one feeds an unclean
      body, the more one harms it.'
86   See Bos/Langermann, "Introduction of Sergius of Resh'aina," p. 190, and n. 26.
87   Cf. aphorism 2.8 (60) above.

البدن وتولّد الدم فلا تقدر أن ينضج من الغذاء المقدار الذي يحتاج إليه البدن ولذلك ينبغي أن يعاد إلى الخصب في زمان طويل.

(2.8)

[٦٠] قال أبقراط: الناقه من المرض إذا كان ينال من الغذاء وليس يقوى فذلك يدلّ على أنّه يحمّل بدنه منه أكثر ممّا يحتمل. وإذا كان ذلك وهو لا ينال منه دلّ على أنّ بدنه يحتاج إلى استفراغ.

٥ قال المفسّر: بيّن العلّة بالفصل الذي أعلمنا فيه بأنّ البدن الغير نقي كلّما غذوته زدته شرًّا.

(2.9)

[٦١] قال أبقراط: كلّ بدن تريد تنقيته فينبغي أن تجعل ما تريد إخراجه منه يجري فيه بسهولة.

قال المفسّر: يكون ذلك بأن توسع وتفتح جميع مجاريه وتقطّع وتلطّف وتذيب الرطوبات التي فيه إن كان لها شيء من الغلظ واللزوجة.

(2.10)

[٦٢] قال أبقراط: البدن الذي ليس بنقي كلّما غذوته إنّما تزيده شرًّا.

١٠ قال المفسّر: بيّن العلّة وأكثر ما يكون ذلك إذا كانت المعدة ممتلئة كيموسات رديئة وعند ذلك يعرض منها الذي ذكر أبقراط أنّه يعرض للناقه وهو أن لا يقدر أن ينال من الطعام.

٣-٤ إذا ... على أنّ بدنه: إلى قوله B ٣ يحمّل: على C. add ٥ الغير: غير C ٦ فيه: A C¹ om. ٩ بنقي:
بالنقي C ‖ إنّما: B om. ١١ منها: فيها B

(2.11)

[63] Says Hippocrates: It is easier for a body to be full with drink than with food.

Says the commentator: [With drink] he means liquids and beverages that are nutritious for our bodies. For liquid food, especially if it is hot by its nature, is the easiest and fastest food for the body.

(2.12)

[64] Says Hippocrates: Remnants of diseases left behind [in the body] after a crisis usually cause a relapse.

Says the commentator: Those remnants mostly putrefy in the course of time and thereby produce fever because every [remaining] humor that is strange to the nature of the surrounding body cannot feed it and therefore eventually putrefies in most cases. And if, next to this, the site [in the body] in which the humor collects is hot, its putrefaction occurs most rapidly and powerfully.

(2.13)

[65] Says Hippocrates: If a crisis reaches someone, the night before the paroxysm of the fever is difficult for him, but the following night is mostly easier.

Says the commentator: When nature separates bad matter from good matter and prepares it for expulsion and evacuation, [the body] is in [a state of] disturbance. When this disturbance happens, the patient is necessarily restless (anxious) and the illness is difficult for him. People usually sleep at night. If that disturbance prevents a patient from sleeping, it is extremely clear [that this happens because of] his restlessness (anxiety) and because of the severity of his disease. Sometimes, this occurs during the day, when the crisis is about to occur in the following night. He says that [in the night following the paroxysm the crisis] is mostly easier because that crisis mostly results in health (recovery).

(2.11)

[٦٣] قال أبقراط: لأن يملأ البدن من الشراب أسهل من أن يملأ من الطعام.

قال المفسّر: أراد الأشياء الرطبة والأشربة التي لأبداننا فيها غذاء. وذلك أنّ الغذاء الرطب وخاصّة إن كان في طبيعته حارًّا أسهل وأسرع غذاء البدن.

(2.12)

[٦٤] قال أبقراط: البقايا التي تبقى من الأمراض من بعد البحران من عادتها أن تجلب عودة من
٥   المرض.

قال المفسّر: في أكثر الأمر تعفن تلك البقايا على طول الأيّام فتتولّد حمّى لأنّ كلّ رطوبة غريبة من طبيعة الجسم الذي يحويها يمكن أن يغذوه ولا يؤول أمرها إلّا إلى العفونة في الأكثر. فإذا كان مع ذلك الموضع الذي هي مجتمعة فيه حارًّا كان مصيرها إلى العفونة بأسرع ما يكون فأقواه.

(2.13)

[٦٥] قال أبقراط: إنّ من يأتيه البحران قد يصعب عليه مرضه في الليلة التي قبل نوبة الحمّى التي يأتي
١٠   فيها البحران ثمّ في الليلة التي بعدها يكون أكثر ذلك أخفّ.

قال المفسّر: عند تمييز الطبيعة للشيء الرديء من الشيء الجيّد وتهيئتها له للاندفاع والخروج يحدث اضطراب. وواجب ضرورة عند هذا الاضطراب أن يقلق المريض ويصعب عليه مرضه. ومن عادة الناس أن يناموا بالليل فإذا منع ذلك الاضطراب من النوم تبيّن قلق المريض وصعوبة مرضه بيانا واضحا. وقد يكون ذلك بالنهار إذا كان البحران متهيّئا لأن يكون في الليلة التي تأتي بعده. وقوله يكون
١٥   أكثر ذلك أخفّ لأنّ أكثر البحران يؤول إلى السلامة.

---

١ لأن (t =) أن (BCV): أن ‖ أسهل: خير B ‖ تجلب: إلى قوله B ‖ عادتها: شأنها AB عادته V   ٩ قد:
om. A   ٩–١٠ قد ... يكون: إلى قوله B   ١٠ أكثر: C¹ ‖ أكثر ذلك: على الأمر الأكثر B

(2.14)

[66] Says Hippocrates: In the case of looseness of the bowels, a change in the various kinds of the stools may be beneficial, unless they change into bad ones.

Says the commentator: This is so, because many different kinds [of stools] indicate the evacuation of many different kinds of humors. The bad kinds [of stools] are those in which there is some indication of the dissolution of the body, namely fatty stools, or [some] indication of putrefaction, namely a bad smell.

(2.15)

[67] Says Hippocrates: If a person suffers from pain in the throat, or if pustules or abscesses appear on the body, he should examine and look at that which is excreted from the body. If bile prevails therein, then[88] the [rest of the] body is affected in addition to that [spot]. But if that which is excreted from the body resembles that which is excreted by the body of a healthy person, one should feel safe to resort to feeding the body.

Says the commentator: Galen says that the throat also receives the humors that descend from the brain[89] and that pustules and abscesses indeed occur when the blood is heated through the yellow bile. Then one should examine and look whether nature has expelled all the superfluities to the diseased parts. You will know [that this is the case] if that which is excreted from the [diseased] body resembles that which is excreted from the body when it is healthy. In that case, there is no danger in feeding [the patient]. But if one has not completely cleansed the body of the humor, one will find bile prevailing in the excretion of the body. In that case, one should cleanse and purge [the body of the patient] before feeding him, because the more one feeds a body that is not clean, the more one harms it.[90]

---

88   "then the [rest of the] body is affected in addition to that [spot]": Cf. Galen, *In Hippocratis Aphorismos commentarius* 2.15, ed. Kühn, vol. 17b, p. 471: τὸ σῶμα ξυννοσέει; Hippocrates, *Aphorisms*, trans. Littré, vol. 4, p. 475: "le corps entier est malade;" trans. Jones, p. 113: "the whole body is affected."

89   Cf. Galen, ibid., p. 472: πολλάκις δὲ ἥ τε φάρυγξ ὑποδεχομένη τοὺς ἐκ τῆς κεφαλῆς καταρρέοντας χυμοὺς ἐνοχλεῖται (in many cases the throat is affected after receiving the humors that stream down from the head). In using the term ﺥﻠﺲ (lit., 'brain') for Greek κεφαλή, Maimonides follows Ḥunayn's translation (E).

90   Galen, ibid., ed. Kühn, pp. 472–473.

(2.14)

[٦٦] قال أبقراط: عند استطلاق البطن قد ينتفع باختلاف ألوان البراز إذا لم يكن تغيّره إلى أنواع منه رديئة.

قال المفسّر: لأنّ كثرة ألوانه تدلّ على استفراغ أصناف كثيرة من الكيموسات والأنواع الرديئة هو أن يكون فيه شيء من علامات ذوبان البدن وهو البراز الدسم أو من علامات العفونة وهو خبث
٥ الرائحة.

(2.15)

[٦٧] قال أبقراط: متى اشتكى الحلق أو خرجت في البدن بثور أو خراجات فينبغي أن ينظر ويتفقّد لما يبرز من البدن فإنّه إن كان الغالب عليه المرار فإنّ البدن مع ذلك عليل وإن كان ما يبرز من البدن مثل ما يبرز من البدن الصحيح فكن على ثقة من التقدّم على أن تغذو البدن.

قال المفسّر: قال جالينوس: الحلق أيضا يقبل الكيموسات التي تنحدر من الدماغ. والبثور والخراجات
١٠ إنّما تكون عندما تسخّن الدم من قبل المرار الأصفر. فينبغي أن يفتقد وينظر هل قذفت الطبيعة جميع الفضول إلى تلك الأعضاء التي اعتلّت وتعلم ذلك بأن يكون ما يبرز من البدن مثل ما يبرز من البدن الصحيح فليس في تغذيته حينئذ خطر. وإن لم تكن استنظفت البدن من الخلط عن آخره وجدت الأغلب على ما يبرز من البدن المرار فينبغي حينئذ أن ينقّى ويستفرغ قبل أن يغذا لأنّ البدن الذي ليس بالنقاء كلّما غذوته زدته شرّا.

١ قد ... أنواع: إلى قوله B || إذا: ما add. C || تغيّره add. A || إلى: ألوان add. A || منه: تغيّره add. A ٣ على: om.
A ٦-٨ أو ... التقدّم: إلى قوله B ٦ خرجت: خرج A || خراجات: خروجات A ٩ الدماغ: E =
١٢ الصحيح: وإن كان ذلك B add. || تكن: C¹ || آخره: فإن add. B ١٣ أن: C .om

(2.16)

[68] Says Hippocrates: When a person is hungry, he should not tire himself out.

Says the commentator: With a small intake of food, one should avoid physical exercise. The reason for this is clear.

(2.17)

[69] Says Hippocrates: If the body receives an amount of food, which is much larger than it is natural [for that body], it produces disease, as the recovery shows.

Says the commentator: It seems to me that his intention in this aphorism is to tell [us] that if the intake of food is much larger than is natural, whether in quantity or in quality, it produces disease. The severity of the illness is according to the degree of deviation [of the intake of food from what is natural]. If the deviation is large, it produces a severe illness. But if the deviation [that produces] the illness is small, then the illness will be light. He [also said] that the degree of deviation is indicated by observing its recovery (i.e., that of the body): If the deviation is small, the recovery is quick.

(2.18)

[70] Says Hippocrates: Foods that nourish quickly and all at once are also quickly excreted.

Says the commentator: That which nourishes most quickly and suddenly is wine. The meaning of the term "quickly" is a short time after ingestion. The term "suddenly" means that once one starts to feed [the body], it uses up (assimilates) all the food all at once and does not attract it little by little.

(2.19)

[71] Says Hippocrates: To predict either death or recovery in the case of acute diseases is not quite safe.

(2.16)

[٦٨] قال أبقراط: متى كان بإنسان جوع فلا ينبغي أن يتعب.

قال المفسّر: مع قلّة الغذاء ينبغي اجتناب الرياضة وعلّة ذلك بيّنة.

(2.17)

[٦٩] قال أبقراط: متى ورد على البدن غذاء خارج عن الطبيعة كثير فإنّ ذلك يحدث مرضا ويدلّ على ذلك بروءه.

قال المفسّر: يبدو لي أنّ غرضه في هذا الفصل أن يخبر أنّ إذا كان الغذاء الوارد خارج عن الطبيعة خروجا كثيرا كان ذلك الخروج في الكمّيّة أو في الكيفيّة فإنّه يحدث مرضا ومبلغ ما يحدث من المرض على قدر خروجه إن خرج خروجا عظيما أحدث مرضا عظيما وإن كان خروجه للمرض خروجا يسيرا كان المرض يسيرا قال ويستدلّ على مقدار خروجه بما يشاهد من بروئه فإنّه إن كان الخروج يسيرا برأ سريعا.

(2.18)

[٧٠] قال أبقراط: ما كان من الأشياء يغذو سريعا دفعة نخروجه أيضا يكون سريعا.

قال المفسّر: أبلغ الأشياء كلّها في أن يغذو سريعا دفعة النبيذ. ومعنى سريعا بعد تناولها بزمان يسير وقوله دفعة أن يكون بعد أن يبتدىء يغذو ويستوفي البدن غذاءها كلّه ولا يجذبه قليلا قليلا بل دفعة واحدة.

(2.19)

[٧١] قال أبقراط: إنّ التقدّم بالقضيّة في الأمراض الحادّة بالموت كانت أو بالبروء ليست تكون على غاية الثقة.

---

٣ خارج ... مرضا: إلى قوله B ‖ عن: من C   ٨ مقدار: om. B   ١١ ومعنى: ويعني A   ١٤ في ... تكون: إلى قوله B ‖ ليست (t =): فليست A   ١٥ غاية: من add. A

Says the commentator: Galen says that fever in the case of an acute illness is most often continuous, for only a small number of acute illnesses, such as apoplexy, occur without fever.[91]

(2.20)

[72] Says Hippocrates: He who has loose bowels when he is young will have constipated ones when he grows old, and he who has constipated bowels when he is young will have loose bowels when he grows old.

Says the commentator: When I tried to verify this [statement] I found that it is not universal and therefore it is a false assertion without any doubt. In my opinion, the truth is that Hippocrates saw one or two persons in whom this happened and turned that into an indefinite[92] verdict, as was his habit in the major part of his book *Epidemics*, because on the basis of the investigation of the condition of one or two persons his assertion turns into a judgment regarding [the whole] category (species). These are, in my opinion, the true facts. If you do not want [to acknowledge] this, but prefer to give this incorrect statement a semblance of truth [by] attaching certain conditions and prerequisites to it, then you should look into what Galen said in [his commentary to] this aphorism.[93]

(2.21)

[73] Says Hippocrates: Drinking *sharāb*[94] alleviates (cures) hunger.

Says the commentator: With *sharāb* he means "wine" and with "hunger" overhere he means "canine appetite," for the drinking of wine, which has a strong warming effect relieves this hunger. Canine appetite originates either from a cold temperament of the stomach alone or from an acid humor that has been absorbed by its substance. Wine, as mentioned, cures both [conditions] together.[95]

---

91   Cf. ibid. 2.19, p. 490.

92   "indefinite verdict" (*qaḍīya muhmila*): For this term, belonging to the field of logic, see Lameer, *Al-Fārābī and Aristotelean Syllogistics*, pp. 75–77.

93   Cf. Galen, *In Hippocratis Aphorismos commentarius* 2.20, ed. Kühn, vol. 17b, pp. 492–498.

94   "*sharāb*" (شراب): The Arabic term, which can mean 'beverage in general' or more specifically 'wine,' represents the Greek θώρηξις; cf. Liddel/Scott, *Greek-English Lexicon*, p. 814: "drinking to intoxication;" Hippocrates, *Aphorisms* 2.21, trans. Littré, vol. 4, p. 477: "vin;" trans. Jones, p. 113: "Strong drink." See also aphorism 7.48 (400) below.

95   Cf. Maimonides, *Medical Aphorisms* 23.81, trans. Bos, vol. 5, p. 59: "A bad craving for food, if unusually severe, is called 'canine appetite.' It happens when a detrimental acid humor burns the stomach or when the entire body suffers from excessive dissolution. *De [morborum] causis et symptomatibus* 4."

قال المفسّر: قال جالينوس: الحمّى في المرض الحادّ تكون مطبقة دائمًا على الأمر الأكثر فإنّ القليل من الأمراض الحادّة يكون من غير حمّى كالفالج.

(2.20)

[٧٢] قال أبقراط: من كانت بطنه في شبابه لينة فإنّه إذا شاخ يبس بطنه ومن كان في شبابه يابس البطن فإنّه إذا شاخ لان بطنه.

٥   قال المفسّر: إذا طلبت التحقيق علمت أنّ هذا الأمر غير مطّرد فهو إذًا قضية كاذبة لا شكّ. والصحيح عندي أنّ أبقراط رأى شخصًا أو شخصين جرى حالهما هكذا فجعلها قضية مهملة كما جرت عادته في معظم كتاب أبيذيميا لأنّه باستقراء حال شخص واحد أو شخصين يصير عنده القضية حكمًا على النوع. هذا هو عندي الإنصاف. فإن لم ترد ذلك وآثرت أن تجعل لهذا القول الغير صحيح وجوه صحّة وتشترط له اشتراطات وتفرض له فرضات فعليك بما ذكر جالينوس في هذا الفصل.

(2.21)

١٠   [٧٣] قال أبقراط: شرب الشراب يشفي الجوع.

قال المفسّر: يريد بالشراب النبيذ وهذا الجوع يريد به الشهوة الكلبيّة فإنّ شرب الخمور التي لها إسخان قوي يشفي هذا الجوع لأنّ الشهوة الكلبيّة إنّما تكون إمّا من برد مزاج المعدة فقط وإمّا من كيموس حامض قد تشرّبه جرمها والنبيذ الذي وصفنا يشفي الأمرين جميعًا.

(2.22)

[74] Says Hippocrates: Illnesses that arise from repletion are cured by depletion and those that arise from depletion are cured by repletion. All diseases are
cured by opposites.

Says the commentator: This is clear.

(2.23)

[75] Says Hippocrates: Acute diseases come to a crisis in fourteen days.

Says the commentator: Galen says that none of the acute diseases that have
a uniform movement and continuous pace (progress) goes beyond this limit.
In many acute diseases, the crisis may come on the eleventh, ninth, seventh,
or fifth [day]. In some of them it may occur on the sixth [day], but this is not
[a] good [crisis]. Hippocrates is used to generally call those illnesses that have
a complete crisis on the fourteenth day or earlier, "acute diseases." As for diseases in which there is an incomplete crisis on one of the first days of the crisis
and in which there remains a part [of the crisis] and which complete their crisis on one of the subsequent days, up to the fortieth day, he calls them "acute
[diseases] whose crisis occurs on the fortieth day."[96]

(2.24)

[76] Says Hippocrates: The fourth day is indicative of the seventh; the eighth
day is the beginning of the second week; the[97] eleventh day is indicative [of
the fourteenth] because it is the fourth day of the second week. The seventeenth day is also a day of prognostic indication since it is the fourth day from
the fourteenth and the seventh day from the eleventh.

Says the commentator: Galen says that the seventeenth day is indicative of
the twentieth because the twentieth day is a day of crisis and it is the end of
the third week.[98]

---

96   Cf. Galen, *In Hippocratis Aphorismos commentarius* 2.23, ed. Kühn, vol. 17b, pp. 506–507.

97   "the eleventh day is indicative [of the fourteenth]": Cf. trans. Ibn Tibbon: והמורה ליום
      הארבעה עשר יום האחד עשר.

98   Cf. Galen, *In Hippocratis Aphorismos commentarius* 2.24 ed. Kühn, vol. 17b, p. 511.

(2.22)

[٧٤] قال أبقراط: ما كان من الأمراض يحدث من امتلاء فشفاؤه يكون بالاستفراغ وما كان منها يحدث من الاستفراغ فشفاؤه يكون بالامتلاء وشفاء سائر الأمراض يكون بالمضادّة.

قال المفسّر: هذا واضح.

(2.23)

[٧٥] قال أبقراط: إنّ البحران يأتي في الأمراض الحادّة في أربعة عشر يوما.

قال المفسّر: قال جالينوس: لا يجاوز شيء من الأمراض الحادّة التي حركتها حركة حادة وسرعة متّصلة ٥ هذا الحدّ. وقد يأتي البحران في كثير من الأمراض الحادّة في الحادي عشر وفي التاسع والسابع والخامس. وقد يأتي بعضهم في السادس لكنّه ليس بمحمود. فالأمراض التي يأتي فيها البحران التامّ في اليوم الرابع عشر أو قبله فمن عادة أبقراط أن يسمّيها أمراض حادّة بقول مطلق. فأمّا الأمراض التي يكون فيها بحران ناقص في أحد أيّام البحران الأوّل ثمّ يبقى منها بقية يتمّ كون بحرانها في أحد ١٠ أيّام البحران التي بعد إلى اليوم الأربعين فيقول فيها الحادّة التي يأتي بحرانها في الأربعين.

(2.24)

[٧٦] قال أبقراط: الرابع منذر بالسابع وأوّل الأسبوع الثاني اليوم الثامن والمنذر يوم الحادي عشر لأنّه الرابع من الأسبوع الثاني واليوم السابع عشر أيضا يوم إنذار لأنّه اليوم الرابع من اليوم الرابع عشر واليوم السابع من اليوم الحادي عشر.

قال المفسّر: قال جالينوس: السابع عشر منذر بالعشرين لأنّ يوم العشرين هو يوم بحران وهو انقضاء ١٥ الأسبوع الثالث.

---

١ من: C¹ ‖ ٢–١ فشفاؤه ... الأمراض: إلى قوله B ٣ هذا: بين B add. B ٤ أربعة: أربع C ٥ يجاوز: يجوز AC ‖ شيء: في شيء C¹ ٦ والسابع: والرابع B add. B ٧ بعضهم ... يأتي: om. A ١٠–٩ الأوّل ... البحران: om. B ١٣–١١ وأوّل ... من اليوم الرابع عشر واليوم السابع: إلى قوله B

(2.25)

[77] Says Hippocrates: The summer quartan fevers are mostly short and the autumn ones long, especially those [contracted] when winter is near.

Says the commentator: Not only quartan fever is short in summer, but all other diseases, because the humors liquefy and are dispersed throughout the whole body and dissolve. As a result, all summer diseases are of short duration. However, Hippocrates only speaks about the longest disease, as an example. And in winter, the opposite is the case, that is to say that the humors remain in the depth of the body as if they were petrified and their strength retains its vehemence. The diseases do not end since the humors that produce them are still there. The patients do not die since their strength remains and does not dissolve.

(2.26)

[78] Says Hippocrates: It is better that the fever occurs after the spasm than the spasm after the fever.

Says the commentator: A spasm occurs either because of overfilling or of evacuation. If the spasm occurs because of overfilling, the nerves are filled with cold, viscous humor, with which they are nourished, and if fever occurs after the spasm, the fever often heats, dilutes, liquefies, and dissolves the humor. But if a person is affected by ardent fever, it dries his whole body and his nerves, and then the spasm occurs because of the dryness, and the affliction is severe.

(2.27)

[79] Says Hippocrates: One should not be deceived by[99] alleviation [of a disease] occurring to a patient, when it is illogical (irregular), nor should one fear a deterioration when it is illogical (irregular), because most such occurrences are uncertain and are hardly ever permanent and protracted.

Says the commentator: When a serious disease occurs and then there is an alleviation all of a sudden without previous concoction or evacuation [of the humors that produce the illness], one should not rely thereon, because the humors have become slow and subsided and their movements have diminished; that's all. Likewise, if a clear concoction precedes and then there occurs bad (difficult) breathing and mental confusion (delirium) and the like, one should not be afraid, because it is not permanent and often indicates a beneficial crisis.

---

99   "by alleviation [of a disease]": Cf. trans. Ibn Tibbon: בקלות החולי.

(2.25)

[٧٧] قال أبقراط: إنّ الربع الصيفيّة في أكثر الأمر تكون قصيرة والخريفيّة طويلة لا سيّما متى اتّصلت بالشتاء.

قال المفسّر: ليس الربع فقط تكون في الصيف قصيرة لكن سائر الأمراض لأنّ الكيموسات تذوب وتنتشر في البدن كلّه وتتحلّل فيجب من ذلك أن لا يطول شيء من الأمراض الصيفيّة.

٥ لكنّ أبقراط جعل كلامه في أطول الأمراض فصيّره مثالا. ويعرض في الشتاء ضدّ ذلك أعني أن تسكن الكيموسات في عمق البدن كأنّها تتحجّر وتبقى القوة على شدّتها فلا الأمراض تنقضي إذ كانت الكيموسات المولّدة لها باقية ولا المرضى يموتون لأنّ قوّتهم تبقى ولا تنحلّ.

(2.26)

[٧٨] قال أبقراط: لإن تكون الحمّى بعد التشنّج خير من أنْ يكون التشنّج بعد الحمّى.

قال المفسّر: التشنّج يكون من امتلاء ومن استفراغ فإذا عرض التشنّج من امتلاء وإنّما يمتلئ العصب ١٠ من الكيموس اللزج البارد الذي منه غذاؤه وحدثت الحمّى بعد هذا التشنّج فكثير ما تسخن ذلك الكيموس وتذيبه وتلطّفه وتحلّله الحمّى. وإذا عرضت للإنسان حمّى محرقة فجفّفت بدنه كلّه وعصبه ثمّ عرض له التشنّج من قبل اليبس فالآفة في ذلك عظيمة.

(2.27)

[٧٩] قال أبقراط: لا ينبغي أن يغترّ بخفّة يجدها المريض بخلاف القياس ولا أن تهولك أمور صعبة تحدث على غير القياس فإنّ أكثر ما يعرض من ذلك ليس بثابت ولا يكاد يلبث ولا تطول مدّته.

١٥ قال المفسّر: متى حدث مرض قويّ ثمّ خفّ بغتة دون تقدّم نضج ولا استفراغ فلا يعتمد على ذلك لأنّ الأخلاط تبلّدت وخمدت ونقصت حركتها لا غير. وكذلك إن تقدّم النضج البيّن ثمّ عرض بعده نفس رديء واختلاط ذهن ونحوه فلا يهولك ذلك لأنّه لا يلبث وكثير ما يدلّ ذلك على بحران محمود.

---

١ إنّ: om. B ‖ في ... متى: إلى قوله B ‖ لا: ولا C ٥ لكنّ: om. B ٦ تسكن: تسخن B ١٣ بخفّة: بخف C ١٣–١٤ بخفّة ... يلبث: إلى قوله B

(2.28)

[80] Says Hippocrates: If someone suffers from a fever that is not very light and his body remains as it is and it does not lose any [weight] and does not waste more than necessary, it is a bad [sign], because the former indicates a long disease and the latter indicates that the strength [of the body] is weak.

Says the commentator: Emaciation of the body is always a bad sign and indicates weakness of the strength [of the body], regardless whether the fever is not very light (mild) or is very strong.

(2.29)

[81] Says Hippocrates: If you think that you can move[100] something, do so, as long as the disease is in the beginning. But if the disease reaches its culmination, the patient should rest and repose.

Says the commentator: The reason for this is given by him in the next aphorism. [With the statement]: "If you think that you can move something, do so," he especially means bleeding and sometimes one may also apply purgation. But none of these should be applied in the time that the disease reaches its culmination, because the concoction of the disease takes place at that time and the psychical faculty is mostly exhausted at the time of the climax. To apply evacuation in the beginning of the disease is the best help for a concoction as quickly as possible, so that the [superfluous] matter [causing the disease] is diminished. The vital faculty and the natural faculty retain their strength at the time of the climax.

Says the commentator: He has already stated before that one should not purge in the beginning [of a disease] except for diseases that flare up.[101] For this reason here he remarks that if you think that you can move something you should do so.

(2.30)

[82] Says Hippocrates: All things are weaker at the beginning and end of the disease, but stronger at its culmination.

---

100   "move" (حرّك) (= Greek κινέω): As ed. Jones remarks in Hippocrates, *Aphorisms* 2.29, p. 115 n. 3, the Greek term "often means to administer a purge, an enema, or an emetic."
101   Cf. aphorism 1.24 (51) above.

(2.28)

[۸۰] قال أبقراط: من كانت به حمّى ليست بالضعيفة جدّا فإن يبقى بدنه على حاله ولا ينتقص شيئا أو يذوب بأكثر ممّا ينبغي رديء لأنّ الأوّل ينذر بطول من المرض والثاني يدلّ على ضعف من القوة.

قال المفسّر: هزال البدن أبدا علامة رديئة ودالّ على ضعف القوة سواء كانت الحمّى ليست بالضعيفة جدّا أو كانت حمّى قويّة جدّا.

(2.29)

٥ [۸۱] قال أبقراط: ما دام المرض في ابتدائه فإن رأيت أن تحرّك شيئا فحرّك فإذا صار المرض إلى منتهاه فينبغي أنْ يستقرّ المريض ويسكن.

قال المفسّر: سيعطي علّة ذلك في الفصل الذي بعده. وقوله فإن رأيت أن تحرّك شيئا فحرّك يريد به الفصد خاصّة وربّما استعمل أيضا الإسهال. وليس ينبغي أن يستعمل واحد من هذين وقت منتهى المرض لأنّ نضج المرض في ذلك الوقت يكون. والقوة النفسانية تكون في وقت المنتهى في أكثر

١٠ الأمر قد كلّت. والأجود في المعونة على أن يكون النضج أسرع هو أن يستعمل الاستفراغ في ابتداء المرض حتّى تقلّ مادّته. وفي وقت المنتهى القوة الحيوانية والقوة الطبيعية باقيتين على قوّتهما.

قال المفسّر: قد تقدّم لك أنّه لا ينبغي أن تسهل في الابتداء إلّا في الأمراض الهائجة ولذلك قال هنا فإن رأيت أن تحرّك شيئا فحرّك.

(2.30)

[۸۲] قال أبقراط: إنّ جميع الأشياء في أوّل المرض وآخره أضعف وفي منتهاه أقوى.

٢-١ جدّا ... يدلّ على: إلى قوله B   ٥-٦ فإن ... المريض: إلى قوله B   ٦ ويسكن: ويستكن C   ٩ والقوة:
بالقوة A   ١١ والقوة: C²

Says the commentator: With things he means symptoms, because these, that is to say the fever attacks, sleeplessness, pain, distress, and thirst, are milder at the beginning and end of the disease. The condition, from which these symptoms originate, namely the disease, is necessarily at its best at the time of the culmination when the patient is one of those who are saved.

(2.31)
[83] Says Hippocrates: If the convalescent has a good appetite, but his body does not put on any weight, it is a bad sign.

Says the commentator: [This] is clear and the matter has already been mentioned before.[102]

(2.32)
[84] Says Hippocrates: In most cases, if someone with a bad constitution has a good appetite at the beginning [of a disease], but does not put on any weight, he will lose his appetite in the end. However, if someone has a strong aversion of taking food in the beginning, but has a good appetite in the end, he will be better off.

Says the commentator: He is speaking here about a convalescent. It is clear that, because of a bad temperament or because of a remnant of [superfluous] humors, his organs are not nourished, although he has a strong appetite [in the beginning]. And [when] he eats, his humors increase and his bad temperament becomes worse, so that he loses his appetite. But if he does not have an appetite in the beginning, because nature is busy with the concoction [of the food], one should know that from the time when he starts to have an appetite, his humors have been concocted and his condition will mostly continue to improve.

(2.33)
[85] Says Hippocrates: A healthy [state of] mind is a good sign in every illness, and likewise a good appetite. The opposite is a bad sign.

Says the commentator: This is clear. I have explained the reason for this in the aphorisms, which I composed.[103]

---

102   Cf. aphorism 2.8 (60) above.
103   Cf. Maimonides, *Medical Aphorisms* 6.94, ed. and trans. Bos, vol. 2, pp. 20–22.

قال المفسّر: يريد بالأشياء الأعراض لأنّها في أوّل المرض وآخره أضعف يعني نوائب الحمّى والأرق والوجع والكرب والعطش. فأمّا الحال التي تكون منها هذه الأعراض وهي المرض فيجب ضرورة أن يكون في وقت المنتهى أجود إذا كان المريض من المرضى الذين يسلمون.

(2.31)

[٨٣] قال أبقراط: إذا كان الناقه يحظا من الطعام فلا يتزيّد بدنه شيئا فذلك رديء.

٥ قال المفسّر: بيّن وقد تقدّم هذا المعنى.

(2.32)

[٨٤] قال أبقراط: إنّ في أكثر الحالات جميع من حاله رديئة ويحظا من الطعام في أوّل الأمر فلا يتزيّد بدنه شيئا فإنّه يؤول أمره بآخره إلى أن لا يحظا من الطعام. فأمّا من يمتنع عليه في أوّل أمره النيل من الطعام امتناعا شديدا ثمّ يحظا منه بآخره كحاله تكون أجود.

قال المفسّر: الكلام هنا في الناقه وبيّن هو أنّه من أجل رداءة مزاجه أو بقيّة الأخلاط لم تغتذ أعضاؤه ١٠ وشهوته قويّة وهو يأكل فتزداد الأخلاط أو يقوى سوء المزاج فتستبطل الشهوة. وإذا كان أوّلا لا يشتهي لاشتغال الطبيعة بالنضج فمنذ يبدئ يشتهي يعلم أنّ قد نضجت أخلاطه فتستمرّ حاله على الصلاح في الأكثر.

(2.33)

[٨٥] قال أبقراط: صحّة الذهن في كلّ مرض علامة جيّدة وكذلك الهشاشة للطعام وضدّ ذلك علامة رديئة.

١٥ قال المفسّر: هذا بيّن وقد بيّنت علّة ذلك في فصول ألفتها.

---

٣ الذين: الذي B   ٤ يحظا ... رديء: om. B   ٦ جميع: في add. C¹   ٨-٦ جميع ... ثمّ يحظا منه بآخره: إلى قوله B   ٧ يتزيّد (= E): يزيد A   بآخره (= E): om. A   يؤول: ditt. A   ١١ يبدئ: يبتدئ B   ١٤-١٣ في ... علامة رديئة: om. B   ١٥ علّة ذلك: علّته A

(2.34)

[86] Says Hippocrates: When the illness corresponds to the nature, age, and complexion of the patient and to the current time of the year, the danger is less than when the illness does not correspond to one of these factors.

Says the commentator: This is clear, because if it does not correspond, it indicates [that the temperament of] the patient is very unbalanced.

(2.35)

[87] Says Hippocrates: In all diseases it is best that the parts around the navel and the lower abdomen keep their fullness. If they are very thin [and] emaciated, it is [a] bad [sign]. Moreover, if the latter is the case, purgation is dangerous.

Says the commentator: The lower abdomen is the [area] between the genitals and the navel. The abdomen has three parts: the hypochondrium and the [parts] around the navel and the lower abdomen. If these regions are fuller, it is better, but if they are leaner, it is worse. The latter is a bad sign and a bad cause [for the illness]. It is a bad sign, because it indicates the weakness of those parts that are emaciated and dissolved. It is a bad cause, because the digestion of the food in the stomach and the production of the blood in the liver are not as they should be in this condition. These two organs benefit from the thick and fat [layer] that covers them because it warms them.

(2.36)

[88] Says Hippocrates: If someone with a healthy body is treated with a purgative or[104] emetic, he will quickly faint. The same [occurs to] someone who feeds himself with bad food.

Says the commentator: "The same [occurs to] someone who feeds himself with bad food." This means that if he is treated with an emetic or purgative, he will quickly faint because his body contains a surplus [of bad superfluities]. If the remedy only irritates it a little bit, then the bad condition [of his body] becomes clear and apparent. This is Galen's argumentation.[105] But in my opinion it is caused by the fact that, if someone constantly takes bad foods, his blood becomes extremely bad and its quality is corrupted. And if the medicine [that

---

104   "or emetic": Missing in the Greek text.

105   Maimonides' statement is not entirely correct, since in the following section, Galen speaks about the bad blood produced in the body of someone who takes bad food.

(2.34)

[٨٦] قال أبقراط: إذا كان المرض ملائمًا لطبيعة المريض وسنّه وسحنته والوقت الحاضر من أوقات السنة نخطره أقلّ من خطر المرض الذي ليس بملائم لواحد من هذه الخصال.

قال المفسّر: هذا بيّن لأنّه إذا لم يكن ملائمًا فهو دليل على خروج كثير عن اعتدال ذلك الشخص.

(2.35)

[٨٧] قال أبقراط: إنّ الأجود في كلّ مرض أن يكون ما يلي السرّة والثنّة له تخن ومتى كان رقيقا

٥ جدًّا منهوكا فذلك رديء وإذا كان أيضا كذلك فالإسهال معه خطر.

قال المفسّر: الثنّة هو ما بين الفرج وبين السرّة فيكون أقسام البطن ثلاثة: المواضع التي في ما دون الشراسيف وما يلي السرّة والثنّة. ومتى كانت تلك المواضع أثخن فالحال أجود ومتى كانت أهزل فالحال أردأ وذلك أنّها علامة رديئة وسبب رديء. أمّا علامة رديئة فلأنّها تدلّ على ضعف تلك الأعضاء التي انتهكت وذابت. وأمّا سبب رديء فلأنّ استمراء الطعام في المعدة وتولّد الدم في الكبد

١٠ لا يكونان عند هذه الحال على ما ينبغي لأنّ هذين العضوين جميعا ينتفعان بثخن ما يغشيهما وسمنه بتسخينه لهما.

(2.36)

[٨٨] قال أبقراط: من كان بدنه صحيحا فأسهل أو قيّئ بدواء أسرع إليه الغشي وكذلك من كان يغتذي بغذاء رديء.

قال المفسّر: وكذلك من كان يغتذي بغذاء رديء فإنّه إن قيّئ أو أسهل أسرع إليه الغشي لأنّ في أبدانهم فضل رديء. فإذا أثاره الدواء أدنى إثارة تبيّنت رداءته وانكشفت. هذا هو تعليل جالينوس.

١٥ والذي يبدو لي في علّة ذلك أنّ الذي داوم الأغذية الرديئة دمه دم مذموم جدًّا فاسد الكيفيّة. فإذا

١-٢ لطبيعة ... بملائم: إلى قوله B ‖ ٢ الذي: اذا كان C ‖ لواحد: لواحدة C ‖ ٤-٥ أن ... كذلك: إلى قوله B ‖ ٦ المواضع: الموضع C ‖ التي: الذي AC ‖ ١٠-١١ لأنّ ... بتسخينه: om. A ‖ ١٢-١٣ أو ... رديء: om. B ‖ ١٥ فضل: خلط B

he takes] attracts [the bad blood] through its attractive power, it moves all the blood in [his body] and attempts to cleanse it of all its corrupt parts. These are extremely numerous and amalgamated; moreover, they are the vessel[106] of the life of this person with this corrupt regimen. Fainting necessarily occurs because of the power of the attraction and because of the large quantity [of amalgamated, mixed bad blood] that the medicine attempts to attract.

(2.37)
[89] Says Hippocrates: If someone is in a good bodily condition, it is hard to purge him.

Says the commentator: If a healthy person takes an emetic or purgative, he will suffer from dizziness, colic and a difficult evacuation. He will also faint easily because the medication attempts to attract the appropriate humor. If it does not find so, it attracts the blood and the flesh and forces from them the extraction of that which is appropriate to it.

(2.38)
[90] Says Hippocrates: With regard to food and drink one should prefer something that is slightly inferior but tastes better above something that is better but tastes worse.[107]

Says the commentator: This is clear, because something that is more pleasant is better digested.

(2.39)
[91] Says Hippocrates: In most cases old[108] people fall ill less often than the young, but when they contract chronic ailments they mostly die while still suffering from them.

---

106   I.e., that, which carries the life of this person, on which his life depends.
107   Cf. Maimonides, *Medical Aphorisms* 20.5, trans. Bos, vol. 4, p. 63: "We as physicians focus especially on the benefit that foods should provide, not on the pleasure to be derived from them. But since some foods are distasteful and their distastefulness hinders their digestion, the physician should make efforts to season such food so that it can be well digested. However, cooks [usually] season food [to such a degree] that it contributes to a bad digestion. *De alimentorum facultatibus* 2."
108   "old people" (كهول): Lit., "adults, people of middle age." My translation is based on the Greek; cf. Galen, *In Hippocratis Aphorismos commentarius* 2.39, ed. Kühn, vol. 17b, p. 538: οἱ πρεσβῦται.

جذب الدواء بقوّته الجاذبة حرّك كلّ دم فيه ورام أن يستخلص منه جميع فساداته وهي كثيرة جدّا
ومتّحدة بل هي مركب حياة هذا الشخص الفاسد التدبير. فحدث الغشي ضرورة لقوّة الجذب وكثرة
ما يرام جذبه وهو متّحد مختلط.

(2.37)

[٨٩] قال أبقراط: من كان بدنه صحيحا فاستعمال الدواء فيه يعسر.

٥   قال المفسّر: الأصحّاء إذا استعملوا القيء أو الإسهال يعرض لهم دوار ومغص ويعسر خروج ما يخرج
منهم ويسرع إليهم مع ذلك الغشي لأنّ الدواء يتوق لاجتذاب الكيموس الملائم له فإذا لم يجده
جذب الدم واللحم واستكرههما لينتزع منهما ما فيهما ممّا يلائمه.

(2.38)

[٩٠] قال أبقراط: ما كان من الطعام والشراب أخسّ قليلا إلّا أنّه ألذّ فينبغي أن يختار على ما هو
منهما أفضل إلّا أنّه أكره.

١٠   قال المفسّر: هذا بيّن لأنّ انضمام الألذّ أجود.

(2.39)

[٩١] قال أبقراط: الكهول في أكثر الأمر يمرضون أقلّ ممّا يمرض الشباب إلّا أنّ ما يعرض لهم من
الأمراض المزمنة على أكثر الأمر يموتون وهي بهم.

---

١ الجاذبة: الحارّة A ‖ فساداته: فسادته B   ٤ فاستعمال ... يعسر: om. B   ٦ له: om. A   ٨-٩ والشراب
... أكره: om. B   ١١ أكثر: أوّل A   ١١-١٢ يمرضون ... بهم: om. B

Says the commentator: Old people are stricter in their regimen than young people. However, their bodily strength is weak and unable to quickly concoct the diseases. All chronic ailments are cold and therefore lead necessarily to their death.

(2.40)

[92] Says Hippocrates: Hoarseness and catarrhs are not concocted (do not ripen) in the very old.

Says the commentator: This holds good not only for these ailments but with all other ailments [caused by] cold humors.

(2.41)

[93] Says Hippocrates: If someone suffers from frequent and severe fainting without obvious cause, he will die suddenly.

Says the commentator: If someone suffers from fainting under the following three conditions: there is no apparent cause, it is severe, and it [occurs] often, it will happen to him because of a weakness of the vital faculty.

(2.42)

[94] Says Hippocrates: If a stroke is severe, it is impossible for the patient to recover, and he will not recover easily if it is a mild one.

Says the commentator: A stroke only occurs when the psychical pneuma is unable to stream into that [part] of the body, which is below the head. This happens either because of a type of swelling occurring in the brain or because the ventricles of the brain are filled with phlegmatic moisture. If a stroke patient is unable to move his chest (cannot breathe), it is a stroke that is most severe and most[109] dangerous. If he breathes with extreme coercion (difficulty), the stroke is also severe [but not as severe as the previous one]. If he breathes without exertion and coercion (difficulty), but the breathing is unequal and irregular, the stroke is also severe, but less [severe] than the previous one. If the [stroke] patient breathes regularly, the stroke [he suffers from] is light. If you proceed cautiously in the matter in all that is necessary to do, you may cure him.[110]

---

109   "most dangerous." (أوحا): Lit., "very quick," i.e., leading to death.
110   Cf. Maimonides, *Medical Aphorisms* 6.94, ed. and trans. Bos, vol. 2, p. 21.

قال المفسّر: الكهول أضبط لأنفسهم في التدبير من الشباب والقوة في أبدان الكهول ضعيفة لا تقدر أن تنضج الأمراض سريعا والأمراض المزمنة كلّها باردة ولذلك يلزمهم للممات.

(2.40)

[٩٢] قال أبقراط: إنّ ما يعرض من البحوحة والنزل للشيخ الفاني ليس تنضج.

قال المفسّر: ليس هذه الأمراض فقط بل سائر ما يعرض من الأمراض من الأخلاط الباردة.

(2.41)

٥ [٩٣] قال أبقراط: من يصيبه مرارا كثيرة غشي شديد من غير سبب ظاهر فهو يموت فجأة.

قال المفسّر: من يصيبه الغشي بهذه الشرائط الثلاث وهو أن يكون من غير سبب ظاهر وشديد ومرارا كثيرة وإنّما يصيبه ذلك من قبل ضعف القوة الحيوانية.

(2.42)

[٩٤] قال أبقراط: السكتة إن كانت قوية لم يمكن أن يبرأ صاحبها منها وإن كانت ضعيفة لم يسهل أن يبرأ.

١٠ قال المفسّر: كلّ سكتة إنّما تكون إذا لم يمكن الروح النفساني أن يجري إلى ما دون الرأس من البدن إمّا العلّة من جنس الورم حدث في الدماغ وإمّا لأنّ بطون الدماغ امتلأت من رطوبة بلغمية. فإن عدم المسكوت حركة الصدر فذلك ما أشدّ ما يكون من الاستكراه وأوحا ما يكون منها. ومتى تنفّس بأشدّ ما يكون من الاستكراه فسكتته قوية أيضا. ومتى كان تنفّسه من غير مجاهدة واستكراه إلّا أنه يختلف غير لازم لنظام واحد فسكتته قوية أيضا إلّا أنّها أنقص من الثانية. ومتى كان صاحبها يتنفّس تنفّسا لازما لنظام فسكتته ١٥ ضعيفة. وإن أنت تأتّيت في أمره بجميع ما ينبغي أن يفعله فلعلّك أن تبرّئه.

---

٣ والنزل ... تنضج: om. B ٥ شديد ... فجأة: om. B || ظاهر: بين A ٧ وإنّما: فإنّها B ٨ السكتة إن كانت قوية: السكتة إذا كانت قوية A¹ ٩–٨ لم ... أن يبرأ: om. B ١٠ النفساني: النفسانية B ١١ حدث: حدثت C ١٤–١٣ ومتى ... أيضا: om. B ١٥ بجميع: لجميع BC

(2.43)

[95] Says Hippocrates: Those who are strangled [by hanging] and lose consciousness, but are not dead yet, will not recover if they have foam at the mouth.

Says the commentator: Galen mentions that some of those who were strangled [by hanging] or who strangled themselves (committed suicide) and foam appeared in their mouth, yet recovered. But that this is exceptional.[111]

(2.44)

[96] Says Hippocrates: If someone is naturally very fat, he is apt to die earlier than someone who is lean.

Says the commentator: The reason for this is clear, namely the narrowness of the vessels and their width as [Galen] explained in *De temperamentis*.[112] Galen further states: "If the body is well-fleshed [and] balanced so that it is neither fat nor lean it is best, [for then] a person will possibly live long and reach extreme old age."[113]

(2.45)

[97] Says Hippocrates: If someone suffering from epilepsy is young, he is above all cured from it by a change in age, place, and regimen.

Says the commentator: Epilepsy and apoplexy are both produced by a cold, thick humor. If someone's age, place, and regimen change into one that is hot and dry, and if there is also a change in the bad diet, which produced this humor to the opposite thereof, he may recover.[114]

(2.46)

[98] Says Hippocrates: If someone suffers from two pains at the same time, but not in the same place, the stronger one obscures the other.

---

111   Galen, *In Hippocratis Aphorismos commentarius* 2.43, ed. Kühn, vol. 17b, p. 546.
112   Cf. idem, *De temperamentis* 2.4, ed. Kühn, vol. 1, p. 605; trans. Singer, p. 246: "... it is thus natural that narrowness of veins for the most part goes together with a fatty, thick condition, while thin conditions tend to be found in the wide-veined."
113   Cf. idem, *In Hippocratis Aphorismos commentarius* 2.44, ed. Kühn, vol. 17b, p. 547.
114   Cf. Maimonides, *Medical Aphorisms* 9.1, ed. and trans. Bos, vol. 2, p. 59.

(2.43)

[٩٥] قال أبقراط: الذين يختنقون ويصيرون إلى حال الغشي ولم يبلغوا إلى حدّ الموت فليس يفيق منهم من ظهر في فيه زبد.

قال المفسّر: وذكر جالينوس أنّ بعض من خنق أو اختنق وظهر في فيه الزبد أفاق وذلك ندرة.

(2.44)

[٩٦] قال أبقراط: من كان بدنه غليظا جدّا بالطبع فالموت إليه أسرع منه إلى القضيف.

٥ قال المفسّر: علّة ذلك بيّنة لضيق العروق وسعتها كما بيّن في المزاج. وقال جالينوس: إن يكون البدن حسن اللحم معتدلا حتّى لا يكون غليظا ولا مهزولا أفضل وأمكن أن يعمر ويبلغ من الشيخوخة غايتها.

(2.45)

[٩٧] قال أبقراط: صاحب الصرع إذا كان حدثا فبروؤه منه يكون خاصّة بانتقاله في السنّ والبلد والتدبير.

١٠ قال المفسّر: الصرع والسكتة الكيموس المولّد لهما جميعا بارد غليظ. وإذا انتقل في البلد والسنّ والتدبير إلى الحرارة واليبس وانتقل أيضا عن التدبير الرديء الذي ولّد هذا الخلط لضدّ ذلك التدبير لعلّه يبرأ.

(2.46)

[٩٨] قال أبقراط: إذا كان بإنسان وجعان معا وليس هما في موضع واحد فإنّ أقواهما يخفي الآخر.

١-٢ ويصيرون ... زبد: om. B   ١ حال: حدّ C   ٢-٩ من ... والتدبير: C¹   ٤-١٣.ه١١٥ قال أبقراط ... إلى ما لم يعتده: C¹   ٤ جدّا ... القضيف: om. B   ٨-٩ إذا ... والتدبير: om. B   ٨ منه: om. C   ١٠-١١ قال ... يبرأ: om. C   ١٠ غليظ: om. B   ١٢ قال ... الآخر: C¹   بإنسان: om. B   معا ... الآخر: om. B   وليس هما: ليس C¹

Says the commentator: When nature turns towards the organ in which there is the pain that is more severe, the sensation [of pain] in the other place becomes less, [so that the patient] may not feel that pain [any more].

(2.47)

[99] Says Hippocrates: Pain and fever occur when pus is forming rather than when it has been formed.

Says the commentator: This happens because then the site of the swelling stretches more and more and the pain gets worse. The heat tends towards [the pus] in order to concoct it and spreads more and more and the fever intensifies.

(2.48)

[100] Says Hippocrates: In every movement of the body, rest at the beginning of pain[115] will prevent further pain.

Says the commentator: This is clear.

(2.49)

[101] Says Hippocrates: If a person is used to a certain labor, even if he has a weak body or is old, he is better able to bear it than someone who is not used to it, even if the latter is strong and young.

Says the commentator: This is clear.

(2.50)

[102] Says Hippocrates: If someone has been used to something for a long time, even if it is more harmful than something to which he has not been used, it will be less harmful to him. But sometimes it may be necessary to change to things one is not used to.

---

115 "pain" (اعياء): Cf. Galen, *In Hippocratis Aphorismos commentarius* 2.48, ed. Kühn, vol. 17b, p. 552: πονεῖν; Hippocrates, *Aphorisms*, trans. Littré, vol. 4, p. 485: "souffrir;" trans. Jones, p. 121: "pain." In the sense of "pain," Arabic اعياء is a non-attested semantic borrowing from Greek πονεῖν, c.q. πονέσθαι, which can mean both 'to toil, labor' and 'to suffer pain;' cf. Liddell/Scott, *Greek-English Lexicon*, p. 1447.

قال المفسّر: إذا اتّجهت الطبيعة نحو العضو الذي فيه الألم الأعظم نقص حسّ الموضع الآخر فلا يحسّ بما فيه ممّا يؤلم.

(2.47)

[٩٩] قال أبقراط: في وقت تولّد المدّة يعرض الوجع والحمّى أكثر ممّا يعرضان بعد تولّدها.

قال المفسّر: لأنّ حينئذ يتمدّد موضع الورم أكثر فيشتدّ الوجع وتميل الحرارة نحو الخلط لتنضجه

٥ فينبسط أكثر فتشتدّ الحمّى.

(2.48)

[١٠٠] قال أبقراط: في كلّ حركة يتحرّكها البدن فإراحته حين يبتدىء به الإعياء تمنعه من أن يحدث له الإعياء.

قال المفسّر: هذا بيّن.

(2.49)

[١٠١] قال أبقراط: من اعتاد تعبا ما فهو وإن كان ضعيف البدن أو شيخا فهو أحمل لذلك التعب

١٠ الذي اعتاده ممّن لم يعتده وإن كان قويّا شابّا.

قال المفسّر: هذا بيّن.

(2.50)

[١٠٢] قال أبقراط: ما قد اعتاده الإنسان منذ زمان طويل وإن كان أضرّ ممّا لم يعتده فأذاه له أقلّ فقد ينبغي أن ينتقل الإنسان إلى ما لم يعتده.

١-٢ قال ... يؤلم: C om.   ٣ قال ... تولدها: C¹ || يعرض ... تولّدها: B om.   ٤-٥ قال ... الحمّى: C om.
٥ أكثر: A om.   ٦-٧ قال ... أن يحدث له الإعياء: C¹ || فإراحته ... أن يحدث له الإعياء: B om.   ٨ قال
المفسّر: هذا بيّن: C om.   ٩-١٠ قال ... شابّا: C¹   ٩ من اعتاد: من كان قد اعتاد C¹   ٩-١٠ فهو ... شابّا:
B om.   ١١ قال المفسّر: هذا بيّن: C om.   ١٢-١٣ قال ... إلى ما لم يعتده: C¹ || منذ ... إلى ما لم يعتده: B om.

Says the commentator: He has laid down a correct premise and has drawn conclusions from it. [This premise] also implies that regarding the preservation of health in all circumstances one should accustom oneself to change from habit to habit, but only gradually so.[116]

Galen says that it is best for everyone to attempt to try everything [to which he is not accustomed], so that when he encounters something unusual—which inevitably happens—, it will not cause him severe harm. He should do so by not always adhering to the same habits but by sometimes attempting [to do] the opposite.

(2.51)

[103] Says Hippocrates: It is dangerous to suddenly fill the body excessively, or to empty it, or to heat it, or to cool it, or to move it with any type of movement. Everything that is excessive is hostile to nature. But that which is [done] gradually is safe, [especially] if you want to change from one thing to another or if you want something else.

Says the commentator: This is clear.

(2.52)

[104] Says Hippocrates: If you do everything that should be done [according[117] to the medical rules], but do not get the result [which[118] you should have according to the medical rules], do not change to another [treatment] as long as your original [diagnosis] remains.

---

116   On Maimonides' concept of habit, cf. *On the Regimen of Health* 4.26, trans. Bos, p. 142: "Habit is fundamental for the preservation of health and the cure of diseases. No one should give up his healthy habits all at once, either in eating, drinking, sexual intercourse, going to the bathhouse, or exercise. In all these [activities] one should observe one's habits, even if the thing one is accustomed to is contrary to the medical rules. One should not abandon it for what is required by [these] rules except gradually and over a long time, so that one does not notice the change. If someone changes his habit [in any of these] all at once, he will perforce fall sick. As for sick people, they should not change their habit in any way, that is to say, that one should not [even] start at the time of illness to change one's habit, [even] for the better." See also idem, *On Asthma* 10.1, ed. and trans. Bos, vol. 1, pp. 51–52, 132 n. 3; and Bos, "Maimonides on the Preservation of Health," p. 220.

117   "[according to the medical rules] (على ما ينبغي)": Cf. Galen, *In Hippocratis Aphorismos commentarius* 2.52, ed. Kühn, vol. 17b, p. 557: κατὰ λόγον; Hippocrates, *Aphorisms*, trans. Littré, vol. 4, p. 485: "conforme à la règle;" trans. Jones, p. 121: "according to rule." See also Barry, *Syriac Medicine*, pp. 163–167 (a reference to this particular aphorism is missing).

118   "[which you should have according to the medical rules]": Cf. Galen, ibid.: κατὰ λόγον; Hippocrates, ibid., trans. Littré: "selon la règle;" trans. Jones: "according to rule."

قال المفسّر: قدّم مقدمة صحيحة وألزم عنها وعمّا يلزم من استدامة الصحّة في جميع الحالات أن يعوّد الإنسان نفسه الانتقال من عادة إلى عادة وعلى تدريج.

قال جالينوس: إنّ الأجود لكلّ واحد من الناس أن يحمل نفسه على تجربة كلّ شيء كيما لا يصادفه عند الضرورة شيء لم يعتده فيناله ضرر عظيم. وإنّما يكون ذلك بأن لا يبقى الإنسان على ما قد اعتاده

٥   دائمًا لكنّ يحمل نفسه في بعض الأوقات على ضدّه.

(2.51)

[١٠٣] قال أبقراط: استعمال الكثير بغتة ممّا يملأ البدن أو يستفرغه أو يسخنه أو يبرّده أو يحرّكه بنوع آخر من الحركة أيّ نوع كان خطر. وكلّ ما كان كثيرا فهو مقاوم للطبيعة. فأمّا ما يكون قليلا قليلا فأمون متى أردت إنتقالا من شيء إلى غيره ومتى أردت غير ذلك.

قال المفسّر: هذا بيّن.

(2.52)

١٠   [١٠٤] قال أبقراط: إن أنت فعلت جميع ما ينبغي أن تفعل على ما ينبغي فلم يكن ما ينبغي أن يكون فلا تنتقل إلى غير ما أنت عليه ما دام ما رأيته منذ أوّل الأمر ثابتا.

١-١١ قال ... فلا تنتقل: .om C   ٢ نفسه الانتقال: .om B || عادة: أخرى A   ٦-٨ ممّا ... إلى غيره: .om B
٧ خطر: رديء A   ١٠-١١ أن ... الأمر: إلى قوله B   ١١ ثابتا: تامّا C

Says the commentator: This aphorism comprises a major rule regarding medical treatment. In his commentary [on this rule], Galen does not go far enough (does not cover everything necessary). The meaning [of this aphorism] is as follows: If the symptoms tell you, for instance, that one should apply [heating medications], and you did so for a long time but the patient did not recover, you should not change to [another] regimen, but continue to apply heating medications as long as the symptoms suggesting these medications remain. This is the meaning of his statement: "as long as your original [diagnosis] remains." And this is the meaning of his statement: "[do not change to another [treatment]," that one should not change from one type of treatment [to another type of treatment]. However, it is certainly appropriate to change from one heating medication to another heating medication and to alternate between all simple and compound medications that have a heating effect, because when a body becomes used to one and the same medicine that has been taken constantly, its effect [on the body] becomes less. Moreover, to alternate between different types of medications that have the same quality is extremely appropriate for every temperament of every singular person and of every singular organ, and for the afflictions [coming with] every singular disease. This is a major principle of the secrets of treatment. Exactly the same method should be applied with regard to nutrition, the different kinds of evacuation of the humor that causes the illness, and with regard to [medications that] dissolve, refine, concoct, or thicken matter, or [medications] that are astringent. Always adhere to the type of therapy that is indicated by symptoms that remain [the same] and alternate between the different medications and nutrients that are of the same kind. Understand this.

(2.53)
[105] Says Hippocrates: If someone has loose bowels, as long as he is young his condition will be better than that of someone who has hard bowels. But when he gets old his condition will be worse, because his bowels will be hard as is mostly the case [in old people].

قال المفسّر: هذا فصل يتضمّن قانونا عظيما من قوانين العلاج ولم يبلغ جالينوس في شرحه ما ينبغي. ومعنى هذا أنّه إذا دلّتك العلامات أنّه مثلا ينبغي أن يسخّن فداومت التسخين فلم يبرأ المريض فلا ينبغي لك أن تنتقل للتدبير بل تدوم على التسخين طال ما ترى الأمور الدالّة على استعمال التسخين ثابتة وهو معنى قوله ما دام ما رأيته منذ أوّل الأمر ثابتا. هذا معنى قوله يعني أن لا تنتقل عن نوع

٥ التدبير لكنّ ينبغي ضرورة أن تنتقل من دواء مسخن إلى دواء آخر مسخن وتتقلب في الأدوية المفردة والمركّبة التي هي كلّها مسخنة لأنّ متى ألف الجسم دواءا واحدا دائما فيقلّ تأثيره له. وأيضا أنّ في اختلاف أنواع الأدوية التي كيفيّتها واحدة موافقة عظيمة لمزاج شخص شخص ولمزاج عضو عضو ولأعراض مرض مرض. هذا أصل عظيم من أسرار العلاج. وهذا النحو بعينه يخي في التغذية وفي أنواع ما يستفرغ به الخلط الممرّض أو في تحليل أو تلطيف أو إنضاج أو تغليظ مادّة أو تقبيض

١٠ داوم أبدا نوع التدبير الذي دلّت عليه الدلائل الثابتة وانقلب في أنواع الأدوية والأغذية التي هي كلّها من قبيل واحد فافهم هذا.

(2.53)

[١٠٥] قال أبقراط: من كانت بطنه ليّنة فإنّه ما دام شابّا فهو أحسن حالا ممّن بطنه يابسة ثمّ يؤول حاله عند الشيخوخة إلى أن يصير أردأ وذلك أنّ بطنه تجفّ إذا شاخ على الأمر الأكثر.

---

٢ المريض:المرض AB   ٦ تأثيره:تأثيره AC   ٨ مرض:C¹   ١٠ أبدا:C¹ || الثابتة:الثلثة A   ١٢-١٣ فإنّه الأكثر:om. B ...

Says the commentator: He has already spoken before about looseness and hardness of the stool during youth and during old age.[119] Galen attempts to give the reasons for this [repetition].[120] I have already given my opinion about [this statement by Hippocrates].[121] Moreover, loose bowels are always, in all ages, one of the reasons for lasting health and hard bowels are bad both for healthy and for ill people.[122]

(2.54)

[106] Says Hippocrates: A large body is not unpleasing when one is young, on the contrary it is desirable, however, when one is old, it is a burden and hard to use (inconvenient). It is worse than a body that is less [in size].

Says the commentator: Galen holds the opinion that with the term "largeness of the body," [Hippocrates] means its length so that this proposition is not merely a presumption (supposition).[123]

This is the end of the second part of the commentary on the *Aphorisms*.

---

119   Cf. aphorism 2.20 (72) above.

120   Galen, *In Hippocratis Aphorismos commentarius* 2.20, ed. Kühn, vol. 17b, p. 492.

121   Cf. aphorism 2.20 (72) above.

122   Cf. Maimonides, *On the Regimen of Health* 3.1, trans. Bos, p. 86: "The physicians agree that the first [thing to look after] in the regimen of health is that the stools be soft. When the stools become dry, let alone if they are retained, very bad vapors develop, ascend to the heart and the brain, corrupt the humors, make the pneumas turbid, produce depression, evil thoughts, stupefaction, and indolence, and prevent all the superfluities of the digestions from being expelled. Therefore, one should take utmost care to soften the stools;" see also idem, *On Asthma* 9.40, ed. and trans. Bos, vol. 1, p. 40.

123   Galen, *In Hippocratis Aphorismos commentarius* 2.54, ed. Kühn, vol. 17b, pp. 559–560.

قال المفسّر: قد تقدّم له هذا الرأي في لين البطن ويبسه في سنّ الشباب والشيخ وجالينوس يروم إعطاء علل ذلك وقد قلت ما عندي ولين الطبع أبدا في جميع الأسنان من أسباب دوام الصحّة وكلّ يبس في الطبع رديء للأصحّاء والمرضاء.

(2.54)

[١٠٦] قال أبقراط: عظم البدن في الشبيبية ليس يكره بل يستحبّ إلّا أنّه عند الشيخوخة يثقل ويعسر

٥ استعماله ويكون أردأ من البدن الذي هو أنقص منه.

قال المفسّر: جالينوس يزعم أنّه يريد بقوله هنا عظم البدن طوله حتّى لا تكون هذه القضية وهم محض.

تمّت المقالة الثانية من شرح الفصول.

---

٢ الطبع B¹ البطن B ٤–٥ ليس ... منه: om. B ٤ أنّه: om. A ٧ من شرح الفصول: وشرحها A ولله الحمد add. B والحمد لله واهب العقل كما هو أهله ومستحقّه add. A

In the name of God, the Merciful, the Compassionate
The third part of the commentary on the *Aphorisms*

(3.1)
[107] Says Hippocrates: Especially the changes of the seasons of the year produce diseases and in [every] singular season, the great changes in cold or in
heat, and similarly all other [changes in the weather] follow the same rule.

Says the commentator: [With] a change in the nature of the seasons he
means that for instance the winter season is hot or the summer season cold
and the like. Similarly, a change in [every] singular season means that a big
change in its [normal] temperament produces diseases, even though the other
seasons do not change.

(3.2)
[108] Says Hippocrates: There are [some people whose] natures are in a better
condition in summer and in a worse condition in winter, and there are others
whose natures are in a better condition in winter and in a worse condition in
summer.

Says the commentator: With the term "natures," he means the temperaments
of people and this is clear because in winter, the condition of people with a hot
[temperament] is better and in summer the condition of people with a cold
[temperament]. In this way one should draw an analogy.

(3.3)
[109] Says Hippocrates: The condition of every singular disease is better or
worse in relation to another. Similarly, someone's age is better or worse in relation to the seasons of the year, the places [where one lives], and the kinds of
regimen [one adheres to].

Says the commentator: If you properly arrange the words of this aphorism, it
will be very clear. Similarly, [if] you arrange every singular illness, its condition
in relation to every particular age, or place, or season of the year, or regimen will
be better or worse. For instance, [the condition of] someone suffering from a
cold disease will be better when he is young, when it is summer, when [he lives]

بسم الله الرحمن الرحيم
المقالة الثالثة من شرح الفصول

(3.1)

[١٠٧] قال أبقراط: إنّ انقلاب أوقات السنة ممّا يعمل في توليد الأمراض خاصّة وفي الوقت الواحد منها التغيير الشديد في البرد أو في الحرّ وكذلك في سائر الحالات على هذا القياس.

٥ قال المفسّر: يعني تغيّر طبائع الفصول مثل أن يكون فصل شتاء حارّا أو فصل صيف باردا ونحوهما. وكذلك تغيّر الوقت الواحد عن مزاجه إذا كان شديدا وإن كانت بقيّة الفصول لم تتغيّر فإنّه يولّد أمراضا.

(3.2)

[١٠٨] قال أبقراط: إنّ من الطبائع ما يكون حاله في الصيف أجود وفي الشتاء أردأ ومنها ما تكون حاله في الشتاء أجود وفي الصيف أردأ.

١٠ قال المفسّر: يعني بقوله من الطبائع من أمزجة الأشخاص وذلك بيّن لأنّ في الشتاء تحسن حالات المحرورين وفي الصيف تحسن حالات المبرودين وعلى هذا فقس.

(3.3)

[١٠٩] قال أبقراط: كلّ واحد من الأمراض فحاله عند شيء دون شيء أمثل وأردأ. وأسنان ما عند أوقات من السنة وبلدان وأصناف من التدبير.

قال المفسّر: هذا الفصل إذا رتّبت ألفاظه تبيّن بيانا واضحا وهكذا يرتّب كلّ واحد من الأمراض
١٥ فحاله عند سنّ دون سنّ أو عند بلد دون بلد أو عند وقت من السنة دون وقت أو عند تدبير دون تدبير أمثل وأردأ. مثاله أنّ صاحب المرض البارد عند سنّ الشباب وفي وقت الصيف وفي البلد الحارّ

---

١ بسم الله الرحمن الرحيم: om. ABP ٢ شرح الفصول: كتاب الفصول لأبقراط وشرحها A ٣-٤ ممّا ... الحالات: إلى قوله B ٤ البرد أو في الحرّ: الحرّ أو في البرد A ٨-٩ في ... أردأ: om. B ١٢-١٣ عند ... التدبير: om. B

in a hot place, and [follows] a hot regimen. But in the opposite [conditions], it will be worse. In general, something is better for something else, when they are opposites. And something similar and unbalanced is very bad for something else that is similar to it and unbalanced in the same aspect. But for someone, whose temperament is balanced because of his age, a moderate regimen, temperate season and place are most appropriate. Only the condition of someone with such a temperament is improved by similar things. For those, whose temperament is unbalanced, opposite places, seasons, and kinds of regimen are most appropriate.

(3.4)

[110] Says Hippocrates: If during any season of the year now heat and now cold occurs on the same day, you must expect the occurrence of autumnal diseases.

Says the commentator: This is clear.

(3.5)

[111] Says Hippocrates: The south wind causes hardness of hearing, dimness of vision, heaviness of the head, indolence and relaxation[124] (weakness). When this wind becomes strong and prevails, these symptoms occur to those who suffer from diseases. The north wind causes cough, a sore throat, dryness of the abdomen (constipation), dysuria, shivering, pain in the ribs (sides) and chest. When this wind becomes strong and prevails, one should expect these symptoms to occur in illnesses.

Says the commentator: The south wind is hot and moist and therefore it produces dimness of the senses and moistens the origin of the nerves. As a result, indolence and difficulty of moving occur. The north wind is cold [and] dry and thus causes rawness of the throat (hoarseness) and chest (cough), dryness of the abdomen (constipation), thickness (obstruction) of the passages, and consequently all [the symptoms] mentioned above occur.

(3.6)

[112] Says Hippocrates: When the summer is similar to the spring, expect much sweating during fevers.

---

124   "relaxation (weakness)" (استرخاء): Cf. Galen, *In Hippocratis Aphorismos commentarius* 3.5, ed. Kühn, vol. 17b, p. 569: διαλυτικοί; Hippocrates, *Aphorisms*, trans. Littré, vol. 4, p. 489: "résolvent;" trans. Jones, p. 123: "are relaxing;" cf. Liddell/Scott, *Greek-English Lexicon*, p. 402, s.v. διαλύω: "to relax, to weaken."

وبالتدبير الحارّ أمثل وفي أضداد هذه أردأ. وبالجملة فالحال عند الضدّ أصلح والمثل الخارج عن الاعتدال عند المثل الخارج عن الاعتدال في تلك الجهة أردأ. أمّا صاحب سنّ معتدلة المزاج فإنّ التدبير المعتدل والوقت والبلد المعتدلان أوفق له. فإنّ صاحب هذا المزاج وحده هو الذي تصلح حاله بما يشابهه. فأمّا أصحاب المزاج المجاوز للاعتدال فالبلدان والأوقات وأصناف التدبير المضادّة لهم هي

٥ لهم أوفق.

(3.4)

[١١٠] قال أبقراط: متى كان في أيّ وقت من أوقات السنة في يوم واحد مرّة حرّ ومرّة برد فتوقّع حدوث أمراض خريفية.

قال المفسّر: هذا بيّن.

(3.5)

[١١١] قال أبقراط: الجنوب تحدث ثقلا في السمع وغشاوة في البصر وثقلا في الرأس وكسلا

١٠ واسترخاء. فعند قوّة هذه الريح وغلبتها تعرض للمرضى هذه الأعراض. وأمّا الشمال فتحدث سعالا ووجع الحلق والبطون اليابسة وعسر البول والاقشعرار ووجع في الأضلاع والصدر فعند غلبة هذه الريح وقوّتها ينبغي أن يتوقّع في الأمراض حدوث هذه الأعراض.

قال المفسّر: ريح الجنوب حارّة رطبة فلذلك تكثّر الحواسّ وترطّب مبدأ العصب فيحدث الكسل وعسر الحركة وريح الشمال باردة يابسة فتخشّن الحلق والصدر وتجفّف البطن وتكثّف المجاري

١٥ فيحدث ما ذكر.

(3.6)

[١١٢] قال أبقراط: إذا كان الصيف شبيها بالربيع فتوقّع في الحمّيات عرقا كثيرا.

---

٢ عند ... الاعتدال: om. B   ٤ المزاج om. A   ٦–٧ في ... خريفية: om. B   ٩ السمع: الرأس A
٩–١٢ السمع ... في الأمراض: om. B   ٩ وثقلا في الرأس: om. A   ١٦ فتوقّع ... كثيرا: om. B

Says the commentator: When the summer is severely dry, perspiration necessarily evaporates and moisture dissolves. When [the summer] resembles spring the moisture is necessarily drawn towards the area of the skin, because of its heat, but it (i.e., the summer) cannot dissolve [the moisture] in the way of vapor because of its fluidity. Since the moisture is evacuated suddenly during the crisis of the illness, much sweating occurs from it.

(3.7)

[113] Says Hippocrates: During droughts, acute fevers occur and if the year is extremely dry and[125] a dry condition of the air is produced, these diseases and their like should be expected most of all.

Says the commentator: It is clear that during droughts, the humors become dry and sharp and that consequently fevers are less frequent but qualitatively more acute.

(3.8)

[114] Says Hippocrates: If the seasons of the year are regular and come with the things that are [proper] to them, the illnesses that occur in them are regular[126] and have an easy crisis. But if the seasons of the year are irregular, the illnesses occurring in them are irregular and their crises are bad.

Says the commentator: This is clear.

(3.9)

[115] Says Hippocrates: In autumn, illnesses are most acute and, in general, most fatal. Spring is the most healthy season and least fatal.

Says the commentator: Spring is moderate and [in] autumn [the weather] is extremely dissimilar (variable).

(3.10)

[116] Says Hippocrates: Autumn is bad for those who suffer from phthisis.

Says the commentator: Because [autumn] is cold and dry [and] variable in temperament, it is very harmful for those who suffer from phthisis.

---

125   "and a dry condition of the air is produced": Cf. Galen, ibid. 3.7 p. 573: ὁκοίην καὶ τὴν κατά-
στασιν ἐποίησεν; Hippocrates, ibid., trans. Littré: "telle elle aura fait la constitution;" trans.
Jones, pp. 123, 125: "according to the constitution it has produced."

126   "regular" (والنظام الثبات حسن): Galen, ibid. 3.8, p. 574: εὐσταθέες; Hippocrates, ibid., trans.
Littré: "réglées;" trans. Jones, p. 125: "normal."

قال المفسّر: واجب متى كان الصيف يابسا قوي اليبس أن تبهى وتحلّل الرطوبة ومتى كان شبيها بالربيع أن تجتذب الرطوبة لحرارته إلى ما يلي الجلد ولا يمكن أن يحلّلها بطريق البخار لرطوبته فمن قبل أنّ تلك الرطوبة في وقت بحران الأمراض تستفرغ دفعة يكون منها عرق كثير.

(3.7)

[١١٣] قال أبقراط: إذا احتبس المطر حدثت حمّيات حادّة وإن كثر ذلك الاحتباس في السنة ثمّ

٥ حدّث في الهواء حال يبس فينبغي أن يتوقّع في أكثر الحالات هذه الأمراض وأشباهها.

قال المفسّر: بيّن هو أنّ بعدم المطر تجفّ الأخلاط وتحتدّ فتكون الحمّيات أقلّ عددا وأحدّ كيفية.

(3.8)

[١١٤] قال أبقراط: إذا كانت أوقات السنة لازمة لنظامها وكان في كلّ وقت ما ينبغي أن يكون فيه كان ما يحدث فيها من الأمراض حسن الثبات والنظام حسن البحران. وإذا كانت أوقات السنة غير لازمة لنظامها كان ما يحدث فيها من الأمراض غير منتظم سمج البحران.

١٠ قال المفسّر: هذا بيّن.

(3.9)

[١١٥] قال أبقراط: إنّ في الخريف تكون الأمراض أحدّ ما تكون وأقلّ في أكثر الأمر وأمّا الربيع فأصحّ الأوقات وأقلّها موتا.

قال المفسّر: الربيع معتدل والخريف في غاية الاختلاف.

(3.10)

[١١٦] قال أبقراط: الخريف لأصحاب السلّ رديء.

١٥ قال المفسّر: لكونه باردا يابسا مختلف المزاج فهو يضرّ للمسلولين جدّا.

---

١ تبهى: تفنى B ٣ الأمراض: وأمراض AC ٤-٥ حدثت ... وأشباهها: om. B ٦ المفسّر: أبقراط A
٧-٩ وكان ... منتظم: إلى قوله B ١١-١٢ تكون ... موتا: om. B ١٥ المسلولين: للمنهوكين BC

(3.11)

[117] Says Hippocrates: As for the seasons of the year, if the winter comes with little rain and [the wind] is northerly and the spring is wet [and the wind]' southerly, acute fevers, ophthalmia, and dysentery[127] necessarily occur in the summer. Dysentery mostly affects women and those with moist natures (constitutions).

Says the commentator: This is clear once you know the principles of the [medical] art.

(3.12)

[118] Says Hippocrates: If the winter comes with south [winds]; [if it is] rainy and [mild][128] and the spring comes with little rain and north [winds], women whose [term of] delivery happens to be around spring will have a miscarriage from the slightest cause, while those who do deliver give birth to children that are weak[129] and sickly, so they (i.e., these children) either die immediately, or, if they survive, are emaciated and sickly all their lives. The rest of the population is affected by dysentery and dry ophthalmia, while old people suffer from catarrhs that quickly are fatal.

(3.13)

[119] Says Hippocrates: If the summer comes with little rain and with north [winds] and the autumn is wet with south [winds], severe[130] headache, cough, hoarseness, and rheums occur in the winter. Some people suffer from phthisis.

(3.14)

[120] Says Hippocrates: But if the [autumn] comes with north [winds] and is dry, it is beneficial to those whose nature (constitution) is moist and to women. Others suffer from dry ophthalmia, acute fevers, chronic rheums and some of them suffer from melancholic delusion caused by black bile.

---

127 "dysentery" (اختلاف دم): Galen, ibid. 3.11, p. 578: δυσεντερίας; Hippocrates, ibid., trans. Littré, p. 491: "des dysenteries;" trans. Jones: "dysentery;" cf. Ullmann, Wörterbuch, pp. 210–211; Barry, Syriac Medicine, pp. 80–81.

128 "[mild]" (دفئا): Lit., "warm," cf. Galen, ibid. 3.12, p. 585: εὔδιος; Hippocrates, ibid., trans. Littré: "calme;" trans. Jones: "calm."

129 "weak" (ضعاف الحركة): Cf. Galen, ibid.: ἀκρατέα; Hippocrates, ibid., trans. Littré: "chétifs;" trans. Jones: "weak."

130 "severe headache" (صداع شديد): Cf. Galen, ibid. 3.13, p. 590: κεφαλαλγίαι; Hippocrates, ibid., trans. Littré, p. 493: "des céphalalgies;" trans. Jones, p. 127: "headaches."

(3.11)

[١١٧] قال أبقراط: فأمّا في أوقات السنة فأقول إنّه متى كان الشتاء قليل المطر شماليا وكان الربيع
مطيرا جنوبيا فيجب ضرورة أن يحدث في الصيف حمّيات حادّة ورمد واختلاف دم وأكثر ما
يعرض اختلاف الدم للنساء ولأصحاب الطبائع الرطبة.

قال المفسّر: هذا بيّن بعد معرفة أصول الصناعة.

(3.12)

٥ [١١٨] قال أبقراط: ومتى كان الشتاء جنوبيا مطيرا دفئا وكان الربيع قليل المطر شماليا فإنّ النساء
اللواتي تتّفق ولادتهنّ نحو الربيع يسقطن من أدنى سبب. واللواتي يلدن منهنّ أطفالا ضعاف
الحركة مسقامة حتّى أنّها إمّا أن تموت على المكان وإمّا أن تبقى منهوكة مسقامة طول حياتها. وأمّا سائر
الناس فعرض لهم اختلاف الدم والرمد اليابس وأمّا الكهول فيعرض لهم من النزل ما يفني سريعا.

(3.13)

[١١٩] قال أبقراط: فإن كان الصيف قليل المطر شماليا وكان الخريف مطيرا جنوبيا عرض في الشتاء
١٠ صداع شديد وسعال وبحوحة وزكام وعرض لبعض الناس السلّ.

(3.14)

[١٢٠] قال أبقراط: فإن كان شماليا يابسا موافقا لمن كانت طبيعته رطبة وللنساء. وأمّا سائر الناس
فيعرض لهم رمد يابس وحمّيات حادّة وزكام مزمن ومنهم من يعرض له الوسواس السوداوي
العارض من السوداء.

(3.15)

[121] Says Hippocrates: Of the conditions of the weather during the year, less rain is, in general, more healthy and less deadly than more rain.

(3.16)

[122] Says Hippocrates: The illnesses, which mostly occur during a lot of rain, are chronic fevers, diarrhea, putrefaction, epilepsy, apoplexy, and angina. The illnesses that occur during a lack of rain are phthisis, ophthalmia, arthritis, strangury, and dysentery.

Says the commentator: All that Hippocrates mentions in these five apho- risms concerning certain diseases, which occur to certain people under certain weather [conditions], is not [the rule] by any means. For this reason, it is not necessary to give the causes [for these diseases] as is well known to someone who studies philosophy (logic). However, Galen attempts to give the cause for all these [diseases] and [to inform us] that, in general, with the knowledge regarding the natures of the seasons and the individual persons and regard- ing the causes of the diseases, which is fundamental in the art of medicine, and [with the knowledge] that moisture is the substance of putrefaction and that heat activates it, it is easy to give the causes of all [the diseases], which he (Hippocrates) mentions, when they occur.[131]

(3.17)

[123] Says Hippocrates: As for the daily conditions of the weather: a north [wind] braces the body, makes it vigorous and strong, improves its movement and complexion, clarifies one's hearing, dries up the bowels, and causes sting- ing of the eyes. If there is a pre-existing pain in the region of the chest, it is stimulated and aggravated by it. However, a south [wind] makes[132] the body loose and relaxed, moistens it, causes heaviness of the head, hardness of hear- ing and vertigo, [and] difficulty of movement of the eyes and of the whole body, and looseness of the bowels.

Says the commentator: It has already been noted that the north wind is cold and dry and that the south wind is hot and moist.[133] All this is clear.

---

131   Cf. Galen, ibid. 3.12–16, pp. 585–609.

132   "makes ... loose and relaxed" (يحلّ ... ويرخي): Cf. Galen, ibid. 3.17, p. 609: διαλύουσι; Hip- pocrates, *Aphorisms*, trans. Littré, vol. 4, p. 495: "résolvent;" trans. Jones, p. 129: "relax."

133   Cf. aphorism 3.5 (111) above.

(3.15)

[۱۲۱] قال أبقراط: إنّ من حالات الهواء في السنة بالجملة قلّة المطر أصحّ من كثرة المطر وأقلّ موتا.

(3.16)

[۱۲۲] قال أبقراط: فأمّا الأمراض التي تحدث عند كثرة المطر في أكثر الحالات فهي حمّيات طويلة واستطلاق البطن وعفن وصرع وسكات وذبحة. وأمّا الأمراض التي تحدث عند قلّة المطر فهي سلّ ورمد ووجع المفاصل وتقطير البول واختلاف الدم.

٥ قال المفسّر: كلّ ما ذكره أبقراط في هذه الخمسة فصول من كون الأمراض الفلانية تحدث بالصنف الفلاني من الناس إذا كان الهواء كذلك فليس ذلك أكثري بوجه ولذلك لا يجب أن يعطي أسبابه على ما قد علم من نظر في الفلسفة لكنّ جالينوس يريد أن يعطي سببا لكلّ ذلك. وبالجملة أنّ مع ما تأصّل في الصناعة الطبّية من معرفة طبائع الفصول والأشخاص وأسباب الأمراض وأنّ الرطوبة مادّة العفونة والحرارة فاعلتها يسهل إعطاء أسباب كلّ ما ذكر إنْ وقع.

(3.17)

۱۰ [۱۲۳] قال أبقراط: فأمّا حالات الهواء في يوم يوم فما كان منها شماليا فإنّه يجمع الأبدان ويشدّها ويقوّيها ويجوّد حركتها ويحسّن ألوانها ويصفّي السمع منها ويجفّف البطن ويحدث في الأعين لذغا. وإن كان في نواحي الصدر وجع متقدّم هيّجه وزاد فيه. وما كان منها جنوبيا فإنّه يحلّ الأبدان ويرخيها ويرطّبها ويحدث ثقلا في الرأس وثقلا في السمع وسدرا في العينين وفي البدن كلّه عسر الحركة ويليّن البطن.

۱۵ قال المفسّر: قد علم أنّ الشمال بارد يابس وأنّ الجنوب حارّ رطب وكلّ ذلك بيّن.

---

۱ في ... كثرة المطر: إلى قوله B ۲ حمّيات: om. A ۳ واستطلاق: واستـلاق C ٥ الفلانية: النائبة A

۷ لكنّ: لكون B ۱۰-۱۳ فما ... عسر الحركة: إلى قوله B ۱۱ ويصفّي السمع: om. A

(3.18)

[124] Says Hippocrates: As to the seasons of the year, in spring and the beginning of summer, children and those next to them in age enjoy the greatest well-being and the most perfect health. During the rest of summer and the first part of autumn, old people enjoy the greatest well-being. During the rest of autumn and winter, those of intermediate age enjoy the greatest well-being.

Says the commentator: I have already given the reason for this in the aphorism in which I altered the order of his words.[134]

(3.19)

[125] Says Hippocrates: All diseases occur during all seasons of the year, but some of them are more likely to occur and to flare up in certain [seasons].

Says the commentator: This is clear.

(3.20)

[126] Says Hippocrates: In spring, [the following diseases] may occur: melancholic delusion, madness, epilepsy, hemorrhages, angina, rheum, hoarseness, cough, peeling[135] of the skin, eczema,[136] alphos,[137] many ulcerative eruptions,[138] tumors,[139] and arthritis.

---

134   Cf. aphorism 3.3 (109) above.

135   "peeling of the skin" (العلّة التي يتقشّر فيها الجلد): Lit., "the illness in which the skin peels off," cf.
      Galen, *In Hippocratis Aphorismos commentarius* 3.20, ed. Kühn, vol. 17b, p. 615: λέπραι; Hippocrates, *Aphorisms*, trans. Littré, vol. 4, p. 495: "des lèpres." Ed. Jones, p. 129 n. 1, remarks
      that "It is not possible to translate the Greek terms for the various skin diseases, as the
      modern classification is so different from the ancient." See also Barry, *Syriac Medicine*,
      pp. 122–124, 131.

136   "eczema" (قوابي): Cf. Galen, ibid.: λειχῆνες; Hippocrates, ibid., trans. Littré: "des lichens;"
      Ullmann, *Wörterbuch*, p. 385: "Hautflechte." My translation follows Galen, *On Examination*, ed. Iskandar, p. 123 l. 10, and al-Safandi, *Pathogenese der pluridyskraten Krankheiten*,
      pp. 22–23: "Ekzem (Eczema lichenificatum);" see also Dozy, *Supplément*, vol. 2, p. 416:
      "dartre;" Sontheimer, "Nachricht," p. 251 (97): "Fischschuppenaussatz. Ichtyosis." For the
      Greek term λειχήν, cf. Durling, *Dictionary of Medical Terms*, p. 219: "a lichen-like eruption on the skin of animals;" Barry, *Syriac Medicine*, pp. 129–130: "tetters." For an extensive
      discussion of the different types of eczema in medieval medicine, see Ibn al-Jazzār, *Zād
      al-musāfir wa-qūt al-ḥāḍir* 7.19, ed. and trans. Bos, p. 105, for the term "eczema" (qūbā'), see
      esp. n. 182.

137   "alphos" (بهق): Cf. Galen, *In Hippocratis Aphorismos commentarius* 3.20, ed. Kühn, vol. 17b,
      p. 615: ἀλφοί; Hippocrates, ibid., trans. Littré: "des alphos;" Ullmann, ibid., p. 97: "weiße
      Hautflecken;" Barry, ibid., p. 31. For an extensive discussion of the different types of *bahaq*
      in medieval medicine, see Ibn al-Jazzār, ibid. 7.18, p. 108, for the term "alphos" (bahaq), see
      esp. n. 196.

138   "eruptions" (بثور): Cf. Galen, ibid.: ἐξανθήσιες; Hippocrates, ibid., trans. Littré: "éruptions;"
      trans. Jones, p. 129: "eruptions;" Ullmann, ibid., p. 248: "Hautausschlag."

(3.18)

[١٢٤] قال أبقراط: وأمّا في أوقات السنة ففي الربيع وأوّل الصيف يكون الصبيان والذين يتلوّنهم في السنّ على أفضل حالاتهم وأكمل الصحّة. وفي باقي الصيف وطرف من الخريف يكون المشائخ أحسن حالا وفي باقي الخريف وفي الشتاء يكون المتوسّطين بينهما في السنّ أحسن حالا.

قال المفسّر: قد تقدّم لنا علّة ذلك في الفصل الذي غيّرنا تركيب ألفاظه.

(3.19)

٥ [١٢٥] قال أبقراط: والأمراض كلّها تحدث في أوقات السنة كلّها إلّا أنّ بعضها في بعض الأوقات أحرى بأن يحدث ويهيج.

قال المفسّر: هذا بيّن.

(3.20)

[١٢٦] قال أبقراط: قد يعرض في الربيع الوسواس السوداوي والجنون والصرع وانبعاث الدم والذبحة والزكام والبحوحة والسعال والعلّة التي يتقشّر فيها الجلد والقوابي والبهق والبثور الكثيرة التي تتقرّح ١٠ والخراجات وأوجاع المفاصل.

٢-١ ففي ... الخريف: om. B   ٣-٢ يكون ... الخريف: om. A   ٣ المتوسّطين: المتوسّطون A

٥-٦ تحدث ... أحرى: إلى قوله B   ٦ بأن: أن A   ٨ قد: فقد BC   ٨-١٠ والجنون ... والخراجات: إلى قوله B   ٨ والصرع: والسكتة add. A   ١٠ وأوجاع: وأنواع B

---

139 "tumors" (خراجات): Cf. Galen, ibid.: φύματα; Hippocrates, ibid., trans. Littré: "des furoncles;" trans. Jones: "tumors;" cf. Liddell/Scott, *Greek-English Lexicon*, p. 1962, s.v. φῦμα: "growth; tumor; tubercle;" Ullmann, ibid., pp. 747–748: "Gewächs, Geschwulst, Tumor."

Says the commentator: This aphorism explains [in detail] what [has been said] in the previous aphorism, namely that every kind of disease can occur in every season of the year, but that some diseases are more likely to occur during certain [seasons] and those are the ones that mostly occur during that season. He concluded this matter by stating that in spring, which is the most moderate season, [the following diseases] may occur: diseases caused by black bile, such as melancholic delusion and madness; diseases caused by phlegm, such as epilepsy, rheum, hoarseness, and cough; diseases caused by yellow bile, such as ulcerative eruptions and tumors; and diseases related to blood, such as hemorrhages and angina. However, the diseases, which are specific to spring, are those that occur as a result of the dissolution of humors and their excretion and the movement of nature to expel them forcefully. Likewise, the next aphorism is based on our explanation that illnesses sometimes occur contrary to the nature of the season [of the year].

(3.21)
[127] Says Hippocrates: During summer, there occur some of the diseases just mentioned as well as continuous fevers, ardent [fevers], and many tertian [fevers], vomiting, diarrhea, ophthalmia, earache, ulcers in the mouth, putrefaction in the genitals,[140] and heat-spots.[141]

(3.22)
[128] Says Hippocrates: In autumn occur most summer diseases as well as quartan and mixed[142] (irregular) fevers, affections[143] of the spleen, dropsy, phthisis, strangury, dysentery, lientery, pain in the hip (sciatica), angina, asthma, the severe colic, which the Greeks call "ileus," epilepsy, madness, and melancholic delusion.

---

140   "genitals" (فروج): The Arabic MSS read: "tumors" (قروح) (= V, fol. 53ᵇ). The text has been emended on the basis of Galen, ibid. 3.21, ed. Kühn, p. 619: σηπεδόνες αἰδοίων.

141   "heat-spots" (حصف): Cf. Galen, ibid.: ἵδρωα; Hippocrates, *Aphorisms*, trans. Littré, vol. 4, p. 497: "des sudamina;" trans. Jones, p. 129: "sweats;" Liddell/Scott, *Greek English Lexicon*, p. 820: "heat-spots, pustules;" Ullmann, *Wörterbuch*, p. 306: "Hitzblattern." For an extensive discussion of this illness in medieval medicine, see Ibn al-Jazzār, *Zād al-musāfir wa-qūt al-ḥāḍir* 7.24, ed. and trans. Bos, p. 122; for the term "heat-spots," see esp. n. 269.

142   "mixed (irregular) fevers" (حمّيات مختلطة): Cf. Galen, ibid. 3.22, p. 621: πλάνητες; Hippocrates, ibid., trans. Littré: "des fièvres erratiques;" trans. Jones, p. 131: "irregular fevers;" cf. Maimonides, *Medical Aphorisms* 10.34, ed. and trans. Bos, vol. 3, p. 10.

143   "affections of the spleen" (أطحلة): Cf. Galen, ibid.: σπλῆνες; Hippocrates, ibid., trans. Littré: "des engorgements de la rate;" trans. Jones: "enlarged spleen." The Arabic term is a loan translation of Greek σπλῆνες; cf. Liddell/Scott, *Greek English Lexicon*, p. 1628: "affections of the spleen."

قال المفسّر: هذا الفصل مبيّن لما قدمه في الفصل الذي قبله وذلك أنّه ذكر في الفصل المتقدّم أنّ
قد يحدث كلّ نوع من أنواع الأمراض في كلّ فصل من فصول السنة لكنّ بعض الأمراض
ببعض الفصول أحرى وهو الذي يحدث على الأكثر في ذلك الفصل. فتمّم هذا المعنى بأنْ قال:
فإنّه قد يحدث في الربيع الذي هو أعدل الفصول أمراض سوداوية كالوسواس السوداوي والجنون

٥ وأمراض بلغمية كالصرع والزكام والبحوحة والسعال وأمراض صفراوية كالبثور التي يتقرّح فيها الجلد
والخراجات وأمراض دموية كانبعاث الدم والذبحة. ولكنّ الأمراض الخصيصة بالربيع هي التابعة
لذوبان الأخلاط وانبعاثها إلى خارج وحركة الطبيعة لدفعها بقوّة. وكذلك الفصل الذي بعد هذا مبني
على ما يبيّنّاه من كون الأمراض قد تحدث على خلاف طبيعة الفصل.

(3.21)

[١٢٧] قال أبقراط: وأمّا في الصيف فيعرض لهم بعض هذه الأمراض وحمّيات دائمة ومحرقة وغبّ

١٠ كثيرة وقيء وذرب ورمد ووجع الأذن وقروح في الفم وعفن في الفروج وحصف.

(3.22)

[١٢٨] قال أبقراط: وأمّا في الخريف فيعرض أكثر أمراض الصيف وحمّيات ربع ومختلطة وأطحلة
واستسقاء وسلّ وتقطير البول واختلاف الدم وزلق الأمعاء ووجع الورك والذبحة والربو والقولنج
الشديد الذي يسمّونه اليونانيون إيلٰوس والصرع والجنون والوسواس السوداوي.

٩–١٠ فيعرض ... الفم: إلى قوله B   ١٠ الفروج: emendation editor: القروح MSS בית העדוה א
١١ ومختلطة: مخلطة C ‖ وأطحلة: غليطة add. A   ١٢ والذبحة: C¹

Says the commentator: All this is clear from what we said before.

(3.23)

[129] Says Hippocrates: In winter occur pleurisy, pneumonia, rheum, hoarseness, cough, pains[144] in the sides and loins, headache, dizziness, and apoplexy.

Says the commentator: This too is based on what has been stated before, because during winter, diseases occur that are mostly specific to it such as rheum, hoarseness, and apoplexy, but also diseases that are not specific to its nature such as pleurisy.

(3.24)

[130] Says Hippocrates: In the [different] ages, the following diseases occur: small children [and] new-born infants suffer from aphthae, vomiting, cough, sleeplessness, fright (nightmares), inflammation of the navel, and discharge from the ears.

Says the commentator: They suffer from aphthae because of the softness of their bodily parts and the sharpness of the milk, vomiting [occurs to them] because of excessive nursing, the weakness of the retentive faculty since they have too much moisture. [They suffer from] cough because of the moisture of the lungs and the large quantity of moisture streaming to them (i.e., the lungs) from the brain. This is also the cause of the discharge from the ears, because superfluities of the brain stream towards them. [They suffer from] inflammation of the navel because of the shortness of time since it was cut. Fright occurs mostly during sleep because the digestion [of the food] in the stomach is corrupted so that vapors arise to the brain and cause frightening imaginations (illusions). As for sleeplessness, Galen did not know its cause, but said that what is specific to children is that they sleep much.[145] This is correct. However, they often suffer from sleeplessness and cry all night long. The reason for this is their excessive sensitivity due to the softness of their bodies. [Moreover], their powers are weak and not firm and the slightest pain will wake them up. It only happens rarely that they do not suffer from a poor digestion and restlessness caused by [a bad digestion of the food] in their stomach because they suckle too much. The pain [resulting from this] wakes them up and keeps them awake.

---

144   "pains in the sides": Hippocrates (Galen, ibid. 3.23, p. 625) adds: στηθέων (in the chest). Maimonides' omission follows Ḥunayn (cf. V, fol. 54ᵇ).

145   Cf. Galen, ibid. 3.24, ed. Kühn, pp. 627–628.

قال المفسّر: كلّ هذا بيّن ممّا قدّمناه.

(3.23)

[١٢٩] قال أبقراط: وأمّا في الشتاء فيعرض ذات الجنب وذات الرئة والزكام والبحوحة والسعال وأوجاع الجنبين والقطن والصداع والسدر والسكات.

قال المفسّر: هذا مبني أيضا على ما تقدّم لأنّه قد تحدث في الشتاء أمراض خصيصة به على الأكثر ٥ كالزكام والبحوحة والسكات وأمراض ليست من طبيعته كذات الجنب.

(3.24)

[١٣٠] قال أبقراط: فأمّا في الأسنان فتعرض هذه الأمراض أمّا الأطفال الصغار حين يولدون فيعرض لهم القلاع والقيء والسعال والسهر والتفزّع وورم السرّة ورطوبة الأذنين.

قال المفسّر: يعرض لهم القلاع من أجل لين أعضائهم وما في اللبن من الجلاء والقيء لكثرة ما يرضعون وضعف القوة الماسكة فيهم لشدّة الرطوبة. والسعال من أجل رطوبة الرئة وكثرة ما يسيل ١٠ من أدمغتهم لشدّة رطوبتها للرئة وهي العلّة في رطوبة الأذنين لأنّ فضول الدماغ تندفع للأذنين. وورم السرّة لقرب عهدها بالقطع والتفزّع أكثره في النوم لفساد هضم المعدة يتبخّر للدماغ فيحدث خيالات مفزعة. فأمّا السهر فلم يعرف له جالينوس علّة بل قال إنّ الأمر الخاصّ بالصبيان كثرة النوم وذلك صحيح. لكنّ كثيرا ما يعرض لهم السهر والبكاء طول الليل وعلّة ذلك شدّة إحساسهم للين أجسامهم وقواهم كلّها ضعيفة غير متمكّنة فأيسر شيء من الألم ينبّههم. وقلّ أنْ يفقدوا سوء هضم

---

١ كلّ: om. A ٢-٣ فيعرض ... والسدر: إلى قوله B ٦-٧ أمّا ... الأذنين: om. B ٩ من: ومن C
١٠ لأنّ ... للأذنين: om. AB ١١ عهدها: عهد B ١٣ والبكاء: مع add. C

If [the pain] becomes a little bit stronger, they cry. This is what we always see [happening in little children and new-born infants].[146]

(3.25)
[131] Says Hippocrates: When a child gets near to [the time] that he gets teeth, he suffers from irritation in the gums, fevers, cramps, and diarrhea, especially when the canine teeth begin to erupt, [this also happens] in the case of fat children and those who have constipated bowels.

Says the commentator: All this [occurs] because the teeth break through and perforate the flesh of the gums and widen the opening. The [resulting] pain is followed by fever and cramps. Diarrhea occurs because the food is not well digested due to the pain and sleeplessness. Cramps occur mostly to fat children and those who have constipated bowels because of the excess of superfluities in their bodies.

(3.26)
[132] Says Hippocrates: When a child gets older, he is affected by inflammations[147] of the throat, inward[148] thrust (curvature) of the vertebrae of the neck, asthma, stones, round worms, [other] intestinal worms (flat worms), warts,[149] scrofula, and other tumors.

Says the commentator: After dentition until nearly thirteen years of age, children take much food and drink a lot; they take food after food and do

---

146   On the diseases affecting small children as discussed in this and the following aphorism, see al-Rāzī, *On Treatment of Small Children*, eds. and trans. Bos/McVaugh.

147   "inflammations of the throat" (ورم الحلق): Cf. Galen, *In Hippocratis Aphorismos commentarius* 3.26, ed. Kühn, vol. 17b, p. 631: παρίσθμια; Hippocrates, *Aphorisms*, trans. Littré, vol. 4, p. 499: "des amygdalites;" trans. Jones, p. 131: "affections of the tonsils."

148   "inward thrust (curvature)" (دخول): Cf. Galen, ibid.: εἴσω ὤσιες; Hippocrates, ibid., trans. Littré: "des luxations;" trans. Jones, p. 129: "curvature."

149   "warts" (الثواليل المتعلّقة): Lit., "hanging warts;" cf. Galen, ibid.: ἀκροχορδόνες; Hippocrates, ibid., trans. Littré: "des verrues;" trans. Jones: "warts;" cf. Liddell/Scott, *Greek-English Lexicon*, p. 58: "warts with a thin neck." See also Barry, *Syriac Medicine*, pp. 78–79. The Hippocratic text adds: σατυριασμοί; trans. Littré: "des tumeurs auprès des oreilles;" ed. and trans. Jones, p. 133: "swellings by the ears;" but cf. n. 1: "I have adopted this explanation (by Galen), but at the same time I am not at all sure that satyriasis is not referred to." Cf. the addition in Judah ben Samuel Shalom's Hebrew translation (MS Vienna, Österreichische Nationalbibliothek, Cod. hebr. 37, fol. 77ᵇ): זקיפת האמה (erection of the penis) (on this translation, NM 3, p. 77); see also Müller-Rohlfsen, *Lateinische ravennatische Übersetzung*, p. 37: "satiriasis."

وقلق من أجل المعدة لكثرة رضاعتهم فينبّههم ذلك الألم فيسهرون وإن زاد قليلا بكوا وهذا مشاهد دائماً.

(3.25)

[١٣١] قال أبقراط: فإذا قرب الصبي من أن تنبت له الأسنان عرض له مضيض في اللثة وحمّيات وتشنّج واختلاف لا سيّما إذا نبتت له الأنياب وللعبل من الصبيان ولمن كانت بطنه معتقلة.

قال المفسّر: هذا كلّه لكون الأسنان تشقّ وتثقب لحم اللثة وتوسع الثقب فيتبع ذلك الألم الحمّى والتشنّج ولكون الغذاء لا ينهضم جيّدا للألم والسهر يحدث الاختلاف وأكثر ما يحدث التشنّج للعبل والمعتقل البطن لكثرة فضول أبدانهم.

(3.26)

[١٣٢] قال أبقراط: فإذا تجاوز الصبي هذه السنّ عرض له ورم الحلق ودخول خرزة القفاء والربو والحصى والحيّات والدود والثواليل المتعلّقة والخنازير وسائر الخراجات.

قال المفسّر: من بعد نبات الأسنان إلى نحو الثلاث عشر سنة يتناول الصبيان الأغذية الكثيرة ويكثر شربهم ويدخّلوا طعاما على طعام وتكثر حركتهم بعد الطعام وجميع هذا التدبير مفسد للهضوم مكثر

٣-٤ عرض ... معتقلة: om. B ٣ مضيض: مضيض C ٤ له: لهم om. AP ‖ كانت: منهم add. P

٥ الحمّى: والحمّى A ٦ ينهضم: تهضم P ٨ هذه: هذا BC ٩-٨ عرض ... الخراجات: om. B

much exercise after a meal. This whole regimen corrupts the digestions[150] and increases the humors, while their bodies are still moist and their organs soft and all [the afflictions] we mentioned necessarily occur [to these children]. When the muscles of the throat swell, they pull the vertebrae of the neck because of the softness of their ligaments.

(3.27)

[133] Says Hippocrates: As for those who are older than [thirteen] and approach puberty,[151] many of these illnesses occur to them and also fevers that last longer and nosebleeds.

Says the commentator: At this age, the blood increases and flows in these [children] and therefore nosebleeds occur to them when they are ill.

(3.28)

[134] Says Hippocrates: In most cases diseases occurring to children reach the crisis in some in forty days, in some in seven months, in some in seven years, and in some at the approach of puberty. However, those diseases that persist and do not dissolve at the time of puberty[152] [in boys] or at the time of the menstruation in girls, have[153] the property (tend) to become chronic.

Says the commentator: With [the term] diseases he means chronic [diseases].

(3.29)

[135] Says Hippocrates: Young people suffer from hemoptysis, phthisis, acute fevers, epilepsy, and other diseases, but mostly they suffer from [the diseases] we have mentioned.

Says the commentator: Galen has explained that epilepsy is in no way specific to young people, but is [also] one of the diseases [occurring to] children.[154]

---

150 Following Galen, Maimonides distinguishes three digestions, the first taking place in the stomach, the second in the liver, and the third in the rest of the organs, cf. Maimonides, *On Asthma* 2.1, ed. and trans. Bos, vol. 1, p. 8 and p. 124 n. 1.

151 "puberty": Lit., "the growing of pubic hair."

152 "puberty": Lit., "the growing [of pubic hair]."

153 "have the property (tend) to" (من شأنها): Cf. Galen, *In Hippocratis Aphorismos commentarius* 3.28, ed. Kühn, vol. 17b, p. 639: εἴωθεν; Hippocrates, *Aphorisms*, trans. Littré, vol. 4, p. 501: "d'ordinaire;" trans. Jones, p. 133: "are wont to."

154 Cf. Galen, ibid. 3.29, p. 643.

للأخلاط وأجسامهم مع ذلك رطبة وأعضاؤهم ليّنة فيلزم كلّ ما ذكر لأنّ إذا ورم عضل الحلق جذب الخرزة من القفاء للين رباطاتهم.

(3.27)

[١٣٣] قال أبقراط: وأمّا من جاوز هذه السنّ وقرب من أن ينبت له الشعر في العانة فيعرض له كثير من هذه الأمراض وحمّيات أزيد طولا ورعاف.

قال المفسّر: في هذه السنّ يكثر الدم فيجري فيهم ولذلك يحدث لهم الرعاف في أمراضهم.

(3.28)

[١٣٤] قال أبقراط: وأكثر ما يعرض للصبيان من الأمراض أتي في بعضه البحران في أربعين يوما وفي بعضه في سبعة أشهر وفي بعضه في سبع سنين وفي بعضه إذا شارفوا إنبات الشعر في العانة. فأمّا ما يبقى من الأمراض فلا يحلّ في وقت الإنبات أو في الإناث في وقت ما يجري منهم الطمث فن شأنها أن تطول.

قال المفسّر: يعني من الأمراض المزمنة.

(3.29)

[١٣٥] قال أبقراط: وأمّا الشباب فيعرض لهم نفث الدم والسلّ والحمّيات الحادّة والصرع وسائر الأمراض إلّا أنّ أكثر ما يعرض لهم ما ذكرنا.

قال المفسّر: قد بيّن جالينوس أنّه لا وجه لكون الصرع خاصّ بالشباب بل هو من أمراض الصبيان.

---

١ إذا:P om. ٣ هذه: هذا B ٤ الأمراض:الأعراض P ٥ هذه: هذا B ٦-٩ وأكثر...تطول: om. B ١١-١٢ والسلّ ... ذكرنا:om. B ١٣ أنّه:P om. أن B || خاصّ:BP om.

(3.30)

[136] Says Hippocrates: Those who are beyond that age, suffer from asthma, pleurisy, pneumonia, fever[155] associated with sleeplessness, fever associated with mental confusion (phrenitis), ardent fever, cholera, chronic diarrhea, abrasion[156] of the intestines, lientery, and hemorrhoids.[157]

Says the commentator: It is known that in this age, namely that of people past their prime, black bile is mostly very evident and therefore mental confusion (delirium), sleeplessness, and hemorrhoids are peculiar to them during fevers. As to the other illnesses enumerated by him, these are not peculiar to [people of] this age.

Galen maintains that he has given specific reasons[158] [for the illnesses] of this age, but that is not so.

(3.31)

[137] Says Hippocrates: Old people suffer from difficulty of breathing and catarrhs associated with cough, strangury, dysuria, arthritis, nephritis, dizziness, apoplexy, bad[159] tumors, pruritus of the body, sleeplessness, loose bowels, watery discharge from the eyes and nostrils, dim-sightedness, cataract, and hardness of hearing.

Says the commentator: The reasons for these [diseases] are all of them clear from what is known from the condition of the temperament of old people.

This is the end of the third part of the commentary on the *Aphorisms*. Praise be to God alone.

---

155   "fever associated with sleeplessness" (الحمّى التي يكون معها السهر): Cf. Galen, ibid. 3.30, p. 644: λήθαργοι; Hippocrates, *Aphorisms*, trans. Littré, vol. 4, p. 501: "des léthargus (fièvres avec somnolence);" trans. Jones, p. 133: "lethargus." Cf. Barry, *Syriac Medicine*, pp. 58–59.

156   "abrasion of the intestines" (سحج الأمعاء): Cf. Galen, ibid.: δυσεντερίαι; Hippocrates, ibid., trans. Littré: "des dysenteries;" trans. Jones: "dysentery."

157   "hemorrhoids" (انتفاخ أفواه العروق من أسفل) (cf. V, fol. 58ᵃ: انفتاح = CP): Lit., "the swelling of the openings of the vessels from below;" cf. Galen, ibid., ed. Kühn: αἱμορροΐδες; Hippocrates, ibid., trans. Littré: "des hémorrhoïdes;" trans. Jones: "hemorrhoids." The regular term for "hemorrhoids" is بواسير, which is the one featuring in Ullmann, *Wörterbuch*, pp. 82–83, and suppl. 1, p. 75. See also Barry, *Syriac Medicine*, pp. 53–54.

158   "reasons [for the illnesses] of this age": Cf. Galen, ibid., p. 647: τῶν κατειλεγμένων ἁπάντων παθῶν ἡ αἰτία (the reasons for all the enumerated illnesses).

159   "bad tumors" (القروح الرديئة): Cf. ibid. 3.31, p. 648: καχεξίαι; Hippocrates, *Aphorisms*, trans. Littré, vol. 4, p. 503: "des cachexies;" trans. Jones: p. 135: "cachexia;" Liddell/Scott, *Greek-English Lexicon*, p. 9323: "bad habit of the body." See also Ullmann, *Wörterbuch*, p. 338: "schlechte körperliche Verfassung."

(3.30)

[١٣٦] قال أبقراط: فأمّا من جاوز هذه السنّ فيعرض له الربو وذات الجنب وذات الرئة والحمّى التي
يكون معها السهر والحمّى التي يكون معها اختلاط العقل والحمّى المحرقة والهيضة والاختلاف الطويل
وسحج الأمعاء وزلق الأمعاء وانتفاخ أفواه العروق من أسفل.

قال المفسّر: معلوم أنّ هذه السنّ وهي سنّ الكهول الخلط السوداوي فيها أظهر على الأكثر ولذلك
٥   يخصّها اختلاط عقل وسهر في الحمّيات وانتفاخ أفواه العروق. أمّا سائر ما عدّد فليس بخصيص بهذه
السنّ.

وجالينوس يزعم أنّه أعطى أسباب خصيصة بهذه السنّ وليس كذلك.

(3.31)

[١٣٧] قال أبقراط: أمّا المشايخ فيعرض لهم رداءة التنفّس والنزل التي يعرض معها السعال وتقطير
البول وعسره وأوجاع المفاصل وأوجاع الكلى والدوار والسكات والقروح الرديئة وحكّة البدن والسهر
١٠   ولين البطن ورطوبة العينين والمنخرين وظلمة البصر والزرقة وثقل السمع.

قال المفسّر: أسباب هذه كلّها بيّنة لما علم من حال مزاج الشيوخ.

كملت المقالة الثالثة من شرح الفصول والحمد لله وحده.

---

١ هذه: هذا BP ‖ له: لهم P   ١-٣ وذات... أسفل: om.B   ٢ العقل: الذهن والعقل P   ٣ وزلق الأمعاء:
om. P ‖ وانتفاخ: emendation editor وانفتاح MSS   ٤ هذه: هذا B   ٥ وانتفاخ: وانفتاح CP ‖ بهذه:
بهذا BP   ٧ بهذه: بهذا BP   ٨-٩ السعال... وعسره: om. A   ٩ وأوجاع: أوجاع A   ١٢ كملت المقالة
الثالثة من شرح الفصول: كملت المقالة الثالثة من من كتاب الفصول وشرحها A كل شرح المقالة الثالثة من
الفصول أبقراط B كملت المقالة الثالثة P ‖ والحمد لله وحده: والحمد لله وحده: والحمد لواهب العقل كما هو أهله A ولله B والله
الحمد وحده P

In the name of God, the Merciful, the Compassionate
The fourth part of the commentary on the *Aphorisms*

(4.1)

[138] Says Hippocrates: It is proper to[160] administer purgative drugs to pregnant women when[161] the humors in their body flare up, from when the fetus
is four months old until it becomes seven months old. But [in the latter case],
one should proceed to administer [a smaller dose]. When [a fetus] is younger
[than four months] or older [than seven months], one should be very careful
[in the administration of these drugs].

Says the commentator: This is clear because at the beginning [the fetus] is
weak and can be easily aborted, and at the end [of the pregnancy] it is heavy
and large and thus contributes to a miscarriage because of its heaviness.

(4.2)

[139] Says Hippocrates: Drugs should be administered to evacuate from the
body such [substances], which, if spontaneously excreted, would be beneficial.
But [substances] of an opposite character should be stopped.

Says the commentator: This is clear.

(4.3)

[140] Says Hippocrates: If the body is purged from such [substances] as should
be evacuated, it is beneficial and easily borne. But if the opposite is the case, it
is borne with difficulty.

Says the commentator: He tells us this here so that it can serve as a diagnostic
sign through which we know whether our conjecture was correct or whether
we erred, that is to say [whether the patient] bore the evacuation with ease or
with difficulty.

---

160   "to administer purgative drugs" (سقى الدواء): Cf. aphorism 1.22 (49) above.

161   "when the humors ... flare up" (إذا كانت الأخلاط ... هائجة): Cf. Galen, *In Hippocratis Apho-
      rismos commentarius* 4.1, ed. Kühn, vol. 17b, p. 652: ἢν ὀργᾷ; Hippocrates, *Aphorisms*, trans.
      Littré, vol. 4, p. 503: "s' il y a orgasme;" ed. and trans. Jones, p. 135: "should there be orgasm;"
      cf. also p. 108 n. 1 (to aphorism 1.22): "An orgasm is literally a state of excitement, and in
      this aphorism signifies that the humors are 'struggling to get out.'"

بسم الله الرحمن الرحيم

المقالة الرابعة من شرح فصول أبقراط

(4.1)

[١٣٨] قال أبقراط: ينبغي أن تسقي الحامل الدواء إذا كانت الأخلاط في بدنها هائجة منذ يأتي على الجنين أربعة أشهر وإلى أن يأتي عليه سبعة أشهر ويكون التقدّم على هذا أقلّ. فأمّا ما كان أصغر من

٥ ذلك أو أكبر منه فينبغي أن يتوقّى عليه.

قال المفسّر: هذا بيّن لأنّه في أوّله ضعيف فيسهل سقوطه وفي آخره قد ثقل وكبر فيعين على سقوطه بثقله.

(4.2)

[١٣٩] قال أبقراط: إنّما ينبغي أن تسقي من الدواء ما يستفرغ من البدن النوع الذي إذا استفرغ من تلقاء نفسه نفع استفراغه. فأمّا ما كان استفراغه على خلاف ذلك فينبغي أنْ تقطعه.

١٠ قال المفسّر: هذا بيّن.

(4.3)

[١٤٠] قال أبقراط: إن استفرغ البدن من النوع الذي ينبغي أن يبقّى منه نفع ذلك واحتمل بسهولة وإن كان الأمر على ضدّ ذلك كان الأمر عسرا.

قال المفسّر: أخبرنا هنا بذلك على أن تكون هذه علامة نعلم بها هل أصبنا في الحدس أو أخطأنا أعني سهولة احتمال الاستفراغ أو عسره.

---

١ بسم الله الرحمن الرحيم: om. ABP ٢ المقالة الرابعة من شرح فصول أبقراط: شرح المقالة الرابعة من فصول أبقراط B المقالة الرابعة من شرح الفصول لأبقراط A المقالة الرابعة P ٣-٤ إذا ... عليه: إلى قوله B ٦ وكبر: C¹ ٨ ينبغي: لك B ٩ استفراغه: C¹ ٩-٨ ما ... ذلك: إلى قوله B add. A ١١ ينبغي: om. A ١١-١٢ أن ... عسرا: om. B ١٣ هنا: هذا A || هذه علامة: يستعمل الاسافراغ؟ A

(4.4)

[141] Says Hippocrates: Evacuation by drugs should be effected more from above in summer and more from below in winter.

Says the commentator: The yellow bile and the heat, which dominate in summer, cause the humors to move upwards continuously. Therefore, evacuation through emesis is to be preferred. During winter, the opposite is the case.

(4.5)

[142] Says Hippocrates: After[162] the time of the rising of the Dog Star (Sirius), during the time of its ascent, and before it, evacuation through drugs is difficult.

Says the commentator: That is the [hottest] time of summer; the powers [of the body] are extremely weak and the heat of the air opposes the attracting force of the remedy, so that nothing results from it except weakness and disturbance.[163]

(4.6)

[143] Says Hippocrates: Those who have a lean body and [thus] easily vomit, should be evacuated with [emetic] remedies from above, but beware of doing so in winter.

Says the commentator: The condition of lean persons is always similar to that of most people in summer. The prohibition against the application of emesis in winter has already been stated before.[164]

(4.7)

[144] Says Hippocrates: If vomiting is difficult for a person and he is moderately corpulent, one should evacuate him with purgative remedies from below, but beware of doing so in summer.

Says the commentator: This is clear.

---

162   "After the time of the rising of the Dog Star (Sirius), during the time of its ascent, and before it" (بعد وقت طلوع الشعرى العبور وفي وقت طلوعها وقبله): Cf. Galen, ibid. 4.5, p. 664: Ὑπὸ κύνα καὶ πρὸ κυνός; Hippocrates, ibid., trans. Jones, p. 135: "At and just before the dog-star."

163   "disturbance" (اضطراب): This term also features in Maimonides' *Medical Aphorisms* 6.86; 8.26, ed. and trans. Bos, vol. 2, pp. 19, 47, where it is used for Greek ταραχή; cf. Liddell/Scott, *Greek-English Lexicon*, p. 1758: "disorder, physiological disturbance or upheaval."

164   Cf. aphorism 4.4 (141) above.

(4.4)

[١٤١] قال أبقراط: ينبغي أن يكون ما يستعمل من الاستفراغ بالدواء في الصيف من فوق أكثر وفي الشتاء من أسفل.

قال المفسّر: الغالب في الصيف الصفراء والحرارة ألجوا الأخلاط متحركة إلى فوق فلذلك يؤثر الاستفراغ بالقيء وفي الشتاء بالعكس.

(4.5)

٥ [١٤٢] قال أبقراط: بعد وقت طلوع الشعرى العبور وفي وقت طلوعها وقبله يعسر الاستفراغ بالأدوية.

قال المفسّر: هذا الوقت أشدّ ما يكون من الصيف فالقوى ضعيفة جدًّا. وحرّ الهواء يمانع جذب الدواء فلا يحصل منه إلّا ضعف واضطراب.

(4.6)

[١٤٣] قال أبقراط: من كان قضيف البدن وكان القيء يسهل عليه فاجعل استفراغك إيّاه بالدواء ١٠ من فوق وتوقَّ أن تفعل ذلك في الشتاء.

قال المفسّر: حال القضيف دائمًا كحال أكثر الناس في الصيف وقد تقدّم النهي عن استعمال القيء في الشتاء.

(4.7)

[١٤٤] قال أبقراط: فأمّا من كان يعسر عليه القيء وكان من حسن اللحم على حال متوسّطة فاجعل استفراغك إيّاه بالدواء من أسفل وتوقَّ أن تفعل ذلك في الصيف.

١٥ قال المفسّر: هذا بيّن.

١-٢ في ... أسفل: om. B   ٥-٦ وفي ... بالأدوية: om. B   ٩ يسهل: B¹ يغلب B ‖ فاجعل: فافعل P
٩-١٠ فاجعل ... الشتاء: om. B   ١٣-١٤ وكان ... الصيف: om. B

(4.8)

[145] Says Hippocrates: If you evacuate those who suffer from phthisis with purgative remedies, beware of evacuating them from above.

Says the commentator: He means those who are predisposed to [get] phthisis, namely those who have a narrow chest. Since they also have narrow passages in their lungs, you should not convey to them [superfluous] matters.

(4.9)

[146] Says Hippocrates: Those [whose temperament] is dominated by black bile should also be evacuated from below with a remedy that is more solid (i.e., stronger), if one applies the same reasoning to these two opposite cases.

Says the commentator: With a more solid remedy he means a stronger remedy. The yellow bile streams upwards and the black bile sinks downwards. The same reasoning to be applied is to choose one of the two opposites for each of these two humors, since we evacuate each humor from the spot where it is most likely to exit [the body].

(4.10)

[147] Says Hippocrates: In the case of very acute illnesses, one should apply evacuating (purging) remedies from the first day when the humors flare up, because it is bad to delay their application in such cases.

Says the commentator: This is clear. One should be cautious not to leave behind these humors, which stream from site to site and do not rest. One should beware of letting them settle in a noble[165] organ, but hasten to evacuate them before they weaken the strength [of the patient] or settle in the site [of a noble organ].[166]

(4.11)

[148] Says Hippocrates: Those who suffer from colic, pains around the navel, and pain in the loins that are lasting and are not alleviated neither with purgatives nor with something else, will eventually develop dry dropsy.

---

165   "noble organ": I.e., heart, brain, or liver.
166   Cf. Maimonides, *Medical Aphorisms* 8.13, ed. and trans. Bos, vol. 2, p. 45.

(4.8)

[١٤٥] قال أبقراط: فأمّا أصحاب السلّ فإذا استفرغتهم بالدواء فاحذر أن تستفرغهم من فوق.

قال المفسّر: يعني المهيّئين للسلّ وهم الضيّقي الصدور فإنّ رئاتهم أيضا ضيّقة المجاري فلا تجلب لها موادّ.

(4.9)

[١٤٦] قال أبقراط: وأمّا من الغالب عليه المرّة السوداء فينبغي أن تستفرغه أيضا بدواء أغلظ إذ تضيف الضدّين إلى قياس واحد.

٥

قال المفسّر: بدواء أغلظ يعني أقوى والصفراء تطفو لفوق والسوداء ترسب لأسفل فالقياس الواحد هو الذي استعمل في هذا اختيار أحد الضدّين لأحد الخلطين لأنّا نستفرغ كلّ خلط من موضعه القريب نخروجه.

(4.10)

[١٤٧] قال أبقراط: ينبغي أن يستعمل دواء الاستفراغ في الأمراض الحادّة جدّا إذا كانت الأخلاط هائجة منذ أوّل يوم فإنّ تأخيره في مثل هذه الأمراض رديء.

١٠

قال المفسّر: هذا بيّن ويخاف من ترك هذه الأخلاط السائلة من موضع لموضع الغير مستقرّة إياك أن تستقرّ في عضو شريف فيبادر باستفراغها قبل أن تضعف القوة أو تستقرّ في الموضع الشريف.

(4.11)

[١٤٨] قال أبقراط: من كان به مغس وأوجاع حول السرّة ووجع في القطن دائما لا يحلّ لا بدواء مسهل ولا بغيره فإنّ أمره يؤول إلى الاستسقاء اليابس.

---

١ فإذا ... فوق: om. B ٢ الصدور: الصدر BP ‖ ضيّقة: ضعفة A ٦ يعني: أيّ A ‖ لفوق: إلى فوق B ‖ لأسفل: إلى أسفل B ٩-١٠ في ... ردي: om. B ١١ إياك: إيال A ١٢ تستقرّ: تستفرغ A ‖ فيبادر: فبادر BP ١٣ مغس: مغص BP ١٣-١٤ وأوجاع ... اليابس: om. B

Says the commentator: If [those pains] are not alleviated through [medical] treatment, it indicates that a bad temperament prevails in those organs and has settled in them. This results in tympanites and this is the [hydrops], which he calls "dry,"[167] contrary to ascites in which there is water. Ascites originates from excessive cold.

(4.12)

[149] Says Hippocrates: If someone suffers from lientery in winter, it is bad to evacuate him with medications from above.

Says the commentator: This means that even if the lientery is caused by a sharp, thin humor, which floats and requires evacuation by emesis, since it is winter one should not apply emesis, as was mentioned before.[168]

(4.13)

[150] Says Hippocrates: If someone needs to be administered a hellebore (*Helleborus* sp.) potion and evacuation from above does not come to him easily, his body should be moistened with increased food and rest before he is administered the potion.

Says the commentator: This is clear.

(4.14)

[151] Says Hippocrates: If you administer a hellebore potion to someone, your intention should be to make that [person] move his body more and sleep and rest less. Travelling by boat [too] indicates that movement stirs up the body.

Says the commentator: It is known that hellebore is a strong emetic. Movement of the body by local transport is also something that helps emesis, as can be concluded from [the case of] someone travelling by boat.

167　Cf. ibid. 23.50, vol. 5, p. 45: "In his commentary on *Aphorisms* 4, [Galen] says that tympanites is [the illness] that Hippocrates calls 'dry dropsy.'"

168　Cf. aphorism 4.4 (141) above.

قال المفسّر: إذا لم يُخِلّ ذلك بعلاج فهو دليل على سوء مزاج قد استولى على تلك الأعضاء وتمكّن فيها فيحدث الاستسقاء الطبلي وهو الذي سمّاه الياس في مقابل الاستسقاء الزقّي الذي فيه الماء والزقّي يتولّد من برد زائد.

(4.12)

[١٤٩] قال أبقراط: من كان به زلق الأمعاء في الشتاء فاستفراغه بالدواء من فوق رديء.

٥ قال المفسّر: يقول حتّى لو كان الموجب لزلق الأمعاء خلط حادّ لطيف يطفو الذي يوجب ذلك أن يستفرغ بالقيء إذ والوقت شتاء فلا سبيل لاستعمال القيء كما تقدّم.

(4.13)

[١٥٠] قال أبقراط: من احتاج إلى أن يسقى الخربق وكان استفراغه من فوق لا يواتيه بسهولة فينبغي أن يرطّب بدنه من قبل إسقائه إيّاه بغذاء أكثر وبراحة.

قال المفسّر: هذا بيّن.

(4.14)

١٠ [١٥١] قال أبقراط: إذا أسقيت إنسانا خربقا فليكن قصدك لتحريك بدنه أكثر ولتنويمه وتسكينه أقلّ. وقد يدلّ ركوب السفن على أنّ الحركة تثوّر الأبدان.

قال المفسّر: معلوم أنّ الخربق مقيّئ قويّ وتحريك البدن بالنقلة المكانية ممّا يعين على القيء واستدلّ براكب السفن.

---

٢ الطبلي ... الاستسقاء: om. B الاستسقاء الزقّي الذي فيه وهو الذي سمّاه الناس في مقابل A ٤ فاستفراغه ... رديء: om. B ٦ إذ ... القيء: om. A ٧-٨ وكان ... وبراحة: om. B ١٠ أسقيت: سقيت C

(4.15)

[152] Says Hippocrates: When you wish that hellebore has a stronger evacuating effect, move the body, and when you wish it to stop, make the [patient] sleep and do not move him.

Says the commentator: This is clear and repetitious.

(4.16)

[153] Says Hippocrates: The ingestion of hellebore is dangerous to those who have healthy flesh, since it induces spasms.

Says the commentator: This is clear.

(4.17)

[154] Says Hippocrates: If someone has no fever, want of appetite, cardialgia,[169] dizziness, and a bitter taste in the mouth indicate that he should be evacuated by a medication from above.

Says the commentator: Fu'ād[170] means the "cardia of the stomach" and nakhs means "stinging, biting" and sadar (dizziness) means that it seems to the patient as if [everything] he sees is turning around him and he suddenly loses the sense of sight so that he thinks that everything he saw is covered with darkness. These afflictions occur when there are bad humors in the cardia of the stomach, which have a biting effect on it. Therefore, these humors should be evacuated through emesis, when these afflictions appear.

(4.18)

[155] Says Hippocrates: Pains above the diaphragm indicate [a need] for evacuating (purging) through medication from above; pains below the diaphragm indicate [a need for] evacuating (purging) through medication from below.

Says the commentator: To whatever side the humors tend [to stream] and settle, from that side one should evacuate with an emetic from above or purgative from below. During the time that the humors are [actually] flowing, one should attract them to the opposite side.

---

169   "cardialgia" (نَخْس الفؤاد): I.e., palpitation of the heart or heartburn (cf. E, fol. 6ᵃ: نخس في
      الفؤاد) (= C); cf. Galen, In Hippocratis Aphorismos commentarius 4.17, ed. Kühn, vol. 17b,
      p. 676: καρδιωγμός; Hippocrates, Aphorisms, trans. Littré, vol. 4, p. 507: "la cardialgie;" trans.
      Jones, p. 139: "heartburn;" Ullmann, Wörterbuch, p. 325: "Herzstechen."

170   "Fu'ād" (فؤاد): Cf. Ullmann, ibid., suppl. 1, p. 518, s.v. καρδία: "Herz; Magenmund: إنّ القدماء
      كانوا يسمون فم المعدة فؤادا (The ancients called the cardia of the stomach 'fu'ād'; = Gal. Loc.
      Aff. V.6)." See also aphorism 4.65 (202) below.

(4.15)

[١٥٢] قال أبقراط: إذا أردت أن يكون استفراغ الحريق أكثر فحرّك البدن وإذا أردت أن تسكّنه فنوّم الشارب له ولا تحرّكه.

قال المفسّر: هذا بيّن ومكرّر.

(4.16)

[١٥٣] قال أبقراط: شرب الحريق خطر لمن كان لحمه صحيحا وذلك أنّه يحدث تشنّجا.

٥ قال المفسّر: هذا بيّن.

(4.17)

[١٥٤] قال أبقراط: من لم تكن به حمّى وكان به امتناع من الطعام ونخس في الفؤاد وسدر ومرارة في الفم فذلك يدلّ على استفراغه بالدواء من فوق.

قال المفسّر: الفؤاد فم المعدة والنخس اللذع والسدر هو أن يخيّل للإنسان أنّ ما يراه يدور حوله ويفقد حسّ البصر بغتة حتّى يظنّ أنّه قد غشيت جميع ما يراه ظلمة. وهذه الأعراض تكون إذا كان في فم

١٠ المعدة أخلاط رديئة تلدغه فلذلك ينبغي إذا ظهرت هذه الأعراض أن تستفرغ بالقيء.

(4.18)

[١٥٥] قال أبقراط: الأوجاع التي فوق الحجاب تدلّ على الاستفراغ بالدواء من فوق والأوجاع التي من أسفل الحجاب تدلّ على الاستفراغ بالدواء من أسفل.

قال المفسّر: إلى أيّ الجهات مالت الأخلاط وتيقّنت هناك فن ذلك الموضع يستفرغ بدواء مقيّئ من فوق أو مسهل من أسفل. وأمّا في حال انصباب الأخلاط فينبغي أن تجذبها إلى خلاف الجهة.

٢-١ وإذا ... تحرّكه: om. B ٣ ومكرّر: مكرّر P ٤ لمن ... تشنّجا: om. B ٦ ونخس: ولحس AC ٧-٦ ونخس ... فوق: om. B ٦ في: om. C ٨ والنخس: والحس AC ‖ أنّ om. C ٩ فم: om. C ١٢-١١ تدلّ ... بالدواء من أسفل: om. B ‖ على ... تدلّ: om. C ١٤ مسهل: يسهل A

(4.19)

[156] Says Hippocrates: If someone ingests a purging medicine and is being purged but is not thirsty, one should not stop the evacuation (purgation) until he becomes thirsty.

Says the commentator: If thirst after the ingestion of a purgative medication does not result from the heat or dryness of the stomach or from the sharpness of the medication or from the fact that the evacuated humor was hot, [this] indicates that the organs have been cleansed and emptied from that humor, which one wanted to evacuate.

(4.20)

[157] Says Hippocrates: If a person free from fever is affected by colic and heaviness in the knees and pain in the loins, [this] indicates that he needs evacuation through a medication (purgation) from below.

Says the commentator: This is clear.

(4.21)

[158] Says Hippocrates: A black stool, which resembles blood and comes spontaneously, either with or without fever, is one of the worst signs, and the more evil the colors of the stool, the worse the sign. If [such stools] occur after the ingestion of a [purgative] medication, it is a better sign and[171] the more numerous the colors, the less evil it is.[172]

Says the commentator: This is clear.

(4.22)

[159] Says Hippocrates: If, at the beginning of any illness, black bile is evacuated either from below or from above, it is a fatal symptom.

---

171   "and the more numerous the colors, the less evil it is": Cf. Galen, *In Hippocratis Aphorismos commentarius* 4.21, ed. Kühn, vol. 17b, p. 681: καὶ ὁκόσῳ ἂν χρώματα πλείω ᾖ, οὐ πονηρόν; Hippocrates, *Aphorisms*, trans. Littré, vol. 4, p. 509: "et, dans ce cas, la multiplicité des couleurs n'est pas mauvaise;" trans. Jones, p. 139: "and it is not a bad one (i.e., sign) when the colours are numerous."

172   Cf. Maimonides, *Medical Aphorisms* 6.89, ed. and trans. Bos, vol. 2, p. 19.

(4.19)

[١٥٦] قال أبقراط: من شرب دواء الاستفراغ فاستفرغ ولم يعطش فليس ينقطع عنه الاستفراغ حتّى يعطش.

قال المفسّر: العطش بعد شرب الدواء إذا لم يكن من أجل حرارة المعدة أو يبسها أو من أجل حدّة الدواء أو من أجل كون الخلط المستفرغ حارّ فإنّه يدلّ على نقاء الأعضاء وخلوّها من ذلك الخلط الذي يراد خروجه.

٥

(4.20)

[١٥٧] قال أبقراط: من لم تكن به حمّى وأصابه مغص وثقل في الركبتين ووجع في القطن فذلك يدلّ على أنّه يحتاج إلى الاستفراغ بالدواء من أسفل.

قال المفسّر: هذا بيّن.

(4.21)

[١٥٨] قال أبقراط: البراز الأسود الشبيه بالدم الآتي من تلقاء نفسه كان مع حمّى أو من غير حمّى فهو

١٠ من أردأ العلامات. وكلّما كانت الألوان في البراز أردأ كانت تلك علامة أردأ. فإذا كان ذلك مع شرب دواء كانت تلك علامة أحمد. وكلّما كانت تلك الألوان أكثر كان ذلك أبعد من الرداءة.

قال المفسّر: هذا بيّن.

(4.22)

[١٥٩] قال أبقراط: أيّ مرض خرجت في ابتدائه المرّة السوداء من أسفل أو من فوق فذلك علامة دالّة على الموت.

---

١ فليس: فلم A ‏ ١-٢ فليس...يعطش: om. B ‏ ٦ مغص: مغس C ‏ ٩-١١ الآتي الركبتين: الوركين A ‏ ‏ ‏ ‏ ‏ ‏ ‏ ‏ ‏ ‏
...الرداءة: om. B ‏ ٩ من: مع AP ‏ ١٠ أردأ: A ‏ om. ‏ ١١ تلك ... كانت: C¹ ‏ ‏ كان: من C ‏ ١٣-١٤ المرّة
الموت: om. B...

Says the commentator: As long as the disease is in the beginning [stages], nothing from what is excreted from the body of the patient is excreted through the movement of nature (in a natural way), rather, the excretion is an accident, which is closely associated with the unnatural conditions of the body. The black bile [mentioned by Hippocrates] is the coarse humor, which—when it is burned—is similar to the lees of wine and has ceased to be the natural black bile. The excretion of these bad humors before they are concocted indicates that they bite (irritate) the organs because of the strength of their badness and the organs are not capable to hold them until they are concocted.

(4.23)
[160] Says Hippocrates: If someone has become weakened because of an acute or chronic disease or miscarriage[173] or any other [cause] and then passes black bile or something resembling black blood, he will die the next day.

Says the commentator: The nature of someone with such a condition is so weakened that it cannot concoct nor select nor evacuate the humors, bad as they are. And because of the severity and gravity of the illness, they flow and pour forth since nothing can withhold them. His statement "[something] resembling black blood" means "black stools." The difference between black bile and black stools is that black bile is soluble, [that it] has a polishing(?) and biting effect, similar to the biting of vinegar, [and that it] strips (scrapes) off the ground when it falls on it.[174] None of these [characteristics] applies to black stools.

(4.24)
[161] Says Hippocrates: If dysentery begins [with the passage of] black bile, it is a fatal sign.

---

173   "miscarriage" (اِسقَاط) (= E, fol. 8ᵃ) (= τρωσμός; cf. Liddell/Scott, Greek-English Lexicon, p. 1832): Cf. Galen, In Hippocratis Aphorismos commentarius 4.23, ed. Kühn, vol. 17b, p. 686: τρώματα/τραύματα; Hippocrates, Aphorisms, trans. Littré, vol. 4, p. 511: "des blessures;" trans. Jones, p. 141: "wounds."

174   Cf. Maimonides, Medical Aphorisms 2.14, trans. Bos, vol. 1, p. 30: "The difference between black bile and the other melancholic humors which often leave the body through vomiting and diarrhea is that one can taste and smell black bile because it is clearly sour or bitter, or both at the same time, so that flies do not go near to it. If some of it happens to fall on the ground, it has the same effect as very acidic vinegar. Its consistency is thick, and it originates especially in the bodies of ill people. The other melancholic humors cannot be tasted, nor do flies shy away from them, nor do they cause the ground to effervesce ... De atra bile."

قال المفسّر: ما دام المرض في ابتدائه فليس شيء ممّا يبرز من بدن المريض يكون خروجه بحركة من الطبيعة بل يكون خروجه عرض لازم لحالات في البدن خارجة عن الطبيعة. والمرّة السوداء هو الخلط الغليظ الشبيه بالدردي إذا احترق وخرج عن أن يكون السوداء الطبيعية. وبروز هذه الأخلاط الرديئة قبل النضج دليل على لدغها الأعضاء لشدّة رداءتها فلم تطق الأعضاء مسكها حتّى تنضج.

(4.23)

٥ [١٦٠] قال أبقراط: من كان قد أنهكه مرض حادّ أو مزمن أو إسقاط أو غير ذلك ثمّ خرجت منه مرّة سوداء أو بمنزلة الدم الأسود فإنّه يموت من غد ذلك اليوم.

قال المفسّر: الطبيعة في من هذه حاله تكون قد ضعفت حتّى لا تقدر أن تنضج ولا تميّز ولا تستفرغ هذه الأخلاط التي هي من الرداءة على ما هي عليه. فلعظم المرض وتفاقمه تفيض وتنصبّ إذ ليس شيء يحبسها. وقوله أو بمنزلة الدم الأسود يعني البراز الأسود والفرق بين المرّة السوداء والبراز الأسود

١٠ أنّ المرّة السوداء ذاتية معها بريق وتلديغ شبيه بتلديغ الخلّ وتقشر الأرض إذا وقعت عليها وليس من ذلك شيء في البراز الأسود.

(4.24)

[١٦١] قال أبقراط: اختلاف الدم إذا كان ابتداؤه من المرّة السوداء فتلك من علامات الموت.

---

٢ من: om. P ٥ قد: om. A ‖ أنهكه: نهكه B ٥–٦ أو ... اليوم: om. B ٦ الأسود: من فوق أو من أسفل add. P ٧ تكون: om. B ٨–١١ التي ... شيء في البراز الأسود: om. C ١٠ أنّ: لأنّ BP ١٢ قال ... الموت: C¹ ‖ أبقراط: في C ‖ إذا ... الموت: om. B

Says the commentator: If the discharge of yellow bile has come first and abraded and inflamed the intestines and blood comes later, it is possible to cure this abrasion. However, if the black bile has abraded [the intestines] and then inflamed them until [the dysentery] began, it (i.e., the abrasion) cannot be cured, because the intestines will be affected by something similar to cancer that occurs on the surface of the body.

(4.25)

[162] Says Hippocrates: The evacuation of blood from above, whatever it is, is a bad sign; but its evacuation from below is a good sign if black [humors] are evacuated [with it].

Says the commentator: "From above" means through emesis. The [evacuation] from below is only good if nature expels it in the manner of cleansing superfluities as in the case of hemorrhoids, but on the condition that there is only a little.

(4.26)

[163] Says Hippocrates: If someone has dysentery and he discharges something similar to pieces of flesh, it is a fatal sign.

Says the commentator: This is so because it indicates that the tumor settled in (penetrated) the intestines to the point that it pierces its substance, and it is impossible for that flesh to be regenerated.

(4.27)

[164] Says Hippocrates: If someone loses much blood from any site during fevers, he will suffer from loose bowels more[175] than is normal if[176] he is nourished during convalescence.

---

175 "more than is normal": Missing in Hippocrates' text; cf. Galen, *In Hippocratis Aphorismos commentarius* 4.27, ed. Kühn, vol. 17b, p. 692; Hippocrates, *Aphorisms*, ed. and trans. Littré, vol. 4, pp. 512–513; ed. and trans. Jones, pp. 140–141. The addition already features in Ḥunayn's translation of the Hippocratic text, ed. Tytler, p. 32, and in his translation with Galen's commentary (cf. E, fol. 9ᵇ: بأكثر من المقدار المعتدل) and is possibly inspired by Galen's τοῖς τοιούτοις εἰκός ἐστι (ibid.); see the following note.

176 "if he is nourished": Missing in Hippocrates' text; cf. Galen, ibid., ed. Kühn. The addition already features in Ḥunayn's translation of the Hippocratic text, ed. Tytler, p. 32: فيغتذى, and in his translation with Galen's commentary (cf. E, fol. 9ᵇ: فيغذى). Ḥunayn probably added this condition on the basis of the following statement by Galen in his commentary: τῆς ἐμφύτου θερμασίας ἀρρώστου γιγνομένης διὰ τὴν αἱμορραγίαν οὔτε πέπτεσθαι καλῶς τὰ σιτία οὔθ' αἱματοῦσθαι ... καὶ διὰ ταῦτα πάντα τὰς κοιλίας ὑγροτέρας γίνεσθαι τοῖς τοιούτοις εἰκός ἐστι ... (Since the innate heat loses its strength because of a hemorrhage, the food [one takes] cannot be well concocted nor turned into blood ... and therefore the bowels will be looser than reasonable ...).

قال المفسّر: إذا ابتدأ خروج الصفراء فسحجت الأمعاء أو قرّحتها وجاء الدم بعد ذلك فيمكن برء هذا السحج. وأمّا إن كان الخلط السوداوي هو الذي أسحج ثمّ قرّح حتّى جاء الدم فلا بروء له لأن يحدث في الأمعاء شبيه بالسرطان الحادث في سطح الجسم.

(4.25)

[١٦٢] قال أبقراط: خروج الدم من فوق كيف كان فهو علامة رديئة وخروجه من أسفل علامة

٥ جيّدة إذا خرج منه شيء أسود.

قال المفسّر: يعني من فوق بالقيء وإنّما يكون من أسفل جيّد إذا دفعته الطبيعة على جهة نفض الفضلات كما يجري في البواسير وبشرط أن يكون قليلا.

(4.26)

[١٦٣] قال أبقراط: من كان به اختلاف دم نفرج منه شيء شبيه بقطع اللحم فتلك من علامات الموت.

١٠ قال المفسّر: لأنّ ذلك دليل على تمكّن القرحة من الأمعاء حتّى تقطع جرمها ولا يمكن أن يتجبّر ذلك اللحم.

(4.27)

[١٦٤] قال أبقراط: من انفجر منه في الحمّى دم كثير من أيّ موضع كان انفجاره فإنّه عندما ينقه فيغذى يلين بطنه بأكثر من المقدار.

١-٣ قال ... الجسم: om. C ٤ om. C قال ... أسود: C¹ ٥-٤ قال ... كيف: ‖ أسود: om. B ٦-٧ قال ... فهو: om. C ٧ قال ... قليلا: om. C ٨-٩ قال ... الموت: C¹ ٨ دم: الدم C ٩-٨ نفرج: الموت: om. B ٨ فتلك: فذلك C ١٠-١١ قال ... اللحم: om. C ١٢-١٣ قال ... المقدار: om. P C¹ ١٢ أبقراط: om. C ‖ من انفجر منه في الحمّى: من كان به حمّى وانفجر منه C¹

Says the commentator: Because of the weakness of the innate heat in his body through the [loss] of blood, the attraction of the food to the intestines and their digestion in them weakens [as well] and, consequently, he suffers from loose bowels.[177]

(4.28)

[165] Says Hippocrates: If someone who suffers from bilious diarrhea, develops deafness, the diarrhea ceases; and if someone who is deaf is affected by bilious diarrhea, the deafness ceases.

Says the commentator: The reason for this is clear, [namely,] the streaming of the [superfluous] matter in the opposite direction. It is also clear that it is a matter of deafness that occurs all of a sudden during illness, especially when the crisis is[178] near.

(4.29)

[166] Says Hippocrates: If rigor occurs to someone suffering from fever on the sixth day of his illness, the crisis will be hard.

Says the commentator: If a rigor occurs during fevers, especially ardent [fevers], it is usually followed by a crisis. [The matter of] the harmfulness of the crisis on the sixth day is well known and this is what he means with the term "hard."

(4.30)

[167] Says Hippocrates: If someone has a fever [illness] with paroxysms, and if the fever returns on the next day at the very same hour that it left him on the previous day, his crisis will be difficult.

---

177   Cf. Galen's commentary in the previous note.
178   "is near": "departs" BC. Cf. aphorism 4.60 (197) below.

قال المفسّر: لضعف الحرارة الغريزية في بدنه من أجل استفراغ الدم يقلّ جذب الأمعاء للغذاء ويضعف الهضم فيلين البطن.

(4.28)

[١٦٥] قال أبقراط: من كان به اختلاف مرار فأصابه صمم انقطع عنه ذلك الاختلاف. ومن كان به صمم لحدث له اختلاف مرار ذهب عنه الصمم.

قال المفسّر: علّة ذلك بيّنة لسيلان المادّة لخلاف الجهة وبيّن هو أنّ الكلام هنا في الصمم العارض بغتة في الأمراض وبخاصّة عند مقاربة البحران.

(4.29)

[١٦٦] قال أبقراط: من أصابه في الحمّى في اليوم السادس من مرضه نافض فإنّ بحرانه يكون نكدا.

قال المفسّر: متى حدث النافض في الحمّيات وبخاصّة في المحترقة فمن عادته أن يأتي البحران بعده وقد علم رداءة بحران السادس وهو معنى قوله نكدا.

(4.30)

١٠ [١٦٧] قال أبقراط: من كانت لحمّاه نوائب ففي أيّ ساعة كان تركها له إذا كان أخذها له من غد في تلك الساعة بعينها فبحرانه يكون عسرا.

١-٢ قال ... البطن: om. CP ٢ البطن: الطبع B ٣ انقطع عنه: عند A ٤ مرار: om. C¹ || عنه: ذلك

٥-٦ قال ... البحران: om. CP ٥ لسيلان: سيلان C || هنا: om. B ٦ مقاربة: emendation

add. C ٧ قال ... الحمّى: om. B || قال ... نكدا: om. P C¹ || أبقراط: om. C ٨-٩ قال ... نكدا: مفارقة AB editor

١٠-١١ قال ... عسرا: om. P C¹ ١٠ قال ... نوائب: om. B || أبقراط: om. C || كانت: كان C om. CP

١١ فبحرانه: فإنّ بحرانه C

Says the commentator: It is clear that if all the paroxysms of the fever are always the same in their beginning and end, it is an indication that the illness will be prolonged. And this is the meaning of his statement that the crisis will be difficult. [It is] as if he says that it will be difficult for this [kind of] fever to end with a crisis, because a crisis occurs, rather, in acute illnesses, whereas chronic illnesses dissolve over a long time.

(4.31)

[168] Says Hippocrates: If someone with fever suffers from fatigue, abscesses[179] will appear especially in his joints and near to the jaws.

Says the commentator: Because of the heat of the fever and the heat of the organs in a patient with fatigue, the superfluity is expelled to the joints and to the upper part of the body [where] it is absorbed by the soft flesh in the joints of the jaws.

(4.32)

[169] Says Hippocrates: If someone is recovering from an illness and a part of his body suffers[180] pain, he will develop an abscess in that part.

Says the commentator: He states that if a convalescent suffers from fatigue in one of his organs (parts) and develops pain in it, an abscess will form there. The reason [for this] is clear. Galen remarks that the occurrence of pain is also called "fatigue."[181]

(4.33)

[170] Says Hippocrates: But if someone already suffered[182] from pain in any organ (part) before he became ill, the illness will settle (establish itself) in that part.

---

179   "abscesses" (خراج) (= E, fol. 10^b): Cf. Galen, *In Hippocratis Aphorismos commentarius* 4.31, ed. Kühn, vol. 17b, p. 697: ἀποστάσιες; Hippocrates, *Aphorisms*, trans. Littré, vol. 4, p. 513: "les dépôts;" trans. Jones, p. 143: "the abscessions;" cf. Ullmann, *Wörterbuch*, p. 125.

180   "suffers pain" (كلّ): Cf. Galen, ibid. 4.32, p. 699: πονήσῃ; Hippocrates, ibid., trans. Littré: "devient douloureuse;" trans. Jones: "have pain." The Arabic كلّ normally means 'to suffer from fatigue.' In the sense of "to have pain," it is a non-attested semantic borrowing of the Greek πονέω, which means both 'to suffer toil' and 'to suffer pain;' cf. Liddell/Scott, *Greek-English Lexicon*, p. 1447, and the next note.

181   I.e., that the Greek term πονέω has both meanings; cf. Galen, ibid., cf. the previous note.

182   "suffered from pain" (تعب): I.e., semantic borrowing from Greek πονέω, just like كلّ in aphorism 4.32 (169) above.

قال المفسّر: بيّن هو أنّ إذا كانت نوائب الحمّى كلّها ثابتة على حال واحدة في ابتدائها وانقضائها فذلك دليل على طول المرض. وهو معنى قوله بحران عسر كأنّه يقول فإنّه يعسر أن تنقضي هذه الحمّى بحران لأنّ البحران إنّما يكون للأمراض الحادّة فأمّا الأمراض المزمنة فإنّها تتحلّل على طول.

(4.31)

[١٦٨] قال أبقراط: صاحب الإعياء في الحمّى أكثر ما يخرج به الخراج في مفاصله وإلى جانب اللحيين.

٥ قال المفسّر: بسبب حرارة الحمّى وحرارة الأعضاء من صاحب الإعياء يندفع الفضل للمفاصل ولأعلى الجسم فيقبله اللحم الرخو الذي في مفاصل اللحيين.

(4.32)

[١٦٩] قال أبقراط: من انتشل من مرض فكلّ منه موضع من بدنه حدث به في ذلك الموضع خراج.

قال المفسّر: يقول إنّ الناقه إن أتعب عضو من أعضائه فأصابه فيه وجع فإنّه يخرج هناك خراج والعلّة بيّنة. وقد ذكر جالينوس أنّ حدوث الوجع أيضا يسمّى كلال.

(4.33)

١٠ [١٧٠] قال أبقراط: فإن كان أيضا قد تقدّم فتعب عضو من الأعضاء من قبل أن يمرض صاحبه ففي ذلك العضو يتمكّن المرض.

_____

٣-١ قال ... الحادّة: om. P ‖ قال ... طول: om. C ‖ ١ إذا: om. A ‖ فذلك: فإنّ ذلك B ٢ بحران: بحرانه B ٣ البحران: om. A ‖ ٤ قال ... اللحيين: C¹ ‖ أكثر ... اللحيين: om. B ‖ جانب: ناحية A ٥-٦ قال ... اللحيين: om. C ‖ ٥ يندفع: ينرفع P ‖ ولأعلى: ولاعالي P في A add. ‖ ٧ قال ... خراج: om. C ‖ انتشل (t =): انتعش E, fol. 11ª; V, fol. 61ᵇ ‖ من مرض: om. A ‖ فكلّ: فيوهن C ‖ فكلّ ... خراج: om. B ‖ ٨ قال المفسّر: يقول إنّ الناقه: om. C ‖ فيه: به P ‖ والعلّة: وعلّته A ١٠ فإن: من P ‖ فتعب: فأتعب A ١٠-١١ فتعب ... المرض: om. B.

Says the commentator: This is clear. He refers here to the fatigue (i.e., pain) that precedes the illness, until it becomes the cause of the illness. In the previous aphorism, he speaks of the fatigue (i.e., pain) that occurs after leaving the disease behind (i.e., when one is recovering from it). In the third aphorism before [our aphorism][183] he mentions the fatigue (i.e., pain) that occurs during the disease itself. However, one should expect all the abscesses mentioned by him [to occur] in the case of crises that are not accompanied by a clear evacuation.

(4.34)
[171] Says Hippocrates: If someone who is suffering from fever but has no swelling in the throat is suddenly seized by suffocation, it is a deadly symptom.

Says the commentator: A sudden suffocation especially occurs as a result of the closure of the larynx, and the fever patient needs to inhale much cold air. If the air is prevented from passing, he will die without any doubt. He stipulated that there should be no swelling, because fever sometimes happens following a swelling in the throat. In such a case the suffocation develops slowly in relation to the growth of the swelling, and when [the swelling] reaches its acme it may decrease slowly and the patient is saved.

(4.35)
[172] Says Hippocrates: If someone is affected by fever and his neck is twisted around so that he can only swallow with difficulty, but no swelling is visible, it is a fatal sign.

Says the commentator: The twisting of the neck and the difficulty to swallow result from straining a dorsal vertebra. The straining sometimes happens because of a swelling and sometimes because of the domination of dryness. [The type of straining] he means here is the one arising from the domination of dryness, for this indicates that the bad temperament has settled in the organs and that dryness is dominant.

---

183   I.e., aphorism 4.31 (168) above.

قال المفسّر: هذا بيّن ذكر هنا التعب المتقدّم للمرض حتّى يكون هو السبب للمرض وذكر في الفصل الذي قبله التعب الذي يكون بعد الخروج من المرض وذكر في الثالث الذي قبل هذا التعب الذي يكون في نفس المرض وإنّما نتوقّع هذه الخراجات كلّها في البحارين التي لا يكون فيها استفراغ ظاهر.

(4.34)

[١٧١] قال أبقراط: من اعترته حمّى وليس في حلقه انتفاخ فعرض له اختناق بغتة فذلك من علامات الموت.

قال المفسّر: الاختناق بغتة إنّما يكون من قبل انسداد الحنجرة والمحموم يحتاج إلى استنشاق هواء بارد كثير. فإذا منع الهواء مات بلا شكّ. وإنّما اشترط أن لا يكون ثمّ انتفاخ لأنّه قد تكون الحمّى تابعة لورم الحلق ويكون الاختناق جاء قليلا قليلا لتزيّد الورم وعند انتهائه يمكن أن يخطّ أيضا قليلا قليلا ويتخلّص المريض.

(4.35)

[١٧٢] قال أبقراط: من اعترته حمّى فاعوجّت معها رقبته وعسر عليه الازدراد حتّى لا يقدر أن يزدرد إلّا بكدّ من غير أن يظهر به انتفاخ فذلك من علامات الموت.

قال المفسّر: اعوجاج الرقبة وعسر الازدراد يكون من زوال أحد الفقار وزواله قد يكون من أجل ورم وقد يكون لغلبة اليبس. والذي نريده هنا هو الكائن من غلبة اليبس فإنّ ذلك دليل على تمكّن سوء المزاج في الأعضاء واستيلاء اليبس.

---

٢ التعب ... هذا: .A om ٥ فعرض: فيعرض P 9-5.169 الاختناق ... ٦-٥ وليس ... الموت: .B om
نوع واحد: .P om ١٢-١١ معها ... الموت: .B om ١١ أن: .C om

(4.36)

[173] Says Hippocrates: Perspiration is beneficial in a fever patient if it begins on the third day, the fifth, the seventh, the ninth, the eleventh, the fourteenth, the seventeenth, the twentieth, the[184] twenty-fourth, the twenty-seventh, the thirty-first, or thirty-fourth day, because perspiration on these days brings the disease to a crisis. However, perspiration not occurring on these days indicates evil,[185] and a lengthy disease.[186]

Says the commentator: This rule applies not only to perspiration but to all discharges during which there is a crisis. The nature of these critical days became known through experience. Every crisis occurs with perspiration or with another discharge. It has been established through experience that it mostly occurs on these days.

(4.37)

[174] Says Hippocrates: If cold sweat occurs with high fever, it indicates death, but if it occurs with mild fever, it indicates that the disease will be prolonged.

Says the commentator: The severity of the fever extinguishes the innate heat,[187] so that the very cold humors, which are at the outside of the body and from which the cold sweat emerges, cannot be concocted. An indication of the crudeness of these humors and the severity of their cold can be derived from the fact that the high fever cannot heat [those humors] that emerge [from the body].[188]

(4.38)

[175] Says Hippocrates: On whatever part of the body there is sweat, it indicates that the illness is in that part.

Says the commentator: For this reason the sweat only comes from that part where the humor is retained.

---

184   "the twenty-fourth": Missing in Hippocrates' *Aphorisms* 4.36, ed. and trans. Littré, pp. 516–517; ed. and trans. Jones, pp. 144–145, and in Galen, *In Hippocratis Aphorismos commentarius*, ed. Kühn, vol. 17b, p. 711. However, it does occur in Ḥunayn's Arabic translation, ed. Tytler, p. 34, and in his translation with the commentary of Galen (cf. E, 13ᵇ).

185   "evil" (أذًى): Cf. Galen, ibid., ed. Kühn: πόνον; Hippocrates, ibid., trans. Littré, p. 517: "souffrances;" trans. Jones, p. 145: "pain."

186   Hippocrates, ibid., ed. and trans. Littré, pp. 516–517; ed. and trans. Jones adds: καὶ ὑποτροπιασμούς ("relapses") (pp. 144–145), and Galen, ibid.: ὑποτροπιασμόν (cf. E, fol. 13ᵇ: نكس). However, the term is missing in Ḥunayn's Arabic translation, ed. Tytler, p. 34.

187   On the notion of "innate heat," the force sustaining life in living beings, see Galen, *De usu partium*, trans. May: *Usefulness of the Parts of the Body*, vol. 1, pp. 50–53.

188   Cf. Maimonides, *Medical Aphorisms* 6.63, ed. and trans. Bos, vol. 2, p. 14.

(4.36)

[١٧٣] قال أبقراط: العرق يحمد في المحموم إن ابتدأ في اليوم الثالث أو في الخامس أو في السابع أو في التاسع أو في الحادي عشر أو في الرابع عشر أو في السابع عشر أو في العشرين أو في الرابع والعشرين أو في السابع والعشرين أو في الواحد والثلاثين أو في الرابع والثلاثين. فإنّ العرق الذي يكون في هذه الأيّام يكون به بحران الأمراض. وأمّا العرق الذي لا يكون في هذه الأيّام فهو يدلّ على آفة أو على
٥ طول من المرض.

قال المفسّر: ليس هذا الحكم في العرق وحده بل في جميع الاستفراغات التي تكون بها البحران فإنّ طبيعة هذه الأيّام الباحورية قد علمت بالتجربة وكلّ بحران يكون بعرق أو بغيره من الاستفراغات فإنّه وجد بالتجربة يكون على الأكثر في هذه الأيّام.

(4.37)

[١٧٤] قال أبقراط: العرق البارد إذا كان مع حمّى حادّة دلّ على الموت وإذا كان مع حمّى هادئة
١٠ دلّ على طول المرض.

قال المفسّر: شدّة الحمّى تطفئ الحرارة الغريزية فلا تنضج الأخلاط الباردة جدّا التي في ظاهر البدن التي منها برز العرق البارد ودليل لفجاجة هذه الأخلاط وشدّة بردها كون حرارة الحمّى القوية لم تقدر على إسخان ما يبرز منها.

(4.38)

[١٧٥] قال أبقراط: وحيث كان العرق من البدن فهو يدلّ على أنّ المرض في ذلك الموضع.

١٥ قال المفسّر: ولذلك كان العرق من ذلك الموضع وحده الذي فيه الخلط المحتقن.

---

٢ عشر ... الرابع A. om ١٠-٩ إذا ... المرض B. om ١٢ القوية: القوي B ١٤ فهو ... الموضع B. om

(4.39)

[176] Says Hippocrates: Whatever part of the body is hot or cold, the disease is in that part.

Says the commentator: This is clear.

(4.40)

[177] Says Hippocrates: When changes occur in the whole body, if the body is sometimes cold and sometimes hot or [now] has this color and then another color, it indicates a prolonged disease.[189]

Says the commentator: When the illness consists of many different kinds, it always lasts longer than the illness that is of one kind.

(4.41)

[178] Says Hippocrates: Copious sweat occurring after sleep without any obvious cause indicates that someone has burdened his body with more food than it can tolerate. But if it occurs to someone and he is not taking any food, know that his body needs evacuation.[190]

Says the commentator: This is clear.

(4.42)

[179] Says Hippocrates: Copious sweat, whether hot or cold, that flows constantly, indicates when it is cold that the illness is more serious, and when it is hot that the illness is less serious.

Says the commentator: [He means] that when the sweat that occurs during the days of the illness—other than as part of a crisis—is cold, [the illness] is more severe because it indicates coldness of the [superfluous] matter.

---

189   Cf. aphorism 7.62 (414) below.
190   Cf. aphorism 2.8 (60) above.

(4.39)

[١٧٦] قال أبقراط: وأيّ موضع من البدن كان باردا أو حارّا ففيه المرض.

قال المفسّر: هذا بيّن.

(4.40)

[١٧٧] قال أبقراط: وإذا كان تحدث في البدن كلّه تغايير وكان البدن يبرد مرّة ثمّ يسخن أخرى أو يتلوّن بلون ثمّ بغيره دلّ ذلك على طول المرض.

قال المفسّر: المرض الذي هو من أنواع كثيرة هو أبدا أطول مدّة من المرض الذي هو من نوع واحد. ٥

(4.41)

[١٧٨] قال أبقراط: العرق الكثير الذي يكون بعد النوم من غير سبب بيّن يدلّ على أنّ صاحبه يحمل على بدنه من الغذاء أكثر ممّا يحتمل. فإن كان ذلك وهو لا ينال من الطعام فاعلم أنّ بدنه يحتاج إلى الاستفراغ.

قال المفسّر: هذا بيّن.

(4.42)

[١٧٩] قال أبقراط: العرق الكثير الذي يجري دائما حارّا كان أو باردا فالبارد منه يدلّ على أنّ المرض ١٠ أعظم والحارّ منه يدلّ على أنّ المرض أخفّ.

قال المفسّر: يقول إنّ العرق الذي يكون في سائر أيّام المرض لا على طريق البحران ما كان منه باردا كان أرداأ لأنّه يدلّ على برد المادّة.

---

١ كان ... المرض: om. B ٣-٤ وكان ... المرض: om. B ٣ ثمّ يسخن: وسخن A ٦-٨ من ... الاستفراغ: om. B ٧-٨ وهو... الاستفراغ: وهو لا ينال منه دلّ على أنّ بدنه إلى الاستفراغ A ٩-١٢ هذا بيّن ... قال المفسّر: om. B

(4.43)

[180] Says Hippocrates: If the fever is unremitting and grows worse every other day,[191] it is exceedingly dangerous. But if it is intermittent in whatever way, this indicates that it is not dangerous.

Says the commentator: [The fever] that is continuous is the one that grows worse every other day, and which is dangerous is the one [called] "semi-tertian."

(4.44)

[181] Says Hippocrates: If someone is attacked by protracted fever, he will develop tumors or pain[192] in the joints.

Says the commentator: The duration of the fever depends upon the quantity of the [superfluous] matter, or the coldness of the matter or the thickness of the humors. When this is the condition of the [superfluous] matter, it is mostly repelled to an organ where it causes a tumor, or to a joint cavity where it causes pain in the joints.

(4.45)

[182] Says Hippocrates: If someone is afflicted by a tumor or pain[193] in the joints after the fever, he takes more food than he can tolerate.

Says the commentator: "After the fever" means after the complete abatement of the fever, while [the patient] is still recovering.

(4.46)

[183] Says Hippocrates: If a rigor occurs to someone who suffers from unremitting fever and has been weakened, it is a fatal sign.[194]

---

191   I.e., turns into a tertian fever.

192   "pain" (كلال): Cf. aphorism 4.32 (169) above.

193   Arabic كلّ normally means 'to suffer from fatigue.' In the sense of 'to have pain,' it is a non-attested semantic borrowing of the Greek πονέω; cf. aphorism 4.32 (169) above.

194   Cf. Maimonides, *Medical Aphorisms* 6.64, trans. Bos, vol. 2, p. 15: "A frequent occurrence of rigor during a fever is a fatal sign because it shakes the body so much that the body's strength dwindles, irrespective of whether evacuation follows thereafter or not. *In Hippocratis Aphorismos commentarius 4.*"

(4.43)

[١٨٠] قال أبقراط: إذا كانت الحمّى غير مفارقة ثمّ تشتدّ غبّا فهي أعظم خطرا وإذا كانت تفارق على أيّ وجه كانت فهي تدلّ على أنّه لا خطر فيها.

قال المفسّر: هذه التي هي دائمة وتشتدّ غبّا التي فيها خطر هي شطر الغبّ.

(4.44)

[١٨١] قال أبقراط: من أصابته حمّى طويلة فإنّه يعرض له إمّا خراجات وإمّا كلال في مفاصله.

قال المفسّر: طول الحمّى إمّا لكثرة مادّتها أو لبرد المادّة وإمّا لغلظ الخلط والمادّة التي هذه حالها في ٥ الأكثر تدفع إمّا لعضو ما فتحدث فيه خراجا أو لفضاء المفاصل فتحدث وجع المفاصل.

(4.45)

[١٨٢] قال أبقراط: من أصابه خراج أو كلال في المفاصل بعد الحمّى فإنّه يتناول من الطعام أكثر ممّا يحتمل.

قال المفسّر: يعني بعد الحمّى بعد إقلاع الحمّى بالجملة وهو بعد ناقه.

(4.46)

[١٨٣] قال أبقراط: إذا كانت تعرض نافض في حمّى غير مفارقة لمن قد ضعف فتلك من علامات ١٠ الموت.

---

١ ثمّ: كانت P. add ‏ ٢-١ ثمّ ... ثمّ P. add ‏ فيها: om. B ‏ ١ كانت: الحمّى CP. add ‏ ٣ التي: الذي AB ‏ ٤ فإنّه ... مفاصله: om. B ‏ خراجات: جراحات C ‏ كلال: om. B ‏ ٥ طول الحمّى: om. BP ‏ أو لبرد المادّة: om. A ‏ التي: هي BP. add ‏ ٦ خراجا: جراحا C ‏ أو لفضاء: وإمّا إلى فضاء B وإمّا لفضاء P ‏ ٧ خراج: جراح C ‏ ٧-٨ أو ... يحتمل: om. B ‏ ٧ كلال: كل A ‏ ١٠ كانت تعرض: كان عرض C كان يعرض P ‏ ١٠-١١ لمن ... الموت: om. B

Says the commentator: Galen says that [Hippocrates'] words "when it (i.e., a rigor) occurs to someone" indicate that it occurs continuously time and again and that its repeated occurrence, while the fever remains uninterrupted, indicates that nature tries to eject and expel the illness-producing humor, but cannot do so because it is firmly established in the organs and remains in them. The strength [of the body] is damaged and dwindles away more and more because it cannot tolerate the tremor of the rigor and its shaking [effect on] the body.[195]

(4.47)
[184] Says Hippocrates: In unremitting fevers, livid expectorations, which are similar to blood, or are fetid, or bilious, are all bad. But if they are properly expelled they are favorable. The same holds good for feces and urine. If something is excreted from one of these sites[196] from which excretion is not beneficial, it is bad.

Says the commentator: This statement means that, in general, bad things that are evacuated indicate bad conditions in the bodies from which they are evacuated. But sometimes their evacuation is like the evacuation of serum from putrid ulcers, the evacuation of which is not beneficial in that disease. And sometimes their evacuation is like the evacuation of pus from an abscess that has broken [and] results in a beneficial cleansing for the diseased organ. The signs that indicate that the evacuation of a [superfluous matter] is beneficial are above all its concoction, that the body easily tolerates its excretion and that it finds relief through it, and also [that it is according to] the nature of the illness, and hereafter [that it is according to] the current time of the year, the place [of living], and the nature of the patient.

(4.48)
[185] Says Hippocrates: In an unremitting fever, if the external [parts] of the body are cold but the internal [parts] burning hot and it is accompanied by thirst, it is a fatal sign.

---

195   Cf. Galen, *In Hippocratis Aphorismos commentarius* 4.46, ed. Kühn, vol. 17b, pp. 724–725.
196   I.e., the bowels and the bladder; cf. aphorism 7.70 (missing in Maimonides' commentary).

قال المفسّر: قال جالينوس: إنّ قوله إذا كانت تعرض يدلّ على مداومة النافض المرّة بعد المرّة فحدوثه مرّة بعد مرّة والحمّى باقية غير مفارقة دليل على كون الطبيعة تروم نفض الخلط الممرّض وإخراجه ولم تقدر لثبوته وتبقّيه في الأعضاء وتزداد القوة نكاية وذبول بكونها لا تحتمل رعدة النافض وزعزعتها للبدن.

(4.47)

[١٨٤] قال أبقراط: في الحمّى التي لا تفارق النخاعة الكمدة والشبيهة بالدم والمنتنة والتي هي من جنس ٥ المرار كلّها رديئة فإن انتفضت انتفاضا جيّدا فهي محمودة. وكذلك الحال في البراز والبول فإنّ خروج ما لا ينتفع بخروجه من أحد هذه المواضع فذلك رديء.

قال المفسّر: القول العامّ أنّ الأشياء الرديئة التي تُستفرغ تدلّ على حالات رديئة في الأبدان التي تُستفرغ منها إلّا أنّها ربّما كان خروجها بمنزلة خروج الصديد من القروح المتعفّنة فلا ينتفع بخروجها في ذلك المرض وربّما كان خروجها بمنزلة خروج المدّة من خراج ينفجر يكون به نقاء محمود للعضو ١٠ الذي فيه العلّة. والعلامات الدالّة على أنّ خروج ما يخرج جيّد هي نضجه خاصّة واحتمال البدن لخروجه بسهولة وخفّته به ومع ذلك طبيعة المرض ومن بعدها الوقت الحاضر من السنة والبلد والسنّ وطبيعة المريض.

(4.48)

[١٨٥] قال أبقراط: إذا كان في حمّى لا تفارق ظاهر البدن باردا وباطنه يحترق ويصاحب ذلك ١٥ عطش فتلك من علامات الموت.

---

١ لحدوثه: لحدوث A   ٣ وتبقّيه: وثقته C ونتقنه P ‖ رعدة: هذا B ردا P ‖ وزعزعتها: وزعزعته B
٧–٥ والشبيهة ... رديء: om. B   ٦ خروج: خرج CP   ٧ أحد: إحدى A   ٨ الرديئة: om. BP   ٩ أنّها: أنّه P   ١٠ المرض: om. P ‖ خراج: جراح C   ١١ هي: هو A   ١٤–١٥ ظاهر ... الموت: om. B

Says the commentator: Galen says that this occurs only in some unremitting fevers and that it is caused by an inflammation in an internal part of the body, whereby the blood and the pneuma are attracted from the whole body to the diseased part. As a result, the internal [parts] of the body are burning hot but the skin is cold, as happens in the beginning of fever attacks. This is Galen's argumentation.[197] But this is not true, because, if this would follow necessarily, this affliction would inevitably be associated with every inflammation that occurs in the internal parts [of the body]. However, we always see that the skin of those who suffer from pleurisy, pneumonia, and liver complaint, is extremely hot, like the inside of their bodies. It seems to me that the reason for this is that the substances, which are in the external [parts] of the body, are very thick [and] very cold. The heat of the putrid humor that produces the fever that putrefies within the body cannot overcome them. The more this putrid substance becomes heated and its heat rises to the external [parts] of the body as it is looking for openings through which to breath, the more it finds itself up against a cold barrier, which prevents the heat from emerging to the surface of the body. As a result, the heat is reversed and returns with the strongest possible [force] so that the inside of the body is burned [even] more and the thirst gets worse. And then something occurs to the heat, which is similar to what happens when blacksmiths sprinkle water on the fire in a smelting furnace until the internal heat of the fire becomes so strong that it melts the iron. This is without any doubt the real natural cause.

(4.49)
[186] Says Hippocrates: If in an unremitting fever the [patient's] lip, eye, nose, or eyebrow is distorted; if the patient, being already weak, does neither see nor hear, whatever of these [things] occur, death is near.

Says the commentator: This is clear, because when these symptoms occur in combination with a weakness of the strength [of the patient], and when fever preceded, one can learn [from this] that dryness prevails over the origins of the nerves and that this causes the distortion and the other [afflictions] mentioned by him.

(4.50)
[187] Says Hippocrates: When difficulty of respiration and mental confusion (delirium) occur during unremitting fever, it is a fatal sign.

---

197   Cf. Galen, *In Hippocratis Aphorismos commentarius* 4.48, ed. Kühn, vol. 17b, pp. 728–729.

قال المفسّر: قال جالينوس: إنّ هذا العارض لا يوجد أبدا إلّا في بعض الحيّات التي لا تفارق. وعلّته

قال أن يحدث ورم حارّ في بعض الأعضاء الباطنة فينجذب الدم والروح إلى العضو العليل من

البدن كلّه ولذلك يحترق باطن البدن حرارة والجلد بارد كما يعرض في أوّل نوائب الحمّى. هذا تعليل

جالينوس وهو غير صحيح لأنّه لو لزم ذلك لكان هذا العارض لازما لكلّ ورم حارّ يحدث في الأعضاء

٥ الباطنة ونحن نشاهد دائما أصحاب ذات الجنب وذات الرئة وذات الكبد جلودهم حارّة جدّا مثل

أجسادهم. والذي يبدو لي أنّ علّة ذلك كون المواد التي في ظاهر الجسم غليظة جدّا باردة جدّا

لا تقهرها حرارة الخلط العفن المولّد للحمّى الذي عفن في باطن الجسد. فكلّ ما التهب ذلك الشيء

المتعفّن وصعدت حرارته نحو ظاهر الجسد تطلب منفسا تتنفّس منه وجدت حجابا باردا دونها تمنع

تلك الحرارة من البروز لسطح الجسد فتنعكس الحرارة راجعة بأشدّ ما يمكن فيحترق باطن البدن

١٠ أكثر ويشتدّ العطش فتعتري الحرارة حينئذ شبه ما يفعله الحدّادون من رشّ الماء على النار في الكور

حتّى تشتدّ حرارة باطن النار فتذيب الحديد وهذه علّة صحيحة طبيعية لا ريب فيها.

(4.49)

[١٨٦] قال أبقراط: متى التوت في حمّى غير مفارقة الشفة أو العين أو الأنف أو الحاجب أو لم ير

المريض أو لم يسمع أيّ هذه كان وقد ضعف فالموت منه قريب.

قال المفسّر: هذا بيّن لأنّ إذا ظهرت هذه العلامات مع ضعف القوة وتقدّم الحمّى علم أنّ اليبس قد

١٥ استولى على مبادئ العصب ولذلك حدث هذا الالتواء أو غيره ممّا ذكر.

(4.50)

[١٨٧] قال أبقراط: إذا حدثت في حمّى غير مفارقة رداءة في التنفّس واختلاط في العقل فذلك من

علامات الموت.

---

٢ حارّ ... الدم: om. A ٣ أوّل: أوائل BP ‖ تعليل: دليل B ٦ لي: إليّ C ٨ وصعدت: وضعفت

BP ‖ نحو: om. A ٩ يمكن: يكون A ‖ فيحترق: فتحرق P ١٠ الحدّادون: الحدّادين P ١١ حرارة: om.

B ١٢-١٣ الشفة ... قريب: om. BP ‖ هذا: om. BP ١٥ الالتواء: التواء P ‖ ذكر: ذكره BP ١٦ حدثت:

حدث AP ١٦-١٧ واختلاط ... الموت: om. B

Says the commentator: This is clear because the heat has taken possession of the organs to the point that also the nerves that move the chest and the diaphragm have weakened, so that respiration is difficult.

(4.51)
[188] Says Hippocrates: An abscess, which occurs during a fever and is not dissolved at the time of the first crisis, indicates a long illness.

Says the commentator: This is clear.

(4.52)
[189] Says Hippocrates: If tears, which flow during a fever or during other illnesses, [are shed] by a patient of his own will, it is not extraordinary. But if [the tears are shed] involuntarily, it is worse.[198]

Says the commentator: This is clear because of the weakness of the retentive faculty. The word "worse" indicates that the first [case] is also bad, that is to say that although he cries of his own will it is an indication that his heart is weak. For this reason, he is quickly affected [by emotions], which make him cry.

(4.53)
[190] Says Hippocrates: If the teeth of someone suffering from fever are covered with viscous matters, his fever is high.[199]

Says the commentator: These viscous matters especially develop from strong heat, which acts upon phlegmatic moisters until they become dried out.

(4.54)
[191] Says Hippocrates: If someone with ardent fever suffers from a frequent dry cough, which [only] irritates him slightly, he will hardly suffer from thirst.

---

198   "worse" (أردأ): Cf. ibid. 4.52, p. 731: ἀτοπώτερον; Hippocrates, *Aphorisms*, trans. Littré, vol. 4, p. 523: "plus inquiétants."

199   "high" (قوية): Galen, ibid. 4.53, p. 732: ἰσχυροί; cf. Hippocrates, ibid., ed. and trans. Littré, pp. 522–523: ἰσχυρότεροι ("plus fortes"); trans. Jones, p. 149: "more severe." The Arabic translation by Ḥunayn, ed. Tytler, p. 36, also reads: قوية, and is thus based on the same Greek reading as Galen.

قال المفسّر: هذا بيّن لأنّ الحرارة قد تمكّنت من الأعضاء حتّى ضعف أيضا العصب المحرّك للصدر والحجاب فساء التنفّس.

(4.51)

[١٨٨] قال أبقراط: الخراج الذي يحدث في الحمّى ولا يحلّ في أوقات البحرانات الأوّل ينذر من المرض بطول.

قال المفسّر: هذا بيّن.

٥

(4.52)

[١٨٩] قال أبقراط: الدموع التي تجري في الحمّى أو في غيرها من الأمراض إن كان ذلك عن إرادة من المريض فليس بمنكر وإن كان عن غير إرادة فهو أردأ.

قال المفسّر: ذلك بيّن لضعف القوة الماسكة وقوله أردأ دليل على أنّ الأوّل رديء أيضا. وذلك أنّه وإن بكى بإرادة فإنّه دليل على ضعف قلبه ولذلك سرع انفعاله وتأتيه للبكاء.

(4.53)

[١٩٠] قال أبقراط: من غشيت أسنانه في الحمّى لزوجات فحمّاه تكون قوية.

١٠

قال المفسّر: هذه اللزوجات إنّما تحدث من حرارة قوية عملت في رطوبات بلغمية حتّى جفّفتها.

(4.54)

[١٩١] قال أبقراط: من عرض له في حمّى محرقة سعال كثير يابس ثمّ كان تهييجه له يسيرا فإنّه لا يكاد يعطش.

---

٣ الخراج: الجراح C ‏ ٣-٤ ولا ... بطول: om. B ‏ || من المرض بطول: بطول من المرض P ‏ ٥ هذا: ذلك C ‏
٦ التي: الذي A ‏ ٦-٧ أو ... أردأ: om. B ‏ ٦ عن: om. A ‏ || إرادة: باردة A ‏ ٧ عن: من A ‏ ٨-٩ أنّ
... على: om. A ‏ ٨ رديء: om. A ‏ ١٢-١٣ كذا B ‏ سعال ... يعطش: om. B

Says the commentator: Galen says that it is impossible during coughing, even if there is no expectoration, that the trachea should not become moistened through the [moisture] that is attracted to it during coughing, and therefore [the patient] is not thirsty.[200]

(4.55)

[192] Says Hippocrates: Any fever that comes with a[201] swelling in the soft flesh of the groins (i.e., bubo) and the like is bad, unless the fever is ephemeral.

Says the commentator: If the fever is caused by a swelling in the soft flesh of the groins and the like, it is ephemeral fever. However, if the fever is due to another cause and is associated with a swelling in the groins and the like, it is bad because in that case the swelling in the groins is associated with a swelling in one of the intestines. And this internal swelling is the cause of the fever mentioned before, and therefore it is dangerous.

(4.56)

[193] Says Hippocrates: If someone with a fever perspires but the fever does not abate, it is a bad sign for it announces that the disease will be prolonged and it is a sign of excessive moisture.

Says the commentator: This is clear.

(4.57)

[194] Says Hippocrates: If someone suffers from spasms or tetanus and then gets a fever, his illness will dissolve.

Says the commentator: There are three types of spasms: backwards spasm (opisthotonus), forwards spasm (emprosthotonus), and tetanus, in which no cramps are visible in the parts of the body because they are stretched backwards and forwards equally.[202] All types of spasm occur either because of

---

200   Cf. Galen, ibid. 4.54, p. 733.

201   "a swelling in the soft flesh of the groins (i.e., bubo)" (ورم اللحم الرخو الذي في الحالبين): Cf.
      ibid. 4.55: βουβῶνες; Hippocrates, *Aphorisms*, trans. Littré, vol. 4, p. 523: "bubons;" trans.
      Jones, p. 151: "buboes;" see also Ullmann, *Wörterbuch*, p. 167.

202   Cf. Galen, *De tremore, palpitatione, convulsione et rigore*, ed. Kühn, vol. 7, p. 641; trans.
      Sider/McVaugh: "On Tremor, Palpitation, Spasm, and Rigor," p. 210: "You already know
      that all agree that one form of this pathos (i.e., spasm) is forward-pulling and is so called
      ['emprosthotonos'], one backward-pulling ['opisthotonos'], and one tetanos. Whenever
      the parts of the body are stretched forward, it is emprosthotonos; whenever backwards,
      opisthotonos; with equal force in both directions, tetanos;" see also idem, *De locis affectis*
      3.7, ed. Kühn, vol. 8, pp. 167–168; trans. Siegel: *On Affected Parts*, p. 84.

قال المفسّر: قال جالينوس: لا بدّ في السعال ولو لم ينفث شيئا أن تتندّى قصبة الرئة بما ينجلب إليها عند السعال ولذلك لا يعطش.

(4.55)

[١٩٢] قال أبقراط: كلّ حمّى تكون مع ورم اللحم الرخو الذي في الحالبين وغيره ممّا أشبهه فهي رديئة إلّا أن تكون حمّى يوم.

قال المفسّر: إذا كان سبب الحمّى ورم الحالبين ونحوه من اللحم الرخو فتكون حمّى يوم. فأمّا إذا كان للحمّى سبب آخر واقترن معها ورم الحالبين ونحوه فهي رديئة لأنّ سبب تورّم الحالبين حينئذ إنّما يكون تابع لورم أحد الأحشاء وذلك الورم الباطن هو سبب الحمّى المتقدّمة ولذلك هي خطرة.

(4.56)

[١٩٣] قال أبقراط: إذا كانت بإنسان حمّى فأصابه عرق فلم تقلع عنه الحمّى فتلك علامة رديئة وذلك أنّها تنذر بطول من المرض وتدلّ على رطوبة كثيرة.

١٠ قال المفسّر: هذا بيّن.

(4.57)

[١٩٤] قال أبقراط: من اعتراه تشنّج أو تمدّد ثمّ أصابته حمّى انحلّ بها مرضه.

قال المفسّر: التشنّج ثلاثة أصناف التشنّج الذي إلى خلف والتشنّج الذي إلى قدّام والتمدّد وليس ترى فيه الأعضاء تتشنّج لأنّها تتمدّد إلى وراء وإلى قدّام تمدّدا سواء. وجميع أصناف التشنّج إمّا من امتلاء

٣-٤ الذي ... يوم: om. B ٨ كانت: كان BP ٨-٩ فلم ... كثيرة: om. B ١١ أو ... مرضه: om. B
١٢ إلى: P om. ‖ إلى ... قدّام: إلى قدّام والتشنّج الذي إلى خلف A

overfilling or depletion of the neural parts. A spasm following ardent fever is necessarily caused by dryness.[203] A spasm, which occurs first and suddenly, necessarily results from overfilling. If [this spasm] is followed by fever, it dissolves part of the superfluous moisture and[204] concocts part of its coldness.

(4.58)
[195] Says Hippocrates: If someone with ardent fever is affected by rigor, the fever will abate.

Says the commentator: When the bilious humor moves to be evacuated, it causes rigor and this is followed by vomiting of yellow bile and diarrhea to evacuate the superfluity that produces the fever. When the vessels [of the patient] are clean, his fever abates.

(4.59)
[196] Says Hippocrates: A[205] tertian fever comes to a crisis, at the latest, in seven cycles.

Says the commentator: Galen says: We have observed and investigated the crisis in quartan and tertian fevers and found that it occurs according to the number of cycles and not according to the number of days. Thus, the seventh cycle in tertian fever falls on the thirteenth day from its beginning. In most cases, the crisis and end of the illness occur on that day and one does not have to wait for the fourteenth day. Hippocrates is speaking here about simple tertian fever.[206]

(4.60)
[197] Says Hippocrates: If someone with acute fever is afflicted by deafness and blood flows from his nose or he suffers from diarrhea, the illness will subside as a result of that.

---

203   Cf. Galen, *De tremore, palpitatione, convulsione et rigore*, trans. Sider/McVaugh: "On Tremor, Palpitation, Spasm, and Rigor," p. 210: "... in the same manner spasms arise from an excessive dryness caused by disease, which strongly dries out the sinews. This happens in ardent fevers due to dryness alone ..."

204   "and concocts part of its coldness": Cf. P: "and concocts part of the moisture."

205   "A tertian fever": Cf. Galen, *In Hippocratis Aphorismos commentarius* 4.59, ed. Kühn, vol. 17b, p. 737: τριταῖος ἀκριβής; Hippocrates, *Aphorisms*, trans. Littré, vol. 4, p. 523: "Une fièvre tierce légitime;" trans. Jones, p. 151: "An exact tertian."

206   Cf. Galen, ibid., pp. 738–739.

الأعضاء العصبية وإمّا من استفراغها. فما تبع من التشنّج حمّى محرقة فواجب أن يكون حدوثه من اليبس. وما كان من التشنّج يحدث ابتداء ودفعة فواجب أن يكون من الامتلاء فإذا حدث بعده حمّى حلّت بعض الرطوبة الفضلية وأنضجت بعض برودتها.

(4.58)

[١٩٥] قال أبقراط: إذا كان بإنسان حمّى محرقة فعرضت له نافض انحلّت بها حمّاه.

قال المفسّر: إذا تحرّك الخلط الصفراوي للخروج أحدث النافض ويتبعه قيء الصفراء وانطلاق البطن لخروج ذلك الفضل المولّد للحمّى فإذا نقت عروقه انحلّت حمّاه.

(4.59)

[١٩٦] قال أبقراط: الغبّ أطول ما تكون تنقضي في سبعة أدوار.

قال المفسّر: قال جالينوس: قد رصدنا وتفقّدنا البحران في الربع والغبّ ووجدناه يكون على حساب عدد الأدوار لا على حساب عدد الأيّام. من ذلك أنّ الدور السابع في الغبّ يقع في اليوم الثالث عشر من أوّلها. وفي ذلك اليوم في أكثر الأمر يكون بحران المرض وانقضاءه من غير أن ينتظر به الرابع عشر. وكلام أبقراط هنا في الغبّ الخالصة.

(4.60)

[١٩٧] قال أبقراط: من أصابه في الحمّى الحادّة في أذنيه صمم لجرى من منخريه دم أو استطلق بطنه انحلّ بذلك مرضه.

---

٣ برودتها: رطوبتها P ٤ فعرضت ... حمّاه: om. B ‖ بها: به P ٧ تنقضي ... أدوار: om. B ١٠ الأمر: الأيّام BP ١٢-١٣ لجرى ... مرضه: om. B

Says the commentator: The reasons for that have already been mentioned above.[207]

(4.61)

[198] Says Hippocrates: If the fever does not leave the patient on one of the odd days, it usually relapses.

Says the commentator: Galen says that this is an error of the copyist and that Hippocrates is speaking about one of the days of the crisis regardless whether it is an even or an odd day.[208]

(4.62)

[199] Says Hippocrates: If jaundice occurs during a fever before the seventh day, it is a bad sign.[209]

Says the commentator: Sometimes jaundice occurs in the way of a crisis, but a crisis with jaundice does not occur before the seventh [day]. [The only exception is] when it is caused by an affliction of the liver and for this reason it is a bad sign.

(4.63)

[200] Says Hippocrates: If someone with fever suffers from rigor every day, the fever abates every day.

Says the commentator: With the words "abates every day," he means that it leaves him and departs from him every day with the evacuation of the humor that caused the rigor and its movement to be excreted. The same holds good for tertian and quartan fevers.

(4.64)

[201] Says Hippocrates: If jaundice occurs during a fever on the seventh, ninth,[210] or fourteenth day, it is beneficial, unless the right side of the hypochondrium becomes hard. If that is the case, it is not beneficial.

---

207 Cf. aphorism 4.28 (165) above.

208 Galen, *In Hippocratis Aphorismos commentarius* 4.61, ed. Kühn, vol. 17b, p. 741. See also Hippocrates, *Aphorisms*, ed. Littré, vol. 4, p. 524 n. 7.

209 Some Greek MSS add: ἢν μὴ ξυνδόσιες ὑγρῶν κατὰ τὴν κοιλίην γένωνται (cf. Hippocrates, ibid., ed. Littré, p. 524 n. 9; trans. p. 525: "à moins qu'il ne survienne par le bas un flux de liquide;" trans. Jones, p. 151: "unless there be watery discharges through the bowels").

210 Ibid., M adds: ἢ τῇ ἑνδεκάτῃ (cf. ed. Jones, p. 152; trans. p. 153: "on the eleventh"). The addition is also missing in Ḥunayn's Arabic translation, ed. Tytler, p. 38, and in Galen, *In Hippocratis Aphorismos commentarius* 4.64, ed. Kühn, vol. 17b, p. 744 (Arabic trans.: E, fol. 19ᵇ).

قال المفسّر: قد تقدّمت علل ذلك.

(4.61)

[١٩٨] قال أبقراط: إذا لم يكن إقلاع الحمّى عن المحموم في يوم من الأيّام الأفراد فمن عادتها أن تعاود.

قال المفسّر: جالينوس يقول إنّ هذا غلط من الناسخ وأنّ قول أبقراط هو في يوم من أيّام البحران كان ذلك زوجا أو فردا.

(4.62)

[١٩٩] قال أبقراط: إذا عرض اليرقان في الحمّى قبل اليوم السابع فهو علامة رديئة.

قال المفسّر: قد يعرض اليرقان على جهة البحران ولا يكون بحران بيرقان قبل السابع بل إنّما سببه آفة من آفات الكبد ولذلك صار علامة رديئة.

(4.63)

[٢٠٠] قال أبقراط: من كانت تصيبه في حمّاه نافض في كلّ يوم فحمّاه تنقضي في كلّ يوم.

قال المفسّر: يعني بقوله تنقضي في كلّ يوم أنّها تقلع عنه وتفارقه في كلّ يوم عند استفراغ الخلط ١٠ الموجب للنافض عند حركته للخروج وكذلك يجري الأمر في الغبّ والربع.

(4.64)

[٢٠١] قال أبقراط: متى عرض اليرقان في الحمّى في اليوم السابع أو في التاسع أو في الرابع عشر فذلك محمود إلّا أن يكون الجانب الأيمن ممّا دون الشراسيف صلب. فإن كان كذلك فليس أمره بمحمود.

––––––––––––––––––––––––––

٢ عن ... تعاود: om. B   ٥ قبل ... رديئة: om. B   ٨ في ... يوم: om. B   ٩-١٣.١٨٥ يعني ... في أمراض مهلكة: om. P   ١١-١٢ في ... بمحمود: om. B   ١١ في: C¹

Says the commentator: The reason for this is clear from the preceding.[211]

(4.65)

[202] Says Hippocrates: If [someone] with fever has a [sensation] of severe heat in the belly and of cardialgia,[212] it is a bad sign.

Says the commentator: If with [the term] *fuʾād* he means the cardia of the stomach, then *khafaqān* refers to a burning [sensation] in the cardia of the stomach because it is being soaked by bilious humors. If with [the term] *fuʾād* he means the heart, the latter is afflicted by palpitations because the heat has taken possession of it. Both afflictions are extremely bad.[213]

(4.66)

[203] Says Hippocrates: In acute fevers, cramps and pains[214] in the intestines are a bad sign.

Says the commentator: An extremely high fever dries the nerves like fire; it stretches and distends them and, in this manner, fatal cramps occur. Sometimes, also pain in the intestines occurs from precisely this condition, that is to say, from the extreme heat and dryness.

(4.67)

[204] Says Hippocrates: Fear or cramps occurring to [someone] with fever [on waking from] sleep, are bad signs.

Says the commentator: If the body is full with humors, the head becomes filled [therewith] during sleep and the brain becomes heavy. If the dominant humor tends towards black bile, fear ensues from it. But if this is not the case, pain and cramps happen from it. Galen says that he has often observed that fear, pain, and cramps occur as a result of sleep in the case of fatal illnesses and that it is seems that this happens during sleep when the harmful humor reaches the brain.[215]

---

211   Cf. aphorism 4.62 (199) above.

212   "cardialgia" (خفقان في الفؤاد): I.e., palpitation of the heart or heartburn; cf. Galen, *In Hippocratis Aphorismos commentarius* 4.65, ed. Kühn, vol. 17b, p. 745: καρδιωγμός. Galen, ibid., pp. 745–746, remarks that according to the ancients, the term καρδία can mean both the heart and the cardia of the stomach, and that the term καρδιωγμός is explained by some in the sense of heartburn and by others in the sense of palpitation of the heart. See also Maimonides' commentary to this aphorism and to aphorism 4.17 (154) above.

213   Maimonides' statement goes back to Galen, ibid., pp. 745–746; see the previous note.

214   "pains" (أوجاع): Cf. ibid. 4.66, p. 746; Hippocrates, *Aphorisms*, trans. Littré, vol. 4, p. 527: "les violentes douleurs;" trans. Jones, pp. 152–153: "violent pains".

215   Cf. Galen, ibid. 4.67, p. 748.

قال المفسّر: علّة ذلك بيّنة ممّا تقدّم.

(4.65)

[٢٠٢] قال أبقراط: متى كان في الحمّى التهاب شديد في المعدة وخفقان في الفؤاد فتلك علامة رديئة.

قال المفسّر: إن كان يريد بفؤاد فم المعدة فمعنى قوله خفقان لدغ فم المعدة لتشرّبه بالأخلاط الصفراوية. وإن كان يريد بالفؤاد القلب فالخفقان يصيبه لتمكّن الحرارة منه وكلا هذين العرضين رديء جدًّا. ٥

(4.66)

[٢٠٣] قال أبقراط: التشنّج والأوجاع العارضة في الأحشاء في الحمّيات الحادّة علامة رديئة.

قال المفسّر: الحمّى القوية الشديدة تجفّف العصب بمنزلة النار فتمدّده وتجذبه وعلى هذا الوجه يحدث التشنّج المهلك. وربّما عرض في الأحشاء أيضا وجع من هذه الحال بعينها أعني من شدّة الالتهاب واليبس.

(4.67)

[٢٠٤] قال أبقراط: التفزّع والتشنّج العارضان في الحمّى من النوم من العلامات الرديئة. ١٠

قال المفسّر: إذا كان البدن ممتلئا من أخلاط فعند النوم يمتلئ رأسه فيثقل الدماغ. فإن كان الخلط الغالب مائلا إلى السوداء عرض منه التفزّع وإن لم يكن كذلك عرض منه التوجّع والتشنّج. وقال جالينوس إنّه رأى مرارا كثيرة في أمراض مهلكة التفزّع والتوجّع والتشنّج تحدث من النوم ويشبه أن يكون ذلك يعرض عند مصير الخلط المؤذي عند النوم للدماغ.

---

٣ يريد: om. A ٦ العارضة ... رديئة: om. B ٨ الأحشاء: الأجساد B ١٠ من ... الرديئة: om. B

١٢ الغالب: الأغلب B

(4.68)

[205] Says Hippocrates: If[216] the air (i.e., respiration) changes during its passage through the body, it is [a bad sign] because it indicates spasms.

Says the commentator: With "air," he means the air of respiration. If it meets an obstruction during its passage so that it is cut off in its entrance or its exit or both together [it is a bad sign].

(4.69)

[206] Says Hippocrates: If someone's urine is thick, similar to blood clots, and of small quantity, and his body is not free from fever, he will benefit if he urinates a large amount of thin urine. This type of urination happens mostly to someone in whose urine a sediment settles from the beginning of his illness or shortly thereafter.

Says the commentator: Most patients with fever have thin urine in the beginning of the illness. The closer they get to the end, the thicker its consistency. Hippocrates informs us about something rare, namely that sometimes the urine resembles mud and that its quantity is small in the beginning of the disease. The reason for its small quantity is that it only passes through the kidneys with difficulty. When the major part of the bad humor has been evacuated and the remainder thereof concocted, [the patient] urinates thinner urine and in a larger quantity.

(4.70)

[207] Says Hippocrates: If someone with fever urinates turbid urine, similar to that of a beast of burden, he suffers from a headache at that moment or will so later on.

Says the commentator: The urine is only like that when the heat acts on a large amount of thick [superfluous] matter. Especially when matters with this property are acted upon by extraordinary heat, vapors originate from them so that [the urine] becomes turbid like wax, pitch, and pine resin. The thick vapors and the heat quickly ascend to the head. Sometimes one can discern that the headache occurs at the same time as the turbid urine; sometimes earlier and sometimes later.

---

216   "If the air (i.e., respiration) changes during its passage through the body": Cf. Galen, ibid.,
       p. 749: Ἐν τοῖσι πυρετοῖσι τὸ πνεῦμα πρόσκοπτον; Hippocrates, *Aphorisms*, trans. Littré, p. 527:
       "Dans les fièvres, la respiration entrecoupée;" trans. Jones, p. 153: "In fevers, stoppage of the
       breath."

(4.68)

[٢٠٥] قال أبقراط: إذا كان الهواء يتغيّر في مجاريه من البدن فذلك رديء لأنّه يدلّ على تشنّج.

قال المفسّر: يعني بالهواء هواء التنفّس إذا حبسه شيء في مجاريه حتّى ينقطع في حال دخوله أو خروجه أو فيهما جميعا.

(4.69)

[٢٠٦] قال أبقراط: من كان بوله غليظا شبيها بالعبيط يسيرا بدنه ينقى من الحمّى فإنّه إذا بال

٥ بولا كثيرا رقيقا انتفع به وأكثر من يبول هذا البول من كان يرسب في بوله منذ أوّل مرضه أو بعده بقليل سريعا ثفل.

قال المفسّر: الأمر الأكثري في المحمومين أن يكون البول أوّل المرض رقيقا وكلّما قارب الانقضاء غلظ قوامه. فأخبرنا أبقراط بهذا الأمر النادر وهو أنّه قد يكون البول شبيها بالحمأة وقليل أوّل المرض وعلّة قلّته لأنّه لا ينفذ الكلى إلّا بكدّ فإذا استفرغ أكثر ذلك الخلط الرديء ونضج ما تبقّى منه استفرغ

١٠ عند ذلك من البول ما هو أرقّ وكثيرا.

(4.70)

[٢٠٧] قال أبقراط: من بال في الحمّى بولا متثوّرا شبيها ببول الدوابّ فيه صداع حاضر أو سيحدث به.

قال المفسّر: إنّما يكون البول كذلك إذا عملت الحرارة في مادّة غليظة كثيرة. وما كان من الموادّ على هذه الصفة خاصّة إذا عملت فيه الحرارة الخارجة تولّدت منه الرياح حتّى يتثوّر مثل القير والزفت

١٥ والراتينج. والرياح الغليظة مع الحرارة تسرع الصعود إلى الرأس وترى الصداع ربّما كان مع البول المتثوّر وربّما كان قبله وربّما كان بعده.

---

١ من ... تشنّج:om. B ٢ هواء:om. C ٤ بالعبيط:om. C ٤ بالعبيط:بالغبيط:CP² ٦-٤ فإنّه ... ثفل:om. B ٥ به:om. A ‖ من:ما:P ٧ أوّل:om. A ٩ بكدّ:بكذا:C ١٢-١١ شبيها ... به:om. B ١٥ تسرع:وتسرع P واسرع B

(4.71)

[208] Says Hippocrates: If someone has a crisis on the seventh day, a red cloud will appear in his urine on the fourth day. Other symptoms are analogous.

Says the commentator: The fourth [day] is the day that foretells what will happen on the seventh. Every important sign that clearly indicates concoction on [this day], indicates a crisis occurring on the seventh [day]. However, a white cloud is a more appropriate sign for this, and an even more appropriate [sign] is a white cloud suspended in the middle of the urine. If the disease moves quickly, only a change in color and in consistency is a sufficient indication for the crisis to occur on the seventh [day]. Galen says that Hippocrates mentions the red cloud, which is the weakest [sign], so that one can learn from it about the matter of the other signs that are stronger. For they indicate that the crisis is imminent. The signs that appear during the prognostic days in the stool or sputum [can be interpreted] according to the same analogy.[217]

(4.72)

[209] Says Hippocrates: If the urine is transparent [and] white, it is bad, especially in[218] [patients] with fever associated with an inflammation of the brain.

Says the commentator: This urine is extremely far from being concocted and it indicates that the illness will be prolonged. It also indicates that all the yellow bile moves upwards, in the direction of the head.

(4.73)

[210] Says Hippocrates: If the hypochondrium in a [patient] is swollen and if there are rumblings in it, and if he is then affected by pain in the lower[219] back, his bowels will be loose unless many winds escape from him or unless he passes much urine. This occurs in fevers.

---

217   Cf. Galen, ibid. 4.71, p. 757.

218   "in [patients] with fever associated with an inflammation of the brain": Cf. ibid. 4.72, p. 759: ἐν τοῖς φρενιτικοῖσιν; Hippocrates, *Aphorisms*, trans. Littré, vol. 4, p. 529: "dans les phrénitis;" trans. Jones, p. 155: "in cases of phrenitis;" Ullmann, *Wörterbuch*, p. 742.

219   "lower back" (أسفل ظهره) (= E, fol. 22ᵇ): Cf. Galen, ibid. 4.73, ed. Kühn, p. 761: ὀσφῦς; Hippocrates, ibid., trans. Littré, p. 529: "des lombes;" trans. Jones, p. 155: "loins;" Ullmann, ibid., p. 478. The regular Arabic term for "loins" is قطن; cf. De Koning, *Trois traités d'anatomie arabes*, p. 825.

(4.71)

[٢٠٨] قال أبقراط: من يأتيه البحران في السابع فإنّه قد يظهر في بوله في الرابع غمامة حمراء وسائر العلامات تكون على هذا القياس.

قال المفسّر: الرابع يوم إنذار بما يكون في السابع فكلّ علامة ذات قدر تظهر فيه تدلّ على النضج فهي تدلّ على البحران الكائن في السابع. لكنّ الغمامة البيضاء أحرى أن تدلّ على ذلك وأولى منها السحاب الأبيض المتعلّق في وسط البول. وإن كان المرض سارع الحركة كان تغيّر اللون وحده وتغيّر القوام دلالة كافية على البحران الكائن في السابع. وقال جالينوس إنّ أبقراط ذكر الغمامة الحمراء التي هي أضعفها ليفهم أمر سائر العلامات التي هي أقوى فإنّها تدلّ على أنّ البحران مزمع. وكذلك العلامات التي تظهر في أيّام الإنذار في البراز أو في البزاق على هذا القياس.

(4.72)

[٢٠٩] قال أبقراط: إذا كان البول ذا مستشفّ أبيض فهو رديء وخاصّة في أصحاب الحمّى التي مع ورم الدماغ.

قال المفسّر: هذا البول في غاية البعد من النضج فيدلّ على طول المرض ويدلّ مع ذلك أنّ حركة المرّة الصفراء كلّها إلى فوق نحو الرأس.

(4.73)

[٢١٠] قال أبقراط: من كانت المواضع التي فيما دون الشراسيف منه عالية فيها قرقرة ثمّ حدث له وجع في أسفل ظهره فإنّ بطنه يلين إلّا أن ينبعث منه رياح كثيرة أو يبول بولا كثيرا وذلك في الحمّيات.

٥

١٠

١٥

١-٢ فإنّه ... القياس om. B: ٣ قدر om. A: ٤ لكنّ: لأنّ P ٦ أبقراط: بقراط P ٦-٧ التي ... العلامات om. A: ٨ البزاق: البصاق P ١١ فيدل: فدل A ١٢ كلّها om. BP: ١٣-١٥ فيها ... الحمّيات om. B: ١٤ أن: أنّه C

Says the commentator: If the wind descends and moves downwards together with the moisture, which causes the intestinal rumblings, the swelling descends to the region of the lower spine and the parts, which are there are stretched so that pain occurs. Sometimes the moisture reaches the vessels and exits with the urine. In that case, the winds exit alone. Sometimes, the wind and the moisture exit together from the intestines and the bowels become loose. Sometimes,[220] the moisture and wind go into the vessels and then pass easily through to the urinary bladder. Especially in the case of someone with a fever one can rely on these symptoms and be aware that nature is determined to expel the harmful matter through the urine or stool.

(4.74)
[211] Says Hippocrates: If an abscess is expected to develop in someone's joints, he may be saved from that abscess by an abundant flow of thick, white urine, like that which sometimes begins on the fourth day in some people who suffer from fever associated with fatigue. And if he has a nosebleed, his illness ends very quickly.

Says the commentator: This is clear.

(4.75)
[212] Says Hippocrates: If someone urinates blood or pus, it indicates that there is an ulceration in the kidneys or urinary bladder.

Says the commentator: This is clear.

(4.76)
[213] Says Hippocrates: If someone with thick urine passes small pieces of flesh or[221] hair-like substances, they are a discharge from the kidneys.

---

220   "Sometimes, the moisture and wind go into the vessels and then pass easily through to the urinary bladder": Cf. Galen, ibid., p. 762: ἔστι δ ὅτε ἄμφω πρὸς ἀνάδοσιν ὁρμώμενα τὸ ὑγρὸν καὶ τὸ πνεῦμα διεξέρχεται ῥᾳδίως ἐπὶ τὴν κύστιν; trans. Ḥunayn, E: وربما تأدّتا كلتاهما إلى العروق أعني الرطوبة والريح فنفذتا سريعا إلى المثانة.

221   "or": Missing in Hippocrates, *Aphorisms* 4.76, ed. and trans. Littré, vol. 4, pp. 530–531; ed. and trans. Jones, pp. 154–155, but cf. Galen, ibid. 4.76, ed. Kühn, p. 767: ἤ (= E, fol. 24ᵃ: أو), and Hippocrates, ibid., ed. Littré, p. 530 n. 8: "L'addition de ἤ, dans plusieurs manuscrits et quelques éditions, est due uniquement a Galien; il commence par noter que cette particule manque dans *tous* les exemplaires; mais il ajoute qu' elle est indispensable, attendu que de *petites chairs* ne ressemblent pas à des *cheveux*."

قال المفسّر: إذا انحدرت الريح مع الرطوبة الموجبة للقراقر وتحرّكت لأسفل يخطّ الانتفاخ إلى ما

يلي أسفل الصلب فتتمدّد الأعضاء التي هناك فيحدث الوجع. فربّما تأدّت تلك الرطوبة إلى العروق

نخرجت بالبول وخرجت الرياح وحدها. وقد تخرجها جميعا الريح والرطوبة من الأمعاء فيلين البطن.

وقد ينفذان جميعا إلى العروق وينفذان سريعا للمثانة الرطوبة والريح. وفي من به حمّى خاصّة تثق بهذه

٥ العلامات وتعلم أنّ الطبيعة قد عزمت على دفع الشيء المؤذي وإخراجه ببول أو براز.

(4.74)

[٢١١] قال أبقراط: من يتوقّع له أن يخرج به خراج في شيء من مفاصله فقد يتخلّص من ذلك الخراج

بول كثير غليظ أبيض يبوله كما قد يبتدئ في اليوم الرابع في بعض من به حمّى معها إعياء. فإن رعف

كان انقضاء مرضه مع ذلك سريعا جدّا.

قال المفسّر: هذا بيّن.

(4.75)

١٠ [٢١٢] قال أبقراط: من كان يبول دما أو قيحا فإنّ ذلك يدلّ على أنّ به قرحة في كلاه أو في مثانته.

قال المفسّر: هذا بيّن.

(4.76)

[٢١٣] قال أبقراط: من كان في بوله وهو غليظ قطع لحم صغار أو بمنزلة الشعر فذلك يخرج من كلاه.

---

٢ فتتمدّد: فتتمد (!) P فتتمدّد A ‖ om.A :جميعا ٣ وحدها: A om.A ‖ ٥ براز: ببراز BP خراج: جراح C

٦–٨ فقد ... جدّا: om.B ٦ الخراج: الجراح C om.P :مرضه ٨ ١٠ فإنّ ... om.B :مثانته ١٢ وهو:

om.B :كلاه ... قطع A ‖ أو ...

Says the commentator: The small pieces of flesh derive from the very substance of the kidneys. But the hair-like [substance] can neither be from the substance of the kidneys nor from the substance of the bladder. Galen says that he has seen that it happened to people that they urinated this [hair-like substance], some of which was about half a cubit long, because they took foods that produce a thick humor. When the heat acts upon this thick humor until it burns and dries it in the kidneys, this [hair-like substance] originates from it. The[222] cure of this illness confirms the correct deduction of the cause, for those who were affected by this illness were indeed healed by [the application] of refining, diluting medications.[223] Hippocrates' statement that "they are a discharge from the kidneys" informs us about the site where this [hair-like substance] develops.

(4.77)
[214] Says Hippocrates: If someone with thick urine passes [bran-like particles], his urinary bladder is affected by scabs.

Says the commentator: This is clear.

(4.78)
[215] Says Hippocrates: If someone urinates blood without[224] anything preceding it, it indicates that a vessel in the kidneys has burst.

Says the commentator: This is clear.

(4.79)
[216] Says Hippocrates: When someone's urine contains a sandy sediment, a stone will develop in the urinary bladder.

Says the commentator: This is clear.

---

222   "The cure of this illness confirms the correct deduction of the cause": Cf. Galen, ibid., ed. Kühn, p. 769: καὶ μέντοι καὶ ἡ θεραπεία μαρτυρεῖ τῷ λογισμῷ τῆς αἰτίας; trans. Ḥunayn (E, fol. 24ᵃ): وعلاج هذا الداء يشهد على صحة القياس في وجود سببه.

223   Cf. ibid., ed. Kühn, pp. 768–769.

224   "without anything preceding it" (من غير شيء متقدّم): Cf. ibid. 4.78, p. 773: ἀπὸ ταὐτομάτου; Hippocrates, Aphorisms, trans. Littré, vol. 4, p. 531: "spontané;" trans. Jones, p. 157: "spontaneous."

قال المفسّر: أمّا قطع اللحم الصغار فن نفس جوهر الكلى وأمّا ما هو بمنزلة الشعر فلا يمكن أن يكون

لا من جوهر الكلى ولا من جوهر المثانة. وقال جالينوس إنّه رأى من عرض لهم أنْ بالوا هذا الشعر

وبعضه كان طوله نحو من نصف ذراع من قبل أنّهم استعملوا أطعمة تولّد خلطا غليظا. فهذا

الخلط الغليظ إذا عملت فيه الحرارة حتّى تحرقه وتجفّفه في الكلى تولّد منه هذا الشعر. وعلاج هذا

٥ الداء يشهد على صحّة القياس في سببه فإنّ الذين أصابتهم هذه العلّة إنّما برئوا بالأدوية الملطّفة المقطّعة.

فقول أبقراط فذلك يخرج من كلاه أعلمنا بموضع تولّد هذا الشعر.

(4.77)

[٢١٤] قال أبقراط: من خرج في بوله وهو غليظ بمنزلة النخالة فمثانته جربة.

قال المفسّر: هذا بيّن.

(4.78)

[٢١٥] قال أبقراط: من بال دما من غير شيء متقدّم دلّ ذلك على أنّ عرقا في كلاه انصدع.

١٠ قال المفسّر: هذا بيّن.

(4.79)

[٢١٦] قال أبقراط: من كان يرسب في بوله شيء شبيه بالرمل فالحصى يتولّد في مثانته.

قال المفسّر: هذا بيّن.

---

١ الكلى: ولا من جوهر المثانة add. A ٢ لا: الا A || أنْ: om. BP ٤ وتجفّفه: om. BP ٧ غليظ: om.
A || بمنزلة ... جربة: om. B ١١ شيء ... مثانته: om. B

(4.80)

[217] Says Hippocrates: If someone urinates blood with clots[225] and has strangury and if a pain seizes him in the lower part of the abdomen and[226] pubes,
the parts about the urinary bladder are affected.

(4.81)

[218] Says Hippocrates: If someone urinates blood, pus, and scales, and his
urine is foul-smelling, it indicates ulceration of the bladder.

(4.82)

[219] Says Hippocrates: If someone gets a tumor[227] in the urethra, when it suppurates and bursts, the illness comes to an end.[228]

(4.83)

[220] Says Hippocrates: If someone passes much urine during the night, it indicates that the stool will be small.

Says the commentator: All these aphorisms are also clear.

This is the end of the fourth part of the commentary on the *Aphorisms*.

---

225   "clots" (عِيط): Cf. Galen, ibid. 4.80, p. 776: θρόμβους; Hippocrates, ibid., trans. Littré:
      "des grumeaux;" trans. Jones: "clots;" Ullmann, *Wörterbuch*, suppl. 1, p. 472; see also Mai-
      monides, *Medical Aphorisms* 23.36, trans. Bos, vol. 5, p. 39: "*Abīṭ* is a congelation of copious
      blood which is clearly visible. *De tumoribus praeter naturam.*"
226   "and pubes" (وعِانة): Cf. Galen, ibid.: καὶ τὸ περιναῖον; Hippocrates, ibid., trans. Littré: "et
      le périnée;" trans. Jones: "and the perineum;" note however that certain Greek MSS read:
      κτένα (pubes); cf. ed. Littré, p. 532 n. 8.
227   "tumor" (بُرُ): Cf. Galen, ibid. 4.82, p. 778: φῦμα; Hippocrates, ibid., trans. Littré, p. 533: "des
      tumeurs;" trans. Jones, p. 157: "tumours;" cf. Ullmann, *Wörterbuch*, pp. 747–748, and apho-
      rism 3.20 (126) above.
228   Cf. aphorism 7.57 (409) below.

(4.80)

[٢١٧] قال أبقراط: من بال دما عبيطا وكان به تقطير البول وأصابه وجع في أسفل بطنه وعانته فإنّ ما يلي مثانته وجع.

(4.81)

[٢١٨] قال أبقراط: من كان يبول دما وقيحا وقشورا وكان لبوله رائحة منكرة فذلك يدلّ على قرحة في مثانته.

(4.82)

٥ [٢١٩] قال أبقراط: من خرجت به بثرة في إحليله فإنّها إذا تقيّحت وانفجرت انقضت علّته.

(4.83)

[٢٢٠] قال أبقراط: من بال من الليل بولا كثيرا دلّ ذلك على أنّ برازه يقلّ.

قال المفسّر: وكذلك بقيّة الفصول بيّنة.

تمّت المقالة الرابعة من شرح الفصول.

---

١ عبيطا: غليظا BP غبيطا C ‖ وكان ... وجع: om. B ٢ ما: om. A ٥ فإنّها ... علّته: om. B ‖ تقيّحت: انفتحت: AC ٦ من: في A ٧ المفسّر: هذه بيّن add. B ٨ من شرح الفصول om. P: من الفصول وشرحها الحمد لله وحده كما هو أهله A من فصول أبقراط والحمد لله وحده B

In the name of God, the Merciful, the Compassionate
The fifth part of the commentary on Hippocrates' *Aphorisms*

(5.1)

[221] Says Hippocrates: Spasms occurring from hellebore (*Helleborus* sp.) are a sign of death.

Says the commentator: Spasms occur as a result of the ingestion of white hellebore (*Veratrum album*).[229] And this is the one intended here, either because of its excessive evacuation or because of the strong movement of the emesis or because of the biting effect on the stomach. To heal this is difficult.

(5.2)

[222] Says Hippocrates: Spasms occurring as a result of a wound are a sign of death.

Says the commentator: This happens because of the inflammation of the nerves and the pain ascends to the brain. Every time Hippocrates refers to something as a sign of death, he means that it is very dangerous and that [the patient] dies in most cases.

(5.3)

[223] Says Hippocrates: If much blood flows from the body and hiccups or spasms occur, it is a bad sign.

Says the commentator: This is clear.

(5.4)

[224] Says Hippocrates: If spasms or hiccups occur after excessive evacuation, it is a bad sign.

Says the commentator: This is clear.

---

229   Cf. Maimonides, *Medical Aphorisms* 21.33, trans. Bos, vol. 4, p. 109: "We should not use white hellebore [*Veratrum album*] in our times because of the bad [physical condition] of the people. Their bodies are full with phlegm; the hellebore attracts it, and the patient suffers from strangulation ..."

بسم الله الرحمن الرحيم

المقالة الخامسة من شرح فصول أبقراط

(5.1)

[٢٢١] قال أبقراط: التشنّج الذي يكون من الحريق من علامات الموت.

قال المفسّر: يعرض التشنّج من شرب الحريق الأبيض وهو المقصود هنا إمّا لكثرة الاستفراغ أو لشدّة حركة القيء أو للدغه المعدة وهذا يعسر برؤه.

(5.2)

[٢٢٢] قال أبقراط: التشنّج الذي يحدث من جراحة من علامات الموت.

قال المفسّر: هذا يكون لتورّم العصب ويتراقى الألم للدماغ. وكلّما يقول أبقراط عن شيء إنّه من علامات الموت يريد به عظم الخطر وإنّه يهلك في الأكثر.

(5.3)

[٢٢٣] قال أبقراط: إذا جرى من البدن دم كثير فحدث فواق أو تشنّج فتلك علامة رديئة.

قال المفسّر: هذا بيّن.

(5.4)

[٢٢٤] قال أبقراط: إذا حدث التشنّج أو الفواق بعد استفراغ مفرط فهو علامة رديئة.

قال المفسّر: هذا بيّن.

---

١ بسم الله الرحمن الرحيم :om. ABP ‖ ٢ المقالة... أبقراط: شرح المقالة الخامسة B ‖ من شرح فصول أبقراط:
om. P من الفصول وشرحها A ٣ من: شرب A add. A ٤ يعرض: بعض A ٧ العصب :om. P ‖ للدماغ:
إلى الدماغ BP ‖ عن شيء: om. BP ٨ يهلك: مهلك BP ٩ فحدث ... رديئة: om. B ‖ أو تشنّج: التشنّج
A ١١ بعد ... رديئة: om. B

(5.5)

[225] Says Hippocrates: If a drunken man suddenly becomes speechless, he will suffer from spasms and die, unless he gets a fever or recovers his speech when [the effects of] his intoxication disappear.

Says the commentator: The spasms occur because of the filling of the nerves. Wine has the property to fill the nerves quickly because it enters in them [quickly] as a result of its thinness and heat. Therefore, if one drinks too much wine, it brings a spasm upon the nerves because of its large quantity. But through its quality, [wine] can also heal and restore that which was corrupted in the nerves since it can heat and dry them. If it cannot do so, the spasm resulting from [too much wine] will necessarily be followed by death. With the afore-mentioned [property] of wine to heal a spasm, it can also be healed by fever. Intoxication is the damage done to the head by the consumption of [too much] wine.[230]

(5.6)

[226] Says Hippocrates: If someone is attacked by tetanus, he will die in four days, [unless] he survives these, for then he will recover.

Says the commentator: Tetanus is a very acute illness because the nature [of the patient] cannot bear the strain of the stretching [of the muscles caused by it], because it consists of backwards spasm (opisthotonus) and forwards spasm (emprosthotonus). It ends in the first of the cycles of the critical days.[231]

(5.7)

[227] Says Hippocrates: If someone is attacked by epilepsy before the growth of pubic hair (i.e., puberty), he may experience a change[232] [of the disease] (i.e., cure). But if it happens to someone after the age of twenty-five, he will die while still having [this disease].

---

230   Cf. ibid. 17.26, p. 27: "It is not good for [adult] persons to drink more than a moderate amount of wine, because it rapidly brings a person to anger, indecency, and obscene language and makes the rational part of his soul confused and his subtle mind sluggish. *De sanitate tuenda* 1."

231   Cf. aphorism 4.57 (194) above.

232   "change [of the disease] (i.e., cure)" (الاستقال): Cf. Galen, *In Hippocratis Aphorismos commentarius* 5.7, ed. Kühn, vol. 17b, p. 790: μετάστασιν; Hippocrates, *Aphorisms*, trans. Littré, vol. 4, p. 535: "guérison;" trans. Jones, p. 159: "cure." In the sense of "cure," the Arabic term is a non-attested semantic borrowing from the Greek.

(5.5)

[٢٢٥] قال أبقراط: إذا عرض لسكران سكات بغتة فإنّه يتشنّج ويموت إلّا أن تحدث به حمّى أو يتكلّم إذا حضرت الساعة التي يتحلّل فيها خماره.

قال المفسّر: هذا التشنّج يحدث من قبل امتلاء العصب ومن شأن الخمر أن تملأ العصب سريعا لأنّه يغوص للطفه وحرارته. فالشراب إذا أكثر منه فهو بكثرة حجمه يجلب للعصب تشنّج إلّا أنّه بكيفيّته يداوي ويصلح ما أفسد في العصب إذ كان يسخنه ويجفّفه. فتى لم يقدر أن يفعل ذلك فيجب ضرورة أن يلحق التشنّج الحادث منه الموت. وبالقوة التي قلنا إنّ الخمر يبرأ بها التشنّج قد تشفيه أيضا الحمّى. والخمار هو الضرر الحادث في الرأس من شرب الخمر.

(5.6)

[٢٢٦] قال أبقراط: من اعتراه التمدّد فإنّه يهلك في أربعة أيّام فإن جاوز الأربعة فإنّه يبرأ.

قال المفسّر: التمدّد مرض حادّ جدّا إذ كانت الطبيعة لا تحتمل تعب تمديده لأنّه مركّب من التشنّج الذي يكون إلى خلف والتشنّج الذي يكون إلى قدّام فانقضاؤه يكون في أوّل دور من أدوار أيّام البحران.

(5.7)

[٢٢٧] قال أبقراط: من أصابه الصرع قبل نبات الشعر في العانة فإنّه يحدث له انتقال. فأمّا من عرض له وقد أتى عليه من السنين خمس وعشرون سنة فإنّه يموت وهو به.

Says the commentator: Galen says: With "change" he means the end of the illness. This occurs as a result of an improvement of the cold, viscous humor, which produces the epilepsy, that is the moist, phlegmatic [humor], [and this happens] through a change [of his temperament] into dryness because of his age, through physical exercise, and through a drying regimen in combination with appropriate medications. In this aphorism, Hippocrates [only] refers to the change (cure), which occurs because of [advancing] age. The time of the growth of pubic hair (puberty) occurs between the end of the fourteenth year and the twenty-fifth year [of age].[233]

(5.8)
[228] Says Hippocrates: If someone is afflicted by pleurisy and is not cleansed thereof in fourteen days, his condition will lead to empyema.[234]

Says the commentator: Hippocrates calls "cleansing" the evacuation of the humor that produces pleurisy by expectoration.

(5.9)
[229] Says Hippocrates: Phthisis occurs mostly between the ages of eighteen and thirty-five.

Says the commentator: He has already said before that phthisis is an illness of young people.[235] He mentions it [again] since he discusses illnesses of the chest and lung.

(5.10)
[230] Says Hippocrates: If someone is afflicted by angina and is saved from it, but the superfluity [that produced the illness] turns to the lungs, he will die within seven days. If he survives these, he will develop empyema.

Says the commentator: It is likely that he (i.e., Hippocrates) had much experience with these and similar illnesses regarding this kind of change. There is no doubt that this [change] and similar ones are the rule.

233　Cf. Galen, ibid., pp. 790–792; cf. Maimonides, *Medical Aphorisms* 3.2, trans. Bos, vol. 1, p. 34: "The age between fourteen and twenty-five years is that in which the pubic hair grows."

234　"empyema" (تقيح): Cf. Galen, ibid. 5.8, p. 793: ἐμπύημα; Hippocrates, *Aphorisms*, trans. Littré, vol. 4, p. 535: "un empyème;" trans. Jones, p. 159: "empyema." Ullmann, *Wörterbuch*, p. 239, only mentions the Arabic: "الخراجات التي تقيح (= Arist. HA 624 a 17)."

235　Cf. aphorism 3.29 (135) above.

قال المفسّر: قال جالينوس: يريد بالانتقال انقضاء المرض وذلك يكون بإصلاح الخلط البارد اللزج المولّد للصرع وهو بلغمي رطب بانتقال السنّ إلى اليبس وبالرياضة والتدبير المجفّف مع الأدوية الموافقة. وأبقراط ذكر في هذا الفصل التغيير الذي يكون بسبب السنّ ومدّة زمان نبات الشعر في العانة بين انقضاء الأسبوعين وبين خمس وعشرين سنة.

(5.8)

٥   [٢٢٨] قال أبقراط: من أصابته ذات الجنب فلم ينق في أربعة عشر يوما فإنّ حاله يؤول إلى التقييح.

قال المفسّر: أبقراط يسمّي استفراغ الخلط المولّد لذات الجنب بالنفث نقاء.

(5.9)

[٢٢٩] قال أبقراط: أكثر ما يكون السلّ في السنين اللاتي بين ثماني عشرة سنة وبين خمس ثلاثين سنة.

قال المفسّر: قد تقدّم أنّ السلّ من أمراض الشباب ولمّا ذكر أمراض الصدر والرئة ذكر هذا أيضا.

(5.10)

[٢٣٠] قال أبقراط: من أصابته ذبحة فتخلّص منها فمال الفضل إلى رئته فإنّه يموت في سبعة أيّام فإن
١٠   جاوزها صار إلى التقييح.

قال المفسّر: يوشك أنّه كثرت له تجربة هذه الأمراض وأمثالها بهذا النحو من الانتقال ولا ريب أنّ هذا وأشباهه إنّما يريد به أنّه أكثري.

---

٥ فلم ... التقييح: om. B   ٧ في ... ثلاثين سنة: om. B ‖ عشر: عشرة A   ٩-١٠ فتخلّص ... التقييح: om. B
١١ تجربة: التجربة في P

(5.11)

[231] Says Hippocrates: If a person suffers from phthisis and expectorates sputum that is foul-smelling when it is poured on hot coals, and if the hair on his head is falling off, it is a fatal sign.

Says the commentator: The foul smell is evidence of the corruption of the humors and their severe putrefaction. The loss of hair confirms what is [already] indicated by the corruption of the humors and also indicates that the organs lack nutrition.

(5.12)

[232] Says Hippocrates: If a patient with phthisis loses his hair and then suffers from diarrhea, he will die.

Says the commentator: Diarrhea in these [patients] indicates that their strength is weak and this indicates that death is near.

(5.13)

[233] Says Hippocrates: If someone spits up frothy blood, the discharge comes from the lungs.

Says the commentator: It is clear that [when] blood emerges, which is frothy, it hails from the substance and essence of the lungs.

(5.14)

[234] Says Hippocrates: If someone with phthisis gets diarrhea, it is a sign of death.

Says the commentator: Diarrhea in patients with phthisis is an indication of death. If this occurs with foul-smelling sputum and loss of hair, it indicates that [death] is near, as previously mentioned.[236]

(5.15)

[235] Says Hippocrates: If the condition of someone with pleurisy results in empyema, the illness will end if he is cleansed from the pus within forty days from its outbreak. But if he is not cleansed within this period, he will develop phthisis.

---

236   Cf. aphorisms 5.11–12 (231–232) above.

(5.11)

[٢٣١] قال أبقراط: إذا كان بإنسان السلّ فكان ما يقذفه بسعال من البزاق منكر الرائحة إذا ألقي على الجمر وكان شعر الرأس ينتثر فذلك من علامات الموت.

قال المفسّر: نتن الرائحة دليل على فساد الأخلاط وشدّة عفنها وذهاب شعر الرأس ممّا يؤكّد دلالة فساد الأخلاط وأيضا يدلّ على عدم الأعضاء للاغتذاء.

(5.12)

٥ [٢٣٢] قال أبقراط: من تساقط شعر رأسه من أصحاب السلّ ثمّ حدث له اختلاف فإنّه يموت.

قال المفسّر: اختلاف هؤلاء دليل على ضعف القوة فلذلك يدلّ على موت قريب.

(5.13)

[٢٣٣] قال أبقراط: من قذف دما زبديا فقذفه إياه إنّما هو من رئته.

قال المفسّر: بيّن هو أنّ الدم الذي يأتي زبديا فهو من جرم الرئة وجوهرها.

(5.14)

[٢٣٤] قال أبقراط: إذا حدث بمن به السلّ اختلاف دلّ على الموت.

١٠ قال المفسّر: إسهال أصحاب السلّ دليل الموت فإن كان ذلك مع ما نتن رائحة ما ينفث وتساقط الشعر فيدلّ على قربه كما تقدّم.

(5.15)

[٢٣٥] قال أبقراط: من آلت به الحال في ذات الجنب إلى التقييح فإنّه إن استنقى في أربعين يوما من اليوم الذي انفجرت فيه المدّة فإنّ علّته تنقضي. وإن لم يستنق في هذه المدّة فإنّه يقع في السلّ.

---

١ البزاق: البصاق P ٢ الجمر: النار A ‖ الرأس: منه A add. ٥ من ... يموت: .B om. ١٠ دليل: على add.
P ١٢-١٣ فإنّه ... السلّ: .B om. ١٢ استنقى: استسقى C

Says the commentator: If the matter (i.e., pus) that broke forth and occurred in the cavity of the chest is not excreted, it will putrefy and solidify and cause ulceration of the lungs.

(5.16)
[236] Says Hippocrates: Heat has the following harmful effects on those who use it frequently: It softens the flesh, weakens the nerves, benumbs the mind, it causes hemorrhages and fainting, and patients with these [afflictions] are overtaken by death.

Says the commentator: He says that if someone uses heat excessively, it softens his flesh and weakens the nerves, that is to say, it makes them soft through the dissolution of its substance by the heat. Galen says that with the statement "it benumbs the mind," he means that it weakens the mind and takes away its strength by the dissolution of the substance of the nerves. And [that] it is clear that a hemorrhage is followed by fainting and fainting by death.[237]

(5.17)
[237] Says Hippocrates: Cold produces spasms, tetanus, blackening (of flesh from mortification), and rigors, which are accompanied by fever.

Says the commentator: This is clear.

(5.18)
[238] Says Hippocrates: Cold is harmful for the bones, teeth, nerves, brain, and the spinal marrow. Heat, however, is good and beneficial for them.

Says the commentator: This is clear.

(5.19)
[239] Says Hippocrates: Any [part] that is chilled should be heated, unless a hemorrhage has to be feared.

Says the commentator: This is clear.

---

237   Cf. Galen, *In Hippocratis Aphorismos commentarius* 5.16, ed. Kühn, vol. 17b, pp. 801–802.

قال المفسّر: إذا لم تخرج المادّة التي انفجرت وحصلت في فضاء الصدر فإنّها تعفن وتجمد وتقرّح الرئة.

(5.16)

[٢٣٦] قال أبقراط: الحارّ يضرّ من أكثر استعماله هذه المضارّ: يؤنّث اللحم ويفنخ العصب ويخدّر الذهن ويجلب سيلان الدم والغشي ويلحق أصحاب ذلك الموت.

قال المفسّر: يقول إنّ من أفرط في استعمال الحارّ فإنّه يرخي لحمه ويفنخ العصب يعني يرخيه بتحليل

٥ الحرارة لجوهره. وقوله ويخدّر الذهن قال جالينوس: يريد به يضعف الذهن ويذهب بقوّته بتحلّل جوهر العصب وبيّن هو أن يتبع سيلان الدم الغشي ويتبع الغشي الموت.

(5.17)

[٢٣٧] قال أبقراط: وأمّا البارد فيحدث التشنّج والتمدّد والاسوداد والنافض التي يكون معها حمّى.

قال المفسّر: هذا بيّن.

(5.18)

[٢٣٨] قال أبقراط: البارد ضارّ للعظام والأسنان والعصب والدماغ والنخاع. وأمّا الحارّ فهو موافق

١٠ نافع لها.

قال المفسّر: هذا بيّن.

(5.19)

[٢٣٩] قال أبقراط: كلّ موضع قد برد فينبغي أن يسخن إلّا أن يخاف عليه انفجار الدم منه.

قال المفسّر: هذا بيّن.

---

٢ أكثر: من C add. ٣-٢ هذه ... الموت: om.B ٢ اللحم: اللم P ٥ ويخدّر: ويكدر B ٧ والتمدّد ... حمّى: om.B ٩ للعظام: للطعام A ‖ وأمّا الحارّ فهو: والحارّ A ١٠ نافع: om.A ١٢ قد: om.A C¹ ‖ إلّا ... منه: om.B

(5.20)

[240] Says Hippocrates: Cold has a biting effect on ulcers, hardens the skin, causes pain without suppuration, blackens [the flesh from mortification], causes feverish rigors, spasms, and tetanus.

Says the commentator: This is clear.

(5.21)

[241] Says Hippocrates: Sometimes, if one pours a large quantity of cold water in the middle of summer over a fleshy[238] youth, who is suffering from tetanus without a [previous] ulcer, one brings a recovery of much heat, and he is saved by that heat.

Says the commentator: This is clear.

(5.22)

[242] Says Hippocrates: Heat causes suppuration, but not in the case of every wound. When it does, it is one of the best indications that[239] one can be confident and reassured [to recover]. It softens the skin, makes it thin, alleviates pain, annihilates[240] the evil (harm) caused by rigors, spasms, and tetanus, and relieves heaviness occurring in the head. It is most beneficial for broken bones, especially when they are exposed, and above all for bones[241] in the head. Also for everything that is affected by mortification or ulcers because of the cold, for corroding herpes, for [ailments of] the anus, genitals, uterus, and urinary bladder—for those who suffer from these ailments, heat has[242] a beneficial and healing effect, while cold is harmful and fatal for them.

Says the commentator: The formation of pus is a good sign on which one can rely in the case of wounds, because it is a type of concoction, as you know. Not every wound forms pus. All bad wounds and corrosive wounds, which are difficult to heal, do not form pus. The rest of what he mentions is clear because every part of the body with nerves and [every] bone is harmed by cold.

---

238   "fleshy" (حسن اللحم): Cf. ibid. 5.21, p. 807: εὐσάρκος; Hippocrates, *Aphorisms*, trans. Littré, vol. 4, p. 539: "bien en chair;" trans. Jones, p. 163: "muscular;" cf. Liddell/Scott, *Greek-English Lexicon*, p. 731: "fleshy, in good condition."

239   "that one can be confident and reassured [to recover]" (الثقة والأمن): Cf. Galen, ibid. 5.22: ἐς ἀσφαλείην; Hippocrates, ibid., trans. Littré, p. 541: "de salut;" trans. Jones: "of recovery."

240   "annihilates the evil (harm)" (ويكسر عادية): Cf. Galen, ibid.: παρηγορικόν; Hippocrates, ibid., trans. Littré: "calme;" trans. Jones: "soothes."

241   "bones" (عظام): Cf. Galen, ibid., p. 808: ἕλκεα; Hippocrates, ibid., trans. Littré: "les plaies;" trans. Jones: "wounds."

242   "has a ... healing effect" (شاف): Cf. Galen, ibid.: κρῖνον; Hippocrates, ibid., trans. Littré: "décide les crises;" trans. Jones: "conduces to a crisis." See also Barry, *Syriac Medicine*, p. 138.

(5.20)

[٢٤٠] قال أبقراط: البارد لذّاع للقروح ويصلّب الجلد ويحدث من الوجع ما لا يكون معه تقيُّح ويسوّد ويحدث النافض التي تكون معها حمّى والتشنّج والتمدّد.

قال المفسّر: هذا بيّن.

(5.21)

[٢٤١] قال أبقراط: وربّما صبّ على من به تمدّد من غير قرحة وهو شابّ حسن اللحم في وسط من ٥ الصيف ماء بارد كثير وأحدث فيه انعطاف من حرارة كثيرة فكان تخلّصه بتلك الحرارة.

قال المفسّر: هذا بيّن.

(5.22)

[٢٤٢] قال أبقراط: الحارّ مقيّح لكن ليس في كلّ قرحة وذلك من أعظم العلامات دلالة على الثقة والأمن ويبيّن الجلد ويرقّقه ويسكّن الوجع ويكسر عادية النافض والتشنّج والتمدّد ويحلّ الثقل العارض في الرأس. وهو من أوفق الأشياء لكسر العظام وخاصّة المعرّى منها ومن العظام خاصّة لعظام الرأس ولكلّ ما أماته البرد وأقرحه وللقروح التي تسعى وتتأكّل وللمقعدة والفرج والرحم ١٠ والمثانة فالحارّ لأصحاب هذه العلل نافع شاف والبارد لهم ضارّ قاتل.

قال المفسّر: التقيّح علامة موثوق بها في القروح جيّدة لأنّه نوع من النضج كما علمت. وليس كلّ قرحة تتقيّح لأنّ القروح الخبيثة كلّها والعسرة البروء المتأكّلة لا يتولّد فيها قيح. وسائر ما ذكر بيّن لأنّ كلّ عضو عصباني والعظام أيضا يضرّها البارد.

١-٢ ويصلّب ... والتمدّد:om. A ١ من الوجع:من الجلد وجع P ٢ التي:الذي A ٤-٥ من ... الحرارة: om. B ٧ مقيّح:يقيح A ٧-١١ لكن ... شاف:إلى قوله B ٨ عادية:عادة P ١٢-١٣ لأنّه ... القروح: om. A ١٣ لأنّ: كلّ add. BP ‖ والعسرة:أو العسرة C ١٤ والعظام:om. P والقرحة B

(5.23)

[243] Says Hippocrates: Cold should be applied to the following [parts of the body]: [to the parts] where there is a hemorrhage or where it is imminent. One should not apply it to the actual spot from where bleeding occurs, but around [whatever spot] it comes from. [It should also be applied to] inflamed tumors and [other] inflammations,243 which tend to red and to the color of fresh blood,244 because it (i.e., cold) blackens [inflammations] when it is applied to them when245 the blood is old. [It should also be applied] in the case of the swelling called "erysipelas" when there is no ulceration, because it is harmful when ulcers have formed.

Says the commentator: This is clear.

(5.24)

[244] Says Hippocrates: Cold things such as snow and ice are harmful to the chest, provoke cough, cause hemorrhage and catarrhs.

Says the commentator: This is clear.

(5.25)

[245] Says Hippocrates: Swellings in the joints and pains [in the joints] without ulceration, and pains of those who suffer from gout or from bruises, which246 occur in places where there are nerves, and most similar cases, are relieved and reduced if one pours much cold water over them. The pain is relieved because it causes numbness, for also a247 small amount of numbness relieves the pain.

Says the commentator: The pain is relieved in such places because [the cold] puts an end to [the248 pain itself], or because it benumbs one's sensation [of pain].

---

243   "inflammations" (التلدّع): Cf. Galen, ibid. 5.23, p. 811: ἐπιφλογίσματα; Hippocrates, ibid., trans. Littré: "les phlogoses;" trans. Jones, p. 165: "inflamed pustules;" cf. Ullmann, *Wörterbuch*, p. 393.

244   I.e., when these inflammations are recent.

245   "when the blood is old" (فيما قد عتق فيه الدم): Cf. Galen, *In Hippocratis Aphorismos commentarius* 5.23, ed. Kühn, vol. 17b, p. 811: ἐπεὶ τά γε παλαιά; Hippocrates, *Aphorisms*, trans. Littré, vol. 4, p. 541: "les inflammations anciennes;" trans. Jones, p. 163: "old inflammations."

246   "which occur in places where there are nerves": Missing in Hippocrates, ibid., ed. Littré, p. 540; Galen, ibid., p. 813.

247   "a small amount" (اليسير): Galen, ibid. 5.25, p. 814: μέτριος; Hippocrates, ibid., trans. Littré, p. 543: "modéré;" trans. Jones, p. 165: "in moderation."

248   "[the pain itself]": Lit., "that which causes the pain."

(5.23)

[٢٤٣] قال أبقراط: فأمّا البارد فإنّما ينبغي أن يستعمله في هذه المواضع أعني في المواضع التي يجري
منها الدم أو هو مزمع بأن يجري منها. وليس ينبغي أن يستعمل في نفس الموضع الذي يجري منه لكنّ
حوله ومن حيث يجيء وفي ما كان من الأورام الحارّة والتلذّع مائل إلى الحمرة ولون الدم الطري
لأنّه إن استعمل فيما قد عتق فيه الدم سوّده وفي الورم الذي يسمّى الحمرة إذا لم تكن معه قرحة لأنّ

٥   ما كانت معه منه قرحة فهو يضرّه.

قال المفسّر: هذا بيّن.

(5.24)

[٢٤٤] قال أبقراط: إنّ الأشياء الباردة مثل الثلج والجمد ضارّة للصدر مهيّجة للسعال جالبة لانفجار
الدم والنزل.

قال المفسّر: هذا بيّن.

(5.25)

١٠ [٢٤٥] قال أبقراط: الأورام التي تكون في المفاصل والأوجاع التي تكون من غير قرحة وأوجاع
أصحاب النقرس وأصحاب الفسخ الحادث في المواضع العصبية وأكثر ما أشبه هذه فإنّه إذا صبّ عليها
ماء بارد كثير سكّنها وأضرها وسكّن الوجع بإحداثه الخدر والخدر أيضا اليسير مسكّن للوجع.

قال المفسّر: يسكّن الوجع في مثل هذه المواضع بقطعه للسبب المولّد له أو بإخداره للحسّ.

---

١ أعني في المواضع P.om أعني إلى المواضع A   ١-٤ أعني ... قرحة B.om   ٢ منه P.om   ٣ والتلذّع:
والتلكّع AC والتلديغ P   ٤ قد P.om   ٥ فهو يضرّه: فهي قصيرة (مضرة P¹) BP   ٨-٧ ضارّة ... والنزل:
B.om   ١٢-١٠ والأوجاع ... الخدر: إلى قوله B   ١٢ كثير B.om

(5.26)

[246] Says Hippocrates: Water, which quickly gets hot and quickly gets cold, is the lightest.

Says the commentator: It is clear that with "heaviness" and "lightness," he means the rapidity with which it leaves the stomach or its delay there.

(5.27)

[247] Says Hippocrates: If someone desires to drink at night because of intense thirst and if he sleeps after that, it is a good [sign].

Says the commentator: If he sleeps after drinking the water, the humor that caused the thirst will be concocted during the sleep. But drinking [water] during the night should only be allowed in the case of severe thirst.

(5.28)

[248] Says Hippocrates: Fomenting[249] with aromatic herbs brings about menstruation. It would also be beneficial in many other cases, if it did not cause heaviness in the head.

Says the commentator: He says that fomenting[250] with aromatic herbs induces the flow of menstrual blood or the blood of parturition if these are withheld, because it thins the blood if it is thick, or it opens an obstruction if it is there, or it widens the openings of the vessels if they are closed. It would also be beneficial for warming cold places or drying moisture (humors) if it did not fill the head, because everything that is hot ascends and causes headache.

---

249   "Fomenting" (تكميد): The Arabic term تكميد stands for Greek πυρίη; cf. Galen, *In Hippocratis Aphorismos commentarius* 5.28, ed. Kühn, vol. 17b, p. 817; Hippocrates, *Aphorisms*, trans. Littré, vol. 4, p. 543: "Les fumigations;" trans. Jones, p. 165: "vapour baths;" cf. Liddell/Scott, *Greek-English Lexicon*, p. 1556, s.v. πυρία: "vapour-bath;" Ullmann, *Wörterbuch*, pp. 575–576: "Dampfbad, Bähung;" WKAS, vol. 1, p. 452, s.v. كمد , "to make a warm poultice, to apply a warm pack" (cf. Freytag, *Lexicon Arabico-Latinum*, vol. 4, p. 58: "Panno calefacto fovit *membrum* dolens").

250   "fomenting with aromatic herbs induces the flow of menstrual blood": Cf. Maimonides, *Medical Aphorisms* 16.2, trans. Bos, vol. 4, pp. 1, 3: "Four or five days before menstruation the woman should adhere to a thinning diet and then be bled from her legs to stimulate the menstrual blood. Along with this, she should ingest remedies with hydromel, water mint [*Menta aquatica*], and cultivated mint. Stronger than these are savin [*Juniperus sabina*] and Cretan dittany [*Origanum dictamnus*], either in the form of a decoction prepared from one of these or its substance [only]. The best time to take these drugs that stimulate the [menstrual] blood is when the woman has left the bath and dried herself. Similarly, the ingestion of the *hiera* at that time stimulates menstrual flow. *De venae sectione*."

(5.26)

[٢٤٦] قال أبقراط: الماء الذي يسخن سريعا ويبرد سريعا فهو أخفّ المياه.

قال المفسّر: بيّن أنّه يريد هنا بالثقل والخفّة سرعة خروجه عن المعدة أو بطؤه فيها.

(5.27)

[٢٤٧] قال أبقراط: من دعته شهوته إلى الشرب بالليل وكان عطشه شديدا فإنّه إن نام بعد ذلك فذلك محمود.

٥ قال المفسّر: إذا نام بعد شرب الماء أنضج النوم الخلط الموجب للعطش ولا يؤذن في الشرب بالليل إلّا من شدّة العطش.

(5.28)

[٢٤٨] قال أبقراط: التكميد بالأفاويه يجلب الدم الذي يجيء من النساء. وقد كان يستنفع به في مواضع آخر كثيرة لولا اتّه يحدث في الرأس ثقلا.

قال المفسّر: يقول إنّ التكميد بالأفاويه يبعث دم الطمث أو دم النفاس إذا انعاق لأنّ ذلك يرقّق

١٠ الدم إن كان غليظا أو يفتح سدّة إن كانت هناك أو يوسع أفام العروق إن كانت انضمّت. وقد كان يستنفع به أيضا في تسخين المواضع الباردة أو تجفيف الرطوبة لولا كونه يملأ الرأس لأنّ كلّ حارّ يرقّ للعلوّ ويصدّع.

---

١ ويبرد ... المياه: om. B ٢ عن: من P ٣ الشرب: om. A ٤-٣ الشرب: شرب الماء A وكان ... محمود: om. B ٦ إلّا:

om. A ٨-٧ يجلب ... ثقلا: om. A ٧ به: B om. B ٩ يبعث: إن كان غليظا add. A ‖ انعاق: اعتاق A

٩-١٠ يرقّق الدم: رقّق للدم A ١٠ أفام: أفواه A

(5.29)

[249] Says Hippocrates: It is proper to administer purgative drugs to pregnant women when the humors in their body flare up from when the fetus is four months old until it becomes seven months old. But [in the latter case], one should proceed to administer [a smaller dose]. When [a fetus] is younger [than four months] or older [than seven months], one should be careful [in the administration of these drugs].[251]

Says the commentator: This aphorism is either repeated [inadvertently] by him, or he has done so on purpose to lead the discussion to [that] of women's diseases.

(5.30)

[250] Says Hippocrates: If a pregnant woman is bled, she will have a miscarriage, especially if the [fetus] is large.[252]

Says the commentator: This is clear.

(5.31)

[251] Says Hippocrates: If a woman is pregnant and attacked by one of the acute diseases, it is a fatal sign.

Says the commentator: If it is one of the acute diseases which is accompanied by fever it is fatal because of its bad temperament which makes it necessary to inhale much air while the organs are compressed and because of the lack of nutrition. If, for instance, [the disease] is hemiplegia or spasms, she cannot bear the strong pain or the stretching [of the muscles] because of the heavy burden that she carries.

(5.32)

[252] Says Hippocrates: If a woman vomits blood and then begins to menstruate, the vomiting [of blood] will stop.

Says the commentator: This is clear.

---

251   Cf. aphorism 4.1 (138) above.
252   Aphorisms 5.30–31 (250–251) are reversed in some of the Greek manuscripts, cf. Hippocrates, *Aphorisms*, ed. Littré, vol. 4, p. 542.

(5.29)

[٢٤٩] قال أبقراط: ينبغي أن تُسقى الحامل الدواء إذا كانت الأخلاط في بدنها هائجة منذ يأتي على الجنين أربعة أشهر وإلى أن يأتي عليه سبعة أشهر ويكون التقدّم على هذا أقلّ. وأمّا ما كان أصغر من ذلك وأكبر فينبغي أن يتوقّى عليه.

قال المفسّر: إمّا أنّه تكرّر له هذا الفصل أو كرّره بالقصد ليوصل الكلام في أمراض النساء.

(5.30)

٥ [٢٥٠] قال أبقراط: المرأة الحامل إن فُصدت أسقطت وخاصّة إن كان طفلها قد عظم.

قال المفسّر: هذا بيّن.

(5.31)

[٢٥١] قال أبقراط: إذا كانت المرأة حاملا فاعتراها بعض الأمراض الحادّة فذلك من علامات الموت.

قال المفسّر: إن كان من الأمراض الحادّة التي معها حمّى فيقتل بسوء المزاج المحوّج إلى استنشاق ١٠ هواء كثير والأعضاء مضغوطة وبتقليل الغذاء. وإن كان مثل الفالج والتشنّج فهي لا تحتمل شدّة الألم أو التمدّد لما تحمله من الثقل.

(5.32)

[٢٥٢] قال أبقراط: المرأة إذا كانت نتقيّاً دما فإن بعثت طمثها انقطع ذلك القيء.

قال المفسّر: هذا بيّن.

١-٣ إذا ... أكبر: إلى قوله B ٣ أكبر: منه A add. A ٥ وخاصّة: وخصّوصا A ‖ وخاصّة ... عظم: om. B
٧-٨ بعض ... الموت: om. B ٩ التي: om. A ١٠ تحتمل: تحمل B

(5.33)

[253] Says Hippocrates: When menstruation stops, a nosebleed is good.

  Says the commentator: This is also clear.

(5.34)

[254] Says Hippocrates: If a pregnant woman suffers from constant diarrhea, one cannot be free from fear that she will have a miscarriage.

  Says the commentator: If the expulsive faculty becomes strongly active in those parts, which are close to the uterus, it has to be feared that also the expulsive faculty, which is in the uterus, will become active.

(5.35)

[255] Says Hippocrates: If a woman who suffers from an[253] affliction of the uterus or difficult labor has an attack of sneezing, it is a good [sign].

  Says the commentator: With "an affliction of the uterus," he means hysterical suffocation and the sneezing indicates that nature is aroused to carry out its activities. It is also that which causes the organs to get rid of the harmful humors that stick and adhere to them. In a similar manner sneezing cures hiccups.[254]

(5.36)

[256] Says Hippocrates: If the menstrual blood of a woman changes[255] its color and does not always arrive at the [normal] time (i.e., is irregular), it indicates that her body requires cleansing.

  Says the commentator: This is clear.

(5.37)

[257] Says Hippocrates: If the breasts of a pregnant woman suddenly become thin, she will have a miscarriage.

---

253 "an affliction of the uterus" (علّة الأرحام): Cf. Galen, *In Hippocratis Aphorismos commentarius* 5.35, ed. Kühn, vol. 17b, p. 824: ὑστερικῶν; Hippocrates, ibid., trans. Littré, p. 545: "hystérie;" trans. Jones, p. 167: "hysteria."

254 For a discussion of hysterical suffocation and its treatment in medieval Islamic medicine, see Ibn al-Jazzār, *On Sexual Diseases* 12, ed. and trans. Bos, pp. 160–171 (Arabic text); 276–281 (English trans.).

255 "changes its color" (متغيّر اللون): Cf. Galen, *In Hippocratis Aphorismos commentarius* 5.36, ed. Kühn, vol. 17b, p. 825: ἄχροα; Hippocrates, *Aphorisms*, trans. Littré, vol. 4, p. 545: "de mauvaise couleur;" trans. Jones, p. 167: "not of the proper colour."

(5.33)

[٢٥٣] قال أبقراط: إذا انقطع الطمث فالرعاف محمود.

قال المفسّر: هذا أيضا بيّن.

(5.34)

[٢٥٤] قال أبقراط: المرأة الحامل إن لجّ عليها استطلاق البطن لم يؤمن عليها أن تسقط.

قال المفسّر: إذا تحرّكت القوة الدافعة في تلك الأعضاء المجاورة للرحم بقوّة فيخاف أيضا أن تتحرّك

٥ قوّة الرحم الدافعة.

(5.35)

[٢٥٥] قال أبقراط: إذا كان بالمرأة علّة الأرحام أو عسر ولادها فأصابها عطاس فذلك محمود.

قال المفسّر: يريد بعلّة الأرحام اختناق الرحم. والعطاس يدلّ على تنبيه الطبيعة لتفعل أفعالها وهو

أيضا سبب لتنفض الأعضاء ما لزق بها وتشبّث فيها من الأخلاط المؤذية وبهذه الجهة يبرئ العطاس

الفواق.

(5.36)

١٠ [٢٥٦] قال أبقراط: إذا كان طمث المرأة متغيّر اللون ولم يكن مجيئة في وقته دائما دلّ ذلك على أنّ

بدنها يحتاج إلى تنقية.

قال المفسّر: هذا بيّن.

(5.37)

[٢٥٧] قال أبقراط: إذا كانت المرأة حاملا فضمر ثديها بغتة فإنّها تسقط.

---

٢ أيضا: .om B ٦ أو ... محمود: .om B ‖ فأصابها: فافص بها؟ A ١٠-١١ ولم ... تنقية: .om B

Says the commentator: The interrelationship between the breasts and the uterus is well known. When [the breasts] become thin, it indicates that [only] a small amount of food reaches them. If the nutrition that reaches the uterus also decreases, the fetus is aborted.[256]

(5.38)

[258] Says Hippocrates: If a woman is pregnant with twins and one of her breasts becomes thin all[257] at once, she will lose one of the twins. If the right breast becomes thin, she will lose the male child; if the left breast becomes thin, she will lose the female child.

Says the commentator: In most cases, the male child is on the right side.[258]

(5.39)

[259] Says Hippocrates: If a woman, who is not pregnant and has not given birth, [produces] milk, her menstruation has stopped.

Says the commentator: Only rarely during amenorrhea do the vessels connected to the breasts become overfilled resulting in the production of milk due to the excess of blood reaching the breasts. It seems to me that this only happens when the body of the woman is extremely clean[259] and her nourishment extremely good.[260]

(5.40)

[260] Says Hippocrates: When blood congeals in the breasts of a woman, it indicates that[261] her condition is [one of] madness.[262]

---

256   Cf. Maimonides, *Medical Aphorisms* 16.26, trans. Bos, vol. 4, p. 11: "When the breasts of a pregnant woman shrink so much that they become emaciated and thin, you should expect that she will miscarry. If she is pregnant with twins and one of her breasts becomes emaciated and thin, one of her fetuses will be aborted. *De locis affectis* 6."

257   "all at once" (دفعة): Missing in the Greek text (cf. Hippocrates, *Aphorisms*, ed. Littré, vol. 4, p. 544; ed. Jones, p. 166), in Ḥunayn's Arabic translation of Hippocrates' *Aphorisms*, ed. Tytler, p. 46, in the Greek text of Galen's commentary (cf. Galen, *In Hippocratis Aphorismos commentarius* 5.38, ed. Kühn, vol. 17b, pp. 828–829), and in Ḥunayn's translation of Galen's commentary (cf. E, fol. 36ª).

258   Cf. Maimonides, *Medical Aphorisms* 16.25, trans. Bos, vol. 4, p. 11: "Male [fetuses] are mostly conceived [by the woman] on the right side of the uterus and female [ones] on the left side. The reverse of this situation only happens rarely. *De locis affectis* 6."

259   I.e., free from superfluous humors.

260   On the subject of amenorrhea in medieval Islamic medicine, see Ibn al-Jazzār, *On Sexual Diseases* 9, ed. and trans. Bos, pp. 125–143 (Arabic text); 262–269 (English trans.).

261   "that her condition is [one of]": Missing in the Greek text of both Hippocrates (cf. *Apho-*

قال المفسّر: قد علم مشاركة الثديين للرحم فإذا ضمرتا فدلّ ذلك على قلّة الغذاء الواصل إليهما فإذا قلّ

الغذاء الواصل للرحم أيضا سقط الجنين.

(5.38)

[٢٥٨] قال أبقراط: إذا كانت المرأة حاملا فضمر أحد ثدييها دفعة وكان حملها تؤما فإنّها تسقط أحد

طفليها. فإن كان الضامر هو الثدي الأيمن أسقطت الذكر وإن كان الضامر هو الثدي الأيسر أسقطت

٥   الأنثى.

قال المفسّر: الذكر في الجانب الأيمن على الأمر الأكثر.

(5.39)

[٢٥٩] قال أبقراط: إذا كانت المرأة ليست بحامل ولم تكن ولدت ثمّ كان لها لبن فطمثها قد ارتفع.

قال المفسّر: في الندرة عند احتباس الطمث تمتلئ العروق المتّصلة بالثدي امتلاءا كثيرا فيحدث اللبن

لكثرة الدم الواصل إلى الثدي ويبدو لي أنّ هذا لا يصحّ إلّا أن كان بدن المرأة في غاية النقاء وكانت

١٠   أغذيتها في غاية الجودة.

(5.40)

[٢٦٠] قال أبقراط: إذا انعقد للمرأة دم في ثدييها دلّ ذلك من حالها على جنون.

٣-٤ وكان ... الأيسر: إلى قوله B ‖ ٧ ولم ... ارتفع: om. B ‖ ٩ الدم: add. A ‖ هذا: الأمر add. A ‖ أن:

om. A ‖ دم: om. P ‖ في ثدييها: om. P ‖ انعقد: تعقّد P ‖ ١١ دم: om. A

risms 5.40, ed. Littré, vol. 4, p. 544; ed. Jones, p. 168) and Galen (cf. *In Hippocratis Aphoris-mos commentarius*, ed. Kühn, vol. 17b, p. 832), but featuring in both Ḥunayn's translations of Hippocrates' *Aphorisms*, ed. Tytler, p. 47, and of Galen's commentary (cf. E, fol. 36b).

262   Cf. Maimonides, *Medical Aphorisms* 16.38, trans. Bos, vol. 4, p. 15: "The accumulation of blood in the breasts indicates that insanity will occur. *In Hippocratis Epidemiarum librum 2 commentaria* 6."

Says the commentator: It seems to me as most probable that he observed this [only] once or twice and [yet] made a definite statement about it as he usually does in his book *Epidemics*. Galen remarks that he has never seen this, and this is true, that is to say that this (i.e., blood congealed in the breasts) is never a cause of madness.[263] It [must] have happened accidentally once or twice and Hippocrates observed it and thought that it was the cause [of madness].

(5.41)

[261] Says Hippocrates: If you want to know whether a woman is pregnant or not, give her honey water to drink when she wants to go to sleep. If she is attacked by a colic in the stomach, she is pregnant, but if she is not attacked, she is not pregnant.

Says the commentator: He means with his [formulation] "when she goes to sleep" the time when she is rested and satiated with food. It is the honey water that gives rise to winds and receives help thereby from the filling of the stomach. If the winds do not find an outlet, because[264] the uterus constricts their passage, a colic occurs.

(5.42)

[262] Says Hippocrates: If a woman is pregnant with a boy, her complexion is good, but if she is pregnant with a girl, her complexion is pallid.[265]

Says the commentator: All this is clear and applies in most cases.

(5.43)

[263] Says Hippocrates: If a pregnant woman suffers from the swelling called "erysipelas" in her womb, it is a sign of death.

Says the commentator: From the writings of Galen it is manifest that he means the death of the [fetus].[266] The same applies to other[267] hot swellings (inflammations).

---

263   Galen, *In Hippocratis Aphorismos commentarius* 5.40, ed. Kühn, vol. 17b, p. 832.

264   "because the uterus constricts their passage": Cf. ibid. 5.41, p. 834: διὰ τὴν ἀπὸ τῆς μήτρας στενοχωρίαν; trans. Ḥunayn (E, fol. 36ᵇ): بسبب مزاحمة الرحم وتضييقه لطريق تلك الرياح.

265   "pallid" (حائل): Cf. Hippocrates, *Aphorisms* 5.42, ed. and trans. Littré, vol. 4, pp. 546–547: δύσχροος ("mauvaise"); trans. Jones, p. 169: "bad."

266   Cf. Galen, *In Hippocratis Aphorismos commentarius* 5.43, ed. Kühn, vol. 17b, p. 836: ὅτι μὲν γὰρ ἐρυσιπέλατος γινομένου τεθνήξεται τὸ ἔμβρυον ἐξ ἀνάγκας εὔδηλον; trans. Ḥunayn (E, fol. 37ᵃ): والامر في أن الورم الذي يدعا الحمرة اذا حدث مات الطفل ضرورة بين.

267   "other hot swellings (inflammations)": Galen, ibid., ed. Kühn, speaks about ὀξεῖς πυρετοί (acute fevers).

قال المفسّر: الأقرب عندي أنّه رأى ذلك مرّة أو مرّتين فأطلق القضية كما جرت عادته في كتابه في أبيديميا. وقد ذكر جالينوس أنّه لم يشاهد هذا قطّ وهو الصحيح أعني أنّ ليس هذا سبب من أسباب الجنون بوجه. وإنّما اتّفق ذلك بالعرض مرّة أو مرّتين فرآه أبقراط فظنّه سببا.

(5.41)

[٢٦١] قال أبقراط: إن أحببت أنْ تعلم هل المرأة حامل أم لا فأسقها إذا أرادت النوم ماء العسل

٥   فإنْ أصابها مغص في بطنها فهي حامل وإنْ لم يصبها مغص فليست بحامل.

قال المفسّر: يريد بأخذه عند النوم عند السكون والامتلاء من الطعام وماء العسل الذي يولّد رياحا ويعينه على ذلك امتلاء البطن. فإذا لم يجد الريح مخلصا لمزاحمة الرحم لطريق تلك الرياح حدث المغص.

(5.42)

[٢٦٢] قال أبقراط: إذا كانت المرأة حبلى بذكر كان لونها حسنا وإذا كانت حبلى بأنثى كان لونها

١٠   حائلا.

قال المفسّر: كلّ هذا بيّن وهو أكثري.

(5.43)

[٢٦٣] قال أبقراط: إذا حدث بالمرأة الحبلى الورم الذي يدعى الحمرة في رحمها فذلك من علامات الموت.

قال المفسّر: يبدو من كلام جالينوس أنّه يريد موت الطفل وكذلك سائر الأورام الحارّة.

---

٤ هل: حال B   ٥-٤ فأسقها ... فليست: om. B   ٥ مغص: مغس C ‖ مغص: يصيبها CP يصبها ‖ مغص: مغس C   ٧ ذلك: om. A ‖ لمزاحمة: لمزاحمة P ‖ تلك الرياح: تلك الريح om. A BP   ٨ المغص: المغس C   ٩-١٠ كان لونها حائلا: om. B   ١١ كلّ هذا: هذا كلّه A   ١٢-١٣ الذي ... الموت: om. B   ١٢ الحمرة: om. A

(5.44)

[264] Says Hippocrates: If a woman, who is unnaturally thin, becomes pregnant, she will have a miscarriage before she will put on weight.

Says the commentator: He says that if she becomes pregnant while she is extremely thin, the food that reaches the organs will be completely seized by those organs and there is nothing left with which the fetus can be nourished when it grows. Therefore, she miscarries before she reaches the point where she can put on weight, [which would not happen during the time that] she [actually] returns to the natural fatness of her body.

(5.45)

[265] Says Hippocrates: If a woman with a normal body has a miscarriage in the second or third month without any obvious cause, the fundus[268] of the uterus is full of mucus and cannot retain the [fetus] because of its weight and[269] it (i.e., the fetus) breaks off from it (i.e., the uterus).

Says the commentator: This is clear.

(5.46)

[266] Says Hippocrates: If a woman is unnaturally fat and cannot become pregnant, the inner membrane of the abdominal membranes, which is called al-tharb[270] (fat, omentum), presses the mouth of the uterus and she will not become pregnant unless she becomes thinner.

---

268 "fundus" (تقعير): Cf. Dozy, Supplément, vol. 1, p. 382: "creux dans la superficie d'un membre;" cf. Galen, ibid. 5.45, p. 838: αἱ κοτυληδόνες; Hippocrates, Aphorisms, trans. Littré, vol. 4, p. 549: "les cotylédons [de la matrice];" trans. Jones, p. 171: "the cotyledons." In his translation of Hippocrates' Aphorisms, ed. Tytler, p. 47, Ḥunayn translates the Greek term as نقر الرحم (i.e., cotyledons; cf. De Koning, Trois traités d'anatomie arabes, p. 829), and in his translation of Galen's commentary, he has قعر الرحم (fundus of the uterus) (E, fol. 37b). It is clear that Maimonides consulted this text. See also Ibn Janāḥ, K. al-Talkhīṣ 623, eds. and trans. Bos/Käs/Lübke/Mensching (forthcoming): نقر الرحم هي أفواه العروق الضوارب وغير الضوارب التي تجلب الدم إلى الرحم من كتاب الفصول. ("Nuqar al-raḥim (cotyledons, lit., 'cavities of the womb') are the endings of the arteries (lit., 'pulsating vessels;' afwāh al-ʿurūq al-ḍawārib) and the veins (lit., 'non-pulsating vessels;' ġayr al-ḍawārib), which supply the womb with blood—from the Aphorisms (K. al-Fuṣūl).")

269 "and it (i.e., the fetus) breaks off from it (i.e., the uterus)" (ينهتك منها): The Arabic term reflects the Greek ἀπορρήγνυνται (cf. Galen, In Hippocratis Aphorismos commentarius 5.45, ed. Kühn, vol. 17b, p. 838), which refers to the breaking of the cotyledons (cf. Hippocrates, Aphorisms, trans. Littré, vol. 4, p. 549: "ils se rompent;" trans. Jones, p. 171: "and break"). But note that trans. Chadwick/Mann (Hippocrates, Hippocratic Writings, ed. Lloyd, p. 225) translate the Greek as relating to the fetus: "It is thus unable to hold the weight of the fetus which therefore is ejected."

270 "al-tharb (fat, omentum)": Cf. Galen, ibid. 5.46, p. 839: τὸ ἐπίπλοον; cf. Hippocrates, ibid., trans. Littré: "l'épiploon;" Barry, Syriac Medicine, p. 56.

(5.44)

[٢٦٤] قال أبقراط: إذا حملت المرأة وهي من الهزال على حال خارجة من الطبيعة فإنّها تسقط قبل
أنْ تسمن.

قال المفسّر: يقول إنّها إذا حبلت وهي في غاية الهزال فإنّ الغذاء الواصل للأعضاء تأخذه الأعضاء
بجملته فلا يفضل عنها شيء يغتذي به الجنين إذا كبر فلذلك تسقط قبل أنْ تنتهي لحيز السمن لا
٥ لرجوعها لطبيعتها في خصب بدنها.

(5.45)

[٢٦٥] قال أبقراط: متى كانت المرأة وبدنها معتدلا تسقط في الشهر الثاني والثالث من غير سبب بيّن
فتقعير الرحم مملوء مخاطا ولا يقدر على ضبط الطفل لثقله لكنّه ينهتك منها.

قال المفسّر: هذا بيّن.

(5.46)

[٢٦٦] قال أبقراط: إذا كانت المرأة على حال خارجة من الطبيعة من السمن فلم تحبل فإنّ الغشاء
١٠ الباطن من غشائي البطن الذي يسمّى الثرب يزحم فم الرحم منها وليس تحبل دون أنْ تهزل.

۲-۱ على ... تسمن: om. B   ۳ إذا: om. P ‖ في: om. A   ٦ المرأة: حامل add. P   ٧-٦ في ... منها: om.
B   ٩ من: om. A   ١٠-٩ فلم ... تهزل: om. B

Says the commentator: The uterus has a long neck (cervix). The end of the neck, which is close to the vagina, and into which the penis enters, is called "the mouth (orifice) of the neck of the uterus;"[271] it is also [simply] called "the mouth (orifice) of the uterus." But what is really called "the mouth of the uterus" is the beginning of the neck near the uterus,[272] and this is what is pressed by the fat in an extremely obese woman.

(5.47)

[267] Says Hippocrates: When the uterus suppurates in the region where it lies[273] close to the hip joint, it is necessary [to[274] perform] an action.

Says the commentator: With 'amal (activity) he means "the[275] activity of the hand;" namely, the insertion of lints. And when suppuration of an external site [of the uterus] occurs, [also] then one should apply lints.

(5.48)

[268] Says Hippocrates: [In the case of] a male [fetus] it is better when it [grows] on the right side, and for a female [fetus] on the left side.

Says the commentator: This is clear because the right side is warmer. Galen has mentioned that the semen that comes from the woman from the right side, from one of her ovaries, is thick and warm, while that which comes from the left side is thin and watery and colder than the other.[276] I wish I knew whether he received this [knowledge] by divine revelation or by analogical reasoning. If he has defined and formulated this argument through analogical reasoning, it is an astonishing and strange logical conclusion.

---

271   Cf. Maimonides, *Commentary on the Aphorisms of Hippocrates*, trans. Rosner, p. 145 n. 109: "external uterine orifice."

272   Cf. ibid., n. 110: "internal uterine orifice."

273   "lies close to" (يستبطن): The Arabic means lit., "to enter (the belly), to penetrate; to lay within" (Lane, *Arabic-English Lexicon*, p. 220); it is a translation of the Greek ἐγκειμένη (cf. Galen, *In Hippocratis Aphorismos commentarius* 5.47, ed. Kühn, vol. 17b, p. 840); cf. Hippocrates, *Aphorisms*, trans. Littré, vol. 4, p. 549: "appuyée sur;" trans. Jones, p. 171: "near."

274   "[to perform] an action" (*'amal*): The version consulted by Maimonides is corrupt. A has the correct version: فتل ([to use] lints), a translation of Greek ἔμμοτον; cf. Galen, ibid.; Hippocrates, ibid., trans. Littré: "les tentes de charpie;" trans. Jones: "tents;" Ullmann, *Wörterbuch*, suppl. 1, pp. 346–347, s.v. ἔμμοτος: "in Charpie, in einem Tampon verwendet, mit Charpie verbunden." Ḥunayn has the correct فتل, both in his translation of Hippocrates' *Aphorisms*, ed. Tytler, p. 48, and of Galen's commentary (E, fol. 38ᵃ).

275   "'the activity of the hand'" (عمل اليد): This is the regular technical term for 'surgery.'

276   Cf. Galen, *In Hippocratis Aphorismos commentarius* 5.48, ed. Kühn, vol. 17b, p. 841.

قال المفسّر: للرحم رقبة فيها طول فطرف تلك الرقبة الذي يلي الفرج وفي داخله يلج الإحليل يسمّى فم رقبة الرحم وقد يسمّى فم الرحم. والذي يسمّى فم الرحم على الحقيقة هو ابتداء الرقبة ممّا يلي الرحم وهو الذي يزحمه الثرب من المرأة المفرطة السمن.

(5.47)

[٢٦٧] قال أبقراط: متى تقيّح الرحم حيث يستبطن الورك وجب ضرورة أنْ يحتاج إلى العمل.

ه قال المفسّر: يعني بالعمل عمل اليد أي إدخال الفتائل وإذا تقيّح ممّا يلي منه خارج لفينئذ قد يحتاج إلى الفتائل.

(5.48)

[٢٦٨] قال أبقراط: ما كان من الأطفال ذكرا فأحرى أنْ يكون تولّده في الجانب الأيمن وما كان أنثى ففي الأيسر.

قال المفسّر: هذا بيّن لأنّ الجانب الأيمن أحرّ. وذكر جالينوس أنّ المني الذي يأتي من المرأة من الجانب الأيمن من أحد يبضتيها فيه تخانة وحرارة والذي يأتي من الجانب الأيسر رقيق مائي وأبرد من الآخر. ١٠ ويا ليت شعري هل أتاه بهذا وحي أو ودّاه إليه القياس. فإنْ كان حدّد وحرّر هذا التحرير بقياس فهذا قياس عجيب غريب.

١ الذي: التي A ‖ يسمّى: فهي B ٢-٣ والذي ... الرحم: om. A ٤ حيث ... العمل: om. B ‖ العمل: الفتل A ه بالعمل: أيّ A. add ٧ ما: من P ٧-٨ فأحرى ... الأيسر: om. B ٩ من: في C ١٠ أحد: احدى B ١١ بهذا: هذا A ‖ كان: om. P ١٢ عجيب: om. BP

(5.49)

[269] Says Hippocrates: If you want to expel the placenta, put a sternutatory medicine into the nose and keep the nostrils and mouth closed.

Says the commentator: This is in order to produce a stretching and tension in the abdomen, which helps to expel the placenta.

(5.50)

[270] Says Hippocrates: If you want to stop the menstrual bleeding of a woman, apply the largest available cupping glass to each of her breasts.

Says the commentator: This is clear because it attracts the blood to the opposite side.[277]

(5.51)

[271] Says Hippocrates: The mouth of the womb of a pregnant woman is closed.

Says the commentator: This is clear.

(5.52)

[272] Says Hippocrates: If milk flows from the breasts of a pregnant woman, it indicates that the [fetus] is weak, but if the breasts are firm, it indicates that the [fetus] is more healthy.[278]

Says the commentator: The milk of a pregnant woman rather flows because the vessels between the uterus and the breasts are filled to overflowing, and the blood is especially abundant there when the [fetus] is undernourished and is only provided with a very small amount [of food] from those vessels.

---

277   Cf. Maimonides, *Medical Aphorisms* 16.11, trans. Bos, vol. 4, p. 7: "If too much [blood] is evacuated from the uterus all at once, apply cupping glasses next to the breasts and it will stop rapidly ..."

278   Cf. ibid. 16.36, p. 15: "If the milk of a pregnant woman flows copiously, the fetus is weak. Because of its weakness, it does not attract the blood, which recedes to the breasts, and milk is produced. If the breasts are firmer, the fetus is healthier. *In Hippocratis Epidemiarum librum 2 commentaria 6.*"

(5.49)

[٢٦٩] قال أبقراط: إذا أردت أنْ تسقط المشيمة فأدخل في الأنف دواءا معطّسا وامسك المنخرين والفم.

قال المفسّر: لأنْ يحدث للبطن عند ذلك تمدّد وتوتّر فيعين على سقوط المشيمة.

(5.50)

[٢٧٠] قال أبقراط: إذا أردت أنْ تحبس طمث المرأة فألق عند كلّ واحد من ثدييها محجمة من أعظم ما يكون.

قال المفسّر: هذا بيّن لأنّه جذب لخلاف الجهة.

(5.51)

[٢٧١] قال أبقراط: إنّ فم الرحم من المرأة الحامل يكون منضمّا.

قال المفسّر: هذا بيّن.

(5.52)

[٢٧٢] قال أبقراط: إذا جرى اللبن من ثدي الحبلى دلّ ذلك على ضعف من طفلها ومتى كان الثديان مكتنزين دلّ ذلك على أنّ الطفل أصحّ.

قال المفسّر: إنّما يجري اللبن ويسيل من الحبلى لامتلاء العروق التي بين الرحم والثديين بكثرة وإنّما يكثر هناك وجود الدم إذا كان الطفل قليل الغذاء ولا يمتار من تلك العروق إلّا أيسر شيئا.

٢-١ فأدخل ... والفم: om. B ٣ ذلك: العطاس P ‖ سقوط: إسقاط BP ٤ فألق: فعلق A ٥-٤ فألق ... يكون: om. B ٨-٧ قال ... بيّن: om. A ٧ من ... منضمّا: om. B ٩-١٠ دلّ ... أصحّ: om. B ‖ والثديين: والثديان P ‖ بكثرة: الدم add. B

(5.53)

[273] Says Hippocrates: If the condition of the woman is such that it leads to a miscarriage, her breasts become thin. If the opposite is the case, i.e., that her breasts become firm [again], she will suffer from pain in her breasts or in the hips or in the eyes or in the knees but she will not miscarry.

Says the commentator: Thinness of the breasts is an indication of lack of blood, as stated [before]; firmness of the breasts is an indication of a balanced amount [of blood]; hardness [of the breasts] is an indication of abundant, thick blood. For this reason, nature can push this excessive superfluity to another organ, which is close to the uterus or to the breasts and thus pain occurs to that organ. In general, all these indications are neither correct nor do they occur most frequently. In my opinion, all these aphorisms and their like follow from his observation of what happened [only] once or twice, for Hippocrates was [merely] a beginner in the [medical] art.

(5.54)

[274] Says Hippocrates: If the mouth of the womb is hard, it is necessarily closed.

Says the commentator: This is clear.

(5.55)

[275] Says Hippocrates: If a pregnant woman catches a fever and [the[279] fever becomes extremely high] without any obvious cause, her delivery will be difficult and dangerous, or she will have a dangerous miscarriage.

Says the commentator: For an easy delivery it is necessary that both are strong, the body of the mother and the body of the child.

(5.56)

[276] Says Hippocrates: If a spasm and fainting occur after menstruation, it is bad.

Says the commentator: This is clear.

---

279   "[the fever becomes extremely high]" (سخنت سخونة قوية): This version is according to Galen, *In Hippocratis Aphorismos commentarius* 5.55, ed. Kühn, vol. 17b, p. 851: ἰσχυρῶς θερμαίνονται (become exceedingly hot (feverish)), following Greek C and several others and according to both Ḥunayn's translation of Hippocrates' *Aphorisms*, ed. Tytler, p. 49, and his translation of Galen's commentary (E, fol. 40ᵃ). Note however that the standard Greek text has: ἰσχυρῶς ἰσχαίνονται; cf. Hippocrates, *Aphorisms*, trans. Littré, p. 553: "maigrissent considerablement;" trans. Jones, p. 173: "become exceedingly thin."

(5.53)

[٢٧٣] قال أبقراط: إذا كانت حال المرأة تؤول إلى أنْ تسقط فإنّ ثدييها يضمران. فإنْ كان الأمر على خلاف ذلك أعني إنْ كان ثدياها صلبين فإنّه يصيبها وجع في الثديين أو في الوركين أو في العينين أو في الركبتين ولا تسقط.

قال المفسّر: ضمر الثديين دليل قلّة الدم كما ذكر واكتنازهما دليل على اعتدال مقداره وصلابتهما دليل على كثرة الدم وغلظه. ولذلك يمكن أنْ تدفع الطبيعة ذلك الفضل الزائد لعضو آخر قريب من الرحم أو من الثدي فيحدث في ذلك العضو وجع. وبالجملة هذه الدلائل كلّها غير صحيحة ولا أكثرية. وكلّ هذه الفصول وأمثالها عندي تابع لما اتّفق مرّة أو مرّتين فرآه لأنّ أبقراط مبتدىء صناعة.

(5.54)

[٢٧٤] قال أبقراط: إذا كان فم الرحم صلبا فيجب ضرورة أنْ يكون منضمّا.

قال المفسّر: هذا بيّن.

(5.55)

[٢٧٥] قال أبقراط: إذا عرضت الحمّى لمرأة حامل وسخنت سخونة قوية من غير سبب ظاهر فإنّ ولادها يكون بعسر وخطر أو تسقط فيكون على خطر.

قال المفسّر: يحتاج في سهولة الولادة أنْ تكون البدنان جميعا قويين بدن الأمّ وبدن الطفل.

(5.56)

[٢٧٦] قال أبقراط: إذا حدث بعد سيلان الطمث تشنّج وغشي فذلك رديء.

قال المفسّر: هذا بيّن.

---

١ المرأة: om. B ٣-١ فإنّ ... تسقط: om. B ١ يضمران: يظمرن P ٤ ضمر: ضمور B ٧ لأنّ أبقراط: لابن بقراط C ٨ فيجب ... منضمّا: om. B ١٠-١١ وسخنت ... خطر: om. B ١٠ ظاهر: بيّن A

(5.57)

[277] Says Hippocrates: When the menstruation is more copious than necessary, illnesses develop; when menstrual blood does not flow, illnesses occur
from the side of the womb.

Says the commentator: This is clear.

(5.58)

[278] Says Hippocrates: If an inflammation occurs in[280] the rectum (lit., in the
extremity of the anus) or in the uterus, it is followed by strangury. Similarly, if
the kidneys suppurate, strangury results, and if an inflammation occurs to the
liver, hiccups follow.

Says the commentator: Strangury occurs because of a weakness of the retentive force of the urinary bladder or because of the sharpness of the urine. The
weakness of the strength [of the bladder] results from a bad temperament or
from the inflammation that occurs there. The sharpness of the urine [occurs]
because of the admixture therein of biting humor. If there is an inflammation
in one of these organs (i.e., the rectum or uterus) it is harmful for the bladder
because of its proximity and it weakens its strength. If there is an illness in the
kidneys, there is a biting [sensation] during [urination]. An inflammation of
the liver is only followed by hiccups when it is severe.

(5.59)

[279] Says Hippocrates: If a woman does not become pregnant and you want to
know whether she can become pregnant or not, cover her with clothes [and]
then fumigate beneath her. If you see that the smell of the fumigation passes
through her body until it reaches her nostrils and mouth, you[281] should know
that there is no reason why pregnancy is impossible for her.

---

280   "in the rectum (lit., in the extremity of the anus)" (طرف الدبر): The Arabic term features in
      Ḥunayn's translation of both Hippocrates' *Aphorisms* 5.58, ed. Tytler, p. 49, and of Galen's
      commentary (E, fol. 41ᵃ), and stands for Greek ἀρχός (Galen, ibid., ed. Kühn, p. 855), which
      can mean both "rectum" and "anus" (cf. Liddell/Scott, *Greek-English Lexicon*, p. 253). The
      regular Arabic term for "rectum" is المعاء المستقيم, which reflects Greek τὸ ἀπευθυσμένον; cf.
      De Koning, *Trois traités d'anatomie arabes*, p. 828. The reason why Ḥunayn chose to trans-
      late ἀρχός as طرف الدبر is possibly to distinguish between دبر in the sense of "anus" and
      طرف الدبر as "rectum."
281   "you should know that there is no reason why pregnancy is impossible for her": Cf. Galen,
      ibid. 5.59, p. 857: γίνωσκε ὅτι αὐτὴ οὐ δι' ἑαυτὴν ἄγονός ἐστιν; Hippocrates, ibid., trans. Littré,
      vol. 4, p. 555: "sachez qu'elle n'est pas stérile de son fait;" trans. Jones, p. 175: "be assured
      that the woman is not barren through her own physical fault."

(5.57)

[٢٧٧] قال أبقراط: إذا كان الطمث أزيد ممّا ينبغي عرضت من ذلك أمراض وإذا لم ينحدر الطمث
حدثت من ذلك أمراض من قبل الرحم.

قال المفسّر: هذا بيّن.

(5.58)

[٢٧٨] قال أبقراط: إذا عرض في طرف الدبر أو في الرحم ورم تبعه تقطير البول وكذلك إنْ تقيّحت
٥ الكلى تبع ذلك تقطير البول وإذا حدث في الكبد ورم تبع ذلك فواق.

قال المفسّر: تقطير البول يكون لضعف قوّة المثانة الماسكة أو لحدّة البول. وضعف القوة من سوء
المزاج أو من ورم يحدث هناك وحدّة البول لما يخالطها من الخلط اللذّاع. فإذا كان ورم في أحد هذين
العضوين فهو يضرّ المثانة بالمجاورة ويضعف قوّتها. وإذا كانت علّة في الكلى فيحدث لذغ في البول ولا
يتبع ورم الكبد فواق إلّا أنْ يكون عظيما.

(5.59)

١٠ [٢٧٩] قال أبقراط: إذا كانت المرأة لا تحمل فأردت أنْ تعلم هل تحبل أم لا فغطّها بثياب ثمّ بخّر
تحتها. فإنْ رأيت أنّ رائحة البخور تنفذ في بدنها حتّى تصل إلى منخريها وفيها فاعلم أنّه ليس سبب
تعذّر الحبل من قبلها.

١-٢ عرضت ... الرحم: om. B ١ الطمث: على ما ينبغي add. A ٤ الدبر: الذكر B ٤-٥ أو ... فواق:
om. B ‖ وكذلك ... البول om. AP ٤ تقيّحت: emendation editor نفتحت C ١٠ تحمل: تحبل P
١٠-١٢ فأردت ... قبلها: om. B ١١ أنّ: om. C ١٢ الحبل: الحمل Pt

Says the commentator: The fumigation should be [done] with fragrant things that have sharpness such as frankincense, myrrh, and storax.

(5.60)

[280] Says Hippocrates: If a pregnant woman has a regular[282] menstruation, it is impossible that the [fetus] is healthy.

Says the commentator: Galen says that it looks like the menstrual blood in the case of a pregnant woman streams from the vessels in the neck of the uterus because the placenta is attached to the mouths of all the vessels that are within the cavity of the uterus and it is impossible that any [blood] is expelled from there to the cavity of the uterus.[283]

(5.61)

[281] Says Hippocrates: If a woman does not have a regular[284] menstruation and she does not suffer from shivering or fever, but suffers from distress,[285] nausea, and despondency,[286] know that she is pregnant.

Says the commentator: This is clear.

(5.62)

[282] Says Hippocrates: If the uterus of a woman is cold and dense, she will not become pregnant. If it is very moist, she will also not become pregnant because the moisture will[287] drown, extinguish, and quench (destroy) the semen. Furthermore, when it is drier than it should be or when it is burning hot, she will

---

282 "regular" (في أوقاته): This term is missing in the Greek text of Hippocrates, ibid., ed. Littré, p. 554; ed. Jones, p. 174, but features in in Ḥunayn's translation of both Hippocrates' *Aphorisms*, ed. Tytler, p. 50, and of Galen's commentary (E, fol. 41ᵇ).

283 Cf. Galen, *In Hippocratis Aphorismos commentarius* 5.60, ed. Kühn, vol. 17b, pp. 858–859.

284 "regular" (في أوقاته): This term is missing in the Greek text of Hippocrates' *Aphorisms*, ed. Littré, p. 554; ed. Jones, p. 174, but features in Ḥunayn's translation of both Hippocrates' *Aphorisms*, ed. Tytler, p. 50, and of Galen's commentary (E, fol. 41ᵇ).

285 "distress" (كرب): See the note above.

286 "despondency" (خبث نفس): See the note above. The same term features in Maimonides' *Medical Aphorisms* 6.52, ed. and trans. Bos, vol. 2, p. 12, and p. 105 n. 111, as a translation of Greek δυσθυμία (despondency, despair; cf. Liddell/Scott, *Greek-English Lexicon*, p. 457).

287 "will drown, extinguish, and quench (destroy) the semen": Cf. Galen, *In Hippocratis Aphorismos commentarius* 5.62, ed. Kühn, vol. 17b, p. 861: ἀποσβέννυται γὰρ ὁ γόνος; Hippocrates, *Aphorisms*, trans. Littré, vol. 4, p. 557: "car le sperme s'y éteint;" trans. Jones, p. 175: "for the seed is drowned."

قال المفسّر: البخور يكون بأمور طيّبة الرائحة لها حدّة مثل الكندر والمرّ والميعة.

(5.60)

[٢٨٠] قال أبقراط: إذا كانت المرأة الحامل يجري طمثها في أوقاته فليس يمكن أنْ يكون طفلها صحيحا.

قال المفسّر: قال جالينوس: يشبه أنْ يكون الطمث الجاري من الحوامل من العروق التي في رقبة

٥ الرحم لأنّ المشيمة معلّقة بأفواه جميع العروق التي من داخل في تجويف الرحم فليس يمكن أنْ يخرج من ذلك شيء لفضاء الرحم.

(5.61)

[٢٨١] قال أبقراط: إذا لم يجر طمث المرأة في أوقاته ولم يحدث بها قشعريرة ولا حمّى لكنْ عرض لها كرب وغثي وخبث نفس فاعلم أنّها قد علقت.

قال المفسّر: هذا بيّن.

(5.62)

١٠ [٢٨٢] قال أبقراط: متى كان رحم المرأة باردا متكاثفا لم تحبل ومتى كان أيضا رطبا جدّا لم تحبل لأنّ رطوبته تغمر المني وتخمده وتطفئه. ومتى كان أيضا أجفّ ممّا ينبغي أو كان حارّا محرقا لم

٣-٢ في ... صحيحا: om. B ٢ طفلها: طولها P om. A :لم ٧ om. P :داخل ٥ ٨-٧ ولم ... علقت:
om. B ٨ وغثي: وغشي P ١٠-٢.٢٣٣ ومتى ... الولد: om. B

not become pregnant, because the sperm is spoiled through lack of food. When the temperament of the uterus is balanced (in the middle) between these two conditions, the woman can[288] get many children.

Says the commentator: This is clear.

(5.63)
[283][289]

(5.64)
[284] Says Hippocrates: Milk is bad for those suffering from headache; it is also bad for fever patients, and for those whose hypochondrium is swollen[290] and [full of intestinal] rumblings, and for those who are thirsty, and for those in whom the yellow bile prevails in their stool, namely those who suffer from acute fever, and for those who have bloody diarrhea. [Milk] is beneficial for those who suffer from phthisis if they do not have a very high fever, and for those with a chronic, low fever, if it is not accompanied by any of the above-mentioned [symptoms] and their body is wasted more[291] than the illness made necessary.

Says the commentator: Milk is one of the [substances] that is changed quickly. If it is in the stomach, which is cooler, it turns sour, and if it is in the stomach, which is hotter, it becomes gaseous. If it is properly digested, it produces abundant good nutrition. But it may happen that during the process of digestion, flatulence is produced in the hypochondrium and pain in the head. This is its effect in healthy people, in sick people [it effects] all that has been mentioned [above].

(5.65)
[285] Says Hippocrates: If someone suffers from a wound and then develops a swelling because of it, he will hardly ever be attacked by spasms or madness. If the swelling disappears suddenly and the wound is in the posterior part [of the

---

288   "can get many children" (كثيرة الولد): Cf. Galen, ibid.: ἐπίτεχνοι; Hippocrates, ibid., trans. Littré: "sont fécondes" trans. Jones: "prove able to conceive."

289   This Aphorism is missing in all the MSS, and likewise in Ḥunayn's translation of both Hippocrates' *Aphorisms*, ed. Tytler, p. 50, and of Galen's commentary (E, fol. 44ᵃ).

290   "swollen" (مشرف): Lit., "raised;" cf. Galen, *In Hippocratis Aphorismos commentarius* 5.64, ed. Kühn, vol. 17b, p. 872: μετέωρα; cf. Liddell/Scott, *Greek-English Lexicon*, p. 1120: "raised from off the ground;" Hippocrates, ibid., trans. Littré, vol. 4, p. 557: "gonflées;" trans. Jones, p. 177: "swollen."

291   "more than the illness made necessary" (على غير ما توجبه العلّة): Cf. Galen, ibid.: παρὰ λόγον; Hippocrates, ibid., trans. Littré, p. 559: "excessive;" trans. Jones: "excessive."

تحبل لأنّ المني يعدم الغذاء فيفسد. ومتى كان مزاج الرحم معتدلا بين الحالين كانت المرأة كثيرة الولد.

قال المفسّر: هذا بيّن.

(5.63)

[٢٨٣]

(5.64)

٥ [٢٨٤] قال أبقراط: اللبن لأصحاب الصداع رديء وهو أيضا للمحمومين رديء ولمن كانت المواضع التي دون الشراسيف منه مشرفة وفيها قراقر ولمن به عطش ولمن به غالب على برازه المرار ممّن هو في حمّى حادّة ولمن اختلف دما كثيرا. وينفع أصحاب السلّ إذا ما لم تكن بهم حمّى شديدة جدّا ولأصحاب الحمّى الطويلة الضعيفة إذا لم يكن معها شيء ممّا تقدّمنا بوصفه وكانت أبدانهم تذوب على غير ما توجبه العلّة.

١٠ قال المفسّر: اللبن هو من الأشياء التي تسرع إليها الاستحالة إمّا في المعدة التي هي أرد فيحمض وإمّا في المعدة التي هي أسخن فيستحيل إلى دخانية وإمّا الذي يستمرّ على ما ينبغي فيولّد غذاءا غزيرا محمودا إلّا أنّه في حال استمرائه قد يحدث نفخة في ما دون الشراسيف فيصدع الرأس. هذا فعله في الأصحّاء وأمّا المرضاء فكلّ ما ذكر.

(5.65)

[٢٨٥] قال أبقراط: من حدثت به قرحة فأصابه بسببها انتفاخ فليس يكاد يصيبه تشنّج ولا جنون.

١٥ فإنْ غاب ذلك الانتفاخ دفعة ثمّ كانت القرحة من خلف عرض له تشنّج أو تمدّد. وإنْ كانت القرحة

---

٢ الولد: الولادة P ٤ ٥–٨ وهو ... تذوب: إلى This aphorism is missing in the Arabic translation

قوله B ٧ ما: om. P ٨ تقدّمنا: قدمنا P ١٥ خلف: كله P

body], spasms or tetanus will occur to him. If the wound is on the front, he will suffer from madness or severe pain in the side, or suppuration or dysentery if that swelling is red.

Says the commentator: I do not need to repeat that most of these assertions of Hippocrates are either mostly so or evenly so [or not so]; and upon verification, some of the statements are true only in a minority of cases. For if you look into them carefully, [you will see that] only some of his assertions are [valid] for very few cases. Perhaps he saw [a case of illness] once and then ascribed it to a cause by which it was not really caused.

The interpretation of this aphorism according to Galen is that with [the term] "swelling," he means the inflammation and any [other] unnatural thickening. The posterior part of the body contains nerves, but the front part is dominated by pulsating vessels. If the humor that produces the inflammation ascends to the brain, spasms occur, and if it ascends through the vessels to the brain, madness occurs. If that humor goes to the chest, it produces pain in the side. Patients with pain in the side often suffer from suppuration.[292]

(5.66)

[286] Says Hippocrates: When severe, bad wounds occur but no swelling appears there, it is a bad affliction.

Says the commentator: With bad wounds he means those that occur in the beginning or end of muscles or[293] [in] muscles in which nerves dominate. If no swelling develops in wounds in which that is usually the case, one cannot be sure that the humors that stream to the wounds are not carried to a location that is more important than that of the wounds.

(5.67)

[287] Says Hippocrates: Soft [swellings] are good, crude [swellings] are bad.

Says the commentator: Galen says that with [the term] "crude" he means "hard" and "resisting" [cooking]; it is the opposite of soft, because the humor of anything that is hard is not cooked.[294]

---

292   Cf. Galen, ibid. 5.65, pp. 877–879.

293   "or [in] muscles in which nerves dominate" (أو ما كان من العضل الغالب عليه العصب): Maimonides' rendering of Galen's words is not exact; cf. Galen, ibid. 5.66, p. 881: καὶ μάλιστα τῶν νευρωδῶν (especially of those muscles in which nerves dominate); cf. trans. Ḥunayn (S, fol. 109ᵃ): وخاصّة ما كان من العضل الغالب عليه العصب.

294   Cf. Galen, ibid. 5.67, ed. Kühn, p. 882.

من قدّام عرض له جنون أو وجع حادّ في الجنب أو تقيّح أو اختلاف دم إنْ كان ذلك الانتفاخ أحمر.

قال المفسّر: لا أحتاج أنْ أكرّر أنْ أكثر هذه القضايا التي يقولها أبقراط بعضها أكثريّة أو على التساوي وعند التحقيق فتوجد بعض قضاياه على الأقلّ ولعلّ رآها مرّة ونسب الأمر في ذلك لسبب ليس ذلك سببه بالحقيقة. ٥

وتأويل هذا الفصل عند جالينوس أنّه يريد بالانتفاخ الورم وكلّ غلظ خارج من الطبع. وما هو من البدن خلف فهو عصبي وما هو منه قدّام فالغالب عليه العروق الضوارب. فإذا تراقى الخلط المولّد للورم من العصب للدماغ كان التشنّج وإنْ تراقى في العروق إلى الدماغ كان الجنون. وإنْ صار ذلك الخلط إلى الصدر ولّد الوجع في الجنب. وكثير ما يصيب صاحب ذات الجنب التقيّح.

(5.66)

[٢٨٦] قال أبقراط: إذا حدثت جراحات عظيمة خبيثة ثمّ لم يظهر معها ورم فالبليّة عظيمة. ١٠

قال المفسّر: يعني بالجراحات الخبيثة التي تكون في رؤوس العضل أو منتهاها أو ما كان من العضل الغالب عليه العصب. فإذا لم يحدث ورم في ما كانت هذه حاله من الجراحات لا يؤمن أنْ تكون الأخلاط التي تنصبّ إلى الجراحات تنتقل عنها إلى موضع أشرف من مواضع الجراحات.

(5.67)

[٢٨٧] قال أبقراط: الرخوة محمودة والنيئة مذمومة.

قال المفسّر: يقول جالينوس إنّه يعني بالنيئ الصلب المدافع هو ضدّ الرخو لأنّ كلّ صلب نخلطه غير ١٥ نضج.

---

١ أو اختلاف: واختلاف P ٣ أنْ: أو A ٤ الأمر في: om. P || ذلك: مرّة add. A ٦ الطبع: الطبيعة B ٧ خلف: من add. BP ١٠ جراحات: جراحة B خراجات A || خبيثة ... عظيمة: om. B ١١ بالجراحات: بالخراجات AP || الجراحات: الخراجات AP ١٢ لم: يكن add. A ١٣ إلى: om. A || الجراحات: الخراجات AP || موضع: آخر add. A || الجراحات: الخراجات AP ١٤ الرخوة: الأورام الرخوة APt ١٦ نضج: نضيج BP

(5.68)

[288] Says Hippocrates: If someone suffers from pain in the back of his head, he will benefit from an incision in the upright vein in the forehead.

Says the commentator: The attraction [of residues] to the opposite site in the neck is from the back to the front and from the front to the back.

(5.69)

[289] Says Hippocrates: Rigors in women mostly begin in[295] the loins and then ascend through the back to the head. In men too, they begin more often in the back [of the body] than in the front as, for example, those that begin in the forearms and thighs. This is because the skin too, in the front part of the body, is porous, as is shown by the hairs.

Says the commentator: The back is quickly affected by cold because its coldness is due to numerous bones there and to the paucity of flesh. Women are colder than men; he brings proof for the looseness [of the skin] of the front [part of the body] from the fact that the hair grows there.[296]

(5.70)

[290] Says Hippocrates: If someone is afflicted by quartan fever, he is hardly attacked by spasms. If he is attacked by spasms before the quartan fever and then gets a quartan fever, the spasms will abate.

Says the commentator: The interpretation of Galen is that this type of spasm is the one that arises from overfilling.[297] It can be cured by the expulsion or concoction of the humor. In quartan fever it is expelled by the force of the spasm and concocted by the heat of the fever.[298]

---

295   "in the loins" (من أسفل الصلب): Lit., "from the lower part of the back;" cf. ibid. 5.69, p. 883: ἐξ ὀσφύος; Hippocrates, *Aphorisms*, trans. Littré, vol. 4, p. 561: "dans les lombes;" trans. Jones, p. 179: "in the loins;" a synonym of أسفل الصلب for "loins" is قطن; cf. aphorism 4.73 (210) above.

296   Cf. Hippocrates, ibid., ed. Jones, p. 179 n. 3 "Littré thinks that this last sentence (i.e., 'This is because the skin too, in the front part of the body, is porous, as is shown by the hairs') is a separate aphorism, contrasting the bodies of women and of men. Commentators mostly think that there is a reference to the fact that the front parts are more hairy than the back; this shows the less rarity of the latter, i.e. their greater coldness and liability to rigors."

297   Cf. Galen, *In Hippocratis Aphorismos commentarius* 5.70, ed. Kühn, vol. 17b, p. 885: γίνεται δ' ὑπὸ γλίσχρων χυμῶν τε καὶ φλεγματικῶν ἐμπλαττομένων γε τοῖς νευρώδεσι μορίοις; cf. trans. Ḥunayn (S, fols. 110ʳ–110ᵛ): وذلك أن التشنج إنما يكون من أخلاط لزجة بلغمية ترسخ في الأعضاء العصبية (For spasms arise especially from viscous, phlegmatic humors that get settled in the organs that contain nerves).

298   Cf. Galen, ibid., ed. Kühn, pp. 885–886.

(5.68)

[٢٨٨] قال أبقراط: من أصابه وجع في مؤخّر رأسه فقطع له العرق المنتصب الذي في الجبهة انتفع بقطعه.

قال المفسّر: الجذب الذي إلى خلاف الجهة في العنق هو من المؤخّر للمقدّم ومن المقدّم للمؤخّر.

(5.69)

[٢٨٩] قال أبقراط: إنّ النافض أكثر ما يبتدىء في النساء من أسفل الصلب ثمّ يتراقى في الظهر إلى

٥ الرأس. وهي أيضا في الرجال تبتدىء من خلف أكثر ممّا تبتدىء من قدّام مثل ما قد تبتدىء من الساعدين والفخذين. وذلك لأنّ الجلد أيضا في مقدّم البدن متخلخل ويدلّ على ذلك الشعر.

قال المفسّر: البرد يسرع للظهر لكونه أبرد لكثرة العظام هناك وقلّة اللحم والنساء أبرد من الرجال واستدلّ على تخلخل المقدّم من نبات الشعر هناك.

(5.70)

[٢٩٠] قال أبقراط: من اعترته الربع فليس يكاد يعتريه التشنّج وإن كان اعتراه التشنّج قبل الربع ثمّ

١٠ حدثت الربع سكن التشنّج.

قال المفسّر: تأويل جالينوس أنّه قال إنّ هذا النوع من تشنّج هو الكائن من امتلاء وبرؤه يكون بانتفاض الخلط الخارج وبنضجه. وفي حمّى الربع يخرج بشدّة النافض وينضج بحرارة الحمّى.

١-٢ فقطع ... بقطعه B:om. ٣ للمقدم:إلى المقدم P || للمؤخّر:إلى المؤخّر B ٤-٦ ثمّ ... متخلخل:إلى قوله
B ٥ ممّا:ما C ٧ العظام:الطعام CP العظام corr. P¹ ٨ واستدلّ:C¹ A:om. ٩ فليس ٩-١٠ فليس
... سكن التشنّج B:om. ١٢ الخارج:إلى خارج B الخارج AP

(5.71)

[291] Says Hippocrates: If someone's skin is stretched, dry, and hard, he dies without sweat. If someone's skin is soft and porous, he dies with sweat.

Says the commentator: He means those people who are close to death and whose skin is [as described].

(5.72)

[292] Says Hippocrates: If someone suffers from jaundice, he will hardly develop winds (flatulence).

Says the commentator: One of the causes that give rise to winds is the phlegm, which is in the site of their origin. This does not happen in the case of jaundice because of the dominance of bile.

This is the end of the fifth part of the commentary on the *Aphorisms*.

(5.71)

[٢٩١] قال أبقراط: من كان جلده ممتدّا لحلا صلبا فهو يموت عن غير عرق ومن كان جلده رخوا متخلخلا فإنّه يموت مع عرق.

قال المفسّر: يعني من أشرف على الموت ممّن كان جلده بحال هذا.

(5.72)

[٢٩٢] قال أبقراط: من كان به يرقان فليس يكاد يتولّد فيه الرياح.

٥ قال المفسر: من أسباب تولّد الرياح وجود البلغم التي في موضع تولّدها وهذا لا يكون مع اليرقان لغلبة المرار.

تمّت المقالة الخامسة من شرح الفصول.

---

١ ممتدّا: متمددا P ‖ صلبا: om. A ‖ ١-٢ فهو ... عرق: om. B ‖ ١ عن: من DPt ‖ ١-٢ عن ... يموت:
om. A ‖ ٢ فإنّه: فهو Pt ‖ ٣ بحال: om. A ‖ ٧ تمّت المقالة الخامسة من شرح: كلت المقالة الخامسة P كل
شرح المقالة الخامسة B ‖ من شرح الفصول: من فصول أبقراط والحمد لله وحده B من كتاب الفصول وشرحها
والحمد لله وحده كما هو أهله om. P A ‖ الفصول: يتلوها في الصفحة التي تلي هذه الصفحة المقالة السادسة من
شرح فصول أبقراط والحمد لله وحده add. C

In the name of God, the Merciful, the Compassionate
The sixth part of the commentary on Hippocrates' *Aphorisms*

(6.1)

[293] Says Hippocrates: If acid eructations occur during the illness called "lientery" when it has become chronic and when [these eructations] did not happen before, they are a good sign.

Says the commentator: If the cause of the lientery is the weakness of the retentive faculty and [the food] is excreted before it is [properly] digested and acid eructations occur thereupon, it is an indication that the food is staying sufficiently [long] in the stomach for a partial digestion (lit., change) to begin to a degree that it (i.e., the food) turns sour. [It is also an indication] that nature is beginning to return to its [normal] activities.

(6.2)

[294] Says Hippocrates: If a person's nostrils are excessively moist by nature and his semen is very thin (watery), his health leans toward sickness. But if the reverse is true in a person, he has a healthier body.

Says the commentator: These are things that indicate moisture of the brain and dryness of the other organs and therefore his semen is thin.

(6.3)

[295] Says Hippocrates: The[299] abstention from food (i.e., loss of appetite) in chronic dysentery is a bad sign; if it is accompanied by fever, it is worse.[300]

Says the commentator: If dysentery is caused by protracted abrasion of the intestines, it increases the emaciation deep in the intestines and results in a putrid wound. The stomach will also hurt because of the sympathetic affection [between the stomach and the intestines], and the digestion [of food] in it will be harmed. If the illness ascends to the cardia of the stomach, the appetite will be less. This is a sign that the illness has settled (established itself) and that its harm is spreading.

---

299   "The abstention from food (i.e., loss of appetite)": Cf. Galen, *In Hippocratis Aphorismos commentarius* 6.3, ed. Kühn, vol. 18a, p. 11: αἱ ἀποσίτιαι; Hippocrates, *Aphorisms*, trans. Littré, vol. 4, p. 565: "anorexie;" trans. Jones, p. 181: "loathing for food."

300   Cf. Maimonides, *Medical Aphorisms* 6.90, ed. and trans. Bos, vol. 2, p. 19.

بسم الله الرحمن الرحيم
المقالة السادسة من شرح فصول أبقراط

(6.1)

[٢٩٣] قال أبقراط: إذا حدث الجُشاء الحامض في العلّة التي يقال لها زلق الأمعاء بعد تطاولها ولم
يكن كان قبل ذلك فهو علامة محمودة.

قال المفسّر: إذا كان علّة زلق الأمعاء ضعف القوة الماسكة فيخرج قبل أنْ ينهضم ثمّ حدث الجُشاء
الحامض فذلك دليل على أنّ الغذاء قد صار يبقى في المعدة مدّة يمكن معها أنْ يبتدئ تغيّره بعض
تغيير قدر ما يحمض وأنّ الطبيعة بدأت أنْ تراجع أفعالها.

(6.2)

[٢٩٤] قال أبقراط: من كان في منخريه بالطبع رطوبة أزيد وكان منيه أرقّ فإنّ صحّته أقرب إلى
السقم. ومن كان الأمر فيه على ضدّ ذلك فإنّه أصحّ بدنا.

قال المفسّر: هذه أشياء تدلّ على رطوبة الدماغ ويبس سائر الاعضاء ولذلك رقّ منيه.

(6.3)

[٢٩٥] قال أبقراط: الامتناع من الطعام في اختلاف الدم المزمن دليل رديء وهو مع الحُمّى أردأ.

قال المفسّر: اختلاف الدم إذا كان من سحج الأمعاء وطال لبثه يزيد الحفر في عمق الأعضاء وصارت
قرحة فيها عفونة وتألم المعدة بالمشاركة فينال هضمها الضرر. فإذا ترقّت الآفة لفم المعدة سقطت
الشهوة وكان ذلك دليل على تمكّن المرض وامتداد عاديته.

---

١ بسم الله الرحمن الرحيم: om. ABP   ٢ المقالة السادسة من شرح فصول أبقراط: المقالة السادسة من كتاب
الفصول لأبقراط وشرحها A شرح المقالة السادسة من فصول أبقراط B المقالة السادسة P ‖ من شرح فصول
أبقراط: من كتاب الفصول لأبقراط وشرحها A   ٣-٤ بعد ... محمودة: om. B   ٥ كان: om. P ‖ علّة: om.
A   ٨ من ... أزيد: om. B   ٩ فيه: om. P ‖ على ضدّ ذلك: بالعكس A   ١١ في ... أردأ: om. B   ١٢ الدم:
om. A   ١٣ لفم: إلى فم B

(6.4)

[296] Says Hippocrates: If[301] the area around ulcers peels[302] off or falls off, it is bad.

Says the commentator: The fact that the hair around the ulcer falls off and that the skin peels off is an indication for the sharpness of [the humor] that streams into it; for this reason, the surrounding area is corroded eventually.

(6.5)

[297] Says Hippocrates: One should observe about pains that occur in the ribs, in the front part of the chest, and in the other parts, whether they show great differences.

Says the commentator: He means that one should not be content with [observing] the spot where the pain is without looking into the severity and mildness of the disease. One can conclude to that from the severity of the pain and the accompanying sensation of pricking, stinging, convulsive tension, and the like, [that is] from the different symptoms and their severity that come with the pain in that organ.

(6.6)

[298] Says Hippocrates: The illnesses that occur in the bladder and kidneys are difficult to cure in old people.

Says the commentator: This is clear.

(6.7)

[299] Says Hippocrates: Of the pains[303] that occur in the belly, those that are located[304] higher are milder, and those that are not so are more severe.

---

301   "If the area around ulcers peels off or falls off": Cf. Galen, *In Hippocratis Aphorismos commentarius* 6.4, ed. Kühn, vol. 18a, p. 12: Τὰ περιμάδηρα ἕλκεα; Hippocrates, *Aphorisms*, trans. Littré, vol. 4, p. 565: "Les ulcères autour desquels le poil tombe;" trans. Jones, p. 181: "Sores, when the hair about them falls off."

302   "peels off": Lit., "is dispersed."

303   "pains": Hippocrates, *Aphorisms* 6.7, ed. and trans. Jones, pp. 180–181, adds: καὶ οἰδήματα ("and swellings"); it is however omitted by ed. and trans. Littré, vol. 4, pp. 564–565, and also by Galen.

304   "located higher" (أعلى موضعا): Cf. Galen, *In Hippocratis Aphorismos commentarius* 6.7, ed. Kühn, vol. 18a, p. 18: μετέωρα; Hippocrates, ibid., trans. Littré, p. 565: "superficiels;" trans. Jones, p. 181: "superficial."

(6.4)

[٢٩٦] قال أبقراط: ما كان من القروح ينتثر ويتساقط ما حوله فهو خبيث.

قال المفسّر: تساقط ما حول القرحة من الشعر وتقشّر الجلد دليل على حدّة ما ينصبّ لها فلذلك تأكّل ما حولها أخيرا.

(6.5)

[٢٩٧] قال أبقراط: ينبغي أنْ يتفقّد من الأوجاع العارضة في الأضلاع ومقدّم الصدر وغير ذلك
٥ من سائر الأعضاء عظم اختلافها.

قال المفسّر: يريد أنْ لا يقتصر على موضع الألم فقط دون أنْ ينظر في عظم المرض أو ضعفه. والاستدلال على ذلك من شدّة الوجع وما يوجد معه من النخس واللدغ والتمدّد ونحو ذلك من اختلاف الأعراض وشدّتها التابعة لألم ذلك العضو.

(6.6)

[٢٩٨] قال أبقراط: العلل التي تكون في المثانة والكلى يعسر برؤها في المشائخ.

قال المفسّر: هذا بيّن.
١٠

(6.7)

[٢٩٩] قال أبقراط: ما كان من الأوجاع التي تعرض في البطن أعلى موضعا فهو أخفّ وما كان منها
ليس كذلك فهو أشدّ.

١ ما: من P ‖ القروح: الأمراض A ‖ ينتثر: ينتشر t ‖ حوله: من الشعر add. t ‏ ٥-٤ ومقدّم ... اختلافها:
om. B ‏ ٤ الصدر: الرأس P الصدر P¹ ‏ ٦ المرض: المريض C ‏ ١١ موضعا: موضع AB ‏ ١٢-١١ فهو ...
أشدّ: om. B

Says the commentator: Galen says that with "higher located" he means [the pain], which is close to the surface of the abdomen above the abdominal membrane (peritoneum). With his statement "those that are not so" he means [the pain] that is in the intestines and belly.

(6.8)

[300] Says Hippocrates: Ulcers occurring on the body of those suffering from dropsy are not easy to heal.

Says the commentator: Ulcers do not scar over (heal) until they have completely dried, and this is something that is not easy in those whose temperament [is affected by] dropsy.

(6.9)

[301] Says Hippocrates: Broad pustules are[305] hardly ever accompanied by itch.

Says the commentator: When pustules and wounds stretch widely but do not swell, it is a sign that their [substance] is very cold. For that reason itch does not occur because of the coldness of the [substance].

(6.10)

[302] Says Hippocrates: If someone suffers from headache and a severe pain in the head and pus[306] or water flows from his nostrils or ears, his illness will be [cured] by that.

Says the commentator: This is clear.

(6.11)

[303] Says Hippocrates: When hemorrhoids develop in[307] those who suffer from melancholic delusion or phrenitis, it is a good sign.

---

305 "are hardly ever accompanied by itch" (لا يكاد تكون معها حكّة): Cf. Galen, ibid. 6.9, p. 19: οὐ πάνυ τι κνησμώδεα; Hippocrates, ibid., trans. Littré, p. 567: "ne causent guère de prurit;" trans. Jones, p. 183: "are not very irritating."

306 "pus or water": Cf. Galen, ibid. 6.10, p. 20: πῦον ἢ ὕδωρ ἢ αἷμα; Hippocrates, ibid., trans. Littré, p. 567: "de pus, ou d'eau, ou de sang;" trans. Jones, p. 183: "pus, water or blood." Maimonides' version is according to trans. Ḥunayn (S, fol. 116ʳ).

307 "in those who suffer from melancholic delusion" (أصحاب الوسواس السوداوي): Cf. Galen, ibid. 6.11, ed. Kühn, p. 21: Τοῖσι μελαγχολικοῖσι; Hippocrates, ibid., trans. Littré, p. 567: "Dans la mélancolie;" trans. Jones, p. 183: "on melancholic ... affections;" for Arabic waswās, cf. Dols, Majnūn, pp. 285–286.

قال المفسّر: يقول جالينوس إنّه يريد بأعلى موضعا مايلي ظاهر البطن فوق الغشاء الممدود على الأمعاء والمعدة وقوله ما كان منها ليس كذلك يريد به ما كان منها في الأمعاء والمعدة.

(6.8)

[٣٠٠] قال أبقراط: ما يعرض من القروح في أبدان أصحاب الاستسقاء ليس يسهل برؤه.

قال المفسّر: القروح ليست تندمل حتّى تجفّ جفافا كاملا وما يسهل ذلك في مزاج المستسقين.

(6.9)

٥   [٣٠١] قال أبقراط: البثور العراض لا يكاد تكون معها حكّة.

قال المفسّر: كون البثور والقروح تمتدّ عرضا ولا يكون لها شخوص دليل على كون المادّة أبرد. ولذلك لا تحدث حكّة لبرد المادّة.

(6.10)

[٣٠٢] قال أبقراط: من كان به صداع ووجع شديد في رأسه فانحدر من منخريه أو أذنيه قيح أو ماء فإنّ مرضه يخلّ بذلك.

١٠   قال المفسّر: هذا بيّن.

(6.11)

[٣٠٣] قال أبقراط: أصحاب الوسواس السوداوي وأصحاب البرسام إذا حدثت بهم البواسير كان ذلك دليلا محمودا فيهم.

---

١ موضعا: موضع AB   ٣ ليس يسهل برؤه: om. B   ٦ عرضا: عراضا A   ٨ في رأسه: C¹   ٩-٨ فانحدر ... بذلك: om. B   ١٢-١١ وأصحاب ... فيهم: om. B

Says the commentator: Melancholic delusion is the mental confusion (delirium) that occurs as a result of black bile. Its Greek name is *mālankhūliyā* (μελαγχολία).[308] Phrenitis is an inflammation of the membranes in the brain. It is clear that the situation improves if the matter [which causes the illness] goes away to the opposite side and comes with an opening of the orifices of the vessels (arteries).

(6.12)

[304] Says Hippocrates: If someone is treated for chronic hemorrhoids until he is cured and not a single one is left, one cannot be sure that he will not suffer from dropsy or phthisis.

Says the commentator: The reason is that if not one [hemorrhoid] is left from which the turbid blood can be evacuated, that blood will return and become burdensome for the liver and extinguish its heat because of its large quantity and dropsy will occur. Alternatively, [the blood] may be sent through other vessels and a vessel in the lungs may burst and phthisis will occur. That is to say that both illnesses may occur [at the same time] or that either of them may happen.

(6.13)

[305] Says Hippocrates: If a person afflicted with hiccups develops sneezing, the hiccups will subside.

Says the commentator: Hiccups mostly occur because of overfilling. This is cured by sneezing because those [excessive] fluids become less as the sneezing moves and expels them.

(6.14)

[306] Says Hippocrates: If a person suffers from dropsy and water flows through his [blood] vessels to the abdomen, the illness will come to an end.

Says the commentator: This is clear because nature does with these fluids what it does with the illness-producing matter in the crises of acute diseases.

---

308 Cf. Maimonides, *Medical Aphorisms* 23.63, trans. Bos, vol. 5, p. 51: "The 'black bile' illness, that is, melancholy, is [the same as] melancholic delusion. *In Hippocratis Epidemiarum librum 6 commentarius 3*."

قال المفسّر: الوسواس السوداوي هو اختلاط الذهن الكائن من السوداء وهو الذي اسمه باليوناني مالنخوليا والبرسام ورم حارّ في أغشية الدماغ. وبيّن هو أنّ إذا انصرفت المادّة إلى خلاف الجهة وجاءت بانفتاح أفواه العروق صلحت الحال.

(6.12)

[٣٠٤] قال أبقراط: من عولج من بواسير مزمنة حتّى يبرأ ثمّ لم يترك منها واحد فلا يؤمن عليه أنْ

٥   يحدث به استسقاء أو سلّ.

قال المفسّر: لأنّه إذا لم يترك منها واحد يستفرغ منه الدم العكر عاد ذلك الدم وكثر على الكبد فأطفأ حرارتها بكثرته فيحدث الاستسقاء أو تبعثه في عروق أخر فينفتق عرق في الرئة فيحدث السلّ يعني أنّه قد يحدث هذين المرضين وقد يحدث من ذلك غيرهما.

(6.13)

[٣٠٥] قال أبقراط: إذا اعترى إنسان فواق لحدث به عطاس سكن به فواقه.

١٠   قال المفسّر: أكثر ما يكون الفواق من الامتلاء وهو الذي يبرأ بالعطاس لانتقاص تلك الرطوبات بحركة العطاس المزعجة.

(6.14)

[٣٠٦] قال أبقراط: إذا كان بإنسان استسقاء لجرى الماء منه في عروقه إلى بطنه كان بذلك انقضاء مرضه.

قال المفسّر: هذا بيّن لأنّه قد تفعل الطبيعة بتلك المائية ما تفعل في بحارين الأمراض الحادّة بالمادّة

١٥   الممرّضة.

٤-٥ ثمّ ... سلّ: om. B   ٤ واحد: واحدا C   ٦ واحد: om. P   ٧ فينفتق: فينبثق ABP   ٩ لحدث ... فواقه: om. B   ١٠ الرطوبات: الرطوبة: C   ١٢-١٣ في ... مرضه: om. B   ١٤ المائية: المادة P ‖ بالمادّة: بالماء A

(6.15)

[307] Says Hippocrates: If a person suffers from prolonged diarrhea, spontaneous vomiting stops the diarrhea.

Says the commentator: This is clear because nature attracts the matter [that causes the illness] to the opposite side.

(6.16)

[308] Says Hippocrates: If a person is afflicted by pleuritis or pneumonia and then gets diarrhea, it is a bad sign.

Says the commentator: Diarrhea is especially a bad sign in these two illnesses when the illness is so severe that the bowels become loose because of the weakness of the strength [of the body].

(6.17)

[309] Says Hippocrates: If a person suffers from ophthalmia and then gets diarrhea, it is a good sign.

Says the commentator: This is clear.

(6.18)

[310] Says Hippocrates: If[309] a tear occurs in the bladder or the brain or the heart or the[310] kidneys or one of the smaller intestines or the stomach or the liver, it is fatal.[311]

---

309 "If a tear occurs" (إذا حدث ... خرق): Cf. Galen, *In Hippocratis Aphorismos commentarius* 6.18, ed. Kühn, vol. 18a, p. 27: διακοπέντι; Hippocrates, *Aphorisms*, trans. Littré, vol. 4, p. 567: "Les plaies;" trans. Jones, p. 183: "A severe wound."

310 "the kidneys": Cf. Galen, ibid.: κοιλίην; Hippocrates, ibid., trans. Littré, p. 569: "diaphragme;" trans. Jones: "belly." See also Barry, *Syriac Medicine*, pp. 76–77.

311 Cf. Maimonides, *Medical Aphorisms* 24.54, trans. Bos, p. 99: "He says: A deep wound that occurs in the lobes of the liver can be cured. Similarly, if one of the lobes of the liver is cut off. Sometimes we see that the neck of the bladder is healed from a cut made to extract a stone because the neck of the bladder is fleshy. But all these things happen only rarely. Some say that the wound occurring in the stomach can be cured. I have seen a man who suffered from a large deep wound in the brain and was cured, although such a thing happens only rarely. *In Hippocratis Aphorismos commentarius* 6."

(6.15)

[٣٠٧] قال أبقراط: إذا كان بإنسان اختلاف قد طال لحدث به قيء من تلقاء نفسه انقطع بذلك اختلافه.

قال المفسّر: هذا بيّن لأنّ الطبيعة جذبت المادّة لخلاف الجهة.

(6.16)

[٣٠٨] قال أبقراط: من اعترته ذات الجنب أو ذات الرئة لحدث به اختلاف فذلك فيه دليل

٥   سوء.

قال المفسّر: إنّما يكون الاختلاف علامة رديئة في هذين المرضين متى كانت العلّة عظيمة جدًّا حتّى يلين الطبع من ضعف القوة.

(6.17)

[٣٠٩] قال أبقراط: إذا كان بإنسان رمد فاعتراه اختلاف فذلك محمود.

قال المفسّر: هذا بيّن.

(6.18)

[٣١٠] قال أبقراط: إذا حدث في المثانة خرق أو في الدماغ أو في القلب أو في الكلى أو في بعض

١٠   الأمعاء الدقاق أو في المعدة أو في الكبد فذلك قتّال.

٢-١ لحدث ... اختلافه: om. B   ٤-٥ أو ... سوء: om. B   ٤ فيه: هو P   ٨ فاعتراه ... محمود: om. B

١٠ في المثانة: بالمثانة A   ١٠-١١ أو ... قتّال: om. B

Says the commentator: Galen says: Hippocrates uses the term "fatal" for that, which kills necessarily [always] or kills in most cases.[312] I have seen myself a man who was afflicted by a large, deep wound in his brain and [yet] he recovered. However, this only happens rarely.

(6.19)
[311] Says Hippocrates: When a bone, cartilage, nerve, the delicate part of the jaw, or the foreskin is severed, it neither grows back nor unites.

Says the commentator: It does not grow back, this means that [restoration] similar to that in [the case of] a deep wound does not happen. If there was a split (crack), it (i.e., bone, cartilage, etc.) will not grow together again because these are dry organs. Also, when they are torn or cut, [these parts] separate widely.

(6.20)
[312] Says Hippocrates: If blood streams into a cavity in an unnatural way, it must suppurate.

Says the commentator: With "suppurate" he means [that the blood] changes and that its blood-like form is spoiled.

(6.21)
[313] Says Hippocrates: If someone is attacked by madness and then has a widening of the veins, which are known as varicose veins or hemorrhoids, his madness disappears.

Says the commentator: This is clear because of the turning of the matter [that produced the illness] to the opposite side, [but] on the condition that the humors that caused the madness flow to the loins. You [should] also know that his (i.e., Hippocrates') verdicts are not the general rule.

---

312   Cf. Galen, *In Hippocratis Aphorismos commentarius* 6.18, ed. Kühn, 18a, p. 27: Τὸ θανατῶδες ὄνομά πολλάκις εἴρηται ἐν ἄλλοις τε καὶ κατ' αὐτὸ τοῦτο τὸ βιβλίον, ἐπὶ τῶν ἐξ ἀνάγκης τεθνηξο-μένων, πολλάκις δὲ τῶν ὡς ἐπὶ τὸ πολύ; cf. trans. Ḥunayn (S, fol. 118ª): قوله قتال في هذا الكتّاب

وفي غيره قد نجده يقوله وهو يعني به أنّ صاحبه يموت لا محالة يقوله ونجده كثيرا يقوله وهو يعني أنّ صاحبه يموت في أكثر الحالات.

قال المفسّر: قال جالينوس: أبقراط يستعمل قتّال فيما يقتل ضرورة وفيما يقتل على الأكثر. وقد رأيت رجلا أصابته في دماغه جراحة عظيمة غائرة فبرأ إلّا أنّ هذا في الندرة.

(6.19)

[٣١١] قال أبقراط: متى انقطع عظم أو غضروف أو عصبة أو الموضع الرقيق من اللحي أو القلفة لم ينبت ولم يلتحم.

قال المفسّر: لم ينبت يعني لا يحدث مثله في قرحة غائرة وإنْ كان شقّ فلا يلتحم لأنّها أعضاء يابسة وتتباعد أيضا بالشقّ والقطع بعدا كثيرا.

(6.20)

[٣١٢] قال أبقراط: إذا انصبّ دم إلى فضاء على خلاف الأمر الطبيعي فلا بدّ من أنْ يتقيّح.

قال المفسّر: يعني بقوله يتقيّح يتغيّر وتفسد صورته الدمية.

(6.21)

[٣١٣] قال أبقراط: من أصابه جنون لحدث به اتّساع العروق التي تعرف بالدوالي أو البواسير انحلّ

١٠   عنه جنونه.

قال المفسّر: هذا بيّن لانصراف المادّة لخلاف الجهة وبشرط أنْ تكون تلك الأخلاط المولّدة للجنون هي التي مالت إلى الساقين. وقد علمت أيضا أنّ قضاياه ليست كلّية.

---

١ قتّال: om. P   مثل B   ٣-٤ أو ... يلتحم: om. B   ٥ يحدث: بالشقّ والقطع add. P || وإنْ: فإنْ P   ٧ على
... يتقيّح: om. B   ٩-١٠ التي ... جنونه: om. B

(6.22)

[314] Says Hippocrates: Pains[313] that descend from the back to the elbows are relieved by venesection.

Says the commentator: If the causes of those pains are humors, [which] flowed to the elbow, and [these humors] are evacuated from the place they flowed to, it is beneficial without any doubt.

(6.23)

[315] Says Hippocrates: If someone suffers from prolonged fear and despondency, it[314] is caused by black bile.

Says the commentator: If someone is affected by fear and despondency for no apparent reason, the cause is a[315] sort of melancholy, even if those symptoms are not continuous. But when the beginning of these symptoms is for an obvious reason, such as anger, fury, or grief, and then [the symptoms] become lengthy and continuous, their continuity indicates a [real] melancholy.[316]

(6.24)

[316] Says Hippocrates: When one of the small intestines is severed, it does not unite.[317]

(6.25)

[317] Says Hippocrates: When the inflammation known as erysipelas moves from the outside to the inside [of the body], it is not [a] good [sign]; but when it moves from the inside to the outside, it is [a] good [sign].

---

313   "Pains": Cf. Galen, ibid. 6.22, ed. Kühn, p. 34: ῥήγματα; Hippocrates, *Aphorisms*, trans. Littré, vol. 4, p. 569: "Les brisements;" trans. Jones, p. 185: "Ruptures." Some Hippocratic MSS however read ἀλγήματα, which is the reading that Ḥunayn had in front of him in his translation of both Hippocrates, ibid., ed. Tytler, p. 55, and of Galen's commentary (S, fol. 119[b]).

314   "it is caused by black bile" (فعلّته سوداوية): Cf. Galen, ibid. 6.23, ed. Kühn, p. 35: μελαγχολικὸν τὸ τοιοῦτον; Hippocrates, ibid., trans. Littré: "c'est un état mélancolique;" trans. Jones: "means melancholia." See also Barry, *Syriac Medicine*, p. 61.

315   "a sort of melancholy": Cf. Pormann/Joosse, *Commentaries on Hippocratic Aphorisms*, p. 230: "by way of melancholy."

316   For an extensive discussion of the commentaries to this aphorism in the Arabic commentary tradition, see ibid., pp. 218–249. For Maimonides' commentary, see pp. 229–230.

317   This Aphorism is lacking in all Arabic MSS, except for P. It is also missing in the Hebrew tradition, except for the anonymous translation.

(6.22)

[٣١٤] قال أبقراط: الأوجاع التي تنحدر من الظهر إلى المرفقين يحلّها فصد العرق.

قال المفسّر: إذا كان سبب تلك الأوجاع أخلاط ومالت نحو المرفق فاستفرغت من الموضع الذي مالت إليه استنفع بذلك بلا شك.

(6.23)

[٣١٥] قال أبقراط: من دام به التفزّع وخبث النفس زمانا طويلا فعلّته سوداوية.

قال المفسّر: متى عرض لإنسان تفزّع وخبث النفس من غير سبب ظاهر فسبب ذلك من طريق ٥
الوسواس السوداوي وإنْ لم تكن تلك الأعراض دائمة. ومتى كان ابتداء هذه الأعراض من سبب
ظاهر مثل غضب أو غيظ أو حزن ثمّ طالت ودام لبثها فدوامها يدلّ على الوسواس السوداوي.

(6.24)

[٣١٦] قال أبقراط: إذا انقطع بعض الأمعاء الدقاق لا يلتحم.

(6.25)

[٣١٧] قال أبقراط: انتقال الورم الذي يدعى الجمرة من خارج إلى داخل ليس هو بمحمود. وأمّا انتقاله
من داخل إلى خارج فهو محمود. ١٠

---

١ إلى ... العرق: om. B   ٣ إليه: نحوه A   ٤-٥ زمانا ... النفس: om. B   ٥ متى ... النفس: om. P
٦ السوداوي: om. BP ǁ تكن: تكون P   ٨ قال ... يلتحم: om. ABC   ٩ قال أبقراط: om. P   ٩-١٠ من
... محمود: om. B

Says the commentator: He mentions the inflammation of erysipelas [only] as an example. The same applies to any inflammation and any [purulent] matter that emerges from the inside to the outside, for it is a good sign. But if the opposite is the case, it is a bad sign because it indicates that nature is weak.

(6.26)

[318] Says Hippocrates: If someone suffers from tremors during ardent fever, mental confusion (delirium) will relieve him from them.

Says the commentator: Galen has already explained the confusion of what he says in this aphorism, namely that when the matter [that causes] the ardent fever and that is in the vessels moves to the nerves, tremors occur. And[318] when [the matter] settles in the brain, a mental confusion (delirium) develops and this is more dangerous than ardent fever. And in such a case, one should not say (it is not helpful to say) that the fever disappears[319] because that which happens [instead of it][320] is more dangerous and worse.

(6.27)

[319] Says Hippocrates: If someone who suffers from an empyema or dropsy is cauterized or incised and then a large quantity of pus or water flows from him all of a sudden, he will die without any doubt.

Says the commentator: Suffering from an empyema refers to everyone who has pus in the cavity between the chest and lung. Someone with this disease needs cauterization to dry that moisture, when he is unable to expel it through expectoration. Similarly, dropsy patients should be incised. He remarks that this sudden evacuation is fatal. He has [the same] opinion in the case of the other organs: When a large swelling occurs in one of them and then pus develops, the sudden evacuation of the pus from it is dangerous, because the patient will faint immediately and his strength will collapse. And afterwards he will remain in this weak condition that will be difficult to reverse.

---

318   "And when [the matter] settles in the brain, a mental confusion (delirium) develops and
      this is more dangerous than ardent fever": This statement does not feature in Galen, *In
      Hippocratis Aphorismos commentarius* 6.26, ed. Kühn, vol. 18a, pp. 37–38. But cf. Ḥunayn
      وهو أنّ الأسباب التي تحدث عنها هذه الحمى إنّما هي في العروق وإذا انتقلت إلى العصب :(S, fol. 120b)
      أحدثت أوّلا ارتعاشا ثمّ إنّه إذا شاركت العصب في العلّة الأصل الذي منه تنبت وهو الدماغ حدث
      اختلاط الذهن (The causes of the ardent fever are in the vessels; if [these causes] move to
      the nerves they produce first of all tremors, but when the nerves share the illness with the
      root (*aṣl*) from which it (i.e., the illness) originates, namely the brain, delirium occurs).
319   Note that Galen's statement that the fever will disappear is contrary to that of Hippocrates,
      who says that the tremors will disappear.
320   I.e., the supervening delirium.

قال المفسّر: ذكر ورم الجمرة مثال وهو القياس في كلّ ورم وكلّ مادّة تبرز من داخل إلى خارج فإنّها علامة محمودة. وإذا كان الأمر بالعكس فعلامة رديئة لأنّه دليل على ضعف الطبيعة.

(6.26)

[٣١٨] قال أبقراط: من عرضت له في الحمّى المحرقة رعشة فإنّ اختلاط ذهنه يحلّها عنه.

قال المفسّر: قد بين جالينوس اضطراب القول في هذا الفصل وذلك أنّ مادّة الحمّى المحرقة في العروق

٥ فإذا انتقلت المادّة للعصب حدثت الرعشة فإذا تمكّنت من الدماغ اختلط الذهن وهو أشدّ خطرا من الحمّى المحرقة. وليس في مثل هذا يقال إن انحلّت الحمّى لكون الأمر الذي حدث أشدّ خطرا وأردأ.

(6.27)

[٣١٩] قال أبقراط: من كوي أو بطّ من المتقيّحين او المستسقين لجرى منه من المدّة أو من الماء شيء كثير دفعة فإنّه يهلك لا محالة.

قال المفسّر: المتقيّحين يسمّى كلّ من كان به مدّة في الفضاء الذي ما بين الصدر والرئة. ويحتاج إلى

١٠ الكيّ صاحب هذه العلّة لينشف تلك الرطوبة إذا أعيا خروجها بالنفث. وكذلك أصحاب الاستسقاء المائي يبطّون. فذكر أنّ هذا الاستفراغ مهلك دفعة. وقد يرى أيضا في سائر الأعضاء متى حدث في واحد منها ورم عظيم فتقيّح فاستفراغ القيح منه دفعة خطر لأنّه يعرض لصاحبه على المكان الغشي وسقوط القوة ثمّ أنّه فيما بعد يبقى على ضعف يعسر ردّه.

---

١ مثال: مثلا A ‖ تبرز: ثور BP   ٢ فعلامة: علامة A   ٣ ذهنه: om. A   ٥ فإذا ... الرعشة: om. A ‖ خطرا: خطر BP   ٦ خطرا: خطر BP   ٨-٧ لجرى ... محالة: om. B   ٩ من كان: om. B ‖ كان: om. BP   ١١ دفعة: om. P

(6.28)

[320] Says Hippocrates: Eunuchs do not suffer from gout, nor do they become bald.

Says the commentator: This is because they are like women. Just as women do not become bald because of their moist temperament, so too [baldness] does not occur to them. The rare occurrence of gout is as will be explained.

(6.29)

[321] Says Hippocrates: Women do not suffer from gout, unless their menstruation has stopped.

Says the commentator: He has [implicitly] given the reason for the rare occurrence of gout in women, namely the evacuation of their superfluities through the menstrual blood.

(6.30)

[322] Says Hippocrates: A young man does not get gout before sexual intercourse with a woman.

Says the commentator: Galen says that having sexual intercourse has a very strong effect in producing gout, but does not say why. In my opinion, the most probable reason is that feet have very little flesh but many nerves and tendons and are exposed to the air. If sexual intercourse is harmful for the nerves in general, because of the evacuation of pneuma from them and because of their cooling, it is most harmful for the nerves in the feet. We always observe that when the feet are cold, the erection is less. This is an indication for their affinity (i.e., of coitus and gout) with regard to the nerves.

(6.31)

[323] Says Hippocrates: Pains in the eyes are alleviated by drinking pure wine or by bathing or by fomenting[321] or by venesection or by taking a purgative drug.

---

321   "fomenting": The Arabic term (تكميد) stands for Greek πυρίη (vapor bath); cf. aphorism 5.28 (248) above.

(6.28)

[٣٢٠] قال أبقراط: الخصيان لا يعرض لهم النقرس ولا الصلع.

قال المفسّر: لأنّهم كالنساء فكما لا يعرض الصلع للنساء لرطوبة مزاجهنّ كذلك لا يعرض لهؤلاء. وقلّة وقوع النقرس كما تبيّن.

(6.29)

[٣٢١] قال أبقراط: المرأة لا يصيبها النقرس إلّا بأنْ ينقطع طمثها.

٥ قال المفسّر: قد أعطى العلّة في قلّة وقوع النقرس في النساء وذلك لاستفراغ فضولهنّ بالطمث.

(6.30)

[٣٢٢] قال أبقراط: الغلام لا يصيبه النقرس قبل أنْ يبتدئ في مباضعة الجماع.

قال المفسّر: قال جالينوس إنّ لاستعمال الجماع في توليد النقرس قوّة عظيمة جدًّا ولم يبيّن سبب ذلك. والأقرب عندي أنّ سبب ذلك كون الرجلين قليلة اللحم كثيرة الأعصاب والأوتار وهي بارزة للهواء. فإذا أضرّ الجماع بالعصب على العموم لاستفراغ روحه وتبريده إيّاه كان نكاية ذلك في أعصاب الرجلين أشدّ. ونحن نشاهد دائمًا أنّ إذا بردت الرجلان نقص الإنعاظ. فهذا دليل على مشاركتها من ١٠ جهة الأعصاب.

(6.31)

[٣٢٣] قال أبقراط: أوجاع العينين يحلّها شرب الشراب الصرف أو الحمّام أو التكميد أو فصد العرق أو شرب الدواء.

---

٢ مزاجهنّ: مزاجهم BP ٤ طمثها: om. A ٩ كان: من P ١٠ نقص: انقش AC ‖ مشاركتها: مشاركته

ما C ١٢-١٣ الصرف ... الدواء: om. B

Says the commentator: Galen has explained the kind of confusion of this aphorism and that it does not come in the way of teaching what is useful in the art of medicine.[322] He said that if the [superfluous] matters are sharp and[323] the body is clean, then bathing is useful, [for then] the pain is alleviated.[324] And when the [superfluous] matters stop streaming while the body is clean, fomenting with hot water is useful.[325] When the vessels of the eye are full, thick blood got stuck in them while the rest of the body is not full, and the eye is dry, drinking pure wine dissolves that [thick] blood, evacuates it, and removes it from the vessels in which it got stuck.[326]

Galen said that these three kinds of treatment are very dangerous if they are not applied in the right situation.[327] As for venesection, for overfilling with blood, or the evacuation of the prevailing humor through purgation, these are clear [and] correct [methods] that are always applied.[328]

(6.32)
[324] Says Hippocrates: People who lisp are especially attacked by prolonged diarrhea.

Says the commentator: Lisping is mostly caused by a large quantity of moisture and softness. For this reason, young people lisp because of their moisture and softness. [People] with this kind of temperament have mostly loose bowels.

(6.33)
[325] Says Hippocrates: Those who suffer from acid eructations are hardly ever attacked by pleuritis.

---

322   Cf. Galen, *In Hippocratis Aphorismos commentarius* 6.31, ed. Kühn, vol. 18a, p. 45.

323   "and the body is clean" (وكان البدن نقيّا): Cf. ibid., p. 49: οὐ μὴν ἔτι γε πληθωρικὸν εἶναι τὸ σῶμα (and the body is not plethoric any more); cf. trans. Ḥunayn (S, fol. 124ᵃ): وليس في البدن امتلاء.

324   Cf. ibid., ed. Kühn.

325   Cf. ibid., p. 50.

326   Cf. ibid., p. 49.

327   Cf. ibid.: ταυτὶ μὲν οὖν ἀγωνιστικὰ βοηθήματα τῆς κατ᾽ ὀφθαλμοὺς ὀδύνης (These are the agonistic remedies for eye pain); cf. trans. Ḥunayn (S, fol. 124ᵃ): فهاذان النوعان من أنواع علاج وجع العينين عظيمًا المنفعة إن استعملا في مواضعهما وعلى حسب ذلك الخطر فيها إن لم استعملا على الصواب (These are the two kinds of treatment of eye pains that are very beneficial if they are applied in the [right] circumstances; accordingly [great] is their danger when they are not applied correctly).

328   Cf. Galen, ibid., ed. Kühn, p. 50: πληθωρικοῦ μὲν ὄντος αὐτοῦ διὰ φλεβοτομίας, κακοχύμου δὲ διὰ καθάρσεως (When [the body] is plethoric [we cleanse it] through venesection, and if it is full of bad humors [we cleanse it] through purgation).

قال المفسّر: قد بيّن جالينوس وجه اضطراب هذا الفصل وكونه لم يأت على طريق التعليم النافع في صناعة الطبّ. وذكر إنّه إذا كانت الموادّ حادّة وكان البدن نقيّا نفع الحمّام وسكن الوجع. واذا انقطع أيضا تحلّب المادّة مع نقاء البدن نفع التكميد بالماء الحارّ. وإذا كانت عروق العين ممتلئة قد لحج فيها دم غليظ من غير أنّ يكون في البدن كلّه امتلاء وكانت العين جافّة فإنّ شرب الشراب الصرف يذيب

٥ ذلك الدم ويستفرغه ويزعجه من العروق التي لحج فيها.

وذكر جالينوس أنّ هذه الأنواع الثلاثة من العلاج خطرة جدّا إنّ لم يصب بها موضع الاستحقاق. أمّا الفصد إنّ كان الامتلاء من دم أو استفراغ الخلط الغالب عليه بالإسهال فأمر بيّن صحيح وهو المستعمل دائما.

(6.32)

[٣٢٤] قال أبقراط: اللثغ يعتريهم خاصّة اختلاف طويل.

١٠ قال المفسّر: أكثر ما يكون سبب اللثغ من أجل رطوبة كثيرة ولين ولذلك يلثغ الصبيان لرطوبتهم ولينهم ومع هذا المزاج يلين الطبع على الأكثر.

(6.33)

[٣٢٥] قال أبقراط: أصحاب الجشاء الحامض لا يكاد يصيبهم ذات الجنب.

---

٤ الصرف: om. P ‖ ٩ يعتريهم: om. P؛ يعرض A ١٠ ولين: om. P ‖ ولذلك: فلذلك BP

Says the commentator: Pleurisy mostly originates from a thin, sharp humor that flows to the membrane that covers the ribs internally and gets stuck there. But this [kind of] humor only rarely originates in people who suffer from sour eructations.

(6.34)

[326] Says Hippocrates: Bald people do not often have veins that become wide that are known as varicose veins, but if they get varicose veins their hair grows again.

Says the commentator: Galen says that here he (i.e., Hippocrates) means the[329] [specific] baldness caused by sores on the head. If the malignant matter [that caused these sores] moves downward, varicose veins develop and the hair grows [back].[330]

(6.35)

[327] Says Hippocrates: If someone who has dropsy develops a cough, it is a bad sign.

Says the commentator: He means [to say that it is a bad sign] if dropsy is the cause of the cough. For this happens if the watery humors increase until they reach the windpipe and [the patient] is on the verge of being suffocated by that moisture.

(6.36)

[328] Says Hippocrates: Venesection cures dysuria, and the incision should be in [one of] the inner veins.

Says the commentator: Galen has corrected this aphorism by saying that sometimes [venesection] cures dysuria,[331] namely when it is caused by an inflamed tumor (lit., bloody tumor) with an excess of blood. For the rest of the aphorism he adds to the words of Hippocrates: "In that case the venesection should be from the back (hollow) of the knee (popliteal fossa)."[332]

---

329   "the [specific] baldness caused by sores on the head" (القَرع): Cf. Dozy, Supplément, vol. 2, p. 332: "ulcères sur la tête qui font tomber les cheveux;" cf. Galen, ibid. 6.34, p. 55: μαδάρω-σις; trans. Ḥunayn (S, fol. 126b): القرع.

330   Cf. Galen, ibid., ed. Kühn, p. 56.

331   Cf. ibid. 6.36, p. 57: δυσουρίην καὶ φλεβοτομία λύει; cf. S, fol. 127a: فصد العروق قد يحلّ عسر البول.

332   Cf. ibid., ed. Kühn, p. 58.

قال المفسّر: أكثر تولّد ذات الجنب إنّما هو من خلط رقيق حادّ يجري إلى الغشاء المستبطن للأضلاع ويلحج فيه. وأصحاب الجشاء الحامض قلّ أنْ يتولّد فيهم هذا الخلط.

(6.34)

[٣٢٦] قال أبقراط: الصلع لا يعرض لهم من العروق التي تتّسع التي تعرف بالدوالي كثير شيء ومن حدثت به من الصلع من الدوالي عاد شعر رأسه.

قال المفسّر: يقول جالينوس إنّه يريد هنا القرع فإذا انتقلت تلك المادّة الرديئة لأسفل حدثت الدوالي ونبت الشعر. ٥

(6.35)

[٣٢٧] قال أبقراط: إذا حدث بصاحب الاستسقاء سعال كان دليلا رديئا.

قال المفسّر: يعني إذا كان سبب السعال الاستسقاء وذلك بأنْ تكثر الرطوبات المائية إلى أنْ تبلغ قصبة الرئة فيكون قد أشفى على أنْ تخنقه تلك الرطوبة.

(6.36)

[٣٢٨] قال أبقراط: فصد العروق يحلّ عسر البول وينبغي أنْ يقطع العروق الداخلة. ١٠

قال المفسّر: أصلح جالينوس هذا الفصل بأن قال: قد يحلّ عسر البول وذلك إذا كان سببه ورم دموي مع كثرة الدم. وبقية الفصل قال إنّه دخيل في كلام أبقراط والواجب أنْ يكون الفصد حينئذ في مأبض الركبة.

---

١ أكثر: يكون A add. ‖ من: om. C ‖ إلى: في C ‖ ٨ تكثر: تكون A ‖ ٩ تخنقه: تراقي BP ‖ ١٠ العروق: العرق ABP ‖ وينبغي ... الداخلة: om. B ‖ العروق: بالعروق P ‖ ١٢ دخيل: دخل A

(6.37)

[329] Says Hippocrates: If a swelling appears on the outside of the throat in the case of someone suffering from angina, it is a good sign.

Says the commentator: It is clear that it is better when illnesses move from the internal organs to the external ones.

(6.38)

[330] Says Hippocrates: If someone develops a hidden cancer, it is better not to treat him, because if he is treated he[333] will die. If he is not treated he will survive for a long time.

Says the commentator: With "hidden" he means [the illness] that is deep inside the body and that is not visible, or it is visible but not accompanied by ulceration. With "omitting treatment" he means the kind [of treatment] that involves surgery or cauterization but not the [kind of treatment that consists of] alleviating [remedies].

(6.39)

[331] Says Hippocrates: Spasms occur either because of overfilling or because of emptying, likewise hiccups.

Says the commentator: The reason for all this is clear.

(6.40)

[332] Says Hippocrates: If someone suffers from pain in the hypochondrium without inflammation and then gets a fever, it will relieve the pain.

Says the commentator: If that pain is caused by wind or an obstruction, it is relieved by the fever. It is as if he had said: the fever may relieve [the pain]. The assertions of this man constantly follow this pattern. His verdicts are mostly missing the conditions [under which they are valid] or they are extraordinary; some of them are imaginary because they [are based] on chance (coincidence). He thought that because two things are connected by chance one of them is the cause of the other. This is what someone who is not biased would say. But someone who is biased can say anything he wants.

---

333   "he will die" (= S, fol. 127ᵃ): Cf. Galen, ibid. 6.38, ed. Kühn, p. 59: ἀπόλλυνται ταχέως; Hip-
        pocrates, *Aphorisms*, trans. Littré, vol. 4, p. 573: "elles meurent rapidement;" trans. Jones,
        p. 189: "[treatment] causes speedy death."

(6.37)

[٣٢٩] قال أبقراط: إذا ظهر الورم في الحلقوم من خارج في من اعترته الذبحة كان دليلا محمودا.

قال المفسّر: بيّن هو أنّ الأصلح انتقال العلل من الأعضاء الباطنة للظاهرة.

(6.38)

[٣٣٠] قال أبقراط: إذا حدث بإنسان سرطان خفي فالأصلح ألّا يعالج. فإن عولج هلك وإنْ لم يعالج بقي زمانا طويلا.

قال المفسّر: يعني بالخفي الذي يكون في عمق البدن فلا يظهر أو يكون ظاهرا ولا تكون معه قرحة ٥ ويعني بترك العلاج نوع القطع والكيّ لا التسكين.

(6.39)

[٣٣١] قال أبقراط: التشنّج يكون من الامتلاء ومن الاستفراغ وكذلك الفواق.

قال المفسّر: كلّ هذا بيّن العلّة.

(6.40)

[٣٣٢] قال أبقراط: من عرض له وجع في ما دون الشراسيف من غير ورم ثمّ حدثت به حمّى حلّت ١٠ ذلك الوجع عنه.

قال المفسّر: إذا كان ذلك الوجع بسبب ريح أو سدد حلّته الحمّى فكأنّه يقول قد تحلّله الحمّى وقد اطّردت أحكام هذا الرجل فإنّ قضاياه أكثرها ومعظمها محذوفة الشرائط أو نادرة وبعضها وهم لأنّها وقعت بالإتّفاق فظنّ لأنّ الشيئين المقترنين بالإتّفاق أنّ أحدهما سبب الآخر. هكذا يقول من لا يتعصّب وأمّا من يتعصّب فليقل ما أراد.

---

١ من ... محمودا: om. B ٣-٤ فالأصلح ... طويلا: om. B ٣ هلك: سريعا add. t ٥ ظاهرا: ظاهر BP ١٢ أكثرها: om. P ‖ ومعظمها ... نادرة: om. A ١٣ لأنّها: قد add. P ‖ الشيئين: om. A السببين ‖ بالإتّفاق: بالانتقال A C¹

(6.41)

[333] Says Hippocrates: If suppuration occurs in a certain place in the body but the suppuration does not show itself, this is due to the thickness of the pus or [the thickness of] the spot (part).

Says the commentator: It is clear that it is difficult to recognize the [suppurating] substance because of its thickness or because of the thickness of the spot (part).

(6.42)

[334] Says Hippocrates: If the liver is hard in someone suffering from jaundice, it is a bad sign.

Says the commentator: This is clear.

(6.43)

[335] Says Hippocrates: If someone suffering from an illness of the spleen is attacked by dysentery and this becomes chronic, dropsy or lientery supervenes and he dies.

Says the commentator: A splenetic patient is someone whose spleen has been hard for a long time. If he develops dysentery, whereby those thick melancholic humors that got stuck in the body of the spleen are removed, he will benefit therefrom, as he (i.e., Hippocrates) will explain later on.[334] But if the dysentery becomes chronic and excessive, it undermines the powers of the intestines by transporting those bad humors through them and thus produces lientery. And the innate heat is extinguished. Because of the sympathetic affection between the intestines and the liver, the liver is weakened and dropsy occurs.

---

334   Cf. aphorism 6.48 (340) below.

(6.41)

[٣٣٣] قال أبقراط: إذا كان موضع من البدن قد تقيّح وليس تبيّن تقيّحه فإنّما لا يتبيّن من قبل غلظ المدّة أو الموضع.

قال المفسّر: بيّن هو أنّ من أجل غلظ المادّة أو غلظ الموضع يعسر تعرّف المادّة.

(6.42)

[٣٣٤] قال أبقراط: إذا كانت الكبد في من به يرقان صلبة فذلك دليل رديء.

٥   قال المفسّر: هذا بيّن.

(6.43)

[٣٣٥] قال أبقراط: إذا أصاب المطحول اختلاف دم وطال به حدث به استسقاء أو زلق الأمعاء وهلك.

قال المفسّر: المطحول هو الذي في طحاله صلابة مزمنة فإذا حدث اختلاف دم على طريق انتقال تلك الأخلاط الغليظة السوداوية التي كانت تثبّتت في جرم الطحال استنفع بذلك كما يبيّن بعد. فإن ١٠ طال ذلك الاختلاف وجاوز القدر هدّ قوى الأمعاء بمرور هذه الأخلاط الرديئة بها وأحدث زلق الأمعاء فتطفئ الحرارة الغريزية. ولأجل مشاركة الأمعاء للكبد تضعف الكبد ويحدث الاستسقاء.

──────────

١-٢ وليس ... الموضع :om. B   ٦ وطال: فطال P   ٩ تشبّتت: سبب P ‖ جرم: ورم P   ١١ الأمعاء: om.

P

(6.44)

[336] Says Hippocrates: If someone suffers, as a result of strangury, from a[335]
colic known as "ileus," which[336] means "that from which one seeks protection,"
he will die within seven days unless he develops fever and there is an abundant
flow of urine.

Says the commentator: Galen was in doubt about this aphorism and com-
pelled himself to give farfetched interpretations in order to authenticate a
statement that is clearly deficient and the product of those who pursue things
that are vain (useless).[337]

---

335   "a colic known as 'ileus'" (القولنج المعروف بإيلاوس): Cf. Galen, *In Hippocratis Aphorismos
       commentarius* 6.44, ed. Kühn, vol. 18a, p. 68: εἰλεός; Hippocrates, *Aphorisms*, trans. Lit-
       tré, vol. 4, p. 575: "iléus;" trans. Jones, p. 189: "ileus;" Liddell/Scott, *Greek-English Lexicon*,
       p. 486: "intestinal obstruction;" Ullmann, *Wörterbuch*, p. 222, s.v. εἰλεός: "Obstruktion der
       Eingeweide, Darmverschlingung (→ auch κωλικός)." See also Barry, *Syriac Medicine*, pp. 54–
       55.

336   "which means 'that from which ones seeks protection'": Missing in Hippocrates, ibid., ed.
       Littré, p. 574, but featuring in Ḥunayn's translation of both the *Aphorisms*, ed. Tytler, p. 47,
       and of Galen's commentary (S, fol. 129ᵇ); cf. Ibn Janāḥ, *K. al-Talkhīṣ* 98, eds. and trans.
       Bos/Käs/Lübke/Mensching (forthcoming): إيلاوُس تفسيره ربِّ أرْحِم من التقسيم والتشجير
       للرازي، وفي كتاب الفصول لأبقراط: تفسيره السِداد منه، وفي الحاوي: هو القولنج المنتن وهو الذي
       يتقيّاً صاحبه الزبل. ("*Īlāwus* (εἰλεός, ileus). According to al-Rāzī's *Al-Taqsīm wa-l-tashjīr*, this
       word means 'O my lord, have mercy!' (*rabbi arḥim*). In the *Aphorisms* (*K. al-Fuṣūl*) by
       Hippocrates, as quoted in the same book: The meaning of this word is "the obstruction"
       (*sidād*). In his *Ḥāwī* he said: This is the stinking colic (*qawlanj*), that is to say the illness,
       the sufferer from which vomits faeces.")

337   Cf. Galen, *In Hippocratis Aphorismos commentarius* 6.44, ed. Kühn, vol. 18a, p. 70: βέλτιον
       οὖν ἀγνοεῖν ὁμολογεῖν, ὅπως εἴρηται τὰ κατὰ τὸν ἀφορισμὸν τοῦτον ὑφ' Ἱπποκράτους. οὔτε γὰρ
       ὁ λόγος ἐνδείκνυται τὴν ἀλήθειαν αὐτων οὔθ' ἡ πεῖρα διδάσκει, τρίτον δ' οὐδὲν ἔχομεν ἄλλο πρὸς
       πίστιν, εἴ γε μὴ ὦπταί ποτε τοιοῦτος ἄρρωστος οὔθ' ὑφ' Ἱπποκράτους οὔθ' ὑφ' ἄλλου τινός· οὔτε
       γὰρ εἰ γνήσιός ἐστιν ὁ ἀφορισμὸς εἰπεῖν ἔχω. πλῆθος οὖν ὠμῶν καὶ παχέων χυμῶν ἅμα ψύξει
       σφοδρᾷ βέλτιόν ἐστιν ὑποτίθεσθαι τῶν εἰρημένων συμπτωμάτων αἴτιον; cf. trans. Ḥunayn (S,
       fol. 130ᵇ): فإقرار الانسان بأنّه لا يعلم من أين قيل ما قيل في هذا الفصل أجود وذلك أنّه لا القياس
       يدلّ على حقيقته ولا التجربة يجد شيئا ثالثا يصحّ به ما يحتاج إلى تصحيحه فإن كان أبقراط وغيره
       قد رأى مريضا هذه حاله؟ فإنّي لا أدري هل هذا الفصل لأبقراط أو لغيره. فالأجود أن نجعل السبب
       في هذه الأعراض التي ذكرت الأخلاط النِيئة الغليظة مع برد شديد (It is better if one acknowl-
       edges that one does not know the origin of that which was said in this aphorism, because
       neither logic nor experience can point to its truth. One can also not find a third [method]
       by which one might authenticate what needs to be authenticated. And has Hippocrates
       or someone else [ever] seen a patient with this condition? I do not know whether this
       aphorism hails from Hippocrates or from someone else. It is best if we suppose that these
       afflictions mentioned [above] are caused by raw, thick humors in combination with severe
       cold ...).

(6.44)

[٣٣٦] قال أبقراط: من حدث به من تقطير البول القولنج المعروف بإيلاوس وتفسيره المستعاذ منه فإنّه يموت في سبعة أيّام إلّا أنْ تحدث به حمّى فيجري منه بول كثير.

قال المفسّر: قد شكّ جالينوس في هذا الفصل وتكلّف تأويلات بعيدة لتصحيح كلام ظاهر السقم من فعل البطّالين.

(6.45)

[337] Says Hippocrates: If ulcers last for a year or longer, the bone must necessarily exfoliate[338] and, once[339] [the ulcer] has healed, the [scar] must be
depressed.

Says the commentator: Ulcers mostly last a long time because of an affliction that reached the bone. When the corrupted bone has been expelled, [the
ulcer] heals but the site remains hollow.

(6.46)

[338] Says Hippocrates: If someone becomes humpback from asthma or cough
before reaching puberty, he will die.

Says the commentator: If a humpback develops without any initial[340] cause,
it comes from a hard tumor. Because of the [curved spine], tightness of the
lungs necessarily follows. During the growth [of the body], the lungs enlarge
but the chest cavity cannot expand and grow in its totality because of the
humpback and its cause, and therefore [the patient] suffocates and dies.

(6.47)

[339] Says Hippocrates: If someone needs to be bled or to be administered a
purgative drug, he should be administered a purgative drug or bled in spring.

Says the commentator: This is clear in the case of someone who needs that
as a precautionary (prophylactic) measure, as healthy people always do.

(6.48)

[340] Says Hippocrates: If someone suffering from an illness of the spleen
develops dysentery, it is a good [sign].

Says the commentator: This has been explained before.[341]

---

338 "exfoliate" (يَتَبَيَّن): Cf. ibid. 6.45, ed. Kühn, p. 71: ἀφίστασθαι; Hippocrates, *Aphorisms*, trans.
     Littré, vol. 4, p. 575: "s' exfolie;" trans. Jones, p. 189: "come away;" cf. Liddell/Scott, *Greek-
     English Lexicon*, p. 291: "exfoliate;" Ullmann, *Wörterbuch*, suppl. 1, p. 202: "sich entfernen,
     abstehen."

339 "once [the ulcer] has healed, the [scar]" (موضع الأثر بعد أندماﻟﻬا): Cf. Galen, ibid.: τὰς οὐλὰς;
     Hippocrates, ibid., trans. Littré, p. 575: "les cicatrices;" trans. Jones, p. 189: "the scars;" Ull-
     mann, ibid., p. 482.

340 "initial cause" (سبب بادئ): For this concept, cf. Pormann/Joosse, *Commentaries on Hippo-
     cratic Aphorisms*, pp. 232–233.

341 Cf. aphorism 6.43 (335) above.

(6.45)

[٣٣٧] قال أبقراط: إذا مضى بالقرحة حول أو مدّة أطول من ذلك وجب ضرورة أنْ يتبيّن منها عظم وأنْ يكون موضع الأثر بعد اندمالها غائرا.

قال المفسّر: أكثر ما يطول زمان القروح من أجل آفة لحقت العظم وإذا خرج العظم الفاسد برأت وبقي الموضع غائرا.

(6.46)

٥ [٣٣٨] قال أبقراط: من أصابته حدبة من ربو أو سعال قبل أنْ ينبت له شعر في العانة فإنّه يهلك.

قال المفسّر: إذا حدثت الحدبة من غير سبب بادئ فهي عن ورم صلب. فإذا أوجب ذلك ضيق على الرئة لأجل التقويس وفي زمان النشوء تتزيّد الرئة ولا يمكن أنْ يتّسع فضاء الصدر ولا يقبل كلّه النمو من أجل الحدبة وسببها فلذلك يختنق فيموت.

(6.47)

[٣٣٩] قال أبقراط: من إحتاج إلى الفصد أو إلى شرب الدواء فينبغي أنْ يسقى الدواء أو يفصد في ١٠ الربيع.

قال المفسّر: هذا بيّن لمن يحتاج ذلك على جهة الاحتياط كما يفعل الأصحّاء دائما.

(6.48)

[٣٤٠] قال أبقراط: إذا حدث بالمطحول اختلاف دم فذلك محمود.

قال المفسّر: قد تقدّم شرحه.

١-٢ أو ... غائرا: om. B ‖ ١ يتبيّن: يبين P ‖ ٥ أصابته: أصابه C ‖ أو ... يهلك: om. B ‖ في العانة: om.
AC ‖ يهلك: قبل الاحتلام P ٧ الصدر: om. P ‖ ٩-١٠ فينبغي ... الربيع: om. B ‖ ١٣ قد: هذا P

(6.49)

[341] Says Hippocrates: When gout-like illnesses are accompanied by an inflammation, the inflammation subsides within forty days.

Says the commentator: I have already described how he arrives at these [incorrect] definitions (conclusions).[342]

(6.50)

[342] Says Hippocrates: If someone suffers[343] from a gash in the brain, he will unavoidably develop fever and bilious vomiting.

Says the commentator: When the brain becomes swollen because of the gash, it is necessarily followed by fever and bilious vomiting because of the sympathetic affection between the brain and the stomach.

(6.51)

[343] Says Hippocrates: If someone who is healthy suddenly gets a headache and immediately loses his voice and starts[344] to breath stertorously (lit., to snore), he will die within seven days, unless he develops fever.

Says the commentator: The stertorous sound (lit., snoring) is an indication for the strength of the apoplexy, and you know that it is fatal unless fever develops, for sometimes [the fever] dissolves those thick humors or thick winds.

(6.52)

[344] Says Hippocrates: One should observe the[345] hidden part of the eye during sleep, for if part of the white of the eye is visible, while the eyelid is closed, and this does not occur after diarrhea or the ingestion of a purgative medication, it is a bad and exceedingly fatal sign.

---

342   Cf. aphorism 6.40 (332) above.

343   "suffers from a gash" (حدث به قطع): Cf. Galen, *In Hippocratis Aphorismos commentarius* 6.50, ed. Kühn, vol. 18a, p. 84: διακοπῇ; Hippocrates, *Aphorisms*, trans. Littré, vol. 4, p. 577: "Les plaies;" trans. Jones, p. 191: "severe wounds;" cf. aphorism 6.18 (310) above.

344   "starts to breath stertorously (lit., to snore)" (عرض له غطيط): Cf. Galen, ibid. 6.51, p. 87: ῥέγχουσιν; Hippocrates, ibid., trans. Littré, p. 577: "ont la respiration stertoreuse;" trans. Jones, p. 191: "breathing stertorously;" cf. Ullmann, *Wörterbuch*, p. 584.

345   "the hidden part of the eye" (باطن العين): Cf. Galen, ibid. 6.52, p. 89: τὰς ὑποφάσιας τῶν ὀφθαλμῶν; Hippocrates, ibid., trans. Littré: "ce qui se laisse voir des yeux;" trans. Jones: "what is seen of the eyes;" cf. Liddell/Scott, *Greek-English Lexicon*, p. 1901: "a being half seen;" Ullmann, ibid., p. 558, s.v. ὑποφαίνομαι: "sich nur ein wenig zeigen."

(6.49)

[٣٤١] قال أبقراط: ما كان من الأمراض من طريق النقرس وكان معه ورم حارّ فإنّ ورمه يسكن في أربعين يوما.

قال المفسّر: قد تقدّم على أيّ جهة تعطى هذه التحديدات.

(6.50)

[٣٤٢] قال أبقراط: من حدث به في دماغه قطع فلا بدّ من أنْ تحدث به حمّى وقيء مرار.

قال المفسّر: إذا ورم الدماغ من أجل القطع ضرورة تبع ذلك الحمّى وقيء المرار من أجل مشاركة الدماغ للمعدة.

(6.51)

[٣٤٣] قال أبقراط: من حدث به وهو صحيح وجع بغتّة في رأسه وأسكت على المكان وعرض له غطيط فإنّه يهلك في سبعة أيّام إنْ لم تحدث به حمّى.

قال المفسّر: الغطيط دليل قوّة السكتة. وقد علمت أنّها مهلكة إلّا أن حدثت حمّى فقد ربّما حلّت تلك ١٠ الأخلاط الغليظة أو الرياح الغليظة.

(6.52)

[٣٤٤] قال أبقراط: قد ينبغي أنْ يتفقّد باطن العين في وقت النوم. فإنْ تبيّن شيء من بياض العين والجفن مطبق وليس ذلك بعقب اختلاف ولا شرب دواء فتلك علامة رديئة مهلكة جدًّا.

---

٢ يوما: يوم BP   ٤ فلا ... مرار: om. B ‖ من: om. P   ٨-٧ وأسكت ... حمّى: om. B   ١٠ الرياح: om.
A   ١١ قد: om. A   ١٢ والجفن ... جدًّا: om. B

Says the commentator: The white of the eye becomes only visible when the eyelid is not closed. The eyelid does not close because of dryness and [the dryness] quickly affects the eyelids because of their natural dryness or because of the weakness of the strength [of the body] as occurs in patients who are too weak to close their mouths.

(6.53)
[345] Says Hippocrates: When mental confusion (delirium) occurs with laughter, it is safer; but when it is accompanied[346] by anxiety and sorrow, it is more dangerous.

Says the commentator: There is not any type of mental confusion (delirium) that is safe. The worst [kind] is that, which comes with a desire to attack (fight) and aggressive behavior, and this is [called] "madness." The least detrimental is [the type] that comes with laughter and unusual pleasure, as [in the case of] someone who drinks wine. Intermediate is [the type] that comes with worry and fear and thought. All these occur because of a[347] primary illness in the brain or because of the sympathetic affection with another organ. The [type of mental confusion (delirium)] that occurs because of heat (fever) only without [the involvement of] any humor is similar to the mental confusion (delirium) that occurs because of the drinking of wine. The [type of [mental confusion (delirium)] that develops from yellow bile is accompanied by worry and fear. When the [yellow bile] becomes increasingly burnt and tends to black bile, the mental confusion (delirium) turns into madness.[348]

(6.54)
[346] Says Hippocrates: Respiration[349] [that is broken as if by sobbing] in acute diseases accompanied by fever is a bad sign.

---

346   "accompanied by anxiety and sorrow" (مع هَمّ وحُزْن): Cf. Galen, ibid. 6.53, p. 90: μετὰ σπου-
       δῆς; Hippocrates, ibid., trans. Littré: "sérieux;" trans. Jones: "with seriousness."

347   "a primary illness in the brain" (علّة في الدماغ أوّلية): Cf. Galen, ibid., trans. Ḥunayn (S,
       fol. 135ᵇ): كانت العلّة منه ابتدأت ([whether] the illness started from [the brain]).

348   Cf. Maimonides, Medical Aphorisms 6.3, trans. Bos, vol. 2, p. 2: "When mental confusion
       results from heat but without [superfluous] matter, it is similar to the mental confusion
       caused by drinking wine. When it results from yellow bile, it is accompanied by worry and
       fear. When the yellow bile becomes increasingly burnt, the confusion turns into madness.
       In Hippocratis Aphorismos commentarius 6."

349   "Respiration [that is broken as if by sobbing]" (نفس البكاء): Cf. Galen, In Hippocratis Apho-
       rismos commentarius 6.54, ed. Kühn, vol. 18a, p. 92: αἱ κλαυθμώδεες ἀναπνοαί; Hippocrates,
       Aphorisms, trans. Littré, vol. 4, p. 577: "la respiration singultueuse;" trans. Jones, p. 191:

قال المفسّر: إنّما يتبيّن البياض إذا لم ينطبق الجفن وكون الجفن لا ينطبق إنّما هو من أجل اليبس وهو

يسرع للأجفان ليبسها بالطبع أو من أجل ضعف القوة كما تضعف في المرضى المدنفين عن إنطباق

الفم.

(6.53)

[٣٤٥] قال أبقراط: ما كان من اختلاط العقل مع ضحك فهو أسلم وما كان منه مع همّ وحزن فهو

أشدّ خطرا. ٥

قال المفسّر: ليس في أنواع الاختلاط شيء سليم وأردأها ما كان معه إقدام وتهجّم وهو الجنون. وأقلّها

شرّا ما كان مع ضحك وفرح غير معتاد كشارب النجر والذي معه همّ وحرص وفكرة فهو متوسّط.

وجميع ذلك من علّة في الدماغ أوّلية أو من أجل المشاركة لعضو آخر. فالذي يكون من أجل حرارة

فقط من غير خلط فهو شبيه بالاختلاط الذي يكون من شرب النبيذ والذي يكون من المرّة الصفراء

يكون معه همّ وحرص. فإذا تزيّدت احتراقا ومالت إلى السوداء مال الاختلاط إلى الجنون. ١٠

(6.54)

[٣٤٦] قال أبقراط: نفس البكاء في الأمراض الحادّة التي تكون معها حمّى دليل رديء.

---

٢ إنطباق: إطباق C   ٤-٥ وما ... خطرا: om. B   ٧ شرّ: شرّ om. C   مع: من A ‖ كشارب: كشراب

BP   ٨ أوّلية: أولبث BCP   ١٠ تزيّدت: تزايدت P الصفراء add. S, fol. 136ª b

---

"moaning respiration;" Liddell/Scott, *Greek-English Lexicon*, p. 956: "broken as if by sob-
bing;" Ullmann, *Wörterbuch*, p. 348: "weinerlich."

Says the commentator: He means that the respiration of the patient stops and then returns like the respiration of someone suffocating from crying. This happens either because the patient is too weak to breathe fully or because the respiratory organs are so dry and hard that [the patient has not the strength] to expand them or because [his] condition is close to that of [someone suffering from] spasms. All these are bad during acute diseases.

(6.55)

[347] Says Hippocrates: Gouty affections are[350] active (lit., move) mostly in spring and autumn.

Says the commentator: [This happens] in spring because the humors flow increasingly as they dissolve from their winter congelation and in autumn because of the earlier consumption of summer fruit.

(6.56)

[348] Says Hippocrates: In melancholic illnesses, one[351] has to fear that they lead to apoplexy or hemiplegia or spasms or madness or blindness.

Says the commentator: Galen says that apoplexy, hemiplegia, spasms, and blindness sometimes originate from phlegmatic humor and [sometimes] from melancholic humor. However, madness only occurs from the burning of yellow bile to a degree that it turns black.[352]

(6.57)

[349] Says Hippocrates: Apoplexy and[353] hemiplegia occur especially in the case of someone who is between forty and sixty years old.

---

350   "are active (lit., move)" (تَتَحَرَّكُ): Cf. Galen, ibid. 6.55, p. 94: κινέεται; Hippocrates, ibid., trans. Littré, p. 577: "se mettent en mouvement;" trans. Jones, p. 193: "become active."

351   "one has to fear that they lead to" (يُخَاف منها أنْ تَؤول إلى): Cf. Galen, ibid. 6.56, p. 95: ἐς τάδε ἐπικίνδυνοι αἱ ἀποσκήψεες; Hippocrates, ibid., trans. Littré, pp. 577, 579: "les déplacements [de l' atrabile] font craindre des maladies de ce genre;" trans. Jones, p. 193: "the melancholy humour is likely to be determined in the following ways;" for Arabic آل إلى as a translation of Greek ἀποσκήψις εἰς, see Endress/Gutas, GALex, vol. 1, p. 611 [10].

352   Cf. Galen, ibid. In fact, Galen says that madness can always be caused by yellow bile because of its irritating and biting properties, and by black bile only when it is extremely burnt or putrefied and thus acquires bad acridness. See also Maimonides, Medical Apho-risms 6.32, trans. Bos, vol. 2, p. 7: "The madness occurring from melancholic humor is not as bad as that arising from the burning of bilious humor. Phlegmatic humor does not cause any madness at all. In Hippocratis Aphorismos commentarius 6."

353   "and hemiplegia": Missing both in Hippocrates, Aphorisms 6.57, ed. Littré, p. 578, and in Galen, ibid., p. 96; but cf. trans. Ḥunayn (E, fol. 67ᵇ): السكتة والفالج.

قال المفسّر: يعني أنْ يكون نفس المريض ينقطع ويعود كتنفّس من خنقه البكاء وذلك يكون إمّا لضعف القوة عن استيفاء التنفّس أو عن يبس آلات التنفّس وصلابتها حتّى لا تقدر القوة أنْ تبسطها أو من حال قريبة من التشنّج وكلّ هذا في الأمراض الحادّة رديّ.

(6.55)

[٣٤٧] قال أبقراط: علل النقرس تتحرّك في الربيع وفي الخريف على الأمر الأكثر.

٥ قال المفسّر: في الربيع لجريان الأخلاط وتزيّدها لتحلّل جمودها الشتوي وفي الخريف لما تقدّم من أكل فواكه الصيف.

(6.56)

[٣٤٨] قال أبقراط: الأمراض السوداوية يخاف منها أنْ تؤول إلى السكتة أو الفالج أو إلى التشنّج أو إلى الجنون أو إلى العمى.

قال المفسّر: قال جالينوس: السكتة والفالج والتشنّج والعمى قد يكون من الخلط البلغمي ومن الخلط

١٠ السوداوي. وأمّا الجنون فلا يعرض إلّا من احتراق الصفراء حتّى تصير سوداء.

(6.57)

[٣٤٩] قال أبقراط: والسكتة والفالج يحدثان خاصّة بمن كان سنه فيما بين الأربعين سنة وإلى الستّين.

---

٢ استيفاء: استسقاء C   ٣ حال: حالة B   ٤ قال ... الأكثر: om. A || وفي ... الأكثر: om. B   ٦ فواكه الصيف: الفواكه في الصيف BP   ٧ أو: إلى BP   ٧ add. BP   ٨–٧ التشنّج أو إلى الجنون: الجنون أو التشنّج BP   ٨ العمى: الإغماء AC   ٩ والعمى: والإغماء AC   ١١ بمن ... الستّين: om. B || فيما: ما P || الأربعين سنة وإلى الستّين: الأربعين والستّين سنة P

Says the commentator: Galen interprets this aphorism in a way that it is correct by saying: With apoplexy and[354] hemiplegia he (i.e., Hippocrates) means apoplexy and hemiplegia that originate from black bile, because black bile dominates in people of that age.[355] However, the truth [of the matter] is that the occurrence of these two [illnesses] as a result of black bile is extremely rare and that they occur mostly as a result of phlegm, and from [the age of] sixty until the end of life.

(6.58)

[350] Says Hippocrates: If the omentum protrudes, it will necessarily putrefy.

Says the commentator: This is clear.

(6.59)

[351] Says Hippocrates: If someone suffers from pain in the sciatic nerve and the hip joint dislocates and then returns again, mucous moisture is formed.

Says the commentator: Because of the mucous moisture, the ligaments become moist and [the head of] the thigh bone dislocates from [its socket in the] hip [bone].

(6.60)

[352] Says Hippocrates: If someone suffers from chronic pain in the hip and the joint becomes dislocated, the leg wastes away completely[356] and [the patient] becomes lame unless [the part] is cauterized.

Says the commentator: That mucous moisture can be dried through cauterization, but if it is not dried through cauterization [the patient becomes lame], and the leg is not nourished as it is normally so that it wastes away.

This is the end of the sixth part of the commentary on the *Aphorisms*.

---

354 "and hemiplegia": Missing in Galen, ibid., ed. Kühn.
355 Cf. ibid.
356 "completely": Missing both in Hippocrates, *Aphorisms* 6.60, ed. Littré, p. 578, and in Galen, ibid., p. 99.

قال المفسّر: تأوّل جالينوس هذا الفصل حتّى يكون كلاما صحيحا قال: يريد السكتة والفالج اللذين يحدثان من المرّة السوداء لأنّ المرّة السوداء تغلب على أصحاب تلك السنّ. وأمّا على التأويل الحقّ فإنّ حدوث هذين من السوداء نادر جدّا وحدوثهما الأكثري من البلغم ومن الستّين إلى آخر العمر.

(6.58)

[٣٥٠] قال أبقراط: إذا بدا الثرب فهو لا محالة يعفن.

٥ قال المقسّر: هذا بيّن.

(6.59)

[٣٥١] قال أبقراط: من كان به وجع النسا وكان وركه يخلع ثمّ يعود فإنّه قد حدثت به رطوبة مخاطية.

قال المفسّر: من أجل الرطوبة المخاطية تبتلّ الرباطات فيسهل انخلاع عظم الفخذ من الورك.

(6.60)

[٣٥٢] قال أبقراط: من اعتراه وجع في الورك مزمن فكان وركه يخلع فإنّ رجله كلّها تضمر ويعرج إن لم يكو.

١٠ قال المفسّر: تجفّف تلك الرطوبة المخاطية بالكيّ ومتى لم تجفّف تلك الرطوبة بالكيّ حدث العرج ولا تغتذي الرجل على معتادها فتضمر.

تمّت المقالة السادسة من شرح الفصول

---

١ اللذين: الذي P ٢ لأنّ المرّة السوداء: om. P C١ ‖ السنّ: الأسنان B ‖ التأويل: تأويل P ٤ بدا ... محالة: om. P ٦ وجع: عرق add. BP ‖ النسا ... مخاطيّة: om. B ‖ مخاطية ... الرباطات: الرطوبات A ٧ الرباطات add. BP ‖ الفخذ: الفخذين BP ٨-٩ فكان ... يكو: om. B ٩ يكو: يكوى AP ١٢ الفصول: من كتاب الفصول وشرحها والحمد لله وحده كما هو أهله ومستحقّه add. A والحمد لله وحده add. B يتلوها في الورقة التي تلي هذه الورقة المقالة السابعة من شرح فصول أبقراط والحمد لله وحده add. C

In the name of God, the Merciful, the Compassionate
The seventh part of the commentary on Hippocrates' *Aphorisms*

(7.1)

[353] Says Hippocrates: Coldness of the extremities in acute diseases is a bad sign.

Says the commentator: This is, in my opinion, an indication for the weakness of the innate heat and that it does not spread to the extremities, while the illness with which it comes is acute, that is to say "hot." For Hippocrates sometimes calls those acute diseases "hot" that are associated with fever that is continuous. The extremities are the tip of the nose, the ears, hands, and feet.

(7.2)

[354] Says Hippocrates: If a bone is diseased and the color of the flesh is livid, it is a bad sign.

Says the commentator: This color results from the extinction of the innate heat.

(7.3)

[355] Says Hippocrates: The occurrence of hiccups and redness of the eyes after vomiting is a bad sign.

Says the commentator: If spasms[357] do not go away after vomiting, it is an indication that it is caused either by an inflammation in the beginning of the nerves, i.e., the brain, or by an inflammation in the stomach. Redness of the eyes results from these two inflammations.

(7.4)

[356] Says Hippocrates: If sweating is followed by shivering, it is not a good sign.

---

357 "spasms": Read: "hiccups." Our text is possibly elliptic and faulty as it stands; the original text might have read: "If hiccups, whose relation to the stomach is comparable to that of spasms to muscles, do not go away after vomiting;" cf. Galen, *In Hippocratis Aphorismos commentarius* 7.3, ed. Kühn, vol. 18a, p. 104: Οἷον τε πάθος τοῖς μυσὶν ὁ σπασμός ἐστι, τοιοῦτον ἐν τῷ στομάχῳ γίνεται ἡ λύγξ; cf. trans. Ḥunayn (S, fol. 139ª): إنّ حال الفواق من المعدة كحال التشنّج من العضل.

بسم الله الرحمن الرحيم

المقالة السابعة من شرح فصول أبقراط

(7.1)

[٣٥٣] قال أبقراط: برد الأطراف في الأمراض الحادّة دليل رديء.

قال المفسّر: هذا عندي دليل على ضعف الحرارة الغريزية وكونها لم تنتشر للأطراف مع كون

المرض حادًا أعني حارًّا لأنّ أبقراط قد يسمّي أمراضا حادّة الأمراض التي تكون الحمّى فيها مطبقة.

والأطراف هي طرف الأنف والأذنين والكفّين والرجلين.

(7.2)

[٣٥٤] قال أبقراط: إذا كانت في العظم علّة فكان لون اللحم عنها كمدا فذلك دليل رديء.

قال المفسّر: هذا لون تابع لانطفاء الحرارة الغريزية.

(7.3)

[٣٥٥] قال أبقراط: حدوث الفواق وحمرة العينين بعد القيء دليل رديء.

قال المفسّر: إذا لم يرتفع التشنّج بعد القيء فذلك دليل بأنّ سببه إمّا ورم في مبدأ العصب أعني الدماغ

وإمّا ورم في المعدة وحمرة العينين تابعة لهذين الورمين.

(7.4)

[٣٥٦] قال أبقراط: إذا حدث عند العرق اقشعرار فليس ذلك بدليل محمود.

---

١ بسم ... الرحيم: ABP om. ٢ المقالة السابعة من شرح فصول أبقراط: المقالة السابعة من كتاب الفصول
وشرحها A شرح المقالة السابعة من فصول أبقراط B || من ... أبقراط: P om. ٤ الغريزية: الغريزة C
٧ فكان ... رديء: B om. ٩ العينين: العين B ١٢ عند: بعد P || فليس ... محمود: B om.

Says the commentator: Hippocrates has already said that if the symptoms of a crisis do not result in a crisis, [these symptoms] indicate death or a difficult crisis because nature is weakened.[358]

(7.5)

[357] Says Hippocrates: If madness is followed by dysentery, dropsy, or confusion,[359] it is a good sign.

Says the commentator: The dropsy and dysentery cure [the madness] by removing the matter [that produces the illness]. Confusion [cures madness] because when the symptoms (i.e., of confusion) increase and become stronger, they constrain and move nature to expel all that is harmful in the way of a crisis. This is Galen's explanation [of the aphorism].[360]

(7.6)

[358] Says Hippocrates: In a chronic illness loss of appetite and unmixed stools are a bad sign.

Says the commentator: With unmixed stools he means those that are not mixed with any watery moisture, for only [in this way] the illness that is in the body can be expelled, whether it is a type of yellow bile or of black bile. This is an indication that all the natural moisture that was in the body has been burnt by the heat of the fever.[361]

(7.7)

[359] Says Hippocrates: If rigor and mental confusion (delirium) occur from excessive drinking, it is a bad sign.

---

358 Cf. Hippocrates, *Epidemics* 2.1.76, ed. and trans. Smith, pp. 22–23: τὰ κρίσιμα μὴ κρίνοντα τὰ μὲν θανατώδεα, τὰ δὲ δύσκριτα ("Critical symptoms without a crisis: some are fatal, some indicate a bad crisis"); quoted also in Galen, *In Hippocratis Prorrheticum commentarius* 1.3, ed. Diels, pp. 146 l. 21–147 l. 12 (= ed. Kühn, vol. 16, pp. 786–787). I thank Vivian Nutton for this reference.

359 "confusion" (خَرَجَ): Cf. Galen, *In Hippocratis Aphorismos commentarius* 7.5, ed. Kühn, vol. 18a, p. 105: ἔκστασις; Hippocrates, *Aphorisms*, trans. Littré, vol. 4, p. 579: "transport au cerveau;" ed. and trans. Jones, p. 195: "raving" (see also n. 2: "By ἔκστασις is meant an increase of the maniacal symptoms, helping to bring the disease to a crisis"); Ullmann, *Wörterbuch*, p. 228 "Entrückung, Verwirrung."

360 Cf. Galen, ibid., pp. 105–106.

361 And thus there is no moisture with which the matter that produced the illness could be expelled.

قال المفسّر: قد قال أبقراط إنّ أعراض البحران إذا لم يحدث عنها بحران دلّت على موت أو عسر بحران لأنّ الطبيعة تخور.

(7.5)

[٣٥٧] قال أبقراط: إذا حدث بعد الجنون اختلاف دم أو استسقاء أو حيرة فذلك دليل محمود.

قال المفسّر: أمّا الاستسقاء والاختلاف فيبرئان بانتقال المادّة. وأمّا الحيرة فإنّ الأعراض إذا تزيّدت
٥ وقويت أرهقت الطبيعة وحرّكتها لدفع كلّ ما يؤذي بطريق البحران هكذا تأوّل له جالينوس.

(7.6)

[٣٥٨] قال أبقراط: ذهاب الشهوة في المرض المزمن والبراز الصرف دليل رديء.

قال المفسّر: يريد بالبراز الصرف الذي لا يخالطه شيء من الرطوبة المائية وإنّما يخرج الداء الذي في البدن فقط من أنواع الصفراء كان أو من أنواع السوداء. فإنّ ذلك يدلّ على أنّ الرطوبة الطبيعية كلّها قد احترقت من حرارة الحمّى.

(7.7)

١٠ [٣٥٩] قال أبقراط: إذا حدث من كثرة الشرب اقشعرار واختلاط ذهن فذلك دليل رديء.

---

١ موت: الموت P ٥ أرهقت: ارتقت BP ٧ om. B:لا ١٠ واختلاط ... رديء: om. B.

Says the commentator: The combination of rigor and mental confusion (delirium) occurs only rarely, except in the case of some people who are often intoxicated. Then the innate heat is extinguished, rigor occurs, their brain is filled with hot blood or hot vapors so that mental confusion (delirium) develops.

(7.8)

[360] Says Hippocrates: If an abscess breaks internally, it results in a collapse of strength, vomiting and fainting.[362]

Says the commentator: This is clear; with *khurāj*[363] he means *dubayla*[364] (abscess). With "internally" he means "into the stomach."

(7.9)

[361] Says Hippocrates: If mental confusion (delirium) or spasms occur as a result of a flow of blood, it is a bad sign.

Says the commentator: After an evacuation [of blood], a mental confusion (delirium) develops because the brain is disturbed in its movements and is then constantly weak. Hippocrates calls a mild delirium "raving."[365]

(7.10)

[362] Says Hippocrates: If vomiting, hiccups, mental confusion (delirium), or spasms occur as a result of a colic,[366] may[367] God protect us from it, it is a bad sign.

Says the commentator: This is clear.

---

362 "fainting" (ذبول نفس): Cf. Galen, *In Hippocratis Aphorismos commentarius* 7.8, ed. Kühn, vol. 18a, p. 108: λειποψυχίη; Hippocrates, *Aphorisms*, trans. Littré, vol. 4, p. 581: "la lipothymie;" trans. Jones, p. 195: "fainting;" Ullmann, *Wörterbuch*, p. 385, s.v. λειποψυχέω: "ohnmächtig werden."

363 "*khurāj*" (خراج): Cf. Galen, ibid.: φῦμα; cf. aphorisms 3.20 (126), 4.82 (219) above.

364 "*dubayla* (abscess)" (دبيلة): Cf. Galen, ibid.: ἐμπύημα; Liddell/Scott, *Greek-English Lexicon*, p. 549: "gathering, abscess, esp. internal;" cf. aphorism 5.8 (228) above.

365 Cf. Galen, ibid., p. 109: αὐτὸς γὰρ εἴωθεν ὀνομάζειν λῆρον τὴν μετρίαν παρακοπήν; cf. idem, *In Hippocratis Epidemiarum librum commentarius* 3.1, ed. Wenkebach, pp. 1 l. 22–2 l. 1: εἴπερ οὖν ἐλήρησεν ὁ Πυθίων, εὔδηλον ὅτι μετρίως παρεφρόνησεν; see also Maimonides, *Medical Aphorisms* 23.58a, trans. Bos, vol. 5, p. 49: "In the first [book] of his commentary on [Epidemics] 3, [Galen] says that raving is a mild form of delirium." My translation of the Arabic term as "raving" follows Stroumsa, *Maimonides in His World*, pp. 138–152.

366 "colic" (قولنج): Cf. Galen, *In Hippocratis Aphorismos commentarius* 7.10, ed. Kühn, vol. 18a, p. 110: εἰλέος; Hippocrates, *Aphorisms*, trans. Littré, vol. 4, p. 581: "un iléus;" trans. Jones, p. 195: "ileus;" cf. aphorism 6.44 (336) above.

367 "may God protect us from it": Missing in Galen, ibid.

قال المفسّر: اجتماع الاقشعرار مع اختلاط قليل الوقوع إلّا في بعض مكثري السكر فتطفأ الحرارة الغريزية فيحدث الاقشعرار ويمتلئ الدماغ دما حارًّا أو بخارا حارًّا فيختلط الذهن.

(7.8)

[٣٦٠] قال أبقراط: إذا انفجر خراج إلى داخل حدث عن ذلك سقوط قوّة وقيء وذبول نفس.

قال المفسّر: هذا بيّن ويعني بالخراج الدبيلة ويعني بقوله إلى داخل إلى المعدة.

(7.9)

٥ [٣٦١] قال أبقراط: إذا حدث عن سيلان الدم اختلاط في الذهن أو تشنّج فذلك دليل رديء.

قال المفسّر: اختلاط الذهن بعد الاستفراغ يكون لاضطراب الدماغ في حركاته ويكون أبدا ضعيفا وأبقراط يسمّي اختلاط الذهن الضعيف هذيان.

(7.10)

[٣٦٢] قال أبقراط: إذا حدث عن القولنج قيء وفواق واختلاط ذهن وتشنّج فذلك دليل سوء.

قال المفسّر: هذا بيّن.

<hr/>

٢ الغريزية: om. A   ٣ خراج: جراح C ‖ وقيء: والقيء P   ٤ بالخراج: بالجراح C   ٥ في ... رديء: om. AP   ٨ في ... سوء: om. B ‖ سوء: رديء AP

(7.11)

[363] Says Hippocrates: If pneumonia occurs as a result of pleurisy, it is a bad sign.

Says the commentator: If the humor that produces the pleurisy has not enough space, some of it flows to the lungs [and causes pneumonia]. But it is almost impossible that pneumonia leads to (causes) pleurisy.

(7.12)

[364] Says Hippocrates: And [it is a bad sign if] phrenitis [develops] from pneumonia.

(7.13)

[365] Says Hippocrates: And [it is a bad sign if] spasms or tetanus [develop] from severe burns.

(7.14)

[366] Says Hippocrates: And it is [a] bad [sign if] a stupor[368] or mental confusion (delirium) [develops] from a blow on the head.

(7.15)

[367] Says Hippocrates: And [it is a bad sign if] spitting of pus [develops] from hemoptysis.

(7.16)

[368] Says Hippocrates: And [it is a bad sign if] phthisis and flux[369] [develop] from the spitting of pus. When the spitting stops, the patient dies.

(7.17)

[369] Says Hippocrates: And [it is a bad sign if] hiccups [develop] from an inflammation of the liver.

---

368 "stupor" (سُبَات): Cf. Galen, ibid. 7.14, p. 114: ἔκπληξις; Hippocrates, *Aphorisms*, trans. Littré, vol. 4, p. 581: "la stupeur;" trans. Jones, p. 197: "stupor."

369 "flux" (سَيَلان): Cf. Galen, ibid. 7.16, p. 115: ῥύσις; Hippocrates, ibid., trans. Littré: "flux;" ed. and trans. Jones: "flux" (cf. n. 2: "Galen says that ῥύσις means either (*a*) the falling out of the hair or (*b*) diarrhoea"); Ullmann, *Wörterbuch*, pp. 595–596.

(7.11)

[٣٦٣] قال أبقراط: إذا حدثت عن ذات الجنب ذات الرئة فذلك دليل رديء.

قال المفسّر: إذا لم يسع الخلط المحدث لذات الجنب موضعه يفيض منه شيء إلى الرئة. فأمّا ذات الرئة فليس يكاد يتبعها ذات الجنب.

(7.12)

[٣٦٤] قال أبقراط: وعن ذات الرئة برسام.

(7.13)

[٣٦٥] قال أبقراط: وعن الاحتراق الشديد التشنّج والتمدّد.

(7.14)

[٣٦٦] قال أبقراط: وعن الضربة على الرأس البهتة واختلاط الذهن رديء.

(7.15)

[٣٦٧] قال أبقراط: وعن نفث الدم نفث المدّة.

(7.16)

[٣٦٨] قال أبقراط: وعن نفث المدّة السلّ والسيلان فإذا احتبس البصاق مات صاحب العلّة.

(7.17)

[٣٦٩] قال أبقراط: وعن ورم الكبد الفواق.

(7.18)

[370] Says Hippocrates: And [it is a bad sign if] spasms and mental confusion (delirium) [develop] from sleeplessness.

Says the commentator: All [these statements are] clear. Their meaning is that if these illnesses become more severe and grave there may develop such and such conditions [as mentioned]. For instance, if the inflammation of the liver becomes more severe and harms the cardia of the stomach, hiccups develop. It is well known that spasms and mental confusion (delirium) may ·develop from dryness, and that dryness comes after excessive evacuation or the movements[370] of the soul (emotions) and sleeplessness.

(7.19)

[371] Says Hippocrates: And [it is a bad sign if] the swelling called "erysipelas" [develops] from the laying bare of a bone.

Says the commentator: Galen has explained that this inflammation only rarely results from the laying bare of a bone. Therefore he (i.e., Hippocrates) mentions everything that can possibly happen as a result [of the laying bare of a bone], even when it is most rare.[371]

(7.20)

[372] Says Hippocrates: And [it is a bad sign if] putrefaction or suppuration [develops] from the inflammation called "erysipelas."

Says the commentator: This is clear according to what [I said] on different occasions before, that it means that this may be the case.[372]

(7.21)

[373] Says Hippocrates: And [it is a bad sign if] a hemorrhage [develops] from violent throbbing in wounds.

Says the commentator: This is clear because the severe pain causes the vessels to move (pulsate) strongly to expel the harmful [matter].

---

370 "movements of the soul (emotions)": For this concept and their role in the regimen of health, cf. Maimonides, *On Asthma* 8.2–3, ed. and trans. Bos, vol. 1, pp. 37–39; idem, *On the Regimen of Health* 3.10, ed. and trans. Bos, pp. 102–103; idem, *Über die Lebensdauer*, ed. Weil; Arabic text repr. by ed. and trans. Schwartz: *Teshuvat ha-Rambam*, pp. 20 (Arabic text), 28–29 (Hebrew trans.); Bos, "Maimonides on Preservation of Health," pp. 222–224; Eisenman, "Maimonides' Philosophic Medicine," p. 149.

371 Cf. Galen, *In Hippocratis Aphorismos commentarius* 7.19, ed. Kühn, vol. 18a, p. 119.

372 Cf. aphorism 7.18 (370) above.

(7.18)

[٣٧٠] قال أبقراط: وعن السهر التشنّج واختلاط الذهن.

قال المفسّر: كلّ هذا بيّن ومعناه إنّه إذا عظمت هذه العلل وتفاقمت قد يحدث عنها كذا وكذا كما أنّ ورم الكبد إذا عظم وأضرّ بفم المعدة حدث الفواق. وقد علم أنّ التشنّج واختلاط الذهن قد يحدث عن اليبس وليس يتبع كثرة الاستفراغ أو الحركات النفسانية والسهر.

(7.19)

٥ [٣٧١] قال أبقراط: وعن انكشاف العظم الورم الذي يدعى الحمرة.

قال المفسّر: بيّن جالينوس أنّ انكشاف العظم لا يحدث عنه هذا الورم إلّا في الندرة فهو إذًا ذكر كلّما يمكن أنْ يتبع ولو على الأقلّ.

(7.20)

[٣٧٢] قال أبقراط: وعن الورم الذي يدعى الحمرة العفونة والتقيّح.

قال المفسّر: هذا بيّن على ما تقدّم مرّات أنّ معناه قد يحدث.

(7.21)

١٠ [٣٧٣] قال أبقراط: وعن الضربان الشديد في القروح انفجار الدم.

قال المفسّر: هذا بيّن لأنّ لشدّة الألم تتحرّك العروق حركة عنيفة لدفع المؤذي.

---

١ التشنّج ... الذهن: om. B ٤ عن: om. B ‖ يتبع: مع BP ١٠ الضربان: الضرابان C

(7.22)

[374] Says Hippocrates: And [it is a bad sign if] suppuration [develops] from chronic pain in the parts about the belly.

Says the commentator: An inflammation develops from chronic pain and that inflammation suppurates.

(7.23)

[375] Says Hippocrates: And [it is a bad sign if] dysentery [develops] from unmixed stools.

Says the commentator: He means that if the stools only consist of a certain humor, corrosion[373] and wounds may occur in the intestines.

(7.24)

[376] Says Hippocrates: And [it is a bad sign if] mental confusion (delirium) [develops] from the severing of a bone, if it reaches the cavity.

Says the commentator: He (i.e., Galen) says that if the bone of the head (i.e., skull) is severed to a degree that it reaches the cavity that surrounds the brain, mental confusion (delirium) develops.[374]

(7.25)

[377] Says Hippocrates: [If] spasms develop from the ingestion of a purgative drug, it is fatal.

Says the commentator: This is clear.

(7.26)

[378] Says Hippocrates: [If] coldness of the extremities [develops] from severe pain in the parts about the belly, it is [a bad sign].[375]

---

373 "corrosion and wounds may occur in the intestines": Cf. Galen, *In Hippocratis Aphorismos commentarius* 7.23, ed. Kühn, 18a, p. 122: θαυμαστὸν οὖν οὐδὲν ἐπὶ ταῖς τοιαύταις ὑποχωρή-σεσιν ἀναβρωθῆναί τι τῶν ἐντέρων (Thus one should not wonder that as a result of such evacuations one of the intestines is corroded); cf. trans. Ḥunayn (S, fol. 143ᵃ): فليس يعجب (Thus) أن يحدث عن هذا البراز تأكّل في بعض الأمعاء فيكون منه قرحة يعرض بسببها اختلاف الدم one should not wonder that corrosion in one of the intestines develops from these stools and that a wound develops from it which causes dysentery).
374 Cf. Hippocrates, *Aphorisms* 7.24, ed. Jones, p. 197 n. 4: "Galen states that this aphorism applies not to any bone, but to severe fractures of the skull piercing the membranes."
375 Cf. Maimonides, *Medical Aphorisms* 10.11, trans. Bos, vol. 3, p. 4: "Cold in the extremities, especially during fevers, [occurs] either because of a large, inflamed tumor in the viscera; or because of a severe pain in the middle part of the body; or because of fainting or syncope; or because of weakness of the innate heat and its near extinction; or because of its

(7.22)

[٣٧٤] قال أبقراط: وعن الوجع المزمن فيما يلي المعدة التقيّح.

قال المفسّر: الوجع المزمن إنّما يكون عنه الورم وذلك الورم سيتقيّح.

(7.23)

[٣٧٥] قال أبقراط: وعن البراز الصرف اختلاف الدم.

قال المفسّر: يعني إنْ يكون البراز خلط من الأخلاط فقط قد يحدث تأكّل وقرحة في المعاء.

(7.24)

٥ [٣٧٦] قال أبقراط: وعن قطع العظم اختلاط الذهن إن نال الموضع الخالي.

قال المفسّر: يقول إنّ إذا قطع عظم الرأس حتّى يصل القطع للموضع الخالي الحاوي للدماغ حدث اختلاط الذهن.

(7.25)

[٣٧٧] قال أبقراط: التشنّج من شرب الدواء مميت.

قال المفسّر: هذا بيّن.

(7.26)

١٠ [٣٧٨] قال أبقراط: برد الأطراف عن الوجع الشديد فيما يلي المعدة رديء.

٢ سيتقيّح: سيقيح BP ٥ إن نال الموضع الخالي: P om. الخالي B نال الخالي C ١٠ عن الوجع الشديد: om.
B ‖ فيما: مما BP

drowning and choking effect due to a surplus of [superfluous] matters. The extremities are the ears, nose, hands, and feet. *In Hippocratis Aphorismos commentarius* 7."

Says the commentator: This is clear.

(7.27)

[379] Says Hippocrates: If a pregnant woman suffers from tenesmus, it causes a miscarriage.

Says the commentator: This is clear.

(7.28)

[380] Says Hippocrates: If part of a bone or cartilage[376] is cut through, it does not grow [together again].

Says the commentator: Galen has already affirmed that [this aphorism] is a repetition.[377]

(7.29)

[381] Says Hippocrates: If someone dominated by white phlegm is attacked by violent diarrhea, his illness will dissolve.

Says the commentator: The white phlegm is the dropsy of the flesh. Says the author (i.e., Maimonides): I have seen this twice.[378]

(7.30)

[382] Says Hippocrates: If someone suffers from diarrhea and the diarrhea is frothy, the cause of the diarrhea is [moisture] descending from the head.

Says the commentator: The reason for [the diarrhea] to be frothy is that it is strongly mixed with air. Sometimes the[379] [airy] moisture [causing the diarrhea to be frothy] descends from the head; sometimes it comes from the other organs, and sometimes it originates in the stomach and intestines.

---

376   "cartilage": Galen, *In Hippocratis Aphorismos commentarius* 7.28, ed. Kühn, vol. 18a, p. 126, adds: ἢ νεῦρον (or sinew); note, however, that this term is already missing in some MSS in the Hippocratic text itself, ed. Littré, p. 584. The term recurs, however, in Hebrew trans. Anonymous as או מן העצבים.

377   Cf. aphorism 6.19 (311) above.

378   I.e., that a patient suffering from dropsy of the flesh was cured through violent diarrhea.

379   "the [airy] moisture": Cf. Galen, *In Hippocratis Aphorismos commentarius* 7.30, ed. Kühn, vol. 18a, p. 128: ὑγρόν πνευματῶδες (flatulent moisture); cf. Ḥunayn (S, fol. 144ᵇ): رطوبة يخالطها ريح (moisture mixed with wind (flatulence)).

قال المفسّر: هذا بيّن.

(7.27)

[٣٧٩] قال أبقراط: إذا حدث بالحامل زحير كان سببا لأنْ تسقط.

قال المفسّر: هذا بيّن.

(7.28)

[٣٨٠] قال أبقراط: إذا انقطع شيء من العظم أو من الغضروف لم ينم.

٥ قال المفسّر: قد أقرّ جالينوس أنّه تكرّر.

(7.29)

[٣٨١] قال أبقراط: إنْ حدث بمن قد غلب عليه البلغم الأبيض اختلاف قوي انحلّ عنه به مرضه.

قال المفسّر: البلغم الأبيض هو الاستسقاء اللحمي. قال المؤلّف: قد رأيت هذا مرّتين.

(7.30)

[٣٨٢] قال أبقراط: من كان به اختلاف وكان ما يختلف به زبدي فقد يكون سبب اختلافه شيء ينحدر من رأسه.

١٠ قال المفسّر: علّة الشيء الزبدي مخالطة الهواء له مخالطة شديدة. وقد تكون تلك الرطوبة المنحدرة من الرأس أو من أعضاء أخر أو نتولّد في المعدة والأمعاء.

٢-٣ قال ... بيّن: .om A ‖ ٢ لأنْ تسقط: للإسقاط B¹ للإسقاط B ‖ ٤ الغضروف: المعرصوف C ‖ ينم: ينبت Pt ‖ ٦ إنْ: إذا BP ‖ اختلاف ... مرضه: .om B ‖ عنه: .om P ‖ ٨ وكان: فكان AC ‖ ٨-٩ وكان ... رأسه: .om A ‖ ٨ به: .om AC ‖ زبدي: ردي A ‖ ١٠ له: .om A B

(7.31)

[383] Says Hippocrates: If someone with fever has sediments in his urine that[380] resemble coarse meal, it is an indication that his illness will be protracted.

Says the commentator: The humors [of someone whose illness appears to be such] are far from being concocted. For this reason, Hippocrates says that these [patients] mostly die and that he, who escapes, has a protracted illness, as he mentioned here.[381]

(7.32)

[384] Says Hippocrates: If the sediment in the urine is dominated by bile and the upper part is thin (watery), it indicates that the illness is acute.

Says the commentator: This is clear. With "thin" he means that the upper part of the sediment is thin and[382] that its shape is like that of pine nuts.

---

380   "that resemble coarse meal" (شبيه بالسويق الجريش): Cf. Galen, ibid. 7.31, ed. Kühn, p. 130: κριμνώδεες; Hippocrates, *Aphorisms*, trans. Littré, vol. 4, p. 585: "semblables à de la farine grossière;" trans. Jones, p. 199: "like coarse meal." For the term سويق, see also Maimonides, *Medical Aphorisms* 5.16, ed. and trans. Bos, vol. 1, pp. 74, 120 n. 28.

381   Cf. Galen, ibid., p. 131: ὀλέθρια μὲν γάρ ἐστι τὰ κριμνώδη τῶν οὔρων, κἂν τῷ προγνοστικῷ λέλεκται καὶ φθάνουσιν ἀποθνήσκειν οἱ πλεῖστοι πρὶν χρονίσαι τὴν νόσον. ὅσοι δ' ἐξ αὐτῶν ἐσώθησαν, ἐχρόνισαν οὗτοι πάντες, οἷς ἂν πολλῆς τῆς πέψεως δεομένης τῆς διαθέσεως (For the urine [that has a sediment] like coarse meal is fatal; in the *Prognostic* it is said that most patients die before the illness becomes chronic. However, those who escape, will, all of them, be ill for a long time, because the condition [of their humors] is such that they need much cooking); cf. trans. Ḥunayn (S, fol. 145ᵃ): وذلك أنّ البول الذي يرى فيه شيء شبيه بالسويق الجريش

قد يدلّ على الهلاك كما قيل في كتاب تقدمة المعرفة وأكثر من يرى هذا في بوله يموت قبل أن يطول به مرضه فأمّا الذين يسلمون ممّن نرى هذا في أبوالهم فكلّهم يرى فيه هذا المرض الذي يرى فيه هذا البول يحتاج إلى نضج كثير. In the *Prognostic*, trans. Jones, p. 27, Hippocrates remarks: "Sediments in urine which are like coarse meal are bad."

382   "and that its shape is like that of pine nuts": This statement does not feature in Galen's commentary, but is derived from Ḥunayn's additional statement to his translation (S, fols. 145ᵇ–146ᵃ) that it is shaped like a cone (مخرط): إنّ اللفظة التي يسمّي بها أبقراط الرقيق في

هذا الفصل يحتمل أن يكون معناها الرقيق في القوام ويحتمل أن يكون معناها الرقيق في الشكل فقد يجوز على هذا القياس عندي أن يكون أبقراط أراد بقوله أعلاه رقيق أيّ مخرط أعلاه ويميل إلى الدقّة لأنّ الثفل الراسب في البول إذا كان غليظا ثقيلا نيئا كان سطحه الأعلى شبيها بالمسطح وإذا كان رقيقا خفيفا نضيجا كان أعلاه مخرط.

(7.31)

[٣٨٣] قال أبقراط: من كانت به حمّى فكان يرسب في بوله ثفل شبيه بالسويق الجريش فذلك يدلّ على أنّ مرضه طويل.

قال المفسّر: الأخلاط التي يظهر منها هذا بعيدة النضج فلذلك ذكر أبقراط أنّ هؤلاء يموتون في الأكثر. ومن سلم منهم طال مرضه كما ذكر هنا.

(7.32)

٥ [٣٨٤] قال أبقراط: إذا كان الغالب على الثفل الذي في البول المرار وكان أعلاه رقيقا دلّ على أنّ المرض حادّ.

قال المفسّر: هذا بيّن. ويريد بقوله رقيقا أنْ يكون أعلى الثفل رقيق فيكون شكله صنوبري.

---

١ فكان: وكان P   ٢-١ الجريش ... طويل: om. B   ٦-٥ وكان ... حادّ: om. B   ٧ ويريد: يريد BP   ‖ الثفل: البول BP

(7.33)

[385] Says Hippocrates: If someone's urine is heterogeneous,[383] it indicates that there is a violent disturbance in his body.

Says the commentator: It means [urine] consisting of different parts, and this is an indication for the [variant activity] of nature with regard to the humors.

(7.34)

[386] Says Hippocrates: If there are bubbles[384] on the surface of someone's urine, it is an indication that the illness is in the kidneys; it also tells [us] that it will be lengthy.

Says the commentator: [This is so] because [bubbles] indicates thick wind (flatulence) within viscous humors, and[385] this tells [us] that [the illness] will be lengthy.

(7.35)

[387] Says Hippocrates: If someone observes that the surface of his urine is totally covered with a greasy substance, it indicates that there is an acute illness in his kidneys.

Says the commentator: If the greasy substance turns up all at once, it is an indication that it comes from the melting of the fat of the kidneys. This is the meaning of the word "totally." But what turns up from the dissolution of the other organs comes little by little.

---

383 "heterogeneous" (مُشْتَّا): Cf. Galen, *In Hippocratis Aphorismos commentarius* 7.33, ed. Kühn, vol. 18a, p. 133: διεστηκότα; Hippocrates, *Aphorisms*, trans. Littré, vol. 4, p. 585: "pas homogène;" trans. Jones, p. 199: "divided;" cf. Liddell/Scott, *Greek-English Lexicon*, p. 428: οὖρα διεστηκότα: "not homogeneous [urine]."

384 "bubbles" (عنب): Cf. Galen, ibid. 7.34, p. 134: πομφόλυγες; Hippocrates, ibid., trans. Littré, p. 587: "des bulles;" trans. Jones: "bubbles;" cf. Ullmann, *Wörterbuch*, p. 548, s.v. πομφόλυξ: "Blase."

385 "and this tells [us] that [the illness] will be lengthy": Maimonides omits the true reason for the lengthiness of the illness as stated by Galen, namely the coldness of the illness; cf. Galen, ibid.: τὸ γὰρ ψυχρὸν ἅπαν δύσλυτόν τε καὶ δύσπεπτόν ἐστι καὶ διὰ τοῦτο χρόνιον (for what is cold is totally hard to dissolve and to be concocted and therefore it lasts for a long time); cf. trans. Ḥunayn (S, fol. 146ª): لأنّ كلّ مرض بارد فهو عسر الانحلال وعسر النضج ولذلك هو من زمن (for every cold illness is hard to dissolve and hard to be concocted and therefore lasts for a long time).

(7.33)

[٣٨٥] قال أبقراط: من كان بوله متشتّتا فذلك يدلّ على أنّ به في بدنه اضطراب قوي.

قال المفسّر: يعني مختلف الأجزاء وذلك دليل على اختلاف فعل الطبيعة في الأخلاط.

(7.34)

[٣٨٦] قال أبقراط: من كان فوق بوله عنب دلّ على أنّ علّته في الكلى وأنذر منها بطول.

قال المفسّر: لأنّه دالّ على ريح غليظة داخل أخلاط لزجة ولذلك ينذر بطول.

(7.35)

٥ [٣٨٧] قال أبقراط: من رأى فوق بوله دسم جملة دلّ على أنّ في كلاه علّة حادّة.

قال المفسّر: إذا كان الدسم يجيء دفعة واحدة فهو دليل أنّه من ذوبان شحم الكلا وهذا هو معنى قوله جملة. أمّا الذي يجيء من ذوبان سائر الأعضاء فيجيء قليلا قليلا.

---

٢ فعل: في C add. ‏ ٣ بطول: المرض add. A ‏ ٤ دالّ: دلّ BP ‏ ٥ جملة ... حادّة: om. B ‏ ٦-٧ شحم ... ذوبان: om. A

(7.36)

[388] Says Hippocrates: When someone is affected by an illness in his kidneys and suffers from the aforementioned symptoms, and also suffers from pain in the muscles in the back, expect an external abscess, provided that the pain is in the external parts. But if the pain is in the internal parts, [expect] rather that the abscess will be internal.

Says the commentator: This is clear.

(7.37)

[389] Says Hippocrates: If someone vomits blood without fever, it[386] is safe (not dangerous) and he should be treated with[387] astringent ingredients. But if [someone vomits] blood while he has fever, it is [a bad sign].

Says the commentator: He means [to say] that if there is no inflammation in the stomach that would necessarily be followed by fever, and if the vomiting of blood is caused by a burst blood vessel or by a wound that has now developed, it is possible that the patient is cured quickly by means of astringent ingredients.[388]

(7.38)

[390] Says Hippocrates: Catarrhs that descend into the upper cavity suppurate within twenty days.

Says the commentator: The upper cavity is the chest cavity in which the lungs are found. The twentieth day is the day of the crisis because it is the last [day] of the third week. He (i.e., Hippocrates) says that this is the ultimate [day] in which a catarrh can concoct.

386　"it is safe (not dangerous) (سلم)": Cf. Galen, ibid. 7.37, ed. Kühn, p. 139: σωτήριον; Hippocrates, *Aphorisms*, trans. Littré, vol. 4, p. 587: "pas inquiétant;" ed. and trans. Jones, p. 201: "may be cured;" and n. 2: "This meaning of σωτήριον (θεραπευθῆναι δυνάμενον) is vouched for by Galen. The word should mean 'salutary;'" cf. Liddell/Scott, *Greek-English Lexicon*, p. 1751, s.v. σωτήριος: "of symptoms: betokening recovery."

387　"with astringent ingredients": Cf. Galen, ibid.: τοῖσι στυπτικοῖσιν ἢ τοῖσι ψυκτικοῖσιν; Hippocrates, ibid., trans. Littré, p. 589: "par le froid et les astringents;" trans. Jones: "with styptics or refrigerants."

388　Cf. Maimonides, *Medical Aphorisms* 9.89, trans. Bos, vol. 2, p. 78: "When internal ulcers do not come with an inflammation, they can be healed quickly with astringent remedies. But those that come with an inflammation and fever cannot be healed. Rather, their size increases every day."

(7.36)

[٣٨٨] قال أبقراط: من كانت به علّة في كلاه وعرضت له هذه الأعراض التي تقدّم ذكرها وحدث به وجع في عضل صلبه فإنّه إنْ كان الوجع في المواضع الخارجة فتوقّع خراج يخرج به من خارج. وإنْ كان ذلك الوجع في المواضع الداخلة فأحرى أنْ يكون دبيلة من داخل.

قال المفسّر: هذا بيّن.

(7.37)

٥ [٣٨٩] قال أبقراط: الدم الذي يتقيّأ من غير حمّى سليم وينبغي أنْ يعالج صاحبه بالأشياء القابضة والدم الذي يتقيّأ مع حمّى رديء.

قال المفسّر: يريد إنّه إذا لم يكن ثم ورم في المعدة الذي الحمّى تابعة له ضرورة. وكان قيء هذا الدم من أجل عرق انبثق أو قرحة حدثت الآن فيمكن أنْ يبرأ سريعا بالأشياء القابضة.

(7.38)

[٣٩٠] قال أبقراط: النزلات التي تنحدر إلى الجوف الأعلى نتقيّح في عشرين يوما.

١٠ قال المفسّر: الجوف الأعلى فضاء الصدر الذي فيه الرئة ويوم العشرين هو يوم بحران لأنّه آخر الأسبوع الثالث. فيقول إنّ هذا أبعد ما يمكن أنْ تنضج فيه النزلة.

٢-٣ فإنّه ... داخل: om. B   ٢ خراج: خراجا P   ٥-٦ من ... رديء: om. B   ٨ قرحة: قرح P   ٩ إلى ... يوما: om. B

(7.39)

[391] Says Hippocrates: If someone urinates blood with clots and he suffers from strangury and pain in[389] the region of the anus and pubes, it indicates that there is a pain[390] in the region of the bladder.

Says the commentator: This [aphorism] is a repetition.[391]

(7.40)

[392] Says Hippocrates: When the tongue suddenly loses its strength or a limb [of one's body] becomes paralyzed, the illness is caused by black bile.

Says the commentator: Galen has already affirmed that this [condition] does not necessarily and unavoidably result from black bile.[392]

(7.41)

[393] Says Hippocrates: If[393] an elderly person suffers from hiccups because of the emptying [of the body] through purging or emesis, it is not a good sign.

Says the commentator: Hiccups after evacuations are bad because they follow dryness. In old people it is worse because of the dryness of their temperament due to their age.

---

389   "in the region of the anus and pubes" (في نواحي الشرج والعانة): Cf. Galen, *In Hippocratis Aphorismos commentarius* 7.39, ed. Kühn, vol. 18a, p. 141: ἐς τὸν περίναιον καὶ τὸν κτένα; Hippocrates, *Aphorisms*, trans. Littré, vol. 4, p. 589: "la périnée et le pubis;" trans. Jones, p. 201: "in the perineum and pubes;" cf. aphorism 4.80 (217) above.

390   "pain" (وجع): Cf. Galen, ibid.: νόσεειν; Hippocrates, ibid. trans. Littré: "affection;" trans. Jones: "disease."

391   Cf. aphorism 4.80 (217) above.

392   Cf. Galen, *In Hippocratis Aphorismos commentarius* 7.40, ed. Kühn, vol. 18a, p. 143: λοιπὸν οὖν ἐστι λέγειν, ὥσπερ ἐπὶ τεταρταίου πυρετοῦ, μελαγχολικὸν εἶναί φαμεν αἴτιον τὸν τῆς περιόδου χυμόν, οὕτω καὶ τῶν εἰρημένων παθημάτων, τῆς τε κατὰ τὴν γλῶτταν ἀκρατείας καὶ τῆς τοῦ μορίου παραλύσεως. καὶ δυνατόν γε τῷ πάχει τοῦ χυμοῦ τὰ τοιαῦτα ἀκολουθῆσαι παθήματα, καθάπερ τῷ πάχει τε καὶ γλίσχρῳ φλέγματι; trans. Ḥunayn (S, fols. 148ᵃ–148ᵇ): فقد بقي أن

يقال إنّه كما أن يقال في حمّى الربع إنّ السبب في دورها خلط سوداوي كذلك يقال في هذه الأعراض أعني عدم اللسان للقوة واسترخاء بعض الأعضاء وقد يمكن أن تحدث هذه الأعراض بسبب الخلط السوداوي لغلظه ويمكن أيضا أن تحدث بسبب البلغم الغليظ اللزج (It remains to say that, as the cause of an attack of quartan fever, is melancholic humor, so too in the case of these afflictions, i.e., paralysis of the tongue and of any [other] part of the body. These afflictions can happen because of a melancholic humor due to its thickness, but they can also happen because of thick, viscous phlegm).

393   "If an elderly person suffers from hiccups because of the emptying [of the body] through purging or emesis": Cf. Galen, ibid. 7.41, ed. Kühn, p. 144: ὑπερκαθαιρομένων τῶν πρεσβυτέρων; Hippocrates, *Aphorisms*, trans. Littré, vol. 4, p. 589: "Dans les superpurgations chez des personnes âgées;" trans. Jones, p. 203: "If old people, when violently purged."

(7.39)

[٣٩١] قال أبقراط: من بال دما عبيطا وكان به تقطير البول وأصابه وجع في نواحي الشرج والعانة دلّ ذلك على أنّ في ما يلي مثانته وجعا.

قال المفسّر: تكرّر معناه.

(7.40)

[٣٩٢] قال أبقراط: متى عدم اللسان بغتة قوّته واسترخى عضو من اعضائه فالعلّة سوداوية.

٥ قال المفسّر: قد أقرّ جالينوس أنّه لا يلزم أنْ يكون هذا عن السوداء ولا بدّ.

(7.41)

[٣٩٣] قال أبقراط: إذا حدث بالشيخ بسبب استفراغ مشيّ أوقيء فواق فليس ذلك بدليل محمود.

قال المفسّر: الفواق بعد الاستفراغات رديء لأنّه تابع ليبس وفي الشيوخ أردأ ليبس مزاجهم بالسنّ.

---

١ عبيطا: غبيطا CP ٢-١ وكان ... وجعا: om. B ١ الشرج: P¹ السرّة ACP (t S, fol. 148ª =) ٢ في ما

P مما AC: ما (t S, fol. 148ª =) ٤ واسترخى ... سوداوية: om. B ٦ استفراغ: om. P

(7.42)

[394] Says Hippocrates: If a person is attacked by fever that is not caused by bile and one pours much hot water over his head, his fever will be dissolved.

Says the commentator: Galen wants to explain this aphorism by saying that with the phrase "fever that is not caused by bile," [Hippocrates] does not refer to putrid fever but to some kind of ephemeral fever. There is no doubt that bathing is beneficial for it and that the fever is dissolved by it.[394]

(7.43)

[395] Says Hippocrates: A woman does not become ambidextrous.

Says the commentator: Galen says that the reason for that is the weakness of her nerves and muscles, for every ambidextrous person has strong nerves.[395]

(7.44)

[396] Says Hippocrates: If patients with empyema are treated either by cautery or by incision and pure white pus flows out, they will be saved (recover). But if turbid and foul-smelling matter flows out, they will die.

Says the commentator: Patients with empyema are those in whom much pus has accumulated between their chest and lungs. The ancient [physicians] used to cauterize them in order to eliminate that matter.

---

394   Galen does not qualify the kind of fever that can be cured by bathing as some kind of ephemeral fever, but describes it as fever caused by fatigue, heat of the sun, cold, or block-age of the pores of the skin; cf. Galen, ibid. 7.42, p. 145: οἵ τε γὰρ ἐπ᾽ ἐγκαύσει καὶ ψύξει γινόμενοι πυρετοὶ πρὸς τῶν τοιούτων ὀνίνανται λουτρῶν, οἵ τ᾽ ἐπὶ κόποις οὐδὲν ἧττον, οἵ τε διὰ στέγνωσιν πόρων; trans. Ḥunayn (S, fol. 148ᵇ): وذلك أنّ الحمّى إن كانت من حرّ الشمس أو من برد فإنّ صاحبها ينتفع بالاستحمام وصبّ الماء الحارّ على الرأس وإن كانت الحمّى من تعب فليس منفعة صاحبها بذلك دون غيره وكذلك الحمّى التي تكون من ضيق المسامّ (If the fever is caused by the heat of the sun or by cold, the patient benefits from bathing and pouring hot water over his head, likewise if the fever is caused by fatigue or by blockage of the pores [of the skin]).

395   Cf. ibid. 7.43, ed. Kühn, p. 148.

(7.42)

[٣٩٤] قال أبقراط: من أصابته حمّى ليست من مرار فصبّ على رأسه ماءً حارّا كثيرا حازا كثيرا انقضت بذلك حمّاه.

قال المفسّر: جالينوس يروم أنْ يتأوّل هذا الفصل بأنْ يقول إنّ غرضه بقوله حمّى ليست من مرار ليست حمّى عفونة بل بعض أنواع حمّى يوم ولا شكّ أنّ الاستحمام فيها نافع وبه تنحلّ الحمّى.

(7.43)

٥   [٣٩٥] قال أبقراط: المرأة لا تكون ذات يمينين.

قال المفسّر: قال جالينوس إنّ علّة ذلك ضعف أعصابها وعضلها لأنّ كلّ ذي يمينين إنّما سببه قوّة الأعصاب.

(7.44)

[٣٩٦] قال أبقراط: من كوي أو بطّ من المتقيّحين نخرجت منه مدّة نقية بيضاء فإنّه يسلم. فإنْ خرجت منه مادّة كدرة منتنة فإنّه يهلك.

١٠   قال المفسّر: المتقيّحين هم الذين تجتمع مدّة كثيرة بين صدورهم ورئاتهم وهم الذين كانت عادة الأوائل بكيّهم ليستخرجوا تلك المادّة.

١-٢ فصبّ ... حمّاه: om. B ‖ ١ حازا كثيرا: حازّ كثير A ٦ قال المفسّر: om. P ‖ أعصابها: أعضاؤها A ‖ وعضلها: وعضلاتها AP ‖ سببه: ضعف A add. ٧ الأعصاب: هذا وجد في نسخة أخرى قال المفسّر يذكر علّة ذا اليمينين ويقال إنّ المرأة ضعيفة الحرارة بلا شكّ ولا يصل حرّها إلى حيّزيساوي اليمين الشمال وتبسّط القول في ذلك P add. يذكر علّة ذا اليمينين ويقال إنّ المرأة قليلة (ضعيفة B¹) الحرارة بلا شكّ ولا يصل حرّها إلّا حيّزيساوي اليمين الشمال وتبسّط القول في ذلك B add. ٨ أو بطّ: om. BCP ٨-٩ نخرجت ... يهلك: om. B ٩ مادّة: om. P ١٠ الذين: الذي P ‖ كثيرة: om. P ١١ بكيّهم: om. BP

(7.45)

[397] Says Hippocrates: If a patient has pus in the liver and is cauterized and clear white pus flows out, he will recover for that pus is situated in the membrane of the liver. But If it flows similar to lees of oil, he will die.

Says the commentator: If the pus is in the membrane and the substance of the liver is healthy, recovery is possible.

(7.46)

[398] Says Hippocrates: If [someone suffers from] pain in the eyes, administer him pure wine, then let him enter the bathhouse, pour much hot water over his head, and bleed him.

Says the commentator: Galen says that this aphorism was ascribed to Hippocrates without proper authority (was falsely ascribed to him).[396] In short, it is totally incorrect, whoever said it [for the first time].

(7.47)

[399] Says Hippocrates: If a dropsical patient suffers from cough, there is no hope for him.

Says the commentator: This [aphorism] is a repetition.[397]

(7.48)

[400] Says Hippocrates: Strangury and dysuria are alleviated by drinking[398] wine and by venesection; one should open the internal veins.[399]

---

396   Cf. ibid. 7.46, p. 151: Τῶν παραγεγραμμένων εἶναί μοι δοκεῖ καὶ οὗτος ὁ ἀφορισμός, οὐχ ὁμολογῶν ἑνὶ τῶν ἔμπροσθεν εἰρημένων τὸ ὀδύνην ὀφθαλμῶν ἀκρατοποσίαν ἢ λουτρὸν ἢ πυρίην ἢ φλεβοτομίην ἢ φαρμακείην λύειν; trans. Ḥunayn (S, fol. 150ᵃ): هذا الفصل عندي إحدى الفصول التي دلست في هذا الكتاب وذلك أنّ هذا القول لا يوافق قولا قد تقدّم من أبقراط قال فيه أوجاع العينين يحلّها الشراب الصرف أو حمّام أو تكميد أو فصد العروق أو شرب الدواء (In my opinion, this aphorism is one of those that have been falsely ascribed to Hippocrates (interpolated) in this text, since it does not agree to Hippocrates' earlier statement: "Pains in the eyes are alleviated by drinking pure wine, or by bathing, or by fomentation, or by venesection, or by taking a purgative drug"); cf. aphorism 6.31 (323) above.

397   Cf. aphorism 6.35 (327) above.

398   "drinking wine" (شرب الشراب): Cf. Galen, *In Hippocratis Aphorismos commentarius* 7.48, ed. Kühn, vol. 18a, p. 153: θώρηξις; Hippocrates, *Aphorisms*, trans. Littré, vol. 4, p. 591: "le vin pur;" trans. Jones, p. 205: "neat wine;" cf. aphorism 2.21 (73) above.

399   Cf. aphorism 6.36 (328) above.

(7.45)

[٣٩٧] قال أبقراط: من كانت به في كبده مدّة فكوي نخرجت منه مدّة بيضاء نقية فإنّه يسلم. وذلك أنّ تلك المدّة فيه في غشاء الكبد وإنْ خرج منه شبيه بثفل الزيت هلك.

قال المفسّر: إذا كانت المدّة في الغشاء وجرم الكبد سالم فيمكن السلامة.

(7.46)

[٣٩٨] قال أبقراط: إذا كان في العينين وجع فأسق صاحبه شرابا صرفا أدخله الحمّام وصبّ عليه
٥ ماءا حارّا كثيرا ثمّ افصده.

قال المفسّر: جالينوس يقول إنّ هذا الفصل دلّس على أبقراط وبالجملة هو خطاء محض قاله من قاله.

(7.47)

[٣٩٩] قال أبقراط: إذا حدث بصاحب الاستسقاء سعال فليس يرجا.

قال المفسّر: تقدّم معناه.

(7.48)

[٤٠٠] قال أبقراط: تقطير البول وعسره يحلّهما شرب الشراب والفصد وينبغي أن تقطع العروق
١٠ الداخلة.

---

١ مدّة: om. P ‏ ١-٢ نخرجت ... هلك: om. B ‏ ٢ المدّة: المادّة A ‏ ٣ الكبد سالم: om. A ‏ || سالم: سليم
BP ‏ ٤-٥ فأسق ... افصده: om. B ‏ ٤ أدخله: إلى add. P ‏ ٩-١٠ يحلّهما ... الداخلة: om. B

Says the commentator: This aphorism is evidently corrupt. But Galen took it upon himself to give a correct meaning (interpretation) to the first part by saying that if it is caused by cold or an obstruction due to thick blood while there is no overfilling in the body, then the drinking of much wine is beneficial.[400] As for the latter part of this aphorism and likewise an earlier aphorism,[401] where he states that one should open the internal veins, Galen has made it clear that this is not correct and that it is not the opinion of Hippocrates.[402]

(7.49)

[401] Says Hippocrates: If a swelling and redness appear on[403] the front of the chest in the case of someone suffering from angina, it is a good sign because the illness will have been diverted outwards.

Says the commentator: This is clear.

(7.50)

[402] Says Hippocrates: If someone is attacked in the brain by the illness called "sphacelus" (mortification), he will die within three days. But if he outlives these, he will recover.

Says the commentator: This illness consists of a corruption of the substance of the brain for which there is no cure once it has become firmly settled. But here he wants to say that if this illness has begun and last longer than three days and [the patient] has not died, it is a sign that [the illness] is not firmly settled and that nature is powerful and will overcome [the illness].

---

400   Cf. Galen, In Hippocratis Aphorismos commentarius 7.48, ed. Kühn, vol. 18a, p. 153: ἐκ τού-
των ἁπασῶν τῶν διαθέσεων τὴν μὲν ψύξιν ἡ θώρηξις λύει ... καὶ μέντοι τὴν τοιαύτην φλεγμονὴν,
ἥτις δι' ἔμφραξιν παχέος αἵματος ἄνευ πλήθους ἐγένετο; trans. Ḥunayn (S, fol. 151ᵃ): من وأما
هذه العلل كلّها أمّا البرد فقد يشفي منه شرب الشراب ... ويشفي أيضا من الورم إذا كان من سدّة
حدثت مّن دم غليظ من غير امتلاء في البدن (As for all these illnesses: the one that is [caused
by] cold is cured by the drinking of pure wine ... likewise [the one that is caused by] an
inflammation due to the obstruction by thick blood, while there is no overfilling in the
body).
401   I.e., aphorism 6.36 (328) above.
402   Cf. Galen, In Hippocratis Aphorismos commentarius 6.36, ed. Kühn, vol. 18a, p. 58: βέλτιον οὖν ἐστι καὶ τοῦτον τὸν ἀφορισμὸν ἕνα τῶν παρακειμένων ὑπολαβεῖν; trans. Ḥunayn (S,
fol. 127ᵃ): فالأجود عندي أن يتوهّم أنّ هذا الفصل أيضا أحد الفصول التي أدخلت في هذا الكّاب (In
my opinion it is best to assume that also this aphorism is one of those that were [subse-
quently] inserted into this book).
403   "on the front of the chest" (في مقدّم الصدر): Cf. ibid. 7.49, ed. Kühn, p. 154: ἐν τῷ στήθει; Hippocrates, Aphorisms, trans. Littré, vol. 4, p. 591: "à la poitrine;" trans. Jones, p. 205: "on the
breast."

قال المفسّر: هذا الكلام ظاهر الفساد لكنّ جالينوس قد تكلّف أنْ يخرج لأوّل هذا الفصل وجه صواب. فقال إذا كان سبب ذلك بردا أو سدّة حادثة من دم غليظ من غير امتلاء في البدن كان شرب الشراب الكثير ينفع من ذلك. وأمّا قوله في هذا الفصل وينبغي أنْ تقطع العروق الداخلة وكذلك في المقالة التي قبل هذه فقد صرّح جالينوس أنّ ذلك غير صحيح ولا هو رأي أبقراط.

(7.49)

٥   [٤٠١] قال أبقراط: إذا ظهر الورم والحمرة في مقدّم الصدر في من اعترته الذبحة كان ذلك دليلا محمودا لأنّ المرض يكون قد مال إلى خارج.

قال المفسّر: هذا بيّن.

(7.50)

[٤٠٢] قال أبقراط: من أصابته في دماغه العلّة التي يقال لها سفاقيلوس فإنّه يهلك في ثلاثة أيّام فإنْ جاوزها فإنّه يبرأ.

١٠   قال المفسّر: هذه العلّة فساد جوهر الدماغ ولا برء له إذا استحكم. وإنّما يريد أنّه إنْ ابتدأ هذا المرض وجاوز الثلاثة أيّام ولم يهلك فذلك دليل أنّه لم يستحكم وأنّ الطبيعة قاوت فأصلحت.

٥-٦ والحمرة ... خارج: .om B   ٥ كان: فإنّ P   ٦ المرض: المريض P   ٨ سفاقيلوس (= ‏S, fol. 151ª):
اسفا كاللشمّوس C سفافيلوس P اسقا كاليوس A شقاقلوس B ‖ فإنْ: فإنّه C فإنْ هو C¹P   ١١ قاوت: قوات
P ‖ فأصلحت: فاصحلت C

(7.51)

[403] Says Hippocrates: Sneezing arises [from][404] the head when the brain becomes hot and the cavity in the head becomes moist; then the air that is inside descends[405] and [produces] a noise because it passes through a narrow passage.

Says the commentator: Sometimes sneezing occurs when the brain gets hot and the empty space in it becomes moist and that moisture dissolves in vapor. Sometimes, wind rises from below during coughing and when it arrives in the nasal passages it causes sneezing. The nasal passages lead to two places (organs): the mouth and the brain. The opening, which leads to the mouth, is cleansed by the wind that arises from below, while the passages that lead to the brain are cleansed by the wind that descends from it. With the term "the empty space" he means the ventricles of the brain.

(7.52)

[404] Says Hippocrates: If someone suffers from a severe pain in the liver and then develops a fever, it will relieve the pain.

Says the commentator: A severe pain in the liver without fever is caused by thick wind (flatulence). For this reason, if fever supervenes, the wind (flatulence) is dissolved.[406]

(7.53)

[405] Says Hippocrates: If a patient needs venesection, one should bleed him in spring.

Says the commentator: This is one of the aphorisms that are repetitious.[407]

(7.54)

[406] Says Hippocrates: If a person has phlegm confined in the area between the stomach and diaphragm and he suffers from pain because it has no outlet into either of the two cavities, the illness will resolve if the phlegm flows through the vessels into the urinary bladder.

---

404   "[from]": "in" MSS; corrected after Hippocrates, *Aphorisms* 7.51, ed. Tytler, and S, fol. 152ᵃ.
405   "descends" (يدخل): Cf. Galen, *In Hippocratis Aphorismos commentarius*, ed. Kühn, vol. 18a, p. 157: ὑπερχεῖται; Hippocrates, ibid., trans. Littré, vol. 4, p. 593: "est chassé au dehors;" trans. Jones, p. 205: "overflows."
406   Cf. aphorism 6.40 (332) above.
407   Cf. aphorism 6.47 (339) above.

(7.51)

[٤٠٣] قال أبقراط: العطاس يكون في الرأس إذا سخن الدماغ ورطب الموضع الخالي في الرأس فانحدر الهواء الذي فيه فسمع له صوت لأنّ نفوذه وخروجه يكون في موضع ضيّق.

قال المفسّر: قد يكون العطاس إذا سخن الدماغ ورطب الموضع الخالي الذي فيه فانحلّت تلك الرطوبة بخارا. وقد يرتفع مع السعال ريح من أسفل فإذا صارت في مجرى المنخرين كان سببا لحدوث العطاس. ومجاري الأنف تنفذ إلى موضعين الفم والدماغ. فالثقب التي تنفذ إلى الفم ينقى بالريح التي ترتفع من أسفل. وأمّا المجاري التي تنفذ إلى الدماغ فتنقى بالريح التي تنحدر منه. وقوله الموضع الخالي يريد به بطون الدماغ.

(7.52)

[٤٠٤] قال أبقراط: من كان به وجع شديد في كبده فحدثت به حمّى حلّت ذلك الوجع عنه.

قال المفسّر: وجع شديد في الكبد دون حمّى إنّما يكون من ريح غليظة فلذلك إذا حدثت الحمّى انحلّت تلك الريح.

(7.53)

[٤٠٥] قال أبقراط: من احتاج إلى أنْ يخرج من عروقه دم فينبغي أنْ تقطع له العرق في الربيع.

قال المفسّر: هذا من الفصول التي تكرّرت.

(7.54)

[٤٠٦] قال أبقراط: من تحيّز فيه بلغم في ما بين المعدة والحجاب وحدث به وجع إذا كان لا منفذ له ولا إلى واحد من الفضائين فإنّ ذلك البلغم إذا جرى في العروق إلى المثانة انحلّت علّته.

---

١ في: من P، t S, fol. 152ª ‖ ٢-١ ورطب ... ضيّق: om. B ‖ ٤ بخارا: بخار P ‖ ٥ موضعين: om. B ‖ فالثقب التي تنفذ: فالذقب الذي ينفذ P فالثقب الذي ينفذ B ‖ ٦-٢.٣٠٩ بالريح ... واخراجها: om. C ‖ ٨ فحدثت ... عنه: om. B ‖ ١١ فينبغي ... الربيع: om. B ‖ ١٣ في ما: om. A ‖ وجع: وجعا P

Says the commentator: It has been said that this [aphorism] is not by Hippocrates. Galen has said that it is not impossible that this humor can penetrate into the vessels through transudation, because nature is crafty in thinning [superfluous] matters and expelling them through[408] any possible passage, even if it is extremely narrow, as it does to expel the pus accumulated in the area between the lung and chest. In general, what he says only happens rarely; it is therefore of very little benefit.

(7.55)

[407] Says Hippocrates: Is someone's liver is filled with water and this water bursts into the omentum,[409] the belly fills with water and he dies.

Says the commentator: These watery[410] vesicles often occur in the liver. His statement that "someone whose belly fills with water dies" means that this is mostly the case.[411]

(7.56)

[408] Says Hippocrates: Anxiety, yawning, and shivering are cured by wine when it is mixed with an equal part [of water].

Says the commentator: Anxiety mostly hails from harmful moisture in the cardia of the stomach. Drinking [diluted[412] wine] cures, as stated, all this because it washes (cleanses) the vessels and improves the humors.[413]

(7.57)

[409] Says Hippocrates: If someone gets a tumor in the urethra, when it suppurates and bursts, the pain comes to an end.

---

408   "through any possible passage, even if it is extremely narrow" (بكلّ طريق ولو بعد ودقّ):
      Cf. Galen, *In Hippocratis Aphorismos commentarius* 7.54, ed. Kühn, vol. 18a, p. 164: καὶ διὰ
      λεπτῶν ὁδοιποροῦσι πόρων; trans. Ḥunayn (S, fol. 154ª): وكانت المجاري التي في ذلك الموضع دقيقة
      ضيّقة (and the passages over there were thin and narrow).
409   "omentum" (الغشاء الباطن): The standard Arabic term for "omentum" (Greek: ἐπίπλοον; cf.
      ibid. 7.55, ed. Kühn, p. 165) is ثرب; cf. aphorism 5.46 (266) above.
410   "watery vesicles" (نفاخات): Cf. Galen, ibid.: ὑδατίδας; Liddell/Scott, *Greek-English Lexicon*,
      p. 1843, s.v. ὑδατίς: "watery vesicle, hydatid."
411   Cf. Maimonides, *Medical Aphorisms* 9.89, trans. Bos, vol. 2, p. 78: "Watery vesicles occur
      more rapidly in the membrane surrounding the liver than in the other organs."
412   "[diluted wine]": The Arabic text reads: 'slightly diluted wine.'
413   Cf. Maimonides, *Medical Aphorisms* 20.24, trans. Bos, vol. 4, p. 69: "Wine mixed with an
      equal amount of water heats the whole body and rapidly moves to all its limbs. It ame-
      liorates and improves the humors of the body by balancing their temperament and by
      evacuating bad humors."

قال المفسّر: قد قيل إنّ هذا ليس لأبقراط وقال جالينوس إنّه لا يمتنع نفوذ هذا الخلط للعروق بالرشح لأنّ الطبيعة تحتال في تلطيف الموادّ وإخراجها بكلّ طريق ولو بعد ودقّ كما تخرج المدّة المجتمعة في ما بين الرئة والصدر. وبالجملة هو كلام قليل الوقوع قليل الفائدة جدًّا.

(7.55)

[٤٠٧] قال أبقراط: من امتلأت كبده ماءا ثمّ انفجر ذلك الماء إلى الغشاء الباطن امتلأ بطنه ماءا

٥ ومات.

قال المفسّر: قد تحدث هذه النفّاخات كثيرا في الكبد وقوله إنّ من امتلأ بطنه ماءا يموت ذلك على الأكثر.

(7.56)

[٤٠٨] قال أبقراط: القلق والتثاؤب والقشعريرة يبرئه الشراب إذا مزج واحد سواء بواحد سواء.

قال المفسّر: أكثر القلق من رطوبة مؤذية في فم المعدة وشرب النبيذ القليل المزج كما ذكر يبرئ من

١٠ جميع ذلك لغسله العروق وإصلاحه للأخلاط.

(7.57)

[٤٠٩] قال أبقراط: من خرجت به بثرة في إحليله فإنّها إذا تقيّحت وانفجرت انقضى وجعه.

Says the commentator: This [aphorism] is a repetition.[414]

(7.58)
[410] Says Hippocrates: Is someone has a concussion of the brain,[415] he[416] will immediately[417] become paralyzed.

Says the commentator: A concussion of the brain or spinal cord is caused by a fall and the like.

(7.59a–b)
[411][418]

(7.60)
[412] Says Hippocrates: If the flesh [of someone's body] is moist, he should starve because hunger dries the body.

Says the commentator: This is clear.

(7.61)
[413] Says Hippocrates: If changes occur in the whole body and it becomes very cold and then hot or it changes its color, it indicates a protracted disease.

Says the commentator: This [aphorism] is a repetition.[419]

(7.62)
[414] Says Hippocrates: Much sweat that flows constantly, whether hot or cold, indicates that moisture should be evacuated from the body; in a strong person from above[420] and in a weak person from below.[421]

---

414   Cf. aphorism 4.82 (219) above.

415   Hippocrates, *Aphorisms* 7.57, adds: ὑπό τινος προφάσιος (cf. Galen, *In Hippocratis Aphorismos commentarius*, ed. Kühn, vol. 18a, p. 170); Hippocrates, ibid., trans. Littré, vol. 4, p. 595: "par une cause quelconque;" trans. Jones, p. 207: "from any cause."

416   "he will ... become paralyzed" (سكتة ... يصيبه): Cf. Galen, ibid.: ἀνάγκη ἀφώνους γίνεσθαι; Hippocrates, ibid., trans. Littré: "nécessairement on perd la parole;" trans. Jones: "the patients of necessity lose ... the power of speech."

417   "immediately" (في وقته): Cf. Galen, ibid.: παραχρῆμα; Hippocrates, ibid., trans. Jones: "at once."

418   The Hippocratic aphorisms 59a–b are missing in the Arabic MSS, as they are repetitions of aphorisms 4.34–35 (171–172) above. Note however that they are also missing in Greek C (cf. Hippocrates, *Aphorisms*, ed. Jones, p. 208).

419   Cf. aphorism 4.40 (177) above.

420   I.e., through emesis.

421   I.e., through purgation.

قال المفسّر: هذا من المتكرّرات.

(7.58)

[٤١٠] قال أبقراط: من تزعزع دماغه فإنّه يصيبه في وقته سكتة.

قال المفسّر: إنّما يكون تزعزع الدماغ أو النخاع بسقطة أو نحوها.

(7.59a–b)

[٤١١]

(7.60)

٥ [٤١٢] قال أبقراط: من كان لحمه رطبا فينبغي أنْ يجوع فإنّ الجوع يجفّف الأبدان.

قال المفسّر: هذا بيّن.

(7.61)

[٤١٣] قال أبقراط: إذا كانت تحدث في البدن كلّه تغايير ويبرد بردا شديدا ثمّ يسخن أو يتلوّن بلون ثمّ يتغيّر فيحول إلى غيره أنذر بطول من المرض.

قال المفسّر: تكرّر.

(7.62)

١٠ [٤١٤] قال أبقراط: العرق الكثير الذي يجري دائما حارًّا كان أو باردا يدلّ على أنّه ينبغي أن تخرج من البدن رطوبة إمّا في القوي فن فوق وإمّا في ضعيف فن أسفل.

---

٢ فإنّه ... سكتة: om. B   This aphorism is missing in the Arabic MSS, as it is a repetition of ٤

٥ فينبغي ... الأبدان: om. B   aphorisms 4.34–35   ٧ تغايير: تغاير P   ٧–٨ ويبرد ... المرض: om. B

٧ أو: و-AC   ٨ أنذر: add. ذلك P   ١٠–١١ حارًّا ... أسفل: om. B

Says the commentator: His[422] statement that the moisture of strong people should be evacuated through emesis and of weak people through purgation should not always be carried out [in this way]. You already know his (i.e., Hippocrates') approach. Galen doubts whether this aphorism is by Hippocrates or by somebody else.[423]

This is the end of the seventh part of the commentary on the *Aphorisms*; praise be to God alone.

---

422   "His statement ... [in this way]": Cf. Galen, *In Hippocratis Aphorismos commentarius* 7.63, ed. Kühn, vol. 18a, p. 177: ἐι δὲ τοῖς ἰσχυροῖς μὲν ἄνωθεν μόνον ἀεὶ, τοῖς δ' ἀσθενέσι κάτωθεν, ἄξιον εἶναι δοκεῖ μοι σκέψεως. βέλτιον γὰρ ἴσως οὐ ταύτῃ διαιρεῖν τῶν βοηθημάτων τὴν χρείαν, ἀλλ' ὡς ὑμῖν ἐν τῇ θεραπευτικῇ πραγματείᾳ περὶ τῶν τοιούτων ἁπάντων διώρισται; cf. trans. Ḥunayn (F (no foliation); S, fols. 156b–157a): وأما القول بأنه ينبغي أن تستفرغ الرطوبة الفاضلة من القوي من فوق دائماً ومن الضعيف من أسفل ففيه عندي نظر والأجود عندي ألّا تجعل تفسير الحاجة إلى العلاجين على هذا الطريق لكن على الطريق الذي حدّدته في كتابي في علاج الأمراض (His statement that the superfluous moisture should always be evacuated of strong people from above and of weak people from below needs to be examined. In my opinion, it is best, if the [use] of these two [kinds of] treatment is not interpreted in this way, but according to what I stipulated in my book *De methodo medendi*).

423   Cf. ibid., ed. Kühn: καὶ τοῦτον οὖν τὸν ἀφορισμὸν ἐκ τῶν παραγεγραμμένων εἶναι νομίζω; cf. trans. Ḥunayn (F (no foliation); S, fol. 157a): وهذا الفصل في ما أحسب هو من الفصول التي زيدت في هذا الكتاب (In my opinion, this is one of the aphorisms that was added [subsequently] to this book).

قال المفسّر: قوله إنّ رطوبة تستفرغ من القوي بالقيء ومن الضعيف بالإسهال لا يطرد ذلك دائمًا. وقد علمت طريقته قد شكّ جالينوس في هذا الفصل هل هو لأبقراط أو لغيره.

كملت المقالة السابعة من شرح الفصول الحمد لله وحده.

<hr />

Aphorisms 7.63–87 are missing in all Arabic MSS and in ١ دائمًا: أبدا P ٢ لأبقراط: لبقراط P ‖

٣ كملت المقالة السابعة من شرح الفصول الحمد لله وحده: تمّت المقالة السابعة من كتاب الفصول لأبقراط t
وشرحها A كملت المقالة السابعة من شرح فصول أبقراط B كملت المقالة السابعة من شرح الفصول ولله الحمد
وتمّ تمامها الكتاب والحمد لله تعالى واهب العقل كما هو أهله ومستحقّه وصلّى الله على سيّد الأنبياء محمّد وآله P
الطاهرين ربّ اختم بالخير add. A و(ب)تمامها تمّ جميع الكتاب الحمد لله تعالى add. B فرّغ نسخا ومقابله من أصل
المصنّف فصح add. C وبتمامها تمّ جميع الكتاب بعون الله ومنّه ברוך יי לעולם ב'נ'ל' כח ולאין או' עצמה ירבה
add. P

PART 2

Hebrew Translations

∵

Commentary on Hippocrates' Aphorisms: First Hebrew Translation (Ibn Tibbon)

[1] אמר הרב הגדול מרנא ורבנא משה בן עבד האלהים הישראלי: איני חושב אחד מן החכמים
אשר חיברו ספרים חבר ספר במין ממיני החכמות והוא יכוין שלא יובן מה שיכללהו ספרו עד
שיפורש ואילו כוין זה אחד מן מחברי הספרים היה מבטל עליו חבור ספרו אשר חבר כי
המחבר אינו מחבר חבורו להבין לעצמו מה שיכלול החבור אבל יחבר מה שיחבר כדי שיבין
אותו זולתו כדי שיבינו בו אחרים וכאשר היה מה שחבר בלתי מובן כי אם בחבור אחר הנה   5
בטל עליו ספרו.

[2] ואולם הסבות המצריכות האחרונים לבאר ספרי הראשונים ולפרשם הוא אצלי אחת
מארבע סבות. הראשונה שלימות מעלת המחבר שהוא לטוב הבנתו ידבר בעניינים עמוקים
נסתרים רחוקים להשיג בלשון קצר ויהיה זה מבואר אצלו לא יצטרך אל תוספת. וכאשר
יבקש הבא אחריו להבין אותם העניינים מן הלשון ההוא הקצר היה קשה זה עליו מאד והוצרך   10
המפרש אל תוספת מלות במאמר ההוא עד שיובן העניין אשר כוונו המחבר הראשון.

[3] והסבה השנית חסרון הקדמות הספר וזה כי המחבר פעמים יחבר ספר חושב שיהיה
המעיין בו כבר קדם לו ידיעת ההקדמות אשר לא יובן לו דבר בלעדיהם ויצטרך המפרש
לזכור בקצור אותם ההקדמות ולהישיר אליהם ולפי זאת הסבה גם כן יבאר המפרש חכמה
אחת שלא זכר המחבר אותה.   15

[4] והסבה השלישית אופני המאמר וזה כי רוב המאמרים בכל לשון יסבול הסברות ואפשר
יהיה שיובן מן המאמר ההוא עניינים מתחלפים גם קצתם מתהפכים גם סותרים. ויפול החלוק
בין המעיינים במאמר ההוא ויסברהו אדם אחד סברא אחת ויאמר לא רצה בו המחבר כי
אם זה העניין ויסברהו אדם אחר סברא אחרת ויצטרך מפרש המאמר ההוא אל הכרעת אחת
הסברות ולהביא ראיה על אמתתה ולבטל זולתה.   20

---

1 הרב הגדול מרנא ורבנא: السيّد العالم الفاضل الإمام a ‖ הגדול: א om. ‖ בן: א om. ‖ הישראלי: זצ״ל א
add. قدّس الله نفسه (except for B) a   2 ספרים: הספרים אד   3 כוין זה אחד מן מחברי הספרים:
יכוין זה (אחד א¹) באחד מן הספרים יכוין זה ויבין אחר באחד מן הספרים בח כוין זה אחד מן הספרים ג
כוין אחד זה באחד מן הספרים ג¹ ‖ עליו (= عليه) ג¹ ‖ עליו (= عليه): غاية a   6 עליו (= عليه): غاية a ‖ ולפרשם: ולבארה
ד ולבארם ד¹ corr.²   7–8 הוא אצלי אחת מארבע: הם אצלי אחת מארבעה א   8 הראשונה: הסבה
הראשונה א מהם ח add.   12 חושב: מסופק א   13 ההקדמות: الفلانية a add. ‖ אשר לא יובן לו דבר
בלעדיהם: فإذا رام فهم ذلك الكتاب من لا علم له بتلك المقدّمات لم يفهم له شيء a   14 ההקדמות: وتبيينها
أو ينبّه على الكتب التي تبيّنت فيها تلك المقدّمات a add.   14–15 חכמה אחת שלא זכר המחבר אותה:
على ما لم يذكر المؤلّف علّته a   16 אופני: ترجّح a   17 החלוק: החלוף ד   19 אל: א om.

[5] והסבה הרביעית הרעיון הנופל למחבר בלא עיון או הדבור הכפול או מה שאין תועלת בו
כלל ויצטרך המפרש שירמה עליו ויביא ראיה על ביטולו או על היות המאמר הוא בלתי מועיל
או כפול. וזה לא יקרא פרוש לפי האמת כי אם השגה והערה. אבל הלך המנהג אצל האנשים
שייעינו הספר ואם זה היה מה שנאמר בו רובו אמת ימנה ההערה על אותם המקומות המעטים
מכלל הפירוש ויאמר בלי עיון דבר המחבר באמרו כך והאמת הוא כך או זה אין צורך לזכרו   5
או זה מאמר כפול בו ויבאר זה כלו. ואולם אם זה היה מה שנאמר בספר ההוא רובו טעות יקרא
החבור האחרון אשר יגלה אותם הטעויות השגה לא פירוש. וכאשר יזכר בספר ההשגה דבר
מן המאמרים האמתיים אשר נזכרו בחבור הראשון יאמר אמנם אמרו כך הוא אמת.

[6] וכל מה שיפורש מספרי אריסטו' אמנם פורש פירוש לפי הסבה הראשונה והשלישית
במה שנראה לנו. וכל מה שיפורש מספרי הלימודים אמנם יפורש לפי הסבה השנית. והנה   10
יפורשו קצת מהמאמרים הלימודיים לפי הסבה הרביעית גם כן. כי זה ספר המג'סטי עם
קשי חבורו כבר נפל לו בספרו דברים נאמרים בלי עיון העירו עליהם רבים מן האנדלוסיים
וכבר חברו בזה. וכל מה שפורש או יפורש מספרי אבוקראט הנה הוא לפי הסבה הראשונה
והשלישית והרביעית רובו וקצת דבריו יפורש לפי הסבה השנית.

[7] אבל כי ג'אלינוס ימאן זה ואינו רואה בשום פנים שיהיה בדברי אבוקראט דבר נאמר בלי   15
עיון אבל יהיה סובר במה שאינו סובל סברא וישים פירוש המאמר מה שלא יורה המאמר
ההוא על כלום ממנו כמו שתראה אותו שעשה בפירושו לספר הליחות נסתפק אם הוא
לאבוקראט או לזולתו. והביאו לזה מה שבספר ההוא מערבוב העניינים והיותם בדמות חבורי
בעלי הכימיא או יותר פחות מהם. והיותר אמתי שבשמות בו אצלי שיקרא ספר הערבובים.
אבל לפרסום היותו לאבוקראט פירש אותו הפירוש ההוא הנפלא. וכל מה שאמרו גליאנוס   20
בפירוש ההוא הנה הנה הוא כלו דברים אמתיים לפי מלאכת הרפואה אבל אינו מורה המאמר
ההוא על דבר מן דבר זה פירוש ולא יקרא זה פירוש לפי האמת כי הוצאת מה שבמאמר
ההוא בכח עם ההבנה אל הפועל עד שאתה כאשר תשוב ותעיין המאמר המפורש אחר
שהבינות אותו מן הפירוש ראית המאמר ההוא מורה על מה שהבינות אותו מן הפירוש.
זהו אשר יקרא פירוש באמת לא שיבוא האדם במאמרים אמתיים ויאמר זה פירוש מאמר   25
האומר כך כמו שיעשה גאלינוס בקצת מאמרי אבוקראט. וכן גם כן אלו אשר יולידו תולדות
מדברי אדם אחד ויקראו זה פירוש אין זה פירוש אצלי אבל חבור כרוב פירושי אקלידס
ללביורוזי הנה איני קורא זה פירוש.

---

1 הרעיון הנופל למחבר בלא עיון: الأوهام الواقعة للمؤلّف a   4 שייעינו: שיראו בח ‖ הספר: הספרים
א   5 בלי עיון דבר: وهم a   8 המאמרים: הדברים בח   11 זה: א   om. ח   12 קשי חבורו: جلالة
مؤلّفه a ‖ דברים נאמרים בלי עיון: أوهام a ‖ העירו: العيدو א   15–16 דבר נאמר בלי עיון: وهم
a   17 נסתפק: وإن كان قد شكّ جالينوس a   18 או: אם ד   22 הוא: בדח om.   23 ההוא: ד
om. ‖ ותעיין: תעיין בח לעיין ד   24 ראית המאמר ההוא: תראה אותו הדבר ד ‖ שהבינות אותו:
שתבינהו א   25 ויאמר: כי יאמר א   28 ללביורוזי: נירוזי א ללביכוס ב ללביכורו ח للنيريزي a ‖ זה:
add. a كلّه

[8] וכן נמצא גאלינוס גם כן בפרשו ספרי אבוקראט פירש המאמר בהפך הכונה המובנת
שישים המאמר ההוא אמת כמו שעשה בספר השביעיות כאשר אמר אבוקראט כי הארץ
מקפת המים ופירש גאלינוס זה המאמר ואמר: אפשר שרצה במאמרו זה כי המים מקיפים
הארץ. אמר כל זה כדי שלא יאמר כי אבוקראט טעה או דבר בלא עיון בזה המאמר. וכבר גבר
העניין ומצא מאמר שהוא טעות מבואר ולא ימצא לו בו תחבולה ואמר זה מיוחס לאבוקראט			5
והכניסוהו במאמרו או הוא דברי איפוקראט הפלוני לא איפוקראט המפורסם כמו שעשה
בפרשו טבע האדם וכל זה להפך אחר זכות אבוקראט. ואע״פ שהיה אבוקראט מגדולי
האנשים כל שכן מן הרופאים בלא ספק הנה אין רדיפת הזכות בדברי שקר מעלה ואפילו
יהיה זה בדין נכבד וידוע.

[9] וידוע כי כל ספר שפורש או שיפורש אין כל מה שבו צריך פירוש אבל בלא ספק יהיה		10
בו מאמר מבואר לא יצטרך אל פירוש. אבל כונות המפרשים בפירושיהם כדרך המחברים
בחיבורהם כי מן המחברים מי שיכוון הקצור ולא יצא מגדר הקצור בשום עניין עד שאלו היה
אפשר לו הדבור במה שכוון בחבורו במאה מלות דרך משל לא ישימם במאה מלות ואחת. ויש
מי שכוונתו האריכות ורבוי הדברים ולעשות ספר גדול ולהרבות מספר חלקיו ואע״פ שיהיה
המקובץ מכל זה מעט העניינים. כן המפרשים מהם מי שיפרש הדבר הצריך פירוש ביותר קצר		15
שאפשר לו ויעזוב מה שזולת זה. ומהם מי שיאריך ויפרש מה שלא יצטרך פירוש או מה שצריך
פירוש ביותר ממה שהוא צריך.

[10] והנה הייתי חושב כי ג׳אלינוס מן המאריכים בפירושו מאד כרוב חבוריו עד שראיתיו ר״ל
ג׳אלינוס יאמר בתחילת פירושו לספר הנימוסים לאפלטון מאמר זה עניינו אמר: הנה ראיתי
קצת המפרשים פירשו זה המאמר ממאמרי אבקראט והוא זה: וכאשר הגיע החולי לתכליתו		20
אז ראוי שתהיה ההנהגה בתכלית האחרון מן הדקות שפירש אותו ביותר ממאה עורות בלא
עניין ובלא סבה.

[11] אמר משה: וכאשר ראיתי זה המאמר לג׳אלינוס דנתיו לזכות בחיבוריו ופירושיו וידעתי
כי הוא קצר בהם מאד בערך אל חבורי אנשי הדורות ההם. אבל הם על כל פנים יש בהם
אריכות לא יחלוק בזה כי אם מתעקש. ואני אמנם אדבר עם מי שישולל מן התאוות ויכוון		25
האמת בכל דבר. וכבר זכר ג׳אלינוס במאמר הששי מהתחבולת הבריאות כי חבריו האריכו
דברים במאמרים ההם.

---

1 המאמר: המאמרים א ‖ בהפך הכונה: בכונה א   2 שישים: א   שישים: حَتّٰى يَجعل a ‖ השביעיות: הטבעיות
ב   3 שרצה במאמרו: שרצה שאבוקראט באמרו א   4 אמר כל זה: לא אמר כל זה אלא א ‖ דבר
בלא עיון: وهم a   4–5 وכבר גבר העניין: .om ب. وإذا غلب في الأمر a   6 הוא: הם ב   7 טבע: ספר ד²
.add ‖ להפך אחר זכות: تعصّب a   8 רדיפת הזכות בדברי שקר: التعصّب a   10 בלא ספק: لا بدّ a
12 ולא יצא מגדר הקצור בשום עניין: الذي لا يحلّ بالمعنى a   16 ויפרש: לפרש ד   18 מן המאריכים:
יאריך המאריכים א   21 שפירש א   וחשבתי שיפרש א   21–22 בלא עניין ובלא סבה: א .om ללא עניין
וללא סבה א¹   25 מתעקש: متعصّب a

[12] ובעבור שראיתי ספר הפרקים לאבוקראט גדול התועלת יותר מכל ספריו ראיתי
שאפרשם כי הם פרקים ראוי שידעם על פה כל רופא אבל זולת הרופאים מלמדים
אותם על פה לנערים אצל מלמדם עד כי פרקים רבים מהם ילמדם על פה מי שאינו רופא
בלמוד הקטן מן המלמד.

[13] ופרקי אבקראט אלו יש מהם פרקים מסופקים צריכים לפירוש ומהם מבוארים בעצמם 5
ומהם כפולים ומהם מה שלא יועיל במלאכת הרפואות. ומהם רעיון פשוט נאמר בלי עיון אבל
ג'אלינוס כמו שידעת ימאן אלו הדברים ויפרש כמו שירצה. אבל אני אפרשם על דרך פירוש
הקצת וזה כי אני לא אפרש אלא מה שיצטרך אל פירוש ואמשיך בזה כונת ג'אלינוס זולתי
בקצת פרקים שאני אזכור מה שנראה לי בהם מיוחס אלי. אבל כל פירוש שאזכרהו סתם הנה
הוא דברי ג'אלינוס ר"ל עניינו כי אני לא שמתי כונתי ללקוט דבריו במילותיו כמו שעשיתי 10
בקצורים. ואמנם היתה כונתי בזה הפירוש קצור לבד כדי שיקל זכרון עניני אלו הפרקים
הצריכים לפירוש ואכון מיעוט מיעוט הדברים בזה בכל יכולתי זולת בפרק הראשון שאני אאריך
בו מעט לא שהוא על דרך הפירוש האמיתי לפרק ההוא אבל להועיל קצת תועלת הארכתי בו
מעט כוון בהם אבוקרט או לא כוון ועתה אתחיל לפרש.

───────────

3 אצל מלמדם: במלמד ‪א‬ في المكتب a ‖ ילמדם: يحفظها a ‖ בלמוד: ולמוד ‪בח‬ כלמוד ‪א‬ حفظ
a ‖ המלמד: المكتب a   6 מה:‪א‬ om.   ‖ רעיון פשוט נאמר בלי עיון: وهم محض a   8 הקצת: הקצור‪א‬
הקצר ‪בח‬ الإنصاف a   9 אזכור: אזכיר‪א‬   10 עניינו: معانيه a   12 בפרק: הפרק ‪ד‬   14–13 הארכתי
בו מעט: سنحت لي فيه a   14 ועתה אתחיל לפרש:‪א‬ om.   ועתה אתחיל בפרוש ‪בח‬

(המאמר הראשון)

(1.1)

[14] אמר אבוקרט: החיים קצרים והמלאכה ארוכה והעת צר והנסיון סכנה והמשפט קשה.
והנה ראוי לך שלא יספיק לך בהשלימך לבדך לעשות מה שראוי מבלתי שיהיה מה שיעשהו
החולה והעומדים לפניו כן והדברים אשר מבחוץ.

אמר המפרש: ידוע שהקצר והארוך ממאמר המצטרף. ואם היה רוצה באמרו החיים קצרים
בסמיכות אל מלאכת הרפואה הנה אמרו והמלאכה ארוכה כפל מאמר בלתי צריך אליו ואין
הפרש בין זה ובין אמרך ראובן יותר קצר משמעון ושמעון יותר ארוך מראובן. ואם רצה
לומר כי חיי אחד מן האנשים קצרים בסמיכות אל שלמות איזו חכמה שתהיה מן החכמות
ומלאכת הרפואה ארוכה בסמיכות אל שאר המלאכות הנה זאת החזרה מועילה כאילו הוא
יאמר: והשלמות היותר רחוק מן האדם בזאת המלאכה זה כולו כדי להזהיר על ההולך
עליה.

[15] ואמנם היות מלאכת הרפואה יותר ארוכה משאר המלאכות העיוניות והמעשיות
הנה זה מבואר כי היא לא תשלם ותגיע תכליתה כי אם בחלקים רבים לא יספיקו חיי
אחד מן האנשים להקיף אותם החלקים כלם על השלימות. וכבר זכר אבונצר אלפראבי
כי החלקים אשר תצטרך אל ידיעתם מלאכת הרפואה שבעה חלקים. הראשון מה שיתלה
ברופא מידיעת נושא מלאכתו והוא גוף האדם וזהו ידיעת החלוק וידיעת מזג כל אבר מן
האיברים בכלל וידיעת פעולתו ותועלתו וענין עצמו מן הקושי והרכות והעובי והספוגיות
וצורת כל אבר מהם ומקומות האיברים הפנימיים והחיצוניים וחיבור האיברים קצתם
בקצתם. וזה השיעור אי אפשר שיסכל הרופא דבר ממנו ובו מן האריכות מה שלא
יעלם.

[16] והחלק השני ידיעת מה שישיג הנושא מעניין הבריאות והוא ידיעת מיני הבריאות בכלל
לכל הגוף ומיני בריאות אבר ואבר.

והחלק השלישי ידיעת מיני החליים וסבותיהם והמקרים הנמשכים אחריהם בגוף כלו בכלל
או באבר מאיברי הגוף.

3 והנה ראוי: וראוי א ‖ שלא יספיק לך בהשלימך לבדך לעשות מה שראוי: أن لا تقتصر على توفّي
فعل ما ينبغي a 4 החולה: והמשרתים אי add. ‖ והעומדים: והמשרתים בח ‖ כן: א om. 5 אמר
המפרש: הפירוש ד וזה הפירוש בח ‖ המצטרף: בח ‖ הסמיכות: הסמיכות בחח ‖ באמרו: במאמרו א 7 קצר: ארוך
א ‖ ארוך: קצר א 10 והשלמות היותר רחוק מן האדם: فا أبعد كال الإنسان a הוא ד add. ‖ האדם:
הוא ד add. ‖ על ההולך (= على الذاهب): ב om. على الدأب a 13 ותגיע תכליתה: להגיע אל תכליתה ח
14 להקיף: לדעת בח ‖ אבונצר אלפראבי: אבונצר אלפרבי ח אבונאצר אלפאראבי ד 15 תצטרך אל:
تلتم بـ a ‖ ידיעתם: ידיעת ח עיקרי בח ‖ הראשון: החלק הראשון א 24 באבר: אבר ח מאבר ח

והחלק הרביעי ידיעת דרכי הראיה והוא איך ילקח מן המקרים ההם המשיגים הנושא ראיות
על מין ומין ממיני הבריאות ועל מין ומין ממיני החולי היה זה בגוף כלו או באיזה אבר שיהיה
מאיבריו ואיך יבדיל בין חולי וחולי כי הנה יתדמו רוב הראיות.

והחלק החמישי דרכי הנהגת בריאות הגוף בכלל ובריאות כל אבר מאיבריו בכל שנה מן
השנים ובכל פרק מפרקי השנה ולפי כל עיר ועיר עד שיתמיד כל גוף וכל אבר על בריאותו
5   אשר ייחדהו.

והחלק השישי ידיעת הדרכים הכלליים אשר ינהגו בהם החולים עד שישיבו הבריאות הנאבד
אל הגוף כלו או אל האבר אשר נחלה.

והחלק השביעי ידיעת הכלים אשר בהם ישתמש הרופא עד שיתמיד הבריאות הנמצא או
10   שישיב הבריאות הנאבד והוא ידיעת מזונות האדם ורפואותיו עם חלוף מיניהם פשוטיהם
ומורכביהם והסמיכה והחיתול והפעות(?) מן המין הזה. וכן הכלים אשר יבקע בהם ויחתוך
הבשר והחתכות אשר יתלה בהם ושאר הכלים אשר ישתמש בהם בנגעים ובחולי העין כולם
מזה המין. והנה נכלל בזה החלק מן המלאכה ידיעת צורת כל צמח וכל מחצב שיכנס במלאכת
הרפואה כי אתה לא תדע ממנו זולת שמו הנה לא השגת אותו על תכליתו. וכן גם כן יצטרך
15   אל שמותיהם המתחלפים בהתחלף המקומות עד שידע בכל מקום אי זה שם יבקש.

[17] וידוע כי ידיעת אלו החלקים השבעה כלם ולדעת אותם על פה הוא מן הספרים המונחים
לכל חלק מהם לא יגיע בו תכלית פעולת הרופא ולא יגיע בעבור החכמות ההם שלמות
המלאכה עד שיהיה מוחזק שיראה האישים בענין בריאותם וענין חלייהם ויגיע לו קנין מהכרת
המופתים אשר יורו בהם איך יורו ידע בקלות ענין מזג האיש מזג וענין מזג כל אבר מאיבריו באיזה
20   מין הוא ממיני הבריאות או ממיני החולי. וכן ענין כל אבר מאיברי האיש הזה וענין עצם איבריו
וכן ידע בקלות באורך ראיית האישים ובאותם הצורות החקוקות בשכלו איך יתעסק באותם
הכלים ר"ל המזונות והרפואות ושאר הכלים וזה יצטרך אל זמן ארוך מאד.

[18] הנה התבאר לך כי ידיעת אותם החלקים בכלל ולדעת על פה אותם הדרכים עד שלא
יעלם ממנו מהם כלום יצטרך אל זמן ארוך מאד. וכן ראיית האישים עד שישמש בהנהגת
25   רפואת חולי איש אחר איש ובשימוש הכלים ההם שימוש פרטי ר"ל הפרידם פעם והרכיב

---

2 הבריאות ועל מין ומין ממיני: א¹ בח om.   5–4 שנה מן השנים: سنّ من الأسنان a   7 עד שישיבו:
שיתמידו הבריאות הנמצא או שישיב ד   11 והסמיכה: והרחיצה א בח om. والشّدّ a || והפעות(?):
והפטות ח والتنطيل a   12 והחתכות: והמזלגים א || ושאר הכלים אשר ישתמש
בהם: א¹   13 שיכנס: يستعمل a   14 הנה: א om. || וכן גם כן: وגם כן אה וגם כן אם בח   17 בו: ידיעת
ד add. || ולא יגיע: א¹   החכמות: العارف a   18 עד שיהיה מוחזק שיראה: حتّى يباشر a || האישים:
האנשים א || וענין חלייהם: וחולייהם א   20–19 כל ... כל אבר: א¹   20 ענין: فعل a   21 איך: يצرם(?)
ישתמש א²ق || יתעסק: ויתעסק א ישתמש בח   24 כלום: דבר כלום א || שישמש: يرتاض a   25 איש:
وفي تدبير شفاء مرض شخص بعد شخص add. a

קצתם עם קצת פעם אחרת וכן פרט הרפואה הזאת או המזון עם פרט אחר ממינו על רפואה
אחרת ממינה כל זה יצטרך אל זמן ארוך מאד. הנה באמת נאמר כי המלאכה הזאת יותר
ארוכה מכל מלאכה למי שיכוון השלמות בה. ואמר גאלינוס בפירושו בספר טימאוס אמר: אי
אפשר לאדם שיהיה חכם במלאכת הרפואה בשלמותה.

5 [19] אמר המחבר: ועם השתמשו בה ידע כי כל מי שהוא בלתי שלם בה הנה יזיק יותר ממה
שיועיל כי היות האיש בריא או חולה יותר טוב יתנהג בעצת רופא כלל משיתנהג בעצת
רופא יטעה בו ולפי שעור חסרון כל איש יהיה טעותו. ואם יארע ממנו קצת טוב הנה הוא
במקרה. ובעבור זה פתח זה הנכבד ספרו בזרוז על השלמות בזאת המלאכה באמרו: החיים
קצרים והמלאכה ארוכה והעת צר והנסיון סכנה והמשפט קשה. אמנם היות הנסיון סכנה הנה
10 הוא מבואר אבל אוסיף בו באור.

[20] ואמרו שהעת צר יראה לי שהוא רצה בו כי עת החולי הוא צר וקצר מאד מן הנסיון כי
אתה כשלא תדע העינים כלם אשר התאמתו בנסיון אבל כשתבוא עתה ותנסה ענינים בזה
החולה הנה העת צר מזה עם מה שיש בהתחלת הנסיון בחולה זה מן הסכנה. ויהיה המאמר
כלו בזרוז על השלמות במלאכה עד שיהיה כל מה שהוא מנוסה בשנים שעברו עומד בזיכרונך.

15 [21] אולם אמרו והמשפט קשה הנה יראה לי שהוא ירצה בו המשפט על נטיית החולי
להצלה או לאבוד או בהתחדש שינוי מן השינויים. ובכלל הקדמת הידיעה במה שיהיה הנה
זה קשה במלאכת הרפואה מאד להגרת החומר ומיעוט קיומו על עניין אחד. וכבר ידעת
כי הדברים הטבעיים כלם הם ברוב לא תמידיים וכמה פעמים יהיו הראיות בתכלית הרוע
וירפא החולי וכמה פעמים יבשרו על טוב הראיות ולא יתאמת מה שהורו עליו. ולכן יצטרך
20 אל שמוש ארוך בראיית הראיות הפרטיות ואז יוכל לשפוט על מה שיתחדש בחריצות
טוב שיהיה קרוב מן האמת. ויהיה זה המאמר גם כן בזרוז על ההרגל במה שיתחייב לזאת
המלאכה.

[22] ואולם אופן הסכנה בניסיון הוא כפי מה שאספר. דע כי כל גשם טבעי הנה ימצאו בו שני
מינים מן המקרים: מקרים ישיגוהו מצד חמרו ומקרים ישיגוהו מצד צורתו. דמיון זה האדם הנה
25 הוא ישיגהו הבריאות והחולי והשינה והיקיצה מצד חמרו ר"ל מצד שהוא בעל חי. וישיגהו
שיחשוב וישתכל ויפלא ויצחק מצד צורתו. ואלו המקרים אשר ישיגו הגוף מצד צורתו הם
אשר יקראו סגולות כי הם מיוחדות במין ההוא לבדו. וכן כל צמח וכל מחצב וכל אבר מאיברי
בעלי חיים ימצאו לו שני אלו המינים מן המקרים.

---

1 קצתם: קצֺת א ‖ פרט: פרטי א ‖ פרט: ... עם פרט: تَخيَّر شَخص على a פרט: פרטי אה
3–5 ואמר ... אמר המחבר: בהההה om. 5 ועם השתמשו (= التصرف) בה: وعند الإنصاف a 7 קצת
טוב: שום טוב אה إصابة a 11 ואמרו שהעת: באמרו העת בה ואמר העת ה 12 כשתבוא: שתבוא
אבה تَستأنف a 13 החולה: החולי אבהה ‖ בהתחלת: בתחלת אה في استئناف a 16 הנה: הוא ד
17 החומר: العنصر a 19 החולי: المريض a 25 חי: חיים אבהה

[23] וימשך אחר כל מקרה מהם אחת מן הפעולות בגופותינו. והפעולות אשר יעשה אותם
הסם בגופותינו מצד חמרו הוא שיחמם או יקרר או ירטיב או ינגב. ואלו הם אשר יקראום
הרופאים הכוחות הראשונים ויאמרו כי זה הסם יחמם בטבעו או יקרר וכן יאמרו גם כן
יעשה באיכותו. וכן הפעולות הנמשכות אחר אלו הכוחות הראשונות הם אשר יקראו אותם
הרופאים הכחות השניות כמו שיהיה הסם מקשה או מרפה או יעשה ספוגות או יעבה. ושאר
5 מה שמנו כלם יעשה אותם הסם מצד חמרו.

[24] והפעולות אשר יעשה אותם הסם בגופותינו מצד צורתו המינית הם אשר יקראו
אותם הרופאים הסגולות. וג׳אלינוס הנהיג בזה המין מן הפעולות לאמר בו יעשה בכלל
עצמו העניין שהוא יעשה פעולתו מצד צורתו המינית אשר בה נתעצם הגוף ההוא ושב
10 זה אבל לא שהוא פועל נמשך אחר איכותו ויקראו אותם גם כן הכחות השלישיות והם
כמו שלשל הסמנים המשלשלים או נגד אותם או היותם סם ממית או מציל מי ששתה
הסם או מי שנשכו אחד מבעלי הארס. כל אלו הפעולות נמשכות אחר הצורה לא אחר
החומר.

[25] והמזונות ג״כ הם מזה המין ר״ל היות זה המין מן הצמחים יזון המין הפלוני מבעלי החיים
15 אין זה שב לאיכויות הראשונות לבד ולא גם כן למה שיתחייב מהם מן הקושי והרכות והעובי
והספוגות אבל זה פועל בכל העצם כמו שאמר ג׳אלינוס. השתכל איך תזון בדברים הקרובים
מטבע העצים ותפעל בהם האצטומכא שלנו ותשנה אותם כמו ערמונים יבשים וגלאנץ יבשים
והחרוב היבש ולא תשנה אצטומכתינו בשום פנים קליפת גרעין הענבים ולא קליפת התפוחים
ודומה להם אבל כמו שיכנסו בגוף כן יצאו כי אין בעצמם שיקבלו מאצטומ׳ שנוי בשום
20 פנים.

[26] וכבר באר ג׳ליאנוס איך ילקח ראיה על טבעי הסמנים ופעולתם הנמשכות אחר
איכותם מטעמיהם בספרו הידוע המפורסם בסמנים הנפרדים. אמנם ידיעת מה שיפעל הסם
מצד צורתו המינית והם אשר יאמר להם שהוא יעשה אותם בכלל עצמו הנה אין אצלנו
ראיה בשום פנים תלקח ראיה בה על הפועל ההוא ואין לידיעת זה דרך אחרת בשום
25 פנים זולת הנסיון. וכמה סמנים מרים מוסרחים תכלית הסרחון והם סמים מועילים וכמה
פעמים ימצא צמח שיהיה ריחו וטעמו כשאר טעמי המזונות וריחותם והוא סם ממית גם
פעמים ימצא צמח יחשב שהוא ממיני המזונות אלא שהוא מדבריי לבד לא פרדסי והוא
סם ממית. הנה כבר התבאר לך סכנת הנסיון שאין גדולה ממנה ועוצם הצורך אליו עם זה

3 הראשונים: הראשונות א‎ 6 הסם: ד‎ .om 7 המינית: אשר בה נתעצם הגוף ההוא אי‎ 8 הנהיג
بزه המין: يعبّر عن هذا النوع a‎ 10 לא: מה ד בח‎ .om 11 שלשל: שלשול אהב ‖ נגד: א‎ .om נגד
המגידים אותם בח שיעירו הקיא אי ‖ 16 והספוגות: והספוגיות א ‖ היותם: היות ד‎
אבהח ‖ הקרובים: הם קרובים א שהם קרובים בהח‎ 17 וגלאנץ: הם קרובים בהח‎ (O.Occ. for acorn; cf. SHS 1, p. 130)
יבשים: א‎ .om וגלאנס יבשים אי‎ (Bet 2) 18 קליפת: בהח‎ .om ‖ גרעין: גרעיני בהח‎ 21 הסמנים:
הסמים א אדוא מפרדא ח‎ 22 הידוע המפורסם: המפורסם אבה הידוע ח ‖ בסמנים: בסמים א‎
25 סמנים: סמים א‎ 26 וריחותם: וריחם א‎ 28 לך: תכלית אי‎ .add

כי כל המזונות לא נודעו כחותם מאשר הם מזון כי אם בנסיון. וראוי לך שלא תקדים בנסיון
ושתהיה זהיר בזכירת כל מה שנסה אותו זולתך.

[27] ודע כי יש סמנים תהיה פעולתם הנמשכת אחר חמרם בגופותינו היא נגלית מבוארת
ופעולתם הנמשכת אחר צורתם נסתרת מאד עד שלא ישוער בה כרוב הסמנים אשר לא יתואר
להם סגולה ולא יוחדו בפעולה ויש סמנים תהיה פעולתם בגופותינו הנמשכת אחר צורתם 5
נגלית גדולה כסמנים המשלשלים והסמים הממיתים והמצילים ולא יעשו רושם בגופותינו
מצד החימום והקירור כי אם רושם קטן מאד אם מפני מהירות מה שיאכל מהם ואם היו
חמים או קרים או מפני שאין להם איכות גובר נגלה. ואי אפשר מבלתי מצוא שתי הפעולות
בהכרח ר״ל הנמשכת אחר החומר והנמשכת אחר הצורה. ובעבור הפעולה הנמשכת אחר
הצורה היו סמנים מיוחדים לאצטומ׳ וסמנים מיוחדים לכבד וסמנים מיוחדים לטחול וסמנים 10
מיוחדים ללב וסמנים מיוחדים למות. ובעבור הצורה המינית גם כן יתחלפו פעולות הסמנים
ואם היה טבעם אחד. השתכל אתה ותמצא סמנים רבים במדרגה אחת בעינה מן החום
והיובש דרך משל ולכל סם מהם פעולות שאינם לסם האחר. זה כלו הוציאו הנסיון באורך
הזמנים.

[28] ולעוצם מעלת מדות אבקראט צוה בזה הפרק אשר פתח בו שלא יתקצר הרופא 15
בעשותו מה שראוי לבד ויספיק זה לו כי זה בלתי מספיק בהגעת הבריאות לחולה. ואמנם
ישלם התכלית וירפא כשיהיה החולה וכל מי שיעמדו לפניו עושה מה שראוי לעשותו ויסלק
המעיקים כלם אשר מחוץ המונעים בריאות החולה. כאילו הוא יצוה בזה השער שיהיה לרופא
יכלת על הנהגת החולים ויקל מעשה הרפואות עליהם כשתית הסמנים המרים והקלוחים
והחתוך והכויה והדומה להם ושיזהיר החולה ומי שיעמוד לפניו לשמרו שלא יחטא בעצמו 20
וישים העומדים לפניו יבינו בהנהגתו לעשות כמו שהוא ראוי בעת שלא יהיה שם רופא. וכן
יסיר המעיקים אשר מחוץ בכל יכלתו לפי איש איש שיקרהו ואם היה החולה עני והוא במקום
יוסיף חליו ואין לו מקום אחר יעתיקהו הוא ממקום למקום וכן יכין לו המזון והרפואה כאשר
לא יהיה זה אצלו. הנה אלו ודומה להם הם הדברים שהם מחוץ ממה שיתחייב הרופא מצד
מלאכתו כי אמנם הם הכרחיות בהגעת התכלית אשר יתחור הרופא הגעתה לחולה הזה. 25
אבל שיאמר לבד מה שראוי שיעשה וילך לא יעשה זה כי פעמים זה לא יגיע מזה התכלית
המכוון.

1 בנסיון: وكذلك معظم الأدوية ما علمت أفعالها إلّا بالتجربة add. a   3 סמנים: סמים א   4 כרוב:
ברוב בדחה ‖ הסמנים: הסמים א ‖ יתואר: יתבאר א   5 סמנים: סמים א ‖ צורתם: המינית add. ד
6 כסמנים: כסמים א   7 החימום והקירור: inv. ד ‖ מהירות: نزارة a   8 מצוא: מציאות אה
10 סמנים: סמים א ‖ וסמנים: וסמים א ‖ וסמנים: וסמים א ‖ וסמנים: וסמים א   11 וסמנים: וסמים
א ‖ הסמנים: הסמים א   12 סמנים: סמים א ‖ בעינה: בעצמה ד   16 ויספיק זה לו: ويكفّ a
17 וירפא: om. א וירפא החולה א¹   18 מחוץ: בחוץ א ‖ החולה: المرض a   19 הרפאות: הרפואה
אהח ‖ הסמנים: הסמים א   20 לשמרו: ويحذّره a   21 וישמרהו בח ‖ יבינו בהנהגתו לעשות: יכונו
בהנהגתו לעשות א يقومون بتدبيره a   22 שיקרהו: مثاله a   23 חליו: בחליו אבחה   24 הרופא:
לרופא אבח

(1.2)

[29] אמר אבקראט: אם היה מה שיורק מן הגוף בעת הגרת הבטן והקיא אשר יהיו ברצון
מן המין אשר ראוי שינקה ממנו הגוף יועיל זה ויהיה נקל לסבלו ואם לא יהיה כן יהיה הדבר
בהפך. וכן הרקת העורקים הנה אם הורקו מן המין אשר ראוי שיריקו ממנו יועיל זה ויהיה
נקל לסבלו ואם לא יהיה כן יהיה העניין בהפך. וראוי גם כן שיעיין בזמן העומד מזמני השנה
ובארצות ובשנים ובחוליים אם יחייבו ההרקה אשר חשבת להריק אותם אם לא.

אמר המפרש: אמרו וכן הרקת העורקים רוצה לומר הגרת השתן והזיעה ודם הנחירים ופתיחת
פיות העורקים ויהיה זה הפרק כלו במה שיבא ברצון. אמנם ג'אלינוס אמר: רצה בהרקת
העורקים הנקוי אשר יהיה ברפואה ולכן יהיה הפרק האחרון מן המאמר הזה אצלו כפול עד
שהוצרך אליו בו סברות. ואחר כן זכר שאם חשבת בהרקת המין אשר ראוי כאשר התבארו
לך אותות התגבורת שלו הנה ראוי גם כן שתשים לזמני השנה והארץ והשנים וטבע החולי
חלק ותנהיג העניין לפיהו כי הרקת האדומה בסתיו או במקומות הקרים או בשני הזקנה או
בחוליים הקרים יקשה ולא יוכל לסבלו. וכן הרקת הליחה הלבנה בקיץ או במקומות חמים או
בבחורים או בחוליים החמים יקשה ולא יסבל.

(1.3)

[30] אמר אבקראט: שומן הגוף המופלג לבעלי העמל סכנה כאשר הגיעו ממנה בתכלית
האחרון וזה כי בלתי אפשר שיתקיימו על עניינם זה ולא יתישבו. ואחר שהוא נמנע מהם שלא
יתישבו ואי אפשר שיוסיפו טוב הנה נשאר שיטו אל ענין יותר רע. ולכן ראוי שיחסרו שומן
הגוף בלא אחור כדי שישוב הגוף ויתחיל לקבל המזון ולא יפליג בהרקתו התכלית האחרון
כי זה סכנה אבל בשעור מה שיסבול טבע הגוף אשר יכונו להריקו. וכן גם כן כל הרקה
יפליג בה התכלית האחרון הנה הוא סכנה וכל הזנה גם כן שתהיה בתכלית האחרון היא
סכנה.

אמר המפרש: רוצה בבעלי העמל עובדי האדמה והדומים להם מאשר לקחו העמל הקשה
לאומנות וזה כי העורקים שלהם כאשר ימלאו יותר ממה שראוי לא יהיה בטוח שלא יבקעו
או יחנק החום הטבעי בהם ויכבה וימות כי הנה הוא צריך שיהיה בעורקים שלהם רקות לקבל
מה שיגיע אליהם מן המזון.

(1.4)

[31] אמר אבקראט: ההנהגה המופלגת בדקות בכל החוליים הנושנים בלא ספק סכנה
ובחוליים החדים כאשר לא יסבלו אותה וההנהגה אשר יפליגו בה התכלית האחרון מן הדקות
הנה הוא קשה רע בלא ספק.

---

1 היה: א‎² ‖ שיורק: שינקה בח שיריק ב‎² ‖ והקיא: הקיא א או הקיא א‎²   3 שיריקו: שיורקו אב
10 כן: ד om.   15 יתישבו: יתהפכו בדח   15–16 ואחר שהוא נמנע מהם שלא יתישבו: ولا كانوا لا
يستقرّون a   16 יתישבו: יתהפכו בדח יתהפכו יתישבו ח ‖ שיטו אל: שינטו על ד שינטו עליו אל בח
שינטו אל ח   21 עובדי האדמה: المصارعين a   22 שלהם: שלו בדחה

אמר המפרש: ההנהגה אשר בתכלית האחרון מן הדקות הוא עזיבת לקיחת המאכל לגמרי.
וההנהגה אשר היא בתכלית הדקות אבל לא בתכלית האחרון היא לקיחת מי הדבש והדומה
לו. וההנהגה הדקה אשר אינה בתכלית היא מי גריס השעור והדומה לו.

(1.5)

[32] אמר אבקראט: בהנהגה הדקה פעמים יפשעו בה החולים בעצמם פשיעה ירבה הזקה
עליהם וזה כי כל מה שיהיה ממנה יהיה הזקה יותר גדול ממה שיהיה מן המזון אשר יהיה לו   5
עובי מעט ומפני זה היתה ההנהגה המופלגת בדקות בבריאים גם כן סכנה אבל כי סבלם למה
שיקרה מטעותם יותר. ולכן היתה ההנהגה המופלגת בדקות ברוב העינים יותר גדולת הסכנה
מן ההנהגה אשר היא יותר עבה מעט.

אמר המפרש: זה מבואר ונגלה.

(1.6)

[33] אמר אבקראט: היותר טובה שבהנהגות בחליים אשר בתכלית האחרון היא ההנהגה   10
אשר בתכלית האחרון.

אמר המפרש: החליים אשר בתכלית האחרון הם החליים החדים מאד.

(1.7)

[34] אמר אבקראט: וכאשר היה החולי חד מאד הנה הכאבים אשר בתכלית האחרון יבואו
בו בתחילה וראוי בהכרח שתעשה בו ההנהגה אשר בתכלית האחרון מן הדקות. וכאשר לא
יהיה כן אבל יהיה סובל מן ההנהגה מה שהוא יותר עב מזה הנה ראוי שתהיה הירידה לפי   15
רפיון החולי וחסרונו מן התכלית האחרון.

אמר המפרש: הכאבים אשר יהיו בתכלית האחרון הם הכאבים הגדולים ר״ל עונות הקדחת
וכל המקרים והוא תכלית החולי כי אין התכלית דבר זולת היותר גדול מחלקי החולי במקריו
והבין מאמרו בתחילה הארבעה ימים הראשונים או אחריהם מעט.

2 לא: שהיא אינה ב היא שאינה ח   3 הדקה: ד²   4 בעצמם: כי לרוב דקותה יתאוו ויאכלו דברים
רעים וגסים מאד בח .add   5-4 פשיעה ירבה הזקה עליהם וזה כי כל מה שיהיה ממנה יהיה הזקה יותר
גדול: ד [...] .om ד¹   5 וזה כי כל מה שיהיה ממנה יהיה הזקה יותר גדול ממה שיהיה מן המזון: وذلك
أنّ جميع ما يكون منه أعظم ممّا يكون منه في الغذاء a   وذلك أنّ جميع ما يكون منه من الخطاء أعظم ضررا
منه ممّا يكون منه في الغذاء t ‖ שיהיה ממנה יהיה: א .om   שיהיה ממנה יותר מן הראוי א²   6 ההנהגה
המופלגת אפי׳ בבריאים מזקת ג״כ אלא שהם יסבלו הזקה יותר ולכן היתה ההנהגה א² .add   7 יותר:
في التدبير الغليظ أقلّ a   10 בחליים: לחליים א א   15 יותר: א .om

(1.8)

[35] אמר אבקראט: כאשר יגיע החולי אל תכליתו אז ראוי בהכרח שתעשה ההנהגה אשר היא בתכלית האחרון מן הדקות.

אמר המפרש: וזה לעוצם המקרים בעת ההיא ובעבור שיתבשל החולי וזה כי אין ראוי שתטריד הטבע בבשול מזון חדש תכניסהו עליו מבשול הליחות המולידות החולי כי היה בעת ההיא משתדל עליהם בכחותיו כלם ואמנם נשאר לו המעט עד שישלם בתגבורת עליהם.

5

(1.9)

[36] אמר אבקראט: ראוי גם כן שתשקול כח החולה ותדע אם יהיה עד עת תכלית החולי ותעיין אם כח החולה יחלש קודם תגבורת החולי ולא תשאר על המזון ההוא או החולי יחלש קודם ותנוח שנאתו.

אמר המפרש: זה מבואר.

10

(1.10)

[37] אמר אבקראט: ואשר יבוא תכלית חליים בתחילה הנה ראוי שיתנהגו בהנהגה הדקה בתחילה ואשר שיתאחר תכלית חליים הנה ראוי שיושם הנהגתם בתחלת חליים יותר עבה ואחר כן יחסר מעביה מעט מעט על מה שיתקרב מתכלית החולי ובעת תכליתו בשיעור מה שישאר כח החולה בו. וראוי שימנע מן המזון בעת תכלית החולי כי התוספת בו יזיק.

אמר המפרש: זה מבואר.

15

(1.11)

[38] אמר אבקראט: כשיהיו לקדחת סבובים היה מונע מן המזון גם כן בעתות עונותיהם.

אמר המפרש: זה מבואר.

(1.12)

[39] אמר אבקראט: הנה יורה על עונות החולי ומדרגתו החליים עצמם וזמני השנה ותוספת הסבובים קצתם על קצתם הן שיהיה עונתה בכל יום או יום ויום לא או ביותר מן הזמן הזה והדברים גם כן אשר יראו אחר זה. ודמיון זה מה שיראה בבעלי חולי הצד כי הוא אם יראה

20

---

1 אל תכליתו: לתכליתו א תכליתו בח   4 היה: הוא א   5 שישלם: שישתדל ד שישלם בתגבורת
עליהם: וישלם לנצח החולי א[2]   8 ולא תשאר על המזון ההוא (= ولا تبقى على ذلك الغذاء): ولا تبقى على ذلك الغذاء
ההוא): ولا تبقى على ذلك الغذاء   9 שנאתו: رعتم ח عادته a   14 בו: א[2] חח om. عليه a   18 עונות:
מדות א[2] ‖ add. ומדרגתו: ومرتبته ونظامه a   19 הן שיהיה עונתה: אם יהיה עונתו בחח   20 אחר זה:
אחריו א אחר בח ‖ בבעלי חולי הצד: בבעלי (נ״א בחולי) הצד ח

רקיקת הדם מתחיל מראשית החולי יהיה החולי קצר ואם תאחר הראותו יהיה החולי ארוך
והשתן והצואה והזיעה כאשר יראו הנה יורו אותנו על טוב נקיון החולי ורעתו ואורך החולי
וקצורו.

אמר המפרש: מטבע החולי עצמו תדע אם תכליתו ממהר או מתאחר כי חולי הצד וחולי
הריאה ומורסת הראש חליים חדים. והשקוי והוסואס ומוגלת הגוף והשדפון והוא נגע הריאה   5
הם חליים ארוכים ועונות הקדחת רוב מה שיהיו בחלי הצד ומורסת הראש יום ויום לא.
ורוב מה שיהיה במי שבו מורסא שיש בה מוגלא באצטומכתו או בכבדו או במי שבו
השדפון בכל יום עונות אילו יהיו בכל יום וכל שכן בלילה ורוב מה שיהיו עונות הקדחת
למי שחליו מהטחול שלו ובכלל מן המרה השחורה יום ושני ימים לא וכן עתות השנה כי
קדחת רביעית הקיצית קצרה ברוב העניינים והחרפית ארוכה וכל שכן כאשר תתחבר עם   10
הסתיו.

ותוספת העונות מורה על תוספת החולי וקרבת תכליתו ויודע תוספת העונה על העונה
הראשונה משלשה דברים. אחד מהם עת עונת הקדחת והאחרת אורך העונה והאחרת גדלה
ר"צ חזקתה.

(1.13)

[40] אמר אבקראט: הישישים יסבלו הצום יותר מכל האנשים ומאחריהם הזקנים והבחורים   15
סובלים יותר מעט והסובלים אותו יותר מעט מכל האנשים הנערים ומי שהיה מן הנערים יותר
חזק התאוה הנה הוא סובל אותו יותר מעט.

אמר המפרש: אשר זכר בזה השער כבר זכרו בשער אשר אחריו וזה כי כל מה שיהיה החום
הטבעי יותר יצטרך אל מזון יותר והנתך מגופות הנערים בעבור לחותם הוא יותר מזה אשר
זכר מסבול הישישים הצום זכר ג׳אלינוס שהוא הישיש שלא הגיע לגבול ההפסד והחולשה   20
אבל הישישים אשר בתכלית הישישות הנה לא יסבלו המתון מן האכילה אבל יצטרכו שיקחו
אותו מעט מעט פעם אחר פעם לקרבת חמימותם מן הכבוי ויצטרכו אל התמדת מה שימשכה
מעט אחר מעט.

(1.14)

[41] אמר אבקראט: מה שהיה מן הגופות בגדול הנה החום הטבעי בו בתכלית מה שיהיה
מן הרבוי ויצטרך בעבור זה מן המזון ליותר ממה שיצטרך אליו שאר הגופים שאם לא   25
יאכל מן המזון מה שיצטרך אליו ישתדף גופו ויחסר. ואולם הישישים הנה החום הטבעי

---

1 רקיקת הדם: הרקיקה (נ"א רקיקת הדם) ה ‖ מראשית החולי: ואם תמהר הראותה א² .add
5 חדים: والذبحة والهيضة والتشنّج أمراض حادّة جدّا .add a ‖ והוסואס: .om א. والهسعان ממרה שחורה ה
7 באצטומכתו: באצטומכא א   13 עת עונת הקדחת: מהירות עונת הקדחת בה מהירות עונות הקדחת
ה   16 והסובלים אותו יותר מעט: .om א   18 כבר זכרו: قد ذكر علّه a ‖ אשר: שהוא א   20 ההפסד
והחולשה: الهرم a   25 המזון: الوقود a ‖ שאר הגופים: שאר האישים א הישיש בהה من الغذاء .add a

בהם מעט ומפני זה לא יצטרכו מן המזון כי אם מעט כי חמימותם תכבה מן הרב ומפני זה
גם כן לא יהיה הקדחת בישישים חדה כמו שתהיה באשר הם בגדול וזה בעבור כי גופותם
קרים.

אמר המפרש: אמר ג'אלינוס: העצם אשר בו החום בנערים שעורו יותר והוא הענין אשר יאמר
ממנו ג'אלינוס תמיד כי החום יותר נוסף בכמות כמו שבאר בספר המזג.

(1.15)

[42] אמר אבקראט: הגופות בסתיו ובאביב הם יותר חמים שיהיו בטבע והשינה יותר ארוכה
שתהיה וראוי בשני אילו הזמנים שיהיה מה שיאכל מן המזון יותר וזה כי החום הטבעי
בגופות בשני אלו העיתים הרבה ולכן יצטרך אל מזון יותר והראיה על זה ענין הנערים ועובדי
האדמה.

אמר המפרש: אמר ג'אלינוס: וזה כי הנערים בעבור שיהיה החום הטבעי בהם יותר הוצרכו מן
המזון אל מה שהוא יותר ועובדי האדמה גם כן בעבור שחמימותם הטבעית תגדל ברוב עמלם
הם יכולים שיאכלו שעור רב מן המזון.

(1.16)

[43] אמר אבקראט: המזונות הלחים יאותו לכל המחוממים כל שכן הנערים ומי שכבר הרגיל
שיאכל המזונות הלחים.

אמר המפרש: זה מבואר והוא משל ימצא בו הדרך הכולל והוא כי כל חולי יתנגד בהפכו.

(1.17)

[44] אמר אבקראט: ראוי שינתן לקצת החולים מזונם בפעם אחת ולקצתם בשתי פעמים
וישים מה שיתן לו ממנו יותר או פחות וקצתם מעט מעט וראוי גם כן שינתן לעת העומד מזמני
השנה חלקו מזה ולמנהג ולשנים.

אמר המפרש: בעבור שנתן הדרך בכמות המזון תחלה ואחר כן באיכותו לקח לתת בכאן
הדרך בצורת אכילתו והשרש בזה בחינת כח החולה ובחינת החולי ויתן גם כן לשנים והמנהג
ומזג האויר חלקו וזה כי הכח החזק יחייב שיקח המזון בפעם אחת והתלוש יחייב שיקחהו
מעט מעט וחסרון הגוף ורזותו יחייב שינתן לו מזון רב ומלואו יחייב המעיט המזון. ויתחייב

---

1 מן: המזון **א** ‎.add‏ **²א**   2 בישישים: בישישות **בדהח** ‖ חדה: חמה **בדהח**   4 שעורו: ושעורו **דה**
7 וראוי: ולכן ראוי **²א**   9-8 ועובדי האדמה: والصريعين a   10 המפרש: ودليل على ذلك أمر الأسنان
والصريعين a ‎.add‏   11 ועובדי האדמה: والصريعين a   13 הנערים (BE =): وغيرهم a ‎.add‏   14 הלחים:
גם כן יקיים הדרך הכולל והוא הדומה מבריא **ח** ‎.add‏   15 ימצא בו: يُؤخَذ منه a ‖ בהפכו: ויש
שכבר הרגיל המזונות הלחים גם כן יקיים הדרך הכולל והוא הדומה בדומה אל בריא **א** ‎.add‏   16 לקצת:
מקצת **א**   22 יחייב: יחשב **א** ‖ המעיט המזון: במיעוט מן המזון **ד**

מזה שאם יהיה הכח חלוש והגוף בענין החסרון שינתן לו מאכל מעט פעמים רבים ואם היה
הכח חלוש והגוף אינו בענין החסרון הנה ראוי שינתן לו מאכל מעט פעמים מעטים וכן כאשר
היה הכח חזק והליחות רבות. אמנם כאשר היה הכח חזק והגוף בענין חסרון או ענין הפסד
ליחות הנה ראוי שיאכל החולה מאכל רב פעמים רבות כי ענין גופו צריך אל מאכל רב וכחו
5   חזק יכול לבשלו ואם יעיקוהו עונות הקדחת ולא ימצא עתים רבים למזון תן אותו בפעמים
מעטים.

הנה כן לקיחת הראיה לפי הכח והחולי. ואנמם הזמן והשנים והמנהג ומה שילך בדרכיהם
הנה הוא בזה המשל: הקיץ יחייב ברבוי הפעמים ומעוט מה שיאכל בכל פעם והסתיו
יחייב ברבוי המאכל ומיעוט הפעמים ואולם אמצע האביב וכאשר קרב מן הקיץ הנה
10   ראוי שיזונו במזון מעט במה שבין עתים ארוכים כי הזמן הזה אפשר שיהיו הגופות
מלאים כי הליחות אשר היו קפואים בסתו יזובו ויותכו. ואולם החורף מי שיתחמם בו
יצטרך אל תוספת משבעת המזון טוב להפסד הליחות בזמן ההוא וענין השנים ומנהגים
מבואר.

(1.18)

[45] אמר אבקראט: יותר קשה שיהיה סבל המאכל על הגופות הוא בקיץ ובחורף ויותר קל
15   שיהיה סבלו עליהם בסתו ואחריו באביב.

אמר המפרש: אמר ג׳אלינוס: דבריו בזה הפרק בחולים ודבריו הקודמים בבריאים.

(1.19)

[46] אמר אבקראט: כאשר יהיו עונות הקדחת דבקות בסבוביהם אין ראוי שינתן לחולה דבר
בעתותיהם או שיצריכוהו אל דבר אבל ראוי שיחוסר מן התוספת מפני עתות ההפרש.

אמר המפרש: אמר ג׳אלינוס: רצה באמרו מפני עתות ההפרש מפני עתות העונות וכאשר
20   יהיה העת הזה ראוי בו לחסר בו התמרים כדי שלא תגדל הקדחת חלילה לך שתוסיף בה
כלום בהזנה.

(1.20)

[47] אמר אבקראט: הגופות אשר יבא אליהם או שכבר בא להם הנקיון על השלמות אין
ראוי שיוענו ולא שיחודש בהם חדוש לא ברפואה משלשלת ולא בזולתה מן התנועות אבל
יונחו.

---

2 הכח: א || om. א ‖ הנה ראוי: א om.   5 לבשלו: בבשולו א   9–8 הפעמים ומעוט מה שיאכל בכל פעם
והסתיו יחייב ברבוי: אה om.   12 משבעת: سابغة a   18 שיצריכוהו: שיצריכהו אה ‖ מפני: מקודם
בה נ״א קודם א² (قبل =) من قبل a   19 מפני: קודם בהה נ״א קודם א² ‖ מפני: אבה om. קודם א²בהה
332.1–22 יבא ... אמרו: א¹

אמר המפרש: אמרו יבא אליהם ר״ל שהוכנו סיבותיו ונראו אותותיו והוא מזומן שיהיה ואמרו
ולא בזולתה מן התנועות כמו הרחיצה וההזעה והגרת השתן או דם הנדות והחפיפה. והתנה
שיהיה הנקיון שלם אבל הנקיון החסר הנה ראוי שישלימו חסרונו ויוציא מה שנשאר מן הליחה
המחליאה באופן היותר נקל בו. ואמר ג׳אלינוס כי הנקיון השלם הוא מה שקבץ ששה דברים:
הראשון שקדמו בישול. השני שיהיה ביום מימי הנקיון. השלישי שיהיה בהרקת דבר מבואר
יצא מן הגוף לא במורסא. הרביעי שיהיה הדבר המורק הוא הדבר המזיק לבד אשר היה סבת
החולי. החמישי שיהיה הרקתו על יושר מן הצד אשר בו החולי. הששי שיהיה עם מנוחה וקלות
מן הגוף.

אמר ג׳אלינוס: וכאשר חסר אחד מהם או יותר מאחד אין הנקיון טוב ולא שלם.

אמר המפרש: ראוי לך שתשאל בכאן ותאמר איך תתנקה הליחה המחליאה בעצמה אחר
הבשול ביום הנקיון ועל יושר ולא יבא אחריו הקלות והמנוחה מתנה כי ג׳אלינוס מתנה תנאי ששי
והוא שיהיה עם קלות ומנוחה והוא ראיה כי פעמים יגיעו התנאים החמשה ולא תהיה מנוחה
ותשובת זה כי הוא איפשר זה כאשר הפליג הנקוי ואע״פ שהוא מן המין שראוי יציאתו עם
שאר התנאים כי כאשר הפליג לא יבא אחריו קלות ולא יהיה עמו מנוחה אבל חולשה ורפיון
מן הגוף ואפשר שיגיעהו עלוף חזק ודע זה.

(1.21)

[48] אמר אבקראט: הדברים אשר ראוי שינקו ראוי שינקו מן המקומות אשר הם אליהם יותר
נוטים באיברים אשר הם טובים לנקוים.

אמר המפרש: אמר ג׳אלינוס: הדברים אשר ראוי שיונקו הם הליחות המולידות החליים אשר
בא בהם הנקיון בלתי שלם והמקומות אשר הם טובים לנקוי הם הבני מעים והאצטומכא
והמקוה והרחם והעור ועם זה גם כן החך והנחירים כאשר רצינו נקוי המוח וראוי לרופא
שישתכל ויזכור בידיעת נטיית הטבע ואם מצא נטייתה אל צד יאות לנקוי אשר ינקה אותו יכין
לטבע מה שיצטרך לנקוי ויעזור הטבע ואם ראה העין בהפך זה וראה תנועתו תנועה מזקת
ימנע אותה ויעתיקה וימשכה אל הפך הצד אשר נטתה אליו. ואמשיל לך בזה משל כאשר
היה בכבד ליחות חולי הנה הנה הצדדים אשר הם טובים שינטו אליהם שני צדדים:
אחד צד האצטום׳ וכאשר תהיה הנטייה לצד ההוא הנה הנה ההרקה בשלשול יותר טוב משיהיה
בקיא והצד האחר צד הכליות והמקוה ואולם נטיית הליחות ההם אל צד החזה והריאה והלב
אינו טוב.

1 שהוכנו: שהוכרו אב שיוכרו ח   2 התנועות: الشِيِّ a || הרחיצה (= التنقية): التنقية a || וההזעה:
והזעה א   3 שלם אבל הנקיון: א²   13 הנקוי: הנקיון א   16 שינקו: שיורקו א שנקו ח || שינקו:
שיורקו א   18 שינקו: שיורקו א   19–18 אשר בא בהם: אשר כבר בא להם אח   19 שלם: והאיברים
(נ״א והאיברים שראוי שיורקו מהם) ח .add והאיברים שראוי שיורקו מהם א   21 שישתכל ויזכור:
أن يتفقّده a   25 משיהיה: ממה שיהיה א

(1.22)

[49] אמר אבקראט: אמנם ראוי לך שתעשה הרפואה וההנעה אחר שיתבשל החולי אבל כל
זמן שהוא נא ובתחלת החולי אין ראוי זה אם לא שיהיה החולי מסתער ואי אפשר ברוב הענין
שיהיה החולי מסתער.

אמר המפרש: אמרו הרפואה רוצה בו המשלשל והחולי המסתער הוא אשר יהיו הליחות
מסערות החולה הוסיפו אותו בחום יהיה להם והגרה מאבר אל אבר בתחלת החולי ויצערוהו   5
ויחדשו לו סערה ולא יניחו לו לשקוט אבל יתנועעו ויגרו מאבר אל אבר וזה המעט שיהיה.
ואולם ברוב הענין הנה יהיו הליחות נחות קיימות באבר אחד ובאבר ההוא יהיה בשלום במדת
זמן החולי כולו עד שיחסר.

(1.23)

[50] אמר אבקראט: אין ראוי שתקח ראיה על השעור אשר ראוי שיורק מן הגוף מרביו אבל
ראוי שנתמיד ההרקה כל זמן שהדבר אשר ראוי שיורק הוא אשר יצא והחולה סובל אותו   10
במהירות וקלות ובעת שתהיה ראויה תהיה ההרקה עד שיקרה העלוף ואמנם ראוי שיעשה
זה כאשר יהיה החולה סובל אותו.

אמר המפרש: אמר ג'אלינוס: אם היה הדבר הגובר הוא אשר הורק הנה גוף החולה יקל
בהכרח ממה שהיה ואם הורק עם הדבר היוצא מהטבע דבר טבעי הנה החולה ירפה
בהכרח ויחלש כחו ויחוש בכבדות וצער וראוי שתהיה ההרקה עד גבול שיתחדש ממנה   15
העלוף במורסות החמות אשר הם בתכלית הגודל ובקדחות השורפות מאד ובכאבים החזקים
המופלגים ויכניס עצמו על זה השעור מן ההרקה כאשר היה הכח חזק. וכבר נסינו זה פעמים
רבות לא ימנו ומצאנו אותו מועיל תועלת חזקה ולא נודע בכאבים החזקים המופלגים רפואה
יותר חזקה ויותר מופלגת מן ההרקה עד שיקרה העילוף אחר שישמור וידע אם ראוי שיוקז
עורק או יעשה השלשול עד שיקרה העלוף.   20

(1.24)

[51] אמר אבקראט: פעמים יצטרך בחליים החדים דרך זרות לעשות הרפואה המשלשלת
בתחלתם וראוי שיעשה זה אחר שיקדים זה וינהיג הענין כפי מה שראוי.

אמר המפרש: באר לנו שלא נתיר השלשול בהתחלות החליים כי אם בקצת החליים החדים
והם המסתערים כמו שנזכר לפנים ועם כל זה ראוי שיעשה זה בשמירה ובעיון גדול מהכנות
הגוף כל מה שיוכל ואחר ידיעת דקות הליחות.   25

---

1 הרפואה: הרפואות נ״א המשלשלת ח ‖ וההנעה: והתנועה ד והנגעה א וההנהגה בח
2 מסתער: מתעורר א נ״א מסתער א‎¹   5 הוסיפו אותו בחום יהיה להם: הזיקו אותו בחום יהיה להם
בח وآذّه بحرارة تكون لها قوّية a ‖ והגרה: והגרת א הליחות א‎² add.   6–5 ויצערוהו ויחדשו: ויסערוהו
ויחדש ד   6 לשקוט: לנוח בח   10 שנתמיד: أن يستغْم a   11 במהירות וקלות: בנחת במהירות
וקלות ד بسهولة وخفّة a ‖ שתהיה: ההרקה ד add.   22 בתחלתם: בהתחולתם ד   23 ראוי: באר
ד ‖ החליים: מהחליים ד   24 מהכנות: מהכרות א‎¹ מהכרות א מהכנת ח מהכרת בח

אמר ג׳אלינוס: הסכנה בעשיית הרפואה המשלשלת על זולת מה שראוי בחליים החדים גדולה
כי הרפואות המשלשלות כלם חמות יבשות והקדחת מצד מה שהיא קדחת לא תצטרך אל מה
שיחמם וינגב אבל היא צריכה אל הפך זה ר״ל מה שיקרר וילחלח. אמנם נעשה אותם בעבור
הליחה הפועלת אותה וראוי שיהיה התועלת בהרקת הליחה אשר התחדש החולי ממנה יותר
מן הנזק אשר ישיגו הגופות בעניין ההוא בסבת הרפואות המשלשלות ואמנם יהיה התועלת
יותר כאשר הורקה הליחה המזקת כלה בלא נזק והנה ראוי שיעיין תחלה אם גוף החולה מזומן
ומוכן לזה השלשול כי האנשים אשר יהיה תחלת חליים מהפסד בשול מאכלו באצטומכא
הפסד גדול או ממאכלים דבקים עבים ואשר בהם במה שלמטה מן החלצים משיכה או נפח
או חום חזק מופלג או שם בקצת הבני מעיים מורסא אין גוף אחד מהם מוכן לשלשול. וראוי
שלא יהיה דבר מזה נמצא ושיהיו הליחות בגוף החולה על יותר טוב שאפשר שיהיה מקלות
הגרמתם ר״ל שיהיו דקות ולא יהיה בהם כלום מן הדבקות ושיהיו המעברים אשר יהיה מעבר
מה שיצא בשלשול בהם רחבים פתוחים אין בהם כלום מן הסתום. הנה נעשה אנחנו אלו
הדברים ויקדם ויוכן הגוף בזה העניין כאשר רצינו שנשלשל אותו.

(1.25)

[52] אמר אבקראט: אם הורק הגוף מן המין אשר ראוי שינוקה ממנו יועיל זה ויסבל בקלות
ואם היה העניין הפך זה היה קשה.

אמר המפרש: זה הפרק אצלי אינו כפל למה שכולל אותו הפרק השני כי הפרק ההוא היה
במה שירוק מאליו וזה הפרק במה שנריקהו אנחנו ברפואות ובעבור ששם גאלינוס הפרק
השני כולל לשני העניינים יחד השתדל לתת סבה בכפל הפרק הזה.

נשלם המאמר הראשון ולנותן השכל תהלה ללא תכלה.

3 וילחלח: ויתלחלח ד 6 המזקת: א¹ ‖ והנה: והוא א 8 גדול (= كبيرة): كثيرة a 9 הבני מעיים:
בני המעים א בני מעים אׁחׁ 11 שיהיו: שיהיה ד ‖ כלום: כלל ד ‖ הדבקות: من النوع الذي ينبغي أن يبقى
منه نفع ذلك واحتمل بسهولة فإن كانت الأمر على ضدّ ذلك add. a ‖ המעברים: פתוחים א¹ add. ‖ מעבר:
המעבר א² 17 במה: ד .om 19 ולנותן השכל תהלה ללא תכלה: ד .om ונתחיל א

המאמר השני מפרקי אבקראט

(2.1)

[53] אמר אבקראט: כאשר היתה השינה בחולי מן החליים מחדשת כאב הנה זה ממופתי
המות וכאשר היתה השינה מועילה אין זה ממופתי המות.

אמר המפרש: רוצה באמרו כאב נזק כי יש חליים ועתים מן החולי תזיק בהם השינה ולכן
ראוי שיצוה החולה בהם ביקיצה ואם ישן אז ינזק. ויש עתים תועיל בהם השינה ואם ישן   5
בהם החולה והתחדש לו הנזק הנה הוא סימן המות כי כאשר קוינו התועלת בא לו הנזק וזה
אמנם יהיה כאשר יהיו ליחות הגוף רעות מאד או מנצחות החום הטבעי. ואמנם החליים אשר
תזיק בהם השינה תמיד הוא בהתחלת המורסות באיברים הפנימיים או עם הגרת הליחות
אל האצטומכא או בהתחלת עונת הקדחת. וכל שכן כאשר היה עמה קור ופלצות והעתים
אשר תועיל בהם השינה הוא אחר הכלות התחלת העונה או המורסא וכל שכן בעת התכלית   10
והיותר מועילה שתהיה השינה עת היירידה ואם תזיק בעת הזה הוא אות המות ואם תועיל לפי
מה שכבר נודע מתועלת השינה בעת הזאת הנה לא יוסיף לנו בראיה כלום.

(2.2)

[54] אמר אבקראט: כאשר הניחה השינה ערבוב השכל הנה הוא סימן טוב.

אמר המפרש: זה יורה שהחום הטבעי גבר על הליחות ונצחם.

(2.3)

[55] אמר אבקראט: השינה והיקיצה כאשר עבר כל אחד מהם השעור המכוון הוא סימן רע.   15

אמר המפרש: זה מבואר.

(2.4)

[56] אמר אבקראט: לא השבע ולא הרעב ולא זולתם מכל הדברים טובים כאשר יעברו
השעורים הטבעיים.

אמר המפרש: זה מבואר.

(2.5)

[57] אמר אבקראט: היגיעה אשר לא נודע אליה סבה מורה בחולי.   20

---

4 יש: שם א ‖ מן החולי: א² 5-4 ולכן ראוי: וראוי ד 5 החולה: אח om. החולה: אח 6 הנזק: כאב אח
10 תועיל בהם: ד inv. ‖ הכלות: הפנות א הכנות ח 11 תועיל: הועילה א מועילה בח מועילה: הועילה א 12 לנו: ד
om. ‖ בראיה: בראה א בהוראה א² 13 הוא: זה א 15 והיקיצה: והתעורה א add.

COMMENTARY ON HIPPOCRATES' APHORISMS

אמר המפרש: זה יורה שהשליחות כבר התנועעו על זולת דרכם הטבעי ולכן נכאבו מהם האיברים או מרוע איכותם או מרבוי כמותם ולכן יורו בחולי.

(2.6)

[58] אמר אבקראט: מי שיכאב דבר מגופו ולא ירגיש בכאבו ברוב עניניו שכלו מעורבב.

אמר המפרש: רוצה בכאב בכאן סבת הכאב כמו שיהיה בחולה מורסא חמה או חומרא והנגע והרסוק והכתישה ומה שדומה לזה והיה בלתי מרגיש בו שכלו מעורבב.

(2.7)

[59] אמר אבקראט: הגופות אשר ירזו בזמן ארוך הנה ראוי שיהיה השבתם במזון אל השומן במתון והגופות אשר נכחשו במעט זמן יהיה השבתם במהירות.

אמר המפרש: וזה כי הגופות אשר ירזו בזמן מועט אמנם התחדש להם הרזון ההוא והכחש מהרקת הלחויות לא מהתכת האיברים הקפואים ואולם הגופות אשר רזו וכחשו בזמן ארוך הנה כבר נתך מהם הבשר והודק וחלשו מהם שאר האיברים אשר בהם יהיה הבשול והתפזר המזון בגוף והולדת הדם ולא יוכלו שיבשלו מן המזון השעור אשר יצטרך אליו הגוף ולכן ראוי שיושב אל השומן בזמן ארוך.

(2.8)

[60] אמר אבקראט: הקם מן החולי כאשר יקח מן המזון ולא יתחזק הנה זה יורה שהוא אוכל ממנו יותר ממה שיסבול ואם היה זה והוא לא יקח מן המזון יותר מדי סבלו הורה שגופו צריך אל הנקוי.

אמר המפרש: באר הסבה בפרק אשר הודיענו בו כי הגוף שהוא נקי בלתי מה שתזונהו תוסיף בו רעה.

(2.9)

[61] אמר אבקראט: כל גוף שתרצה לנקותו הנה ראוי שתשים מה שתרצה להוציאו ממנו יעבור בו בקלות.

אמר המפרש: יהיה זה בשירחיב ויפתח מעבריו ויחתוך וידק ויזיב הלחויות אשר בו אם היה להם כלום מן העובי והדבקות.

---

1 הטבעי: הנודע ה   3 עניניו: ענינו אבח ב   4 בכאב בכאן: א inv.   .om ב   5 בו: ד   6 במזון: ד
.om   7 במעט זמן: בזמן מועט א   9 הלחויות: הליחות א   10 והודק (= ودق): ודقّ a (= והודקו)
11 יוכלו: יוכל אבחח   20 וידק: .om א   וידקדק א¹

(2.10)

[62] אמר אבקראט: הגוף אשר איננו נקי כל מה שתזונהו תוסיף בו רעה.

אמר המפרש: סבת זה מבוארת ורוב מה שיהיה זה כאשר היתה האצטומכא מלאה מליחות רעות ואז יקרה מהם מה שזכר אבקראט שיקרה לקם מחולי והוא שלא יוכל שיקח מן המזון יותר מדי סבלו.

(2.11)

[63] אמר אבקראט: בשימלא הגוף מן המשקה יותר נקל משימלא מן המאכל. 5

אמר המפרש: רצה במשקה הדברים הלחים והמשקים אשר לגופותינו בהם מזון וזה כי המזון הלח וכל שכן כאשר היה בטבעו חם יותר קל ויותר מהיר להיות מזון לגוף.

(2.12)

[64] אמר אבקראט: השאריות אשר ישארו מן החליים אחר הנקיון ממנהג שיסבבו חזרת החולי.

אמר המפרש: ברוב החליים יתעפשו השאריות ההם באורך הימים והולידו קדחת כי כל לחות 10 נכרי מטבע הגשם אשר יקפהו הנה הוא בלתי אפשר שיזון אותו ולא יסור ענינם כי אם אל העפוש ברוב וכאשר היה עם זה המקום אשר הם מקובצות בו חם יהיה שובם אל העפוש יותר מהיר שאפשר להיות ויותר חזק.

(2.13)

[65] אמר אבקראט: מי שיבא לו הנקיון הנה יכבד עליו חליו בלילה אשר לפני עונת הקדחת אשר יבא בה הנקיון ובלילה אשר אחריו יהיה ברוב יותר קל. 15

אמר המפרש: בהבדל הטבע הדבר הרע מן הדבר הטוב ויכין לו הדחיה והיציאה יתחדש הסתערות. וראוי בהכרח בעת ההסתערות ההוא שיסתער החולה ויכבד עליו חליו וממנהג בני אדם שישנו בלילה וכאשר מגע ההסתערות ההוא מן השינה יתבאר סערת החולה וכבדות חליו ביאור נגלה. ופעמעם היה זה ביום זה כאשר היה הנקיון מוכן שיהיה בלילה אשר יבא אחריו ואמרו יהיה ברוב יותר קל כי רוב הנקיון יביא אל 20 השלום.

---

2 מליחות: ליחות א‎　3 שיקרה לקם מחולי: أنّه يعرض للثقه a‎　4 יותר מדי סבלו: בח‎ om.
5 בשימלא: שימלא אח מי שימלא בח‎　10 החליים: الأَمر a ‖ ההם: ד om. ‖ והולידו: וייולידו
אבח ‖ לחות: שהוא ד add.‎　19 היה זה ביום כאשר היה: יהיה זה ביום כאשר יהיה א‎　20 רוב:
ברוב ד

(2.14)

[66] אמר אבקראט: עם התרת הבטן פעמים יועיל בהתחלף מראות הצואה כשלא יהיה
השתנותו אל מינים רעים ממנו.

אמר המפרש: כי רבוי צבעיו יורה על הרקת מינים רבים מן הליחות. והמינים הרעים הוא שיהיה
בו דבר מאותות התכת הגוף והוא הצואה השמנה או מאותות העפוש והוא סרחון הריח.

(2.15)

[67] אמר אבקראט: כשיקרה כאב בגרון או יצא בגוף שחין או מורסות הנה ראוי שיראה
ויעיין למה שיצא מן הגוף כי אם היה הגובר עליו המרה האדומה הנה הגוף עם זה חולה ואם
היה מה שיצא מן הגוף כמו (מה) שיצא מן גוף הבריא תהיה בבטחון להקדים ולזון הגוף.

אמר המפרש: אמר גאלינוס: הגרון גם כן יקבל הליחות אשר ירדו מן המוח והשחין והמורסות
אמנם יהיו כשיתחמם הדם מפני המרה האדומה וראוי שתעיין ותראה אם השליך הטבע כל
המותרות אל אותם האיברים אשר נחלו וידע זה כשיהיה מה שיצא מן הגוף כמו מה שיצא מן
גוף הבריא ואין בהזנתו אז סכנה. ואם לא יהיה הגוף נקי מן הליחה לגמרי תמצא הגובר על
מה שיצא מן הגוף המרה האדומה וראוי אז שינוקה ויורק קודם שיזון אותו כי הגוף שאיננו נקי
כל מה שתזוננהו תוסיפהו רעה.

(2.16)

[68] אמר אבקראט: כשיהיה האדם רעב אין ראוי שייגע.

אמר המפרש: עם מעוט המזון ראוי להרחיק העמל וסבת זה מבוארת.

(2.17)

[69] אמר אבקראט: כאשר יכנס בגוף מזון יוצא מן הטבע מאד הנה זה יחדש חולי ויורה על
זה התרפאו.

אמר המפרש: נראה כי כונתו בפרק הזה שיספר כי כשיהיה המזון היורד יוצא מן הטבע יציאה
גדולה תהיה היציאה ההיא בכמות או באיכות הנה הוא יחדש חולי והגעת מה שיתחדש מן
החולי לפי שעור יציאתו אם יצא יציאה גדולה יחדש חולי גדול ואם היתה יציאתו המחליאה
יציאה קטנה יהיה החולי קטן אמר ויקח ראיה על שעור יציאתו במה שיראה מהתרפאו כי אם
היתה היציאה קטנה יתרפא מהר.

1 הצואה: היציאה ח ‖ כשלא: ושלא א   4 התכת: התרת ד   7 הגוף: החולה ד   add. ד   11 הגוף: א
²א הגוף: עن آخره a ‖ לגמרי: .om   12 המרה האדומה וראוי אז שינוקה ויורק קודם שיזון אותו כי הגוף: א
16 יוצא: חוץ א   add. 18 היורד: ورد على البدن a   ‖ יוצא: חוץ א   add. 19 חולי: א   add. 20 אם
יצא יציאה: ואם יציאה א

(2.18)

[70] אמר אבקראט: מה שיהיה מן הדברים זן מהר פתאום הנה יציאתו גם כן יהיה מהר.

אמר המפרש: היותר מפליג שבכל הדברים שיזון מהר פתאום היין וענין מהר אחר שיקח אותו בזמן מועט ואמרו פתאום שיהיה אחר לקיחתו משלים הגוף מזונו כלו ולא ימשכהו מעט מעט אלא בפעם אחת.

(2.19)

5 [71] אמר אבקראט: ההקדמה במשפט בחליים החדים הן למות הן לבריאות לא יהיה בתכלית הבטחון.

אמר המפרש: אמר ג׳אלינוס: הקדחת בחולי החד תהיה דבקה תמידית ברוב כי המעוט מן החליים החדים יהיו מבלתי קדחת כמו הפלג׳.

(2.20)

[72] אמר אבקראט: מי שהיה בטנו בבחרותו לח הנה הוא כאשר יהיה ישיש יבש בטנו ומי 10 שהיה בבחרותו יבש הנה כאשר יהיה ישיש יתלחלח בטנו.

אמר המפרש: כאשר בקשתי האמת מצאתי כי זה דבר בלתי נמצא והוא אם כן משפט כזב בלי ספק והאמת אצלי כי אבקראט ראה אדם אחד או שני אנשים אירע להם כן ושם אותו משפט סתום כמו שהלך מנהגו ברוב ספר אפידימיא כי הוא חפש ענין איש אחד או שני אנשים ושב אצלו המשפט דין על המין. זהו אצלי לפי לקיחת החלק ואם לא תרצה לאמר זה ורצית שיושם 15 לזה המאמר הבלתי אמתי אפני אמתות ויונחו לו הנחות קח לך מה שזכר ג׳אלינוס בשער הזה.

(2.21)

[73] אמר אבקראט: שתיית המשקה יסיר הרעב.

אמר המפרש: רצה במשקה היין וזה הרעב רוצה בו התאוה הכלבית כי שתיית היין אשר לו חמום חזק ירפא זה הרעב כי התאוה הכלבית תהיה אם מקור מזג האצטומכא לבד ואם מליחה 20 חמוצה נבלעת בגרמה והיין והיא אשר זכרתי ירפא שני הדברים יחד.

---

1 מה שיהיה מן הדברים זן מהר: המזונות אשר יזונו מהר א ‖ פתאום: נ״א המזונות אשר יגדלו(?) (=
יזונו) מהר פתאום תהיה יציאתם מהר ד ח add. 3-2 ‖ וענין מהר אחר שיקח add. ח 2 פתאום: הוא א²
אותו בזמן מועט: וענין מהר שיבשל הטבע מה שיאכל ראשון ראשון קודם שיתקבץ דח 4 אלא: אבל
אבהח 7 המעוט: המעט אבח 9 יהיה: ח add. a البطن :יבש 10 ח om. אדח ‖ הנה: ד om. 11 בלתי
נמצא: غير مطّرد a 13 סתום: מוחלט אבהח חתוך דח add. ‖ חפש ענין ... ושב: باستقراء حال ... يصير
a ‖ שני אנשים: שנים א שני אישים בדח 14 דין על: כולל א ‖ לפי לקיחת החלק: الإنصاف a 15 קח
לך: فعليك a 19 אם: בדחח om. ‖ ישיבה: ישבה ד add. 20 נבלעת: ישרה ח add.

(2.22)

[74] אמר אבקראט: מה שהיה מן החליים יתחדש מן המלוי הנה רפואתו תהיה בהרקה ומה שיהיה מהם יתחדש מן ההרקה רפואתו תהיה במלוי ורפואת שאר החליים תהיה בהפכם.

אמר המפרש: זה מבואר.

(2.23)

[75] אמר אבקראט: כי הנקיון יבא בחליים החדים בארבעה עשר יום.

אמר המפרש: אמר ג׳אלינוס: לא יעבור אחד מן החליים החדים אשר תנועתם תנועה אחת
ומהירות דבק זה הגבול ופעמים יבא הנקיון בהרבה מן חליים החדים באחד עשר ובתשיעי
ובשביעי ובחמישי ופעמים יבא בקצתם בששי אבל אינו טוב. והחליים אשר יבא בהם הנקיון
השלם ביום הארבעה עשר או לפניו ממנהג אבקראט שיקראם חליים חדים במאמר מוחלט.
אבל החליים אשר יהיה בהם נקיון חסר באחד מימי הנקיון הראשונים עוד ישאר מהם שארית
ישלם נקיונם באחד מימי הנקיון אשר אחריו עד יום הארבעים הנה יאמר בהם החדים אשר
יבא נקיונם בארבעים.

(2.24)

[76] אמר אבקראט: הרביעי מורה לשביעי וראשית השבוע השני היום השמיני והמורה ליום
הארבעה עשר יום האחד עשר כי הוא הרביעי מן השבוע השני ויום השבעה עשר גם כן יום
הוראה כי הוא היום הרביעי מיום הארבעה עשר והיום השביעי מן היום האחד עשר.

אמר המפרש: אמר ג׳אלינוס: השבעה עשר מורה בעשרים כי יום העשרים הוא יום נקיון והוא
תכלית השבוע השלישי.

(2.25)

[77] אמר אבקראט: הרביעית הקיצית ברוב תהיה קצרה והחרפית ארוכה וכל שכן כאשר
תדבק בסתיו.

אמר המפרש: לא הרביעית לבד תהיה בקיץ קצרה אבל שאר החליים גם כן כי הליחות
יזובו ויתפזרו בגוף כלו ויותכו ויתחייב מזה שלא יארך דבר מן החליים הקיציים אבל
אבקראט שם מאמרו בחלי היותר ארוך ושם אותו למשל. ויקרה בסתו הפך זה ר״ל
שינוחו הליחות בעומק הגוף כאלו הם מתאבנות ותשאר הכח בחזקתו והחליים לא יכלו
כל זמן שיהיו הליחות המולידות אותם קיימות ולא החולים ימותו כי כחותם ישאר ולא
יתך.

(2.26)

[78] אמר אבקראט: טוב שתהיה הקדחת אחר הקווץ משיהיה הקווץ אחר הקדחת.

אמר המפרש: הקווץ יהיה ממלוי או מהרקה וכאשר אירע הקווץ ממלוי הנה ימלאו העצבים מן
הליחה הדבקה הקרה אשר ממנה מזונם ובהתחדש הקדחת אחר הקווץ הזה והרבה פעמים
תחמם הליחה ההיא ותזיבה ותדקדקה ותתיכה הקדחת. וכאשר אירע לאדם קדחת שורפת
ותנגב כל גופו ועצביו ואחר כן יקרה לו הקווץ מפני היובש הנה המדוה מזה גדול.

(2.27)

[79] אמר אבקראט: אין ראוי שתבטח בקלות החולי שימצא החולה שלא בדרך ההקש ולא
שיפחידוך ענינים קשים יתחדשו שלא בדרך ההקש כי רוב מה שיקרה מזה אינו קיים ואי
אפשר שיעמוד ולא תאריך עמידתו.

אמר המפרש: כאשר התחדש חולי חזק ואחר כן תקל פתאום מבלתי קדימת בשול או הרקה
לא תסמוך על זה כי הליחות נבהלו ונקפאו ונחסרה תנועתם בלא ספק. וכן אם קדם הבשול
לגוף ואחר כן יקרה אחריו נשימה רעה וערבוב השכל והדומה להם לא יפחידך זה כי לא יעמוד.
והרבה פעמים יורה זה על נקיון טוב.

(2.28)

[80] אמר אבקראט: מי שהיתה בו קדחת בלתי חלושה מאד אם ישאר גופו בעינו ולא יחסר
כלום או שיתך יותר ממה שראוי רע כי הראשון יורה באריכות החולי והשני יורה על חולשת
הכח.

אמר המפרש: רזון הגוף תמיד אות רע ומורה על חולשת הכח בין שהיתה הקדחת בלתי
חלושה מאד או שהיתה קדחת חזקה מאד.

(2.29)

[81] אמר אבקראט: כל זמן שיהיה החולי בהתחלתו אם ראית שיתנועע דבר הניע וכאשר
הגיע החולי אל תכליתו הנה ראוי שישקוט החולה וינוח.

אמר המפרש: הנה יתן סבת זה בפרק אשר אחריו. ואמרו אם ראית שיתנועע דבר הניע רוצה
בו ההקזה לבד ופעמים יעשה השלשול גם כן. ואין ראוי שיעשה אחד מאלו השנים בעת תכלית
החולי כי בשול החולי יהיה בעת ההיא. והכח הנפשית יהיה בעת התכלית ברוב הענינים כבר

5

10

15

20

---

3 ובהתחדש: וכשתתחדש א ותתחדש א ותתחדש בח 4 ותדקדקה: ותרקקה בחה ותנגב: יתנגב ד
6 שתבטח: أَن يَغْتَرَّ a 6–7 ולא שיפחידוך: ושלא יפחידוך א 7–8 ואי אפשר שיעמוד: وَلَا يَكَاد
يَلْبَث a 8 ולא תאריך עמידתו: א‎ 10 נבהלו: تَبَلَّدَت a || בלא ספק: لَا غَيْرَ a 11 לגוף: البِين a
13 בלתי חלושה מאד: א‎ חזקה מאד א 14 שראוי: יהיה זה א‎ add. 17 חלושה: חזקה אה 20 אם:
ד om. || ראית שיתנועע דבר: ראית דבר שיתנועע א

נתך והעזר הטוב כדי שיהיה הבשול יותר מהיר הוא שתעשה ההרקה בהתחלת החולי עד
שימעט חומרו. ובעת התכלית הכח החיוני והכח הטבעי קיימים בכחם.

אמר המפרש: כבר קדם לך שאין ראוי שיעשה השלשול בהתחלה כי אם בחליים המסתערים
ולכן אמר בכאן אם ראית שהתנועע דבר הניע.

(2.30)

5   [82] אמר אבקראט: כל הדברים בתחלת החולי ואחריתו יותר חלושים ובתכליתו יותר חזקים.

אמר המפרש: רוצה בדברים המקרים כי הם בהתחלת החולי ואחריתו יותר חלושים כלומר
עונות הקדחת והצער והכאב והסערה והצמא. ואמנם הענין אשר יהיו ממנו המקרים האלו
והוא החולי יתחייב בהכרח שיהיה בעת התכלית יותר טוב כאשר יהיה החולה מן החולים
אשר ינצלו.

(2.31)

10   [83] אמר אבקראט: כאשר היה הקם מחולי יחטא מרוב האכילה ולא יתוסף גופו כלום הנה
זה רע.

אמר המפרש: זה מבואר וכבר נזכר זה הענין.

(2.32)

[84] אמר אבקראט: הנה ברוב העניינים כל מי שענינו רע ויחטא מרוב המאכל בתחלת הענין
ולא יתוסף גופו כלום הנה הוא בסופו יגיע ענינו אל הירידה מן המאכל. ואולם מי שימנע ממנו
15   בתחלת ענינו הלקיחה מן המאכל מניעה חזקה ואחר כן יחטא ממנו בסופו הנה ענינו יהיה
יותר טוב.

אמר המפרש: הדבור בכאן בקם מחולי ובאר בכאן כי מפני רוע מזגו ושארית הליחות אינם
נזונים איבריו ותאותו חזקה והוא יאכל ויתוספו הליחות או יתחזק רוע המזג ותבטל התאוה.
וכאשר היה בתחלה לא יתאוה התעסק הטבע בבשול ואחר כן יתחיל להתאוות ידע כי כבר
20   נתבשלו ליחותיו וישלם ענינו אל הטוב ברוב.

---

1 הוא: א¹ או א   4 שהתנועע דבר: ד inv.   5 יותר: יהיו א   6 בהתחלת: בתחלת אה ‖ ואחריתו:
וסופו בח   7 והצער: والأرق a ‖ והסערה: והתעורה א   10 יחטא מרוב האכילה: לוקח מן המזון א
ولא יחטא מרוב האכילה א¹ .add   יחטא מרוב מאכל ח يحظا من الطعام a   13 ויחטא מרוב המאכל:ויקח
מן המזון ב ויחטא וירבה מאכלו א¹ וירבה מאכלו ויחטא מרוב המאכל ב יחטא מרוב המאכל ח וירבה
מאכלו ויחטא ברוב המאכל ח ويحظا من الطعام a ‖ בתחלת: ברוב ח   14 אל הירידה מן המאכל: أن
لا يحظا من الطعام a   15 יחטא ממנו בסופו: يقح ממנו באחרונה א יחטא וירבה מננו באחרונה א¹ ירבה
ממנו בסופו בח يحظا منه بآخره a ‖ ענינו: הענין ד   17 בכאן: om. ד   20 וישלם: فتستمر a

(2.33)

[85] אמר אבקראט: בריאות השכל בכל חולי אות טוב וכן התאוה למאכל והפך זה אות רע.

אמר המפרש: זה מבואר וכבר בארנו סבת זה בפרקים חברתים.

(2.34)

[86] אמר אבקראט: כאשר היה החולי נאות לטבעו ולתוכן גופו ושניו ולזמן ההווה מזמני
השנה סכנתו מעוטה מסכנת החולי כאשר הוא בלתי נאות לאחת מאלו המדות.

5 אמר המפרש: זה מבואר כי הוא כאשר איננו ניאות הוא ראיה על יציאה גדולה משווי האיש
ההוא.

(2.35)

[87] אמר אבקראט: הנה הטוב בכל חולי שיהיה עובי למה שקרוב מן הטבור ושפל הבטן
וכאשר היה דק מאד כחוש הנה זה רע וכאשר היה גם כן בשלשול יש בו סכנה.

אמר המפרש: שפל הבטן הוא מה שבין הערוה והטבור ויהיו חלקי הבטן שלשה: המקום אשר
10 למטה מן החלצים ומה שסמוך לטבור ושפל הבטן וכאשר היו המקומות ההם עבים הנה העניין
יותר טוב וכאשר היו כחושים הנה העניין יותר רע וזה כי הוא אות רע וסבה רעה. ואולם אות
רע בעבור שהוא מורה על חולשת האיברים ההם אשר כחשו ונתכו. ואולם סבה רעה בעבור
כי בשול המאכל באצטומכא ותולדת הדם בכבד לא יהיו עם זה העניין כפי מה שראוי כי שני
אילו האברים יחד יקבלו תועלת בעובי מה שיכסם ושמנו בחממו אותם.

(2.36)

15 [88] אמר אבקראט: מי שהיה גופו בריא ושלשלו אותו ברפואה או הקיאוהו ימהר אליו העלוף
וכן מי שהיה נזון במזון רע.

אמר המפרש: וכן מי שהיה נזון במזון רע הנה אם יקיאוהו או ישולשל ימהר אליו העלוף
כי בגופם מותר רע וכאשר תעירהו הרפואה קצת הערה יתבאר הרוע שלו ויתגלה. זה הוא
סבתו לפי דעת גאלינוס. ואשר יראה לי בסבת זה כי אשר התמיד המזונות הרעים הדם

---

1 והפך זה אות רע: והפכו רע דה והפכו אות רע בח	3 לטבעו: لطبيعة المريض a || ולתוכן גופו ושניו:
ולשניו ולמזג ולתוכן גופו א وسنه وسِنته a	7 הבטן: שיהיה עובי א	8 וכאשר היה גם כן
בשלשול: وإذا كان أيضا كذلك فالإسهال معه a	9 הערוה: בית הערוה בח	11 כחושים: أهزل a
14 תועלת: גדול א .add	17 המפרש: לא באר לנו הסבה במקרה העלוף לבריא אחר השלשול אבל
אפלטון הזכיר הטעם מפני שהוא בבריאותו ואין בליחותיו מותר וכאשר הרפואה לא מצאה מותר תנקהו
מהליחות הטבעיות שהם יסוד הגוף ויקרה מזה חולשת הכח ה .add	18 רע: בסבת רוע המזון א .add
19 גאלינוס: א״א: מה שיהיה מן המאכל והמשקה יותר טוב מעט אלא שהוא יותר (...) ולכן ראוי שיובחר
על מה שהוא יותר משובח מהם אלא שהוא יותר נתעב ה .add

שלו נשחת מאד ואיכותו נפסד וכאשר משכה הרפואה בכחה המושך הניע כל דם אשר
בו ורצה שינקה ממנו כל הפסדיו והם רבים מאד ונקשרים והם מרכב חיי זה האיש נפסד
ההנהגה ויתחדש העלוף בהכרח לכח המשיכה ורוב מה שיחשוב למשוך אותו והוא נקשר
ומעורב.

(2.37)

5 [89] אמר אבקראט: מי שהיה גופו בריא הנה עשיית הרפואה בו קשה.

אמר המפרש: הבריאים כשיעשו הקיא או השלשול יקרה להם סבוב הראש וצירים מעשוי
היציאה ויקשה יציאת מה שיצא מהם וימהר אליהם עם זה העלוף כי הרפואה תשתדל למשוך
הליחה הנאותה לה וכאשר לא תמצאה תמשוך הדם והבשר ויעמידם להוציא מהם מה שבהם
ממה שיאות לה.

(2.38)

10 [90] אמר אבקראט: מה שהיה מן המאכל והמשקה פחות מעט אבל שהוא יותר ערב הנה
ראוי שיבחרו אותו על מה שהוא משניהם יותר טוב אבל שהוא בלתי ערב.

אמר המפרש: זה מבואר כי הבישול לערב יותר טוב.

(2.39)

[91] אמר אבקראט: הזקנים ברוב יחלו יותר מעט ממה שיחלו הבחורים אבל כי מה שיקרה
להם מן החליים הנושנים על הרוב ימותו והם בהם.

15 אמר המפרש: הזקנים יותר מושלים בהנהגת עצמם מן הבחורים והכח בגופות הזקנים
חלוש לא שלא יוכל לבשל החליים לבד אלא מה שיקרה להם מן החליים יהיה מן הליחות
הקרות.

(2.40)

[92]

(2.41)

[93] אמר אבקראט: מי שימצאהו פעמים רבות עלוף חזק מבלתי סבה נגלית הנה הוא ימות
20 פתאום.

---

2 מאד: ד .om ‖ מרכב: مركب a   7–6 וצירים מעשוי היציאה: ومغص a   8 ויעמידם: واستكرههما a
10 המאכל והמשקה: المشقة والمأكل بدح a   13 שיחלו: הנערים אˣ .add ²   15 יותר מושלים בהנהגת
עצמם: أضبط لأنفسهم a   16 לא שלא יוכל לבשל: لا تقدر أن تنضج a   החליים: سريعا والأمراض
المزمنة كلّها باردة ولذلك يلزمهم للممات. قال أبقراط: إنّ ما يعرض من البحوحة والنزل للشيخ الفاني ليس
تنضج. قال المفسّر: ليس هذه الأمراض .add a ‖ מה: سائر ما a   18 This aphorism is missing in all
MSS.

אמר המפרש: מי שימצאהו העלוף באלו התנאים השלשה והוא שיהיה מבלתי סבה נגלית וחזק ופעמים רבות אמנם ימצאהו זה מפני חולשת הכח החיוני.

(2.42)

[94] אמר אבקראט: השתוק אם היה חזק אי אפשר שירפא ממנו בעליו ואם היה חלוש אינו נקל להרפא.

אמר המפרש: כל שתוק אמנם יהיה כאשר לא יהיה אפשר לרוח הנפשיי לעבור אל מה שלמטה מן הראש מן סתום אם לסבה מסוג המורסא נתחדשה במוח ואם בעבור שבטני המוח נמלאו מליחות מסוג הליחה הלבנה. ואם מנע השתוק תנועת החזה הנה זה יותר גדול ויותר מסוכן שיהיה מהם וכאשר יתנשם ביותר גדול שיהיה מן הזרות הנה שתוקו חזק גם כן וכאשר היה התנשמו מבלתי מלחמה וזרות אבל שהוא מתחלף בלתי דבק לסדר אחד אחד הנה שתוקו חלוש. ואם אתה תבא על ענינו בכל מה שנשאר כלומר שתעשהו אפשר לך שתרפאהו.

(2.43)

[95] אמר אבקראט: אשר יתנקו ויגיעו אל גבול העלוף ולא הגיעו אל גבול המות הנה לא ינצל מהם מי שנראה קצף בפיו.

אמר המפרש: הנה זכר גאלינוס כי ראה קצת מאשר נחנקו או חנק עצמו ונראה בפיו הקצף ונצל וזה יהיה מעט.

(2.44)

[96] אמר אבקראט: מי שהיה גופו עב מאד בטבע המות יותר מהירה לבוא אליו מאשר היא אל הכחושים.

אמר המפרש: סבת זה מבוארת לצרות העורקים ורחבם כמו שבאר בספר המזגים. ואמר גאלינוס שיהיה הגוף בריא בשר ממוצע עד שלא יהיה עב ולא רזה יותר טוב ויותר אפשר שיחיה אל ימי הזקנה.

(2.45)

[97] אמר אבקראט: בעל חולי הנופל כשיהיה חדש הנה רפואתו תהיה לבד בהעתקתו בשנים הארץ וההנהגה.

---

3 השתוק: הנקרא אפוקלוקשיאה א add. ‖ 6 מן סתום: من البدن a add. ‖ אם: ד om. ‖ 7 החזה: והעדירה ממנו א¹ 9 אחד: فسكته قريّة أيضاً إلّا أنّها أنقص من الثانية. ومتى كان صاحبها يَتنفّس تنفّسا لازما لنظام add. a 10 שנשאר: שאפשר א يَنبغي a ‖ שתעשהו: كفي الرواي א² add. ‖ שתרפאהו: אמר אבוק': מן האסכרה והירידה לישיש המופלג לא יתבשל. אמר המפרש: זה מבואר א add. ‖ 11 גבול (حَدّ = C): حال a 18 גאלינוס: מי א add. ‖ בשר: בבשר א² ‖ 19 הזקנה: غايتها a add.

אמר המפרש: חולי הנופל והשתוק הליחה המולידה אותם יחד קרה עבה וכאשר יעתק בארץ
ובשנים ובהנהגה אל החום והיובש ויעתק גם כן מן ההנהגה הרעה אשר הולידה הליחה ההיא
בהפך ההנהגה ההיא ירפא.

(2.46)

[98] אמר אבקראט: כשיהיו שני כאבים יחד ואינם במקום אחד הנה היותר חזק מהם יסתיר
האחר.   5

אמר המפרש: כאשר ימשך הטבע אל האבר אשר בו הכאב היותר גדול יחסר הרגש המקום
האחר ולא ירגיש במה שבו ממה שיכאיב.

(2.47)

[99] אמר אבקראט: בעת הולד המוגלא יקרה הכאב והקדחת יותר ממה שיקרו אחר הולדם.

אמר המפרש: כי אז ימשך מקום המורסא יותר ויתחזק הכאב ויטה החום אצל הליחה כדי
שיבשלה ויתפשט יותר ויתחזק הקדחת.   10

(2.48)

[100] אמר אבקראט: בכל תנועה יניע אותה הגוף הנה מנוחתו בעת שהתחיל בו היגיעה
תמנעהו מהמשך אליו היגיעה.

אמר המפרש: זה מבואר.

(2.49)

[101] אמר אבקראט: מי שהרגיל עמל אחד הנה הוא ואע״פ שיהיה חלוש הגוף או זקן יותר
טוב לעשות העמל ההוא אשר הרגיל אותו ממי שלא הרגילו ואע״פ שיהיה חזק בחור.   15

אמר המפרש: זה מבואר.

(2.50)

[102] אמר אבקראט: מה שכבר הרגיל האדם מזמן ארוך ואם היה יותר מזיק ממה שלא
הרגילו הנה הזיקו אותו יותר מעט והנה ראוי שיעתק האדם אל מה שלא הרגיל אותו.

אמר המפרש: הקדים הקדמה אמתית וחייב ממנה מה שיתחייב בהתמדת הבריאות בכל
העניינים שירגיל האדם עצמו להעתק ממנהג אל מנהג ועל מדרגות. אמר גאלינוס כי טוב   20

---

١ יחד: א om.   3 ירפא: لعلّه يبرأ a   4–7 אמר ... שיכאיב: ד om.   5 האחר: האחד א   6 כאשר:
ואשר א   12 מהמשך (= من أن يجذب): من أن يحدث a   14–15 יותר טוב לעשות: أحمل a   15 ממי:
מאותו א   19 וחייב ממנה מה שיתחייב: وألزم عنها وعمّا يلزم m a   20 ועל מדרגות: על המדרגות א

לכל אחד מהאנשים שישא עצמו לנסות כל דבר כדי שלא יעותהו בעת ההכרח דבר שלא
הרגיל אותו ויגיעהו נזק גדול ויהיה זה בשלא ישאר האדם במה שהרגילו תמיד אבל ישים
עצמו בקצת העתים בהפכו.

(2.51)

[103] אמר אבקראט: עשות הרב פתאום ממה שימלא הגוף או יריקהו או שיחממהו או
יקררהו או שיניעהו במין אחר מן התנועה אי זה מין שיהיה סכנה. וכל מה שהוא רב הנה
הוא מתנגד לטבע ואולם מה שיהיה מעט מעט הוא בטוח וכן כשתרצה להעתק מדבר אל
זולתו וכאשר רצית זולת זה.

אמר המפרש: זה מבואר.

(2.52)

[104] אמר אבקראט: כשאתה תעשה כל מה שראוי לעשות וכפי מה שראוי ולא יהיה מה
שראוי להיות לא תעתק אל זולת מה שאתה בו כל זמן שהתמיד מה שראית אותו בתחלת
העניין קיים.

אמר המפרש: זה פרק כולל סדר גדול מסדרי הרפואה ולא הגיע גאלינוס בפרושו אל מה
שראוי ור״ל זה כי כאשר ראית האותות שהוא דרך משל ראוי שיחממו אותו והתמדת החמום
ולא ירפא החולה הנה אין ראוי לך שתעתק לקרר אבל תתמיד בחמום כל זמן שתראה העניינים
המורים לעשות החמום קיימים והוא עניין אמרו כל זמן שהתמיד מה שראית אותו מתחלת
העניין קיים. זה עניין מאמרו כלומר שלא יעתק ממין ההנהגה אבל ראוי בהכרח שיעתק
מרפואה מחממת אל רפואה אחרת מחממת ויחליף הרפואות הנפרדות והמורכבות אשר
הם כלם מחממות כי כאשר הרגיל הגוף רפואה אחת תמיד תמעט פעולתו בו. ועוד כי בחלוף
מיני הרפואות אשר איכותם אחת עניין נאות מאד למזג איש איש ולמזג אבר אבר ולמקרי חולי
חולי וזה שורש גדול מסודות הרפואה וזה המין בעצמו יעשה במזון ובמיני מה שירקקו הליחה
המחליאה או בהתוך או בהדק או בבשול או בעבות חומר או בקבץ. יתמיד תמיד מין ההנהגה
אשר הורו עליו המופתים הקיימים ויהפך במיני הרפואות והמזונות אשר הם ממין אחד והבן
זה.

(2.53)

[105] אמר אבקראט: מי שהיה בטנו לח הנה הוא כל זמן שיהיה בחור יהיה עניינו יותר טוב
ממי שבטנו יבש ואחר כן יגיע עניינו בזמן הישישות שיהיה יותר רע וזה כי בטנו ייבש כשיהיה
ישיש ברוב.

1 שישא: שישיא א ‖ יעותהו: א¹ יתעהו א יעוותותוה ח יעיתהו ב يصادفه a   5 אחר: אחד אח   6 וכן:
om. a   7 וכאשר רצית זולת זה: om. א   12 המפרש: משה א   14 לקרר: للتدبير a ‖ תתמיד: התמיד
אבח   17 אל רפואה אחרת מחממת: א¹   18 פעולתו: א¹   20 שיריקו: تأثيره a   21 add. a به בהתוך:
om. א ‖ בהדק: ברקק א בדקק בח   24 לח: בנערותו א   add.

אמר המפרש: כבר קדמה לו הסברה הזאת ברכות הטבע ויבשותו בשנות הבחרות והישישות. וג׳אלינוס ישתדל לתת סבת זה וכבר אמרתי מה שנראה לי ברכות הטבע תמיד בכל השנים מסבות התמדת הבריאות וכל יובש בטבע רע לבריאים ולחולים.

(2.54)

[106] אמר אבקראט: גודל הגוף בבחרות לא יגונה אבל ישובח אלא שהוא בעת הישישות יכבד ויקשה השתמשו ויהיה יותר רע מן הגוף אשר הוא יותר קצר ממנו.

אמר המפרש: ג׳אלינוס סובר שהוא רצה באמרו הנה גודל הגוף ארכו עד שלא יהיה זה המשפט בעביו ושמנותו.

נשלם המאמר השני מפירוש הפרקים.

1 לו: א ‖ .om הטבע: البطن a ‏3 בטבע: בטבעו א ‏4 לא יגונה אבל ישובח: יותר טוב ויותר נאה א ‏5 יותר קצר: أنقص a ‏6 עד: אי דה ‏om. ‏7 המשפט: ההקש א ‖ בעביו ושמנותו: وهم لحض a ‏8 מפירוש הפרקים: מפרקי אבוקרט אה

המאמר השלישי מפירוש הפרקים

(3.1)

[107] אמר אבקראט: התהפך זמני השנה ממה שיעשה בתולדת החליים בפרט ובזמן האחד
מהם השנוי החזק בקור או בחום וכן בשאר העניים בזה ההקש.

אמר המפרש: ר״ל שנוי טבעי התקופות כמו שתהיה תקופת הסתיו חמה או תקופת הקיץ
5   קרה והדומה להם וכן שנוי הזמן ההווה ממזגו כאשר היה חזק ואע״פ ששאר זמני התקופות
לא ישתנו הנה הוא יוליד חליים.

(3.2)

[108] אמר אבקראט: מן הטבעים מי שיהיה עניו בקיץ יותר טוב ובסתיו יותר רע ומהם מי
שיהיה עניו בסתיו יותר טוב ובקיץ יותר רע.

אמר המפרש: ר״ל באמרו מן הטבעים המזגים מעניַן האישים וזה מבואר כי בסתיו יהיה טוב
10   עניַן המחוממים ובקיץ יהיה טוב עניַן המקוררים והקש על זה.

(3.3)

[109] אמר אבקראט: כל אחד מן החליים עניו עם דבר זולת דבר יותר טוב ויותר רע וקצת
שנים עם עתים מן השנה וארצות ומינים מן ההנהגה.

אמר המפרש: זה הפרק כאשר סדרת מילותיו יתבאר באור נגלה וכן יסודר כל אחד מן החליים
הנה עניו עם שנה זולת שנה או עם ארץ זולת ארץ או עם זמן מן השנה זולת זמן או עם הנהגה
15   זולת הנהגה יותר טוב ויותר רע. והמשל כי בעל החולי הקר עם שנות הבחרות ובעת הקיץ
ובארצות החמות ובהנהגה החמה יותר טוב ובהפכי אלו יותר רע. ובכלל הנה ההפך עם ההפך
יותר טוב והנטיה היוצאת מהשווי עם הנטיה היוצאת בצד ההוא יותר רע. אמנם בעל שנים
ממוצעות המזג הנה ההנהגה הממוצעת והזמן והארץ הממוצעים יותר נאות לו כי בעל המזג

1 מפירוש הפרקים: om. א מפרקי אבוקרט ח   3–2 ובזמן האחד מהם: כן שני הזמן האחד מטבעו
א   4 שנוי: התהפכות א   5 שנוי: בשנוי א ‖ ההווה: الواحد a   7 ומהם מי: ויש מהם א   8 בסתיו:
بزمن الⲕور א   9 מעניַן האישים: המזגים מעניַן האישים א من أﻣﺰﺟﺔ الأﺷﺨﺎص a   10 עניַן: עניַנו מן
א ‖ עניַן: עניַנו מן א   11 עם דבר זולת דבר יותר: עם שנה זולת שנה יותר דﺡ עם שנה זולת דבר יותר בﺡ
13 סדרת: תסדר א   15 בעל: בעלי ﺡ   16 טוב: הבעל החולי הקר הנזכר בשנות הזקנה ובעת החורף
ובארצות הקרות ובהנהגה הקרה הוא יותר רע. אמר גאלינו׳: הנה זה ראוי וﺯה שאין שמות עתות השנה
הם הסבות הפועלות לחולים אמנם הסבות הפועלות להם הם הם מזג כל א׳ מאותם העתים כי הם משנים
מזג א׳ מהם וראוי בהכרת שישתנו החליים בשנוניים (= בשנויים). ובאמרו הרפויים (= חרפיים) ר״ל
הדומים לﬣﬧﬥ הﬡ﬛﬩גּﬤ (del. ﺡ) משנים מזג א׳ וראוי בהכרת שישתנו החליים בשנויים. ובאמרו חרפיים
ר״ל הדומים לחלק החורף add. ﺡ   16–17 ובכלל ... רע: om. א ‖ רע: א   17 והנטיה: والﻤﺜﻞ a ‖ עם: הנה ד מן
ﺡ ‖ הנטיה: والﻤﺜﻞ a ‖ היוצאת: عن الاﻋﺘﺪال add. a ‖ שנים: om. ד

הזה כוונתו הוא שיתקן עניינו במה שיתדמה לו. ואולם בעלי המזג היוצא מהשווי הנה הארצות
והזמנים ומיני ההנהגה שהם הפכיהם הם יותר נאותים להם.

(3.4)

[110] אמר אבקראט: כאשר היה באיזה זמן שיהיה מזמני השנה ביום אחד פעם חום ופעם
קור תפחד מהתחדש חוליים חרפיים.

5 אמר המפרש: ‹זה מבואר›.

(3.5)

[111] אמר אבקראט: הרוח דרומי יחדש כבדות בשמע ועכירות בראות וכבדות בראש ועצלה
ורפיון ועם חוזק הרוח הזה והתגבורת שלו יקרו לחולים אלו המקרים. ואולם הרוח הצפוני
יחדש שעול וכאב הגרון ויובש הבטן ועצירת השתן והפלצות וכאב בצלעות והחזה ועם
תגבורת הרוח הזה וחזקתו הנה ראוי שתפחד מהתחדש בחולים אלו המקרים.

---

1 כוונתו: وحده a ‖ שיתדמה: שידמה א   5 ‹זה מבואר›: אמר ג׳אלינוס: הנה זה הראוי וזה שאין
שמות עתות השנה הם סבות הפעולות לחלאים ואמנם הסבות הפועלות להם הם מזג כל אחד מאותם
העתים הם משנים מזג אחד מהם ראוי בהכרח שישתנו החליים בשנוים ד א״ה לא רצה באמרו חליים
חרפיים חלי המרה השחורה המתעוררים בימי החורף אמנם רצה בזה חליים מתחלפים פעמים חמים
פעמים קרים כהתחלפות הזמן ההוא שיתקרר לעתים ויתחמם לעתים וכשיתחזק הקור בו תתחדש
קדחת תדירה ורביעית ועובי באיברים ומורסות וכאשר יתחזק החום תתעורר קדחת שלישית ואדמימות
העור וכשיבא ההתהפכות ביום אחד כאשר יבא בזמן החורף ראוי לחליים המתעוררים שיקראו חרפיים
א¹   6 יחדש: מחדש ד ‖ כבדות: כובד ד ‖ ועכירות: ועכירות ד מטלת(?) בהה ומחשך ח¹ وغشاوة
a ‖ וכבדות: וכובד ד   7 ועם: ובעת ד ‖ הזה: om. ד ‖ והתגבורת שלו: ותגבורתו ד ‖ יקרו: יתחדשו
ד ‖ ואולם: ואמנם ד ‖ הרוח הצפוני: הרוח הצפונית ד   8 יחדש: מחדש ד יחדש שעול וכאב הגרון: خشّن
الحلق والصدر a ‖ הגרון: גרוני ד ‖ הבטן: בטנם ד ‖ ועצירת השתן: om. ד ונעצר השתן ה ועוצר השתן
בח ‖ והפלצות: וסמור ד ‖ ועם: om. ד   9 וחזקתו: וכחו ד ‖ הנה: om. ד ‖ שתפחד מהתחדש
בחולים: שיפול בחליים התחדשות ד ‖ המקרים: אמר המפרש: אלו השני פרקים נגלים מבוארים א
.add מכאן חסר פי׳ הפרק ד add. חסר פי׳ ב¹ אמר פלדיוס: מפני שטבע הרוח הדרומי חמה לחה
ויתיך הליחה אשר בראש ותרד הליחה אל שרשי העצבים ולזה יתחדש כובד בשמע ובראות וזולתם מן
החושים ואמנם העצלה והרפיון מפני שעצבי הגוף כלו ירבה בו מן הליחות שהתיכה הרוח הדרומי כי
כל הווסן(?) הליחות כשיתקבצו יתיכו השמרים והלחות ההוא יזיק ברוח הנפש ותביא העצלה והרפיון.
וכבר זכר אבוקרט מהנעת האויב (= האויר) והתוכו כמו מה שבכלי הים בהנעת המים. ואולם הרוח
הצפוני היא קרה ויבשה ותעיר השיעול וכאב הגרון בסבת נגוב הליחות אשר באברים ותסתום המקומות
הדקים וכשתרד באמה תקרר אשכי(?) הכיס. ויובש הבטן מפני כי חום הבטן יברח מפני הקור ההוא
ויכנס בפנים ותיבש היציאה. והפלצות מפני שהיא תמנע יציאת המרה האדומה ותעורר פלצות בגוף ה
.add قال المفسّر: ريح الجنوب حارّة رطبة فلذلك تكدّر الحواسّ وترطّب مبدأ العصب فيحدث الكسل وعسر
.add الحركة وريح الشمال باردة يابسة فتخشّن الحلق والصدر وتجفّف البطن وتكثّف المجاري فتحدث ما ذكَر
a

(3.6)

[112] אמר אבקראט: כשיהיה הקייץ דומה לאביב ראוי שתתפחד מהתחדש זיעה רבה בקדחות.

אמר המפרש: יתחייב כאשר היה הקייץ יבש חזק היובש שיצא באיד ויתך הלחות וכאשר היה
דומה באביב שימשך הליחות בחומו אל מה שקרוב מן העור ולא יהיה אפשר שיתיכהו בדרך
האד ללחותו והנה בעבור שהלחות ההוא בעת נקיון החליים יתרוקן פתאום יהיה ממנו זיעה
רבה.

(3.7)

[113] אמר אבקראט: כשיעצר המטר יתחדשו קדחות חדות ואם תרבה העצירה ההיא בשנה
ואחר כן נתחדש באויר ענין יובש הנה ראוי שיפחד ברוב מאלו החליים והדומה להם.

אמר המפרש: באר כי בהמנע המטר יתנגבו הליחות ויקפאו ויהיו הקדחות מעט מספר
ובאיכות יותר חדים.

(3.8)

[114] אמר אבקראט: כאשר יהיו זמני השנה דבקים בסדורם ויהיה בכל אחד מהם מה שראוי
שיהיה בו יהיה מה שיתחדש בהם מן החליים טובי הקיום והיושר וטובי הנקיון וכשיהיו זמני
השנה בלתי דבקים בסדרם יהיה מה שיתחדש בהם מן החליים בלתי מסודר רע הנקיון.

אמר המפרש: (זה מבואר).

(3.9)

[115] אמר אבקראט: הנה בחורף יהיו החליים יותר חדים שיהיו ויותר ממיתים ברוב ואולם
האביב הוא יותר בריא מכל הזמנים והמות בו יותר מעט.

אמר המפרש: האביב ממוצע והחורף בתכלית החלוף.

(3.10)

[116] אמר אבקראט: החורף לבעלי השדפון רע.

אמר המפרש: להיותו קר יבש מתחלף המזג הנה הוא יזיק המושחתים מחולי מאד.

---

4 נקיון החליים: הנקיון והחליים דה נקיון וחליים בה بحران وأمراض AC   6 תרבה: היתה א הרבתה אי
7 ענין: ד .om   8 באר: אבוקרט א .add || ויקפאו: وتجمد a   9 חדים: חם ד חד בהה   10 דבקים
בסדורם: נוהגין כסדרן א דבקים בסבוביהם בה   11 טובי: טוב א || הקיום והיושר: הקיום א الثبات
والنظام a || וטובי: וטוב א   12 דבקים בסדרם: נוהגין כסדרן א || בהם: מהם ד || רע הנקיון: והנקיון
משונה בדהה   13 (זה מבואר): זה כלו הוא מבואר נגלה א מכאן חסר פיי הפרק ד חסר פיי חיי
14 שיהיו: א .om

(3.11)

[117] אמר אבקראט: ואולם בזמני השנה אומר כי כשיהיה הסתו מעט מטר צפוני ויהיה האביב ממטיר דרומי יתחייב בהכרח שיתחדשו בקיץ קדחות חדות וקצידה בעינים ושלשול דם ורוב מה שיקרה שלשול הדם לנשים ולבעלי הטבע הלח.

אמר המפרש: זה מבואר אחר ידיעת שרשי המלאכה.

(3.12)

[118] אמר אבקראט: כאשר יהיה הסתיו דרומי מטרי חם והיה האביב מעט המטר צפוני הנה   5
הנשים אשר יקרה לידתן אצל האביב הנה יפילו במעט סבה ואשר תלדנה מהם תלדנה ילדים חלושי התנועה עלולים עד שהם אם שימותו מיד ואם שישארו דלים עלולים כל ימיהם. ואולם שאר האנשים הנה יקרה להם שלשול הדם והקצידה היבשה. ואולם הזקנים הנה יקרה להם מן היירידות מה שיכלה מהר.

(3.13)

[119] אמר אבקראט: ואם היה הקיץ מעט המטר ורוחותיו צפוניות והיה החורף רב   10
המטר דרומי יקרה בסתו כאב חזק בראש ושעול ורוקי ורבמאס ויקרה לקצת האנשים השדפון.

(3.14)

[120] אמר אבקראט: ואם היו רוחותיו צפוניות יבשות הנה יהיה נאות למי שהיה טבעו לח ולנשים ואולם שאר האנשים הנה יקרה להם קצידה יבשה וקדחות חדות ורבמאס מתמיד ומהם מי שיקרה להם בלבול השכל מן המרה השחורה.   15

(3.15)

[121] אמר אבקראט: מעניני האויר בשנה בכלל מעוט המטר יותר בריא מרבוי המטר והמות בה יותר מעט.

1 הסתו: בסתו א   2 וקצידה א (O.Occ.: *cassida*, i.e., defluxion of the eyes) בעינים: וקצירה בעינים
בה ورمד a ‖ ושלשול: של א add.   5 מטרי: מטר בדח מעט ה ‖ צפוני: ד om.   6 יקרה: לא יבוא
ד ‖ ילדים: ולדות ד ילדות ח וולדי בח   8 הנה: ד om.   9–8 שלשול הדם והקצידה היבשה. ואולם
הזקנים הנה יקרה להם מן היירידות: א¹   8 והקצידה: והקצירה ב   9 מן היירידות: ד om.   10 אמר:
עוד אמר א   11 דרומי: ד om. ‖ ורוקי: ורוקיטט א ורוקיי: ורוקיירי א וַרְוֹקִיֵר ב ודזקיירי ח ורוקירר ח הוא נמיכת הקול א
‖ ורבמאס (O.Occ. *raumas/reumas*, i.e., cold):ורבמס וזכאם א ורבמוס ה ורבמס בח add.   13 אמר:
ועוד אמר א ‖ היו: היה בד ‖ הנה: ד om.   14 קצידה: קצירה אבה ‖ ורבמאס: ורואמס א ורבמס בחה
16 אמר: ועוד אמר א   17 בה: בו א

(3.16)

[122] אמר אבקראט: ואולם החליים אשר יתחדשו מרב המטר ברוב הענינים קדחות ארוכות
והתרת הבטן ועפוש וחולי הנופל והשתוק והאסכרא. ואולם החליים אשר יתחדשו עם מעט
המטר הם שדפון וקצידה וכאב הפרקים וטפטוף השתן ושלשול הדם.

אמר המפרש: כל מה שזכרו אבקראט באלו החמישה פרקים מהיות החליים הפלוניים
יתחדשו במין הפלוני מהאנשים כאשר היה האויר כן זה על הרוב בשום פנים ולכן אין
ראוי שינתנו סבותיו לפי מה שנודע למי שעיין בפילוסּפיא אבל גאלינוס רצה שיתן סבה לכל זה
ובכלל הנה עם ידיעת שרשי מלאכת הרפואה מידיעת טבעי התקופות והאישים וסבות החליים
ושהלחות חומר העפוש והחום פועל בהם נקל לתת סבות לכל מה שזכר כאשר יתחדש.

(3.17)

[123] אמר אבקראט: ואולם עניני האויר בכל יום ויום מה שהיה מהם צפוני הנה הוא יקבץ
הגופות ויאמצם ויחזקם ויחזק תנועותיהם ויפה מראיהם ויזכך השמע להם וייבש הבטן ויחדש
בעינים עקיצה ואם קדם להם בצדדי החזה כאב יעירהו ויוסיף בו. ומה שהיה מהם דרומי הנה
הוא יתיך הגופות וירפם וילחלחם ויחדש כובד בראש וכבדות בשמע וסבוב בעינים עד שלא
יראה ובגוף כלו קשי התנועה ורכות הטבע.

אמר המפרש: כבר נודע כי הרוח הצפוני קר ויבש והדרומי חם ולח וכל זה מבואר.

(3.18)

[124] אמר אבקראט: ואולם בזמני השנה באביב ובתחלת הקיץ יהיו הנערים והקרוב
מאחריהם בשנים ביותר טוב שבעניניהם ובבריאות יותר שלם ובנשאר מן הקיץ ובראשית
החורף יהיו הזקנים ביותר טוב שבעניניהם ובנשאר מן החורף ובסתיו יהיו הממוצעים ביניהם
בשנים ביותר טוב שבעניניהם.

אמר המפרש: כבר קדם לנו סבת זה בפרק אשר החלפנו הרכבת מלותיו.

(3.19)

[125] אמר אבקראט: החליים כלם יתחדשו בכל זמני השנה אבל כי קצתם בקצת הזמנים יותר
ראויים שיתחדשו ויתעוררו.

אמר המפרש: זה מבואר.

---

1 אמר: עוד אמר א   3 וקצידה: וקצירה בח   4 החליים: הם דה   add. 5 במין: בקיץ ד ‖ הפלוני: א
om. הפלוני בפלוני א²   7 עם: זה א   add. 8 בהם: בדחח .om   9 מהם: א   add. 10 ויחזק: ويحذ a
11 יעירהו: מּקּדّם a .add   12 וסבוב: א¹ וסתום וחולשה א ‖   13 ובגוף: א¹ ויתחדש
בגוף א ‖ ורכות הטבע: ורפיון הבטן א   16–15 והקרוב מאחריהם: והסמוכים להם א   17–16 ובנשאר
מן הקיץ ובראשית החורף יהיו הזקנים ביותר טוב שבעניניהם: ד .om   20 כי קצתם: שקצתם א   22 זה
מבואר: הנה זה כלו מבואר נגלה א

(3.20)

[126] אמר אבקראט: פעמים יקרה באביב בלבול הראש השחור והשטות וחולי הנופל והגרת
הדם והאסכרא והרבמאס והרבקיי והשעול והחולי אשר יתקלף בו העור והקואבי והבהק
והשחין הרב אשר יפתח ויתנגע והמורסות וכאבי הפרקים.

אמר המפרש: זה הפרק מבואר למה שהקדים בפרק אשר לפניו וזה כי הוא זכר בפרק הקודם
כי פעמים יתחדש כל מין ממיני החליים בכל פרק מפרקי השנה אבל קצת החליים בקצת פרקי   5
השנה יותר ראויים והם אשר יתחדשו על הרוב בפרק ההוא. והשלים זה העניין במה שאמר
כי יתחדש באביב אשר הוא יותר ממוצע מכל הפרקים חליים שחוריים כמו הוסואס השחורי
והשטות וחליים מליחה לבנה כחולי הנופל והרבמאס והבחוחה הוא רוקאג׳י והשעול וחליים
ממרה אדומה כמו השחין אשר יתנגע בהם העור והמורסות וחליים שהם מדם כהגרת הדם
והאסכרא אבל החליים המיוחדים באביב הם הנמשכים אחר התכת הליחות והגרתם לחוץ   10
ותנועת הטבע תדחה אותם בחזקה. וכן הפרק אשר אחר זה נבנה על מה שביארנוהו מהיות
החליים פעמים יתחדשו בחלוף טבע הפרק.

(3.21)

[127] אמר אבקראט: ואולם בקיץ הנה יקרה קצת אלו החליים וקדחות מתמידות והשורפות
ושלישית הרבה וקיא ושלשול וקצידה וכאב באזן ונגעים בפה ועפוש בנגעים.

(3.22)

[128] אמר אבקראט: ואולם החורף הנה יקרה בו רוב חליי הקיץ וקדחות רבעיות מעורבות   15
וחליי הטחול ושקוי ושדפון וטפטוף השתן ושלשול הדם וקלוח המעים וכאב הירך והאסכרא
והרבקיי והקולון החזק אשר יקראוהו היונים אילאוס והחולי הנופל והשטות והוסואס השחורי.

אמר המפרש: כל זה מבואר במה שהקדמנו.

(3.23)

[129] אמר אבקראט: ואולם בסתו יקרה מדוה הצד ומדוה הריאה והרובמאס והבחוחה
והשעול וכאבי הצדדים ושפל השדרה וכאב הראש והסבוב והשתוק.   20

1 פעמים: ואשר א לפעמים א' ‖ הראש השחור: השכל מן המרה השחורה א ‖ הנופל: והשתוק א .add
2 והרבקיי: ורוקיי א והרבקיגי א' ‖ והקואבי: والقواني a   6 הרוב: הדם א   8 והרבמאס: והרומאס
א ‖ רוקאג׳י: רוקיי אבחרובבקנא ה   10 התכת: התרת ד   11 שביארנוהו: שביארנו א   13 מתמידות:
מדם דה דה הדם ב   14 ושלשול: .om בדחה ‖ וקצידה: וקצירה: ה ‖ בנגעים (= الفروج a): בית הערוה
א الفروج emendation editor והנגע הנקרא חסף א .add וحصف א .add   15 אמר: ועוד אמר א
17 והרבקיי: והרוקיי א והרוק בחהובחוחה ה ‖ אילאוס: אילאוה ד אליאוס בח ‖ הנופל: המחשבה הרעה
דה .add ‖ והוסואס: השעמוס א'   18 כל זה מבואר במה שהקדמנו: כל מה שאמר באלו שני הפרקים
הוא מבואר במה שהקדמנוהו א   19 והרובמאס: והרומאס א והרבמס בחה

אמר המפרש: נבנה זה גם כן על על מה שקדם כי פעמים יתחדש בסתו חליים מיוחדים בו על
הרוב כמו הרובמאס והבחוחה והשתוק וחליים שאינם מטבעו כמו חולי הצד.

(3.24)

[130] אמר אבקראט: ואולם בשנים הנה יקרו אלו החליים: בילדים הקטנים בעת שיולדו יקרה
להם השחין אשר בפה והקיא והשעול והיקיצה והפחד ומורסת הטבור ולחות האזנים.

אמר המפרש: יקרה להם שחין הפה העבור רכות איבריהם ומה שבחלב מן הנגוב והקיא   5
לרוב מה שינקו וחולשת הכח המחזיק לחוזק הלחות והשעול בעבור ליחות הריאה ורוב מה
שיגר ממוחם לחוזק לחות לריאה והיא הסבה בליחות האזנים כי מותרי המח ידחו לאזנים
ומורסת הטבור לקרוב הזמן מן החתוך והפחד רובו בשינה להפסד בשול האצטומכא יעלה
עשנו אל המוח ויחדש דמיונים מפחידים. ואולם היקיצה הנה לא ידע לו גאלינוס סבה אמר
כי הענין המיוחד בנערים רבוי השינה וזה אמת אבל הרבה פעמים תקרה להם היקיצה והבכי   10
כל הלילה וסבת זה חוזק הרגשתם לרכות גופותם וכחותם כלם חלושות בלתי קיימות ומעט
דבר מן הכאב יקיצם ומעט שיקרם מהפסד בשול וצער מפני האצטומכא לרוב יניקתם ויעירם
הכאב ההוא ואם נוסף מעט יבכו וזה נראה תמיד.

(3.25)

[131] אמר אבקראט: וכאשר קרב היד שיצמחו לו השנים יקרה לו חיכוך בחניכים וקדחות
וקווץ ושלשול כל שכן כאשר יצמחו השנים אשר כנגד העינים ולשמן מן הנערים ולמי שבטנו   15
עצור.

אמר המפרש: זה כלו בעבור כי השנים יבקעו וינקבו בשר החניכים וירחיבו הנקב ותמשך
אחר זה הכאב והקדחות והקווץ ולהיות המזון בלתי מתבשל בשול טוב בעבור הכאב והיקיצה
יתחדש השלשול ורוב מה שיתחדש הקווץ לשמן ולעצור הבטן לרבוי מותרי גופותם.

(3.26)

[132] אמר אבקראט: וכאשר עבר היד אלו אלו השנים יקרה לו מורסת הגרון והכנסת   20
חוליות הצואר והרנפלי והאבן והתולעים הגדולים והקטנים והיבלת הנתלית והחזירים ושאר
הנגעים.

---

2 הרובמאס: הרומאס אבהה‎ 5 הנגוב: الجلاء‎ a 6 שינקו: מהחלב א² add. 9 היקיצה: עניין‎
היקיצה א || אמר: א om. بل قال‎ a 12 שיקרם: שיקעו א שיקדים ח שיקדים א ואפשר שיקרב‎
להם רוע עכול והערה מפני האצ' א¹ أَنْ يَفْقُدوا‎ a 14–15 בחניכים וקדחות וקווץ ושלשול כל שכן‎
כאשר יצמחו השנים אשר כנגד: א¹ 15 העינים: הפנים ח || ולשמן: העב א add.² 17 החנכים: החנך‎
בדח החיך ח 19 לשמן: העב א² add. 20 והכנסת: והכנס א 21 חוליות: חליי ד || והרנפלי‎
(cf. French ronflar, O.Occ. ronflar, i.e., to snore, to grumble):והרנפלי ח והרינפלי ח || והתולעים‎
הגדולים והקטנים: والحيّات والدود‎ a

אמר המפרש: אחר צמיחת השנים עד קרוב לשלוש עשרה שנה יאכלו הנערים המזונות
הרבות וירבו השתיה ויכניסו מאכל אחר מאכל וירבו תנועתם אחר המאכל וכל ההנהגה
הזאת מפסדת הבשול מרבה הליחות וגופותם עם זה לחים ואיבריהם רכים. ויתחייב
כל מה שזכרנו בעבור כי כאשר התנפח מיתר הגרון משך החוליה מן הצואר לרכות
קשריהם.

(3.27)

[133] אמר אבקראט: ואולם מי שעבר אלו השנים וקרב שיצמח לו השער סביב הערוה הנה
יקרו לו רבים מאלו החליים וקדחות יותר ארוכות וצאת דם הנחירים.

אמר המפרש: באלו השנים ירבה הדם וירוץ בהם ולכן יתחדש להם צאת דם הנחירים.

(3.28)

[134] אמר אבקראט: ורוב מה שיקרה לנערים מן החליים יבא בקצתו הנקיון בארבעים יום
ובקצתו בשבעה חדשים ובקצתו בשבע שנים ובקצתו כאשר גמרו לצמח השער בשפל הבטן.
ואולם מה שישאר מן החליים שלא יתך בזמן הצמיחה או בנקבות בעת שיגר מהן דם הנדות
הנה מדרכם שיאריכו.

אמר המפרש: ר״ל מן החליים הנושנים.

(3.29)

[135] אמר אבקראט: ואולם הבחורים הנה יקרה להם רקיקת הדם והשדפון והקדחות החדות
וחולי הנופל ושאר החליים אבל כי רוב מה שיקרה להם מה שזכרנוהו.

אמר המפרש: כבר ביאר ג׳אלינוס כי אין פנים להיות חולי הנופל מיוחד בבחרות אבל הוא
מחלי הנערים.

(3.30)

[136] אמר אבקראט: ואולם מי שעבר אלו השנים הנה יקרה לו הרנפלי וחלי הצד וחלי
הריאה והקדחת אשר תהיה עמה היקיצה והקדחת אשר יהיה עמה ערבוב השכל והקדחת
השורפת והשפיכה והשלשול הארוך וחמרמרות המעים וקלוח המעים ופתיחת פיות העורקים
מלמטה.

---

4 משך: ימשוך א 7 יקרו: יקרה א 8 השנים: ד om. 10 ובקצתו: ובקצתם א || ובקצתו: ובקצתם
א || גמרו: شارفوا a 11 דם: א om. 12 שיאריכו: וישארו עם האדם כל זמן שהוא נשאר add. א
15 אבל כי: אלא ש- א || להם: הוא ד add. 20 והשפיכה: אלהיצ׳ה א¹ || ופתיחת (= وانفتاح): وانفتاخ
emendation editor

אמר המפרש: ידוע שאלו השנים והם שנות הזקנים הליחה השחורה בהם נראית על הרוב ולכן ייוחד בהם בלבול השכל והיקיצה בקדחות ופתיחת פיות העורקים. ואולם שאר מה שמנה אינם מיוחדים באלו השנים וגאלינוס חושב שהוא נתן סבות מיוחדות באלו השנים ואיננו כן.

(3.31)

[137] אמר אבקראט: ואולם הישישים הנה יקרה להם רוע הנשימה והירידה אשר יקרה עמה

5 השעול וטפטוף השתן ועצירתו וכאבי הפרקים וכאבי הכליות והסבוב והשתוק והנגעים הרעים וחכוך הגוף והיקיצה ורכות הטבע ולחות בעינים והנחירים וחושך הראות ולובן העינים וכבדות השמע ואלזרקה פירו׳ מראה החשמל.

אמר המפרש: סבות אלו כלם מבוארות למי שידע ענין מזג הישישים.

נשלם המאמר השלישי מפרוש הפרקים.

---

1 שנות: ד .om   2 ייוחד: נתיחד א ‖ ופתיחת (= وانفتاح): ופתיחת א וلنفاخ emendation editor   3 וגאלינוس: ואולי ד   4 והירידה: הנזילה אי   6–7 ולובן העינים וכבדות השמע ואלזרקה פירו׳ מראה החשמל: ולובן העינים פי׳ מראה החשמל וכבדות ואלזרקה הוא כעין תבלת א וכבדות השמע בח والزرقة وثقل السمع   a 9 נשלם המאמר השלישי מפרוש הפרקים: נשלם המאמר השלישי א ה .om

המאמר הרביעי מפ׳ הפרקים לאבקראט

(4.1)

[138] אמר אבקראט: ראוי שתנתן הרפואה למעוברת כאשר יהיו הליחות מתעוררות אחר
שיעבור על הולד ארבעה חדשים עד שיעברו עליו שבעה חדשים ויכניס עצמו בזה מעט ואולם
המעט מזה והיותר הנה ראוי שישמור ממנו.

אמר המפרש: זה מבואר כי ⟨הוא⟩ בתחלתו חלוש ויקל הפלתו וסופו כבר הכביד וגדל ויעזור
5   על נפילתו בכבדותו.

(4.2)

[139] אמר אבקראט: אמנם ראוי שישקוה מן הרפואה מה שיריק מן הגוף המין אשר אם יורק
מעצמו תועיל הרקתו ואולם מה שהיתה הרקתו בחלוף זה הנה ראוי שיפסיקהו.

אמר המפרש: זה מבואר.

(4.3)

[140] אמר אבקראט: אם הורק מן הגוף מן המין אשר ראוי שינוקה ממנו יועיל ויסבול בקלות
10   ואם היה הענין בהפך זה היה קשה.

אמר המפרש: ספר לנו הנה בזה כדי שיהיה זה אות יודע בו אם הישרנו בסברא או טעינו ר״ל
קלות סבל ההרקה או קשיו.

(4.4)

[141] אמר אבקראט: ראוי שיהיה מה שיעשה מן ההרקה ברפואה בקיץ מלמעלה יותר ובסתו
מלמטה.
15

אמר המפרש: הגובר בקיץ המרה האדומה והחום ישים הליחות מתנועעות למעלה ולכן יעשה
ההרקה בקיא ובסתו ההפך.

(4.5)

[142] אמר אבקראט: אחר זמן עליית הכלב ובעת עלייתו ולפניו קשה ההרקה ברפואה.

<hr>

אמר המפרש: הזמן הזה החזק שיהיה מן הקיץ והכחות חלושות חלושות מאד וחום האויר ימנע משיכת הרפואה ולא יגיע ממנה כי אם חולשה והסתערות.

(4.6)

[143] אמר אבקראט: מי שהיה רזה הגוף יהיה הקיא נקל עליו ושים הרקתו אם כן ברפואה מלמעלה והשמר שלא תעשה זה בסתו.

אמר המפרש: ענין הכחוש תמיד כענין רוב האנשים בקיץ וכבר קדמה האזהרה מעשות הקיא 5 בסתו.

(4.7)

[144] אמר אבקראט: מי שיהיה קשה עליו הקיא והיה מבריאות הבשר על ענין ממוצע שים הרקתו ברפואה מלמטה והשמר שלא תעשה זה בקיץ.

אמר המפרש: זה מבואר.

(4.8)

[145] אמר אבקראט: בעלי השדפון כאשר תריק אותם ברפואה השמר שלא תריקם 10 מלמעלה.

אמר המפרש: ר״ל המוכנים לשדפון והם צרי החזה כי מעברי ריאתיהם צרים גם כן ולא ימשך אליהם חמרים.

(4.9)

[146] אמר אבקראט: מי שיגבר עליו המרה השחורה הנה ראוי שתריקהו מלמטה ברפואה יותר עבה כאשר תחבר שני ההפכים אל הקש אחד. 15

אמר המפרש: ברפואה יותר עבה ר״ל יותר חזקה והמרה האדומה צפה למעלה והשחורה צוללת למטה וההקש האחד הוא אשר יעשה בזה בחר אחד משני ההפכים לאחת משתי הליחות כי אנחנו נריק כל ליחה ממקומה הקרוב ליציאתה.

---

1 וחום: emendation editor ואז חום א או חום **בדהח**   4 בסתו: אמנם מי שיקשה הקיא והיה מרבוי הבשר על הענין הממוצע תשים הרקתך אותו ברפואה מתחת ותשמר שלא תעשה כן בקיץ א .add   9 מבואר: נגלה א .add   12 צרים: الجَارِي .add. a ‖ ולא: ולא יאות א ואין ראוי א¹ ‖ ימשך: שימשוך א   15 תחבר: א¹ תלוה א   16 והמרה: כי המרה א   17 בחר: לבחור א בחם(!) **בח**

(4.10)

[147] אמר אבקראט: ראוי שתעשה רפואת ההרקה בחליים החדים מאד כאשר יהיו הליחות
מתעוררות מן היום הראשון כי אחורו בכמו החליים האלה רע.

אמר המפרש: זה מבואר ויפחד מלכת אלו הליחות הנגרות הבלתי נחות ממקום למקום
וחלילה שינוחו באבר נכבד ולכן יתחיל בהרקתם קודם שיחלש הכח או שינוחו במקום
נכבד.   5

(4.11)

[148] אמר אבקראט: מי שהיו בו צירים וכאב תחת הטבור וכאב בשפל הבטן תמיד ולא יסורו
ברפואה משלשלת ולא בזולתה הנה עניינו יבוא אל השקוי היבש.

אמר המפרש: כאשר לא יותך זה ברפואה הנה הוא ראיה על הפסד מזג שגבר על האיברים
ההם ונשתקע בהם ויחדש השקוי התופי והוא אשר קראו כנגד השקוי הנאדי אשר בו
המים והנודי יתחדש מקור נוסף.   10

(4.12)

[149] אמר אבקראט: מי שהיה בו קלוח המעים בסתו הנה הרקתו ברפואה מלמעלה רע.

אמר המפרש: יאמר שאפילו יהיה מביא לקלוח המעים ליחה חדה דקה תצוף אשר יחייב זה
שתורק בקיא בעבור שהזמן סתו הנה אין דרך לעשות הקיא כמו שקדם.

(4.13)

[150] אמר אבקראט: מי שהוצרך לקחת הליבורוס הוא אלחרבק והיתה הרקתו מלמעלה ולא
ישמע לו בקלות ראוי שירטיב גופו קודם שיקח אותו במזון יותר ובמנוחה.   15

אמר המפרש: זה מבואר.

(4.14)

[151] אמר אבקראט: כאשר השקית לאדם לברוס תהיה כונתך להניע גופו יותר ולישן ולנוח
פחות והנה יורה ההליכה בספינות על שהתנועה תעורר הגופות.

אמר המפרש: ידוע כי הליברוס מביא הקיא בחזקה והניע הגוף תנועה מקומית ממה שיעזור
על הקיא והביא ראיה מרכיבת הים.   20

(4.15)

[152] אמר אבקראט: כשתרצה שתהיה הרקת הליברוס יותר הניע הגוף וכאשר תרצה שתתפסיקהו צוה לישן השותה ולא תניעהו.

אמר המפרש: זה מבואר וכפול.

(4.16)

[153] אמר אבקראט: שתיית הליברוס סכנה למי שהיה בשרו בריא וזה כי הוא ימשוך קווץ.

5 **אמר המפרש:** זה מבואר.

(4.17)

[154] אמר אבקראט: מי שלא תהיה בו קדחת והיה בו מניעה מן המאכל ונשיכה במוראה וסבוב ומרירות בפה הנה זה יורה על שהרקתו ברפואה מלמעלה.

אמר המפרש: המוראה ר״ל פי האצטומכא והנשיכה והסבוב ר״ל שידמה לאדם שיסבוב מה שסביבו ויאבד חוש הראות פתאום עד שיחשוב שכסה כל מה שהיה רואה חושך ואלו 10 המקרים יהיו כשיהיה בפי האצטו׳ ליחות רעות עוקצות אותה ולבן ראוי כשיראו אלו המקרים שיורק בקיא.

(4.18)

[155] אמר אבקראט: הכאבים אשר יהיו למעלה מהיותרת יורו על שההרקה ברפואה מלמעלה והכאבים אשר מלמטה מן היותרת יורו על שההרקה ברפואה מלמטה.

אמר המפרש: אל אי זה צד מן הצדדים נטו הליחות ונתישבו שם הנה מן המקום ההוא יורקו ברפואה מקיאה מלמעלה או משלשל מלמטה ואולם בעת השפך הליחות הנה ראוי שימשכו 15 אל הפך הצד.

(4.19)

[156] אמר אבקראט: מי ששתה רפואת ההרקה והורק ולא צמא אין ראוי להפסיק ממנו ההרקה עד שיצמא.

אמר המפרש: הצמא אחר שתיית הרפואה כאשר לא יהיה בעבור חום האצטומכא ויבשה או בעבור חדוד הרפואה או בעבור היות הליחה המורקת חמה הנה הוא יורה על נקיון האיברים 20 ורקותם מן הליחה ההיא אשר נרצה הוצאתה.

1 הליברוס: הליבורוס **אבח** ‖ 4 הליברוס: הליבורוס **אבח** ‖ ימשוך: יולד א يحدث a ‖ 6 במוראה: בוושט **בחח** ‖ והנשיכה: والنخس اللدغ a ‖ 10 יהיו: היה **ד** ‖ 12 מהיותרת: מהטרפשא **א** ‖ 13 מן היותרת: לטרפשא **א** ‖ 15 משלשל: משלשלת א²**בח**

(4.20)

[157] אמר אבקראט: מי שלא היתה בו קדחת ומצאוהו צירים וכבדות בארכובות וכאב בשפל הבטן הנה הנה הוא מורה שהוא צריך אל ההרקה ברפואה מלמטה.

אמר המפרש: זה מבואר.

(4.21)

[158] אמר אבקראט: הצואה השחורה הדומה לדם הבאה מעצמה היה עם קדחת או בלתי קדחת היא מן היותר רעות שבאותות וכל מה שהיו המראים יותר (רעים) בצואה היו אות (יותר) רע וכאשר היה זה זה עם שתיית רפואה יהיה אות יותר טוב וכל מה שיהיו אותם המראים יותר יהיה זה יותר רחוק מן הרוע.

אמר המפרש: זה מבואר.

(4.22)

[159] אמר אבקראט: אי זה חולי תצא בתחלתו המרה השחורה מלמטה או מלמעלה הנה זה בו אות מורה על המות.

אמר המפרש: כל זמן שיהיה החולי בהתחלתו הנה אין דבר ממה שיצא מגוף החולה תהיה יציאתו בתנועה מן הטבע אבל תהיה יציאתו מקרה דבק לעניינים הם בגוף חוץ מן הטבע. והמרה השחורה היא הליחה העבה הדומה בשמרים כאשר נשרפה ויצאה מהיות המרה השחורה הטבעית ויציאת אלו הליחות הרעות קודם הבשול ראיה על היותם נושכים האיברים לחוזק רעתם ולא יוכלו האיברים להחזיק בהם עד שיתבשלו.

(4.23)

[160] אמר אבקראט: מי שכבר החלישו חולי חד או נושן או נפילה או זולת זה ואחר כן יצא ממנו מרה שחורה או כמו דם שחור הנה הוא ימות ממחרת היום ההוא.

אמר המפרש: הטבע במי שעניננו כן כבר חלש עד שלא יוכל שיבשל ולא יבדיל הרע מן הטוב ולא יריק אלו הליחות אשר הם מן הרוע על מה שהם בו. אבל לגודל החולי ויתרונו ישפעו וישפכו כי אין דבר שיחזיק בהם. ואמרו או כמו דם השחור ר"ל הצואה השחורה וההבדל בין המרה השחורה והצואה השחורה כי המרה השחורה זבה ועמה לטישה ועקיצה דומה בחדוד החומץ תחלוק הארץ כשתפול עליה ואין דבר מזה בצואה השחורה.

---

4 הצואה: היציאה ח 5 בצואה: ביציאה ח 6 זה: ד .om 7 יותר: בצואה אבח .add ביציאה ח
.add || יותר: ד .om 9 המרה השחורה: נ"א הצואה אי 11 אין: ראוי דה .add 12 אבל תהיה
יציאתו מקרה דבק לעניינים הם בגוף חוץ מן הטבע: א .om 13 הדומה: החמה דה 14 ויציאת: וצאת
אוצואה בח 17 ממחרת: מחרת ד 18 הרע מן הטוב: a .om 19 אבל: בדה .om || ויתרונו: ויתרוניו
a وتفاقه 20 הצואה: היציאה ח 21–20 וההבדל בין המרה השחורה והצואה השחורה: דה .om
21 לטישה: צהוב בח 22 תחלוק: وتقشر a || בצואה: ביציאה ח

(4.24)

[161] אמר אבקראט: שלשול הדם כשיהיה התחלתו מן המרה השחורה הנה הוא אות המות.

אמר המפרש: כאשר התחיל יציאת המרה האדומה וחמרמרו ממנה המעים ונתנגעו ובא הדם
אחר כן הנה אפשר להרפא החמרמרות. ואולם כשתהיה הליחה המרה השחורה היא אשר
עשתה החמרמרות עד שבא הדם הנה בלא ספק יתחדש במעים דומה בסרטן המתחדש
5   בשטח הגוף.

(4.25)

[162] אמר אבקראט: יציאת הדם מלמעלה באי זה ענין שיהיה הוא אות רע ויציאתו מלמטה
הוא אות טוב וכל שכן כשיצא בו דבר שחור.

אמר המפרש: ר״ל מלמעלה בקיא ואמנם יהיה מלמטה טוב כשידחה אותו הטבע על צד נקיון
המותרות כמו שיגר מן הטחורים ובתנאי שיהיה מעט.

(4.26)

[163] אמר אבקראט: מי שהיה בו שלשול מדם ויצא ממנו דומה בחתיכות הבשר הנה הוא
10   מאותות המות.

אמר המפרש: כי זה ראיה על שקיעת הנגע במעים עד אשר יחתוך גרמם ואי אפשר להחתם
הבשר ההוא.

(4.27)

[164] אמר אבקראט: מי שיצא ממנו בקדחות דם רב מאי זה מקום שיהיה הנה יציאתו כאשר
15   יבריא יאכל דברים שירפה בטנו ביותר מן השיעור.

אמר המפרש: לחולשת החום הטבעי בגופו בעבור הרקת הדם ימעט משיכת האיברים המזון
ויחלש הבשול וירכך הטבע.

(4.28)

[165] אמר אבקראט: מי שהיה בו שלשול המרה האדומה וימצאהו חרשות יפסק ממנו
השלשול ההוא ומי שהיה בו חרשות ויתחדש בו שלשול מרה אדומה יסור ממנו החרשות.

---

2 כאשר: אם כבר א   3 ואולם כשתהיה הליחה: אבל אם תהיה זו הליחה א   4-3 ואולם ...
החמרמרות: ד om.   4 החמרמרות: ثُمَّ قَرَّح ‖ add. a   הדם: فلا برء له add. a ‖ בלא ספק: a om.
6 שיהיה: הנה א add. ‖ אות: ד om.   7 וכל שכן: ד om.   9 שיגר מן הטחורים: يجري في البواسير
a   15-14 כאשר יבריא יאכל דברים שירפה בטנו: כאשר יחלישהו ישוב ברכות הטבע בדחה عندما
ينقه فيغذا يلين بطنه a   15 יאכל דברים שירפה בטנו: ישוב ברכות הטבע א¹   17 וירכך: ולזה ירכך א
18 וימצאהו: ויקרה לו בח

אמר המפרש: סבת זה מבוארת ללכת החומר בחלוף הצד ובאר כי דבורו הנה בחרשות אשר יקרה פתאום בחליים ובפרט בקרוב מן הנקיון.

(4.29)

[166] אמר אבקראט: מי שיקרה לו בקדחת ביום הששי מחליו פלצות הנה נקיונו יהיה קשה.

אמר המפרש: כאשר התחדש הפלצות בקדחות וכל שכן בשורפות ממנהגו שיבוא הנקיון
5 אחריו וכבר נודע רוע נקיון הששי והוא ענין אמרו קשה.

(4.30)

[167] אמר אבקראט: מי שהיה לקדחתו עונות הנה באיזו שעה שתהיה עזיבתה כשתהיה לקיחתה ממחרת בשעה ההיא בעצמה הנה נקיונה יהיה קשה.

אמר המפרש: באר כי כשהיו עונות הקדחת כלם קיימות על ענין אחד בהתחלתם ותכליתם
הנה זה ראיה על אריכות החולי והוא ענין אמרו הנה נקיונה יהיה קשה כאלו יאמר שהוא קשה
10 שתכלה הקדחת הזאת בנקיון כי הנקיון אמנם יהיה לחוליים החדים ואולם החוליים הנושנים
הנה הם יותכו באריכות.

(4.31)

[168] אמר אבקראט: בעל היגיעה בקדחת רוב מה שיצא בו היציאה בפרקיו ואל צד הלחיים.

אמר המפרש: חום הקדחת וחום האיברים מבעל היגיעה ידחה המותר לפרקים ולעליון הגוף
כי יקבלהו הבשר הרפה אשר בפרקי הלחיים.

(4.32)

15 [169] אמר אבקראט: מי שנצל מחולי וחש מקום מגופו יתחדש במקום ההוא יציאה.

אמר המפרש: יאמר כי הקם מחולי כאשר ייגע אבר מאיבריו ויקרה לו בו כאב הנה יצא שם
יציאה והסבה מבוארת וכבר זכר גאלינוס כי התחדש הכאב ג״כ יקרא חש.

(4.33)

[170] אמר אבקראט: ואם היה ג״כ כבר קדם ויגע אבר מן האיברים קודם שיחלה בעליו הנה
באבר ההוא ישתקע החולי.

1 ובאר: ובארנו א‎ 3 שיקרה: שהיה א‎ 5 רוע נקיון הששי: ענין רוע הנקיון בששי א‎ 13 חום: بِسَبِب
حرارة a‎ 15 וחש: فكلّ a‎ 17 חש: كلال a‎

אמר המפרש: זה מבואר זכר הנה היגיעה הקודמת לחולי עד שתהיה היא הסבה לחולי וזכר
בפרק אשר לפניו היגיעה אשר תהיה אחר צאתו מן החולי וזכר בשלישי אשר קודם זה היגיעה
שתהיה מעצם החולי ואולם יפחד מאלו היציאות כלם בנקיונים אשר לא תהיה בהם הרקה
נגלית.

(4.34)

[171] אמר אבקראט: מי שקרה לו קדחת ואין בגרונו נפח וקרה לו חנק פתאום הנה זה מאותות
המות.

אמר המפרש: החנק פתאום אמנם יהיה מפני הסתם השפוי כובע והמוקדח צריך אל שאיפת
אויר קר רב וכאשר ימנע האויר ימות בלא ספק ואולם התנה שלא יהיה שם נפח כי פעמים
תהיה הקדחת נמשכת למורסת הגרון ויהיה החנק בא מעט מעט לתוספת המורסא ועם
תכליתו אפשר שירד גם כן מעט מעט וינצל החולה.

(4.35)

[172] אמר אבקראט: מי שיקרה לו הקדחת ונתעות עמה צוארו ויכבד עליו הבליעה עד שלא
יוכל לבלוע כי עם בקושי מבלתי שיראה בו נפח הנה זה מאותות המות.

אמר המפרש: עוות הצואר ועוצר הבליעה יהיה מסור אחת מן החליות וסורה פעמים יהיה
בעבור מורסא ופעמים יהיה לתגבורת היובש ואשר ירצה בו הנה הוא המתהווה מתגברות
היובש כי הוא ראיה על שקיעת הפסד המזג באיברים ותגבורת היובש.

(4.36)

[173] אמר אבקראט: הזיעה המשובחת במוקדח אם התחילה ביום השלישי או בחמישי או
בשביעי או בתשיעי או באחד עשר או בארבעה עשר או בשבעה עשר או בעשרים או בארבעה
ועשרים או בשבעה ועשרים או באחד ושלושים או ארבעה ושלושים כי הזיעה אשר תהיה
באלו הימים יהיה בה נקיון החליים ואולם הזיעה אשר לא תהיה באלו הימים הנה היא תורה
על חולי או על אריכות החולי.

אמר המפרש: אין המשפט הזה בזיעה לבדה אבל בכל ההרקות אשר יהיה בהם הנקיון כי טבע
אלו הימים להיות בהם הנקיון כבר נודע בנסיון וכל נקיון בזיעה או בזולתה מן ההרקות כבר
נמצא בנסיון בהיותו על הרוב באלו הימים.

---

2 לפניו: קדם א ‖ היגיעה: הטורח א ‖ היציאה א   3 יפחד: יפלו א יפוחד א¹ ‖ בנקיונים:
בנקיונם אד ח om.   7 הסתם: הסתר ד   8 רב: א om.   9–10 ועם תכליתו: ובעמידתה א
13 יהיה מסור אחת מן החליות וסורה פעמים: א om.   14 ירצה: רצה אבהח ‖ הוא המתהווה: יהיה
א   16 השלישי: או ביום הרביעי א add.   17 עשר: או ביום תשעה עשר א add. ‖ או ביום
שלשים א add. ‖ ושלושים: או ביום שבעה ושלשים א add.   18 ועשרים: או ביום

(4.37)

[174] אמר אבקראט: הזיעה הקרה כשתהיה עם קדחת חדה תורה על מות וכאשר תהיה עם
קדחת נחה תורה על אריכות החולי.

אמר המפרש: חוזק הקדחת יכבה החום הטבעי ולא יתבשלו הליחות הקרות מאד אשר
בנראה מן הגוף אשר מהם תצא הזיעה הקרה ותורה על נאות הליחות האלה וחוזק קרירותם
היות חום הקדחת החזקה לא יוכל לחמם מה שיצא מהם.   5

(4.38)

[175] אמר אבקראט: באשר תהיה הזיעה מן הגוף הנה היא תורה על שהחולי במקום ההוא.

אמר המפרש: ולכן היתה הזיעה מן המקום ההוא לבדו אשר בו הליחה הנאצרת.

(4.39)

[176] אמר אבקראט: אי זה מקום מן הגוף היה קר או חם הנה בו החולי.

אמר המפרש: זה מבואר.

(4.40)

[177] אמר אבקראט: כאשר יתחדש בגוף כלו שנויים ויהיה הגוף יתקרר פעם ואחר כך יתחמם   10
פעם אחרת או יהיה במראה אחד ואחר כן ישתנה ממנו יורה על אריכות החולי.

אמר המפרש: החולי אשר הוא ממינים רבים הוא לעולם יותר ארוך מן החולי אשר הוא ממין
אחד.

(4.41)

[178] אמר אבקראט: הזיעה הגדולה אשר תהיה אחר השינה מבלתי סבה מבוארת תורה על
כי בעליו שם בגופו מן המזון יותר ממה שיסבול ואם היה זה זה והוא לא לקח מזון יותר מדאי דע   15
כי גופו צריך אל הרקה.

אמר המפרש: זה מבואר.

(4.42)

[179] אמר אבקראט: הזיעה הרבה אשר תגר תמיד תהיה קרה או חמה הנה הקרה ממנה
מורה שהחולי יותר גדול והחמה ממנה תורה על שהחולי יותר קל.

---

4 וחוזק: לחוזק **א**   6 באשר: במקום **אבח**   7 הנאצרת: הנאסרת **א**   11 ממנו: לזולתו **אי** .add
14 הגדולה: الكثير a

אמר המפרש: יאמר כי הזיעה אשר תהיה בשאר ימי החולי על דרך הנקיון מה שיהיה ממנה
קרה תהיה יותר רע כי היא מורה על קור החומר.

(4.43)

[180] אמר אבקראט: כאשר תהיה הקדחת בלתי נפרדת ואחר כך תתחזק ותשוב שלישית
היא יותר סכנה. וכאשר היתה הקדחת נפסקת על איזה פנים שתהיה הנה הוא מורה שאין
סכנה בה.

אמר המפרש: זאת אשר היא תמידית ותתחזק ותשוב שלישית אשר בה סכנה היא חצי
שלישית.

(4.44)

[181] אמר אבקראט: מי שמצאהו קדחת ארוכה הנה יקרה לו אם יציאות ואם שברון בפרקיו.

אמר המפרש: אורך הקדחת לרוב חומרה ולקור החומר או לעובי הליחה והחומר אשר זה
ענינה על הרוב תדחה אם לאבר אחד ותתחדש בו יציאה או למקום הפנוי בפרקים ותתחדש
כאב בפרקים.

(4.45)

[182] אמר אבקראט: מי שימצאהו יציאה או שברון בפרקים אחר הקדחת הנה הוא לוקח
אוכל מן המאכל יותר ממה שיסבול.

אמר המפרש: ר״ל אחר הקדחת אחר הפרד הקדחת לגמרי והוא עדיין חלוש.

(4.46)

[183] אמר אבקראט: כשיקרה פלצות בקדחת בלתי נפסקת למי שכבר נחלש הנה היא
מאותות המות.

אמר המפרש: אמר ג׳אלינוס כי אמרו כשיקרה מורה על התמדת הפלצות פעם אחר פעם
והתחדשו פעם אחר פעם והקדחת נשארת בלתי נפסקת ראיה על היות הטבע משתדל לנענע
הליחה המחליאה ולהוציאה ולא יוכל להתישבה והשתקעה באברים ויוסיף הכח חולשה
וחסרון להיותו בלתי סובל רעש הפלצות וזעזוע הגוף.

---

3 נפרדת: נפסקת בה ‖ ואחר כך: והיא א ‖ ותשוב שלישית: א¹ ביום השלישי א   4 נפסקת: בעלת
עונה מפסקת א   6 היא: תהיה א ‖ ותשוב שלישית: א¹ בשליש י: א¹ בשלישי א   8 שברון: וחולשה: א add. כלל a
9 חומרה: חומר א ‖ לעובי הליחה: לעוביו והליחה א   12 לוקח: אוכל ד   14 חלוש: ‏‏تﺎ8 a   17 פעם
אחר פעם: בפעם אחר הפעם א   18 והתחדשו: כי התחדשו א   19 והשתקעה: והשקעה א

(4.47)

[184] אמר אבקראט: בקדחות שלא יפסקו הרקיקה חשוכת המראה והדומה בדם והמוסרחת
ואשר היא מסוג המרה האדומה כולם רעות ואם יצאו יציאה טובה הם טובות. וכן הענין בצואה
או בשתן ואם יצא מה שאין תועלת ביציאתו מאחד מאלו המקומות הנה זה רע.

אמר המפרש: המאמר הכולל כי הדברים הרעים אשר יורקו יורו על ענינים רעים בגופות
אשר יורקו מהם אבל שהם פעמים תהיה יציאתם כמו יציאת המוגלא מן הנגעים המעופשים
ולא תהיה תועלת ביציאתם בחולי ההוא ופעמים תהיה יציאתם כמו יציאת המוגלא ממורסא
תפתח תהיה בה נקוי טוב לאבר אשר בו החולי והראיות המורות על היות יציאת מה שיצא
טוב הוא בשולו בפרט וסבול הגוף יציאתו בקלות ומצאו מרגוע בו ועם זה טבע החולי ואחריו
העת ההווה מן השנה והארץ והשנים וטבע החולה.

(4.48)

[185] אמר אבקראט: כשיהיה בקדחת בלתי נפסקת הנראה מן הגוף קר ותוכו שורף ויהיה
עם זה צמא הנה זה מאותות המות.

אמר המפרש: אמר ג'אלינוס כי המקרה הזה לא ימצא תמיד כי אם בקצת הקדחות אשר לא
יפסקו וסבתו אמר כי תתחדש מורסא חמה בקצת האברים הפנימיים ותמשוך הדם והרוח
אל האבר החולה מן הגוף כלו ולכן ישרף פנים הגוף חום והעור קר כמו שיקרה בתחלת עונות
הקדחת. זה סבתו לפי דעת גאלינוס והוא בלתי אמת כי הוא אלו התחייב זה היה המקרה הזה
מתחייב לכל מורסא חמה תתחדש באברים הפנימיים ואנחנו נראה תמיד בעלי חולי הצד
וחולי הריאה וחולי הכבד עורותיהם חמים מאד כמו תוך גופותם. ואשר נראה לי כי סבת זה
היות החמרים אשר בנראה מן הגוף עבים מאד קרים מאד לא ינצחם חום הליחה המעופשת
המולידה הקדחת אשר נתעפש בתוך הגוף וכל מה שהתהלב הדבר ההוא המעופש ועלה
חמימותו אל הנראה מן הגוף מבקש הנקבים יתנשם מהם ימצא מסך קר כנגדה ימנע החום
הוא מעבור שטח הגוף ויתהפך החום חוזר אחורנית ביותר חזק שיהיה אפשר וישרוף פנים
הגוף יותר ויתחזק הצמא ויקרה לחום אז דומה למה שיעשו הנפחים מהזות המים על האש
בכור הברזל עד שיתחזק חום פנים האש ויתיך הברזל וזאת סבה אמיתית טבעית אין ספק בה.

(4.49)

[186] אמר אבקראט: כאשר נתעות בקדחת בלתי נפסקת השפה או העין או החוטם או גביני
העין או לא יראה החולה או לא ישמע אי זה מאלו היה וכבר יחלש הנה המות קרובה ממנו.

אמר המפרש: זה מבואר כי כאשר נראו אלו האותות עם חולשת הכח וקדמה הקדחת נודע
כי היובש כבר גבר על עקרי העצבים ולכן התחדש העוות או זולתו ממה שזכר.

2 בצואה: ביציאה ‏ח‎ ‏8‎ בשולו: בשול ‏א‎ ‖ ומצאו: ומצא ‏א‎ וימצא ‏א‎¹ ‏10‎ הנראה מן הגוף: שטח הגוף
‏א‎ ‏14‎ כלו: om. ‏א‎ ‏22‎ אז: דבר ‏א‎ add. ‏23‎ עד שיתחזק חום פנים: ‏א‎¹ ‖ האש: om. ‏א‎

(4.50)

[187] אמר אבקראט: כאשר נתחדש בקדחת בלתי נפסקת רוע הנשימה וערבוב בשכל הנה זה מאותות המות.

אמר המפרש: זה מבואר כי החום כבר נשקע באברים עד שנחלש גם כן העצב המניע החזה והיותרת ונפסדה הנשימה.

(4.51)

[188] אמר אבקראט: היציאה אשר תתחדש בקדחת ולא תתך בזמני הנקיונים מודיעים מן החולי שיארך.

אמר המפרש: זה מבואר.

(4.52)

[189] אמר אבקראט: הדמע אשר יגר בקדחת או בזולתה מן החליים אם היה זה מרצון מן החולה אין זה מגונה ואם היה מבלתי רצון הנה הוא יותר רע.

אמר המפרש: זה מבואר לחולשת הכח המחזיק ואמרו יותר רע ראיה כי הראשון רע גם כן וזה שהוא אע״פ שיבכה ברצון הנה הוא ראיה על חולשת לבבו ולכן יתפעל מהר ויבואהו הבכי.

(4.53)

[190] אמר אבקראט: מי שנתמלאו שיניו בקדחת מליחות דבקות הקדחת שלו חזקה.

אמר המפרש: אלי הדבקיות אמנם יתחדשו מחום חזק פעלו בלחויות לבנות עד שנגבו אותם.

(4.54)

[191] אמר אבקראט: מי שקרה לו בקדחת שורפת שעול רב יבש ואחר כן יהיה מעורר אותו מעט הנה הוא בלתי אפשר שיצמא.

אמר המפרש: אמר ג׳אלינוס: אי אפשר בשעול ואפילו לא ירוק כלום שלא יתלחלחו קני הריאה ממה שימשך אליו עם השעול ולכן לא יצמא.

(4.55)

[192] אמר אבקראט: כל קדחת תהיה עם מורסת הבשר הרפה אשר באינגש וזולתו ממה שדומה לו הנה היא רעה אם לא שתהיה קדחת יום.

_____

8 מרצון: ברצון א 9 הנה: א .om 12 שנתמלאו: שנתכסו א غشيت a 13 הדבקיות: הליחות הדבקות א ‖ לבנות: לבניות א¹ .add 14 ואחר כן יהיה: ויהיה א 15 הוא: א .om 18 באינגש (= באינגש): cf. Romance inguina/inguines

אמר המפרש: כאשר היתה הקדחת בסבת מורסת האינגש והדומה לו מן הבשר הרפה הנה
תהיה קדחת יום ואמנם כאשר היתה הקדחת בסבה אחרת והתחבר עמה מורסת האינגש
והדומה לה הנה היא רעה כי סבת התנפח האינגש אז אמנם תהיה נמשך למורסת אחת מן
בני המעים וזאת המורסא הפנימית היא סבת הקדחת הקודמת ולכן היא מסוכנת.

(4.56)

[193] אמר אבקראט: כאשר היתה קדחת באדם ומצאתהו זיעה ולא תסור ממנו הקדחת הנה   5
היא אות רע וזה שהיא מורה באריכות מן החולי ותורה על לחות רב.

אמר המפרש: זה מבואר.

(4.57)

[194] אמר אבקראט: מי שקרהו קווץ או משיכה ואחר כן תמצאהו קדחת יותר בה חליו.

אמר המפרש: הקווץ שלשה מינים: הקווץ אשר לאחור והקווץ אשר לפנים והמשיכה ולא יראו
בה האברים מתקוצצים כי הם ימשכו לפנים ולאחור משיכה שווה וכל מיני הקווץ אם ממלוי   10
האברים העצביים ואם מהרקתם. ומה שנמשך מן הקווץ אחר קדחת שורפת הנה הוא מחוייב
שיהיה התחדשו מן היובש ומה שיהיה מן הקווץ יתחדש ראשון ופתאום הנה הוא מחוייב
שיהיה מן המלוא וכאשר התחדש אחריו קדחת תתיך קצת מליחות הנוספות ותבשל קצת
קרירותה.

(4.58)

[195] אמר אבקראט: כאשר תהיה באדם קדחת שורפת וקרה לו פלצות תתך בו קדחתו.   15

אמר המפרש: כאשר התנועעה הליחה האדומה לצאת התחדש הפלצות וימשך אחריו קיא
המרה האדומה ושלשול הבטן לצאת המותר ההוא המוליד לקדחת וכאשר יתרקנו עורקיו
תתך קדחתו.

(4.59)

[196] אמר אבקראט: השלישית היותר ארוכה תכלה בשבעה הקפים.

אמר המפרש: אמר ג'אלינוס: כבר הבטנו והשתכלנו הנקיון בקדחת הרביעית והשלישית   20
ומצאנוהו שהוא לפי חשבון מספר הסבובים לא לפי חשבון מספר הימים מזה כי הסבוב

———————————
3 והדומה לה הנה היא רעה כי סבת התנפח האינגש: א¹ ‖ הנה היא רעה: הוא רעה ד ‖ נמשך: om. א
נמשכת א² ‖ אחת: אחרת א   5 הנה: ד .om   7 מבואר: נגלה א   10 בה: בה: ד .om   11 ומה
שנמשך מן הקווץ אחר קדחת: فَا تبع من التَشنّج حمّى a   12–13 התחדשו מן היובש ומה שיהיה מן
הקווץ יתחדש ראשון ופתאום הנה הוא מחוייב שיהיה: א¹   14 קרירותה: קרירותם ה לחותם ה رطوبتها
21 שהוא לפי חשבון מספר הסבובים: לפי חשבונו שחשבנו מספר הכוכבים ד לפי מה שחשבנו   P
חשבון מספר הכוכבים ה

השביעי בשלישית יפול ביום השלשה עשר מתחלתה וביום ההוא ברוב יהיה נקיון
החולי ותכליתו מבלתי שימתין בו הארבעה עשר ומאמר אבוקראט בכאן הוא בשלישית
הפשוטה.

(4.60)

[197] אמר אבקראט: מי שימצאהו בקדחת החדה באזניו חרשות ויגר מנחיריו דם או שבא
5   לו שלשול יותר בזה חליו.

אמר המפרש: כבר קדמו סבות זה.

(4.61)

[198] אמר אבקראט: כשלא תהיה פרידת הקדחת מן המוקדח ביום מהימים הנפרדים הנה
ממנהגה שתשוב.

אמר המפרש: אמר ג'אלינוס כי זה טעות מן הסופר ושמאמר אבוקראט הוא ביום מימי הנקיון
10 היה זוג או נפרד.

(4.62)

[199] אמר אבקראט: כשיקרה הירקון בקדחת קודם היום השביעי הנה הוא אות רע.

אמר המפרש: פעמים יקרה הירקון על צד הנקיון ולא יהיה נקיון בירקון קודם השביעי אבל
אמנם סבתו שהוא מחוליי הכבד ולכן היה אות רע.

(4.63)

[200] אמר אבקראט: מי שימצאו בקדחתו פלצות בכל יום הנה קדחתו תכלה בכל יום.

אמר המפרש: ר"ל באמרו תכלה בכל יום שהיא תסור ממנו ותפסק ממנו בכל יום עם הרקת
15 הליחה המחייבת הפלצות עם תנועתה לצאת וכן ילך הענין בשלישית וברביעית.

(4.64)

[201] אמר אבקראט: כשיקרה הירקון בקדחת ביום שביעי או בתשיעי או בארבעה עשר הנה
זה טוב אם לא שיהיה הצד הימני ממה שלמטה מן החלצים קשה ואם היה כן הנה אין ענינו
טוב.

אמר המפרש: סבת זה מבוארת ממה שקדם.
20

---

2 ותכליתו: וכלותו א ‖ ומאמר: החכם א   6 זה: אלו א   12 השביעי: היום השביעי א

(4.65)

[202] אמר אבקראט: כשתהיה בקדחת התלהבות גדול באצטו' ודפיקה במוראה הנה זה אות רע.

אמר המפרש: אם היה רוצה במוראה פי האצטומכא הנה ענין אמרו דפיקה ר"ל עקיצה בפי האצטומכא להיותה משוקה בלחות אשר ממרה אדומה ואם היה רוצה באמרו המוראה הלב הנה הדפיקה תמצאהו להיות החום ממנו ושני אלו המקרים רעים מאד. 5

(4.66)

[203] אמר אבקראט: הקווץ והכאבים אשר יקרו בבני המעים בקדחות החדות אות רע.

אמר המפרש: הקדחת החזקה מאד תנגב העצבים כדמות האש ותמשכם ועל האופן הזה יתחדש הקווץ הממית ופעמים יקרה בבני המעים כאב מזה הענין בעצמו ר"ל מחוזק ההתלהבות והיובש.

(4.67)

[204] אמר אבקראט: הפחד והקווץ אשר יקרו בקדחת מן השינה מן האותות הרעים. 10

אמר המפרש: כאשר היה הגוף מלא מליחות הנה עם השינה יתמלא ראשו ויכבד המוח ואם היתה הליחה הגוברת נוטה אל השחורה יקרה ממנו הפחד ואם (לא) יהיה כן יקרה ממנו הכאב והיוץ. אמר ג'אלינוס שהוא ראה פעמים רבות בחליים ממיתים הפחד והכאב והקווץ יתחדשו מן השינה וידמה שיהיה זה עם לכת הליחה המזקת בעת השינה אל המוח.

(4.68)

[205] אמר אבקראט: כשיהיה האויר משתנה במעבריו בגוף הנה זה רע כי הוא יורה על קווץ. 15

אמר המפרש: רוצה באויר אויר הנשימה כאשר אצרו כלום במעבריו עד שיפסק בעת כניסתו או יציאתו או בשניהם יחד.

(4.69)

[206] אמר אבקראט: מי שיהיה שתנו עב דומה לדם הקפוי מעט ואין גופו נקי מן הקדחת הנה הוא כאשר השתין שתן רב דק יקבל תועלת בו ורוב מי שישתין זה השתן מי שהיה צולל בשתנו מהתחלת חליו או אחריו מעט מהר שמרים. 20

---

1 ודפיקה במוראה: ודפיקה בלב ובמוראה א בוושט ב*ח* add. פי האצטו *ח* add. وخفقان في الفؤاد a
4 המוראה: *אי* האלפؤاد א 5 להיות: לَـتَـكّن a 6 רע: הוא א 7 האש: فَتـمدده a add. a
9 והיובש: وروب היובש א 10 בקדחת מן השינה מן האותות הרעים: בקדחת מן השינה אות רע *דה*
16 אצרו כלום במעבריו: אסרו כלום במעבריו א יעצרנו שום דבר במעבריו *אי* حبسه شيء في مجاريه a
17 יחד: לפי שיורה על העצבים המניעים החזה קרה להם קצת קווץ *בח* add. א 18 לדם: כדם *אבח*

אמר המפרש: רוב הענין במוקדחים שיהיה השתן בהתחלת החולי דק וכל אשר יקרב אל
התכלית יתעבה עצמותו. והגיד לנו אבקראט בזה הענין הזר והוא כי פעמים יהיה השתן דומה
לטיט ומעט בתחלת החולי וסבת מיעוטו כי הוא לא יעבור בכליות כי אם בקושי וכאשר הורק
רוב הליחה ההיא הרעה והתבשל מה שנשאר ממנה יורק אז מן השתן מה שהוא יותר דק
5   ויותר רב.

(4.70)

[207] אמר אבקראט: מי שהשתין בקדחות שתן עכור דומה לשתן הבהמות הנה יש לו כאב
הראש או יתחדש לו.

אמר המפרש: אמנם יהיה השתן כן כאשר פעל החום בחמר עב רב ומה שהיה מן החמרים
בתאר הזה לבד כאשר פעל בו החום היוצא מהטבע יתילדו ממנו הרוחות עד שיתעבה
10   ויעכר כמו השעוה והזפת והסרפי והרוחות העבות עם החום ימהרו לעלות אל הראש
ויתחדש כאב הראש ופעמים היה עם השתנת השתן העכור ופעמים יהיה לפניו ופעמים
לאחריו.

(4.71)

[208] אמר אבקראט: מי שיבואהו הנקיון בשביעי הנה יראה בשתנו ענן אדום ושאר המופתים
יהיו על זה ההקש.

15   אמר המפרש: הרביעי יום הוראה למה שיהיה בשביעי וכל אות בעל שיעור יראה בו מורה
על הבישול הנה הוא יורה על הנקיון המתהווה בשביעי אבל הענן הלבן יותר ראוי שיורה על
זה ויותר קודם מן הענן הלבן התלוי באמצע השתן ואם היה החולה מהיר התנועה יהיה שינוי
המראה לבדו ושינוי העצמות ראיה מספקת על הנקיון המתהווה בשביעי. ואמר ג'אלינוס כי
אבקראט זכר העב האדום אשר הוא יותר חלוש כדי שיובן שאר האותות אשר הם יותר חזקים
20   ושהם יורו על שהנקיון מוכן. וכן האותות אשר יראו בימי ההוראה בצואה או ברקיקה על זה
ההקש.

(4.72)

[209] אמר אבקראט: כשיהיה השתן ספירי לבן הנה הוא רע וכל שכן בבעלי הקדחת אשר
עם מורסת המוח.

---

2 והגיד: וספר אבח והזכיר ח ‖ הזר: ד om. ‖ 8 שהיה: כן א .add   9 בו: בחומר ד ‖ מהטבע: ד
והסרף של   10 om.   והסרפי (Catalan serapi, a synonym of Catalan sagapin; i.e., gum resin):
הצנובר א ‖ העבות: הנה ד .add   11 ויתחדש כאב הראש: وترى الصداع a ‖ השתנת השתן העכור:
השתנות השתן העכור בהח البول المثوّر a   16 הענן: העב אבח   17 ויותר קודם מן הענן: وأول منها
السحاب a ‖ החולה: المرض a   19 שאר: שתי א   20 מוכן: مزمع a   22 ספירי: כמראה המים א¹
‖ add. הקדחת: הקדחות א

אמר המפרש: זה השתן בתכלית הרוחק מן הבשול ויורה על אריכות החולי ויורה עם זה כי
תנועת המרה האדומה כלה למעלה אל הראש.

(4.73)

[210] אמר אבקראט: מי שהיו המקומות אשר למטה מחלציו ממנו נפוחים ובהם קרקור ואחר
כן התחדש לו כאב בשפל שדרתו הנה בטנו יתרכך אם לא שיצאו ממנו רוחות רבות או
שישתין שתן רב וזה בקדחות.   5

אמר המפרש: כאשר נתגלגל הרוח עם הליחות המחייב לקרקור והתנועע למטה ירד הנפח אל
מה שקרוב מן הגב וימשכו האיברים אשר שם ויתחדש הכאב ופעמים ילך הלחות ההוא אל
העורקים ויצא השתן לבדו. ופעמים יצאו יחד הרוח והלחות מן המעים ויתרכך הבטן ופעמים
יעברו יחד אל העורקים ויעברו מהר למקוה הלחות והרוח. ובמי שיש בו קדחת לבד יהיה
בטוח באלו האותות וידע כי הטבע כבר חשב לדחות הדבר המזיק ולהוציאו בשתן או בצואה.   10

(4.74)

[211] אמר אבקראט: מי שתפחד שתצא לו יציאה באחד מפרקיו הנה ינצל מן היציאה ההיא
בשתן רב עב לבן יתילד כמו שפעמים יתחיל ברביעי מי שבו קדחת שעמה יגיעה ואם
יצא דם מנחיריו תהיה התכת חליו בו מהר מאד.

אמר המפרש: זה מבואר.

(4.75)

[212] אמר אבקראט: מי שהיה משתין דם ומוגלא הנה זה יורה כי יש נגע בכליותיו ובמקוה.   15

אמר המפרש: זה מבואר.

(4.76)

[213] אמר אבקראט: מי שהיה בשתנו בהיותו עבה חתכות בשר קטנות או כמו השער הנה
זה יוצא מכוליתו.

אמר המפרש: אולם חתכות הבשר הקטנות הם מעצם הכוליא בעצמה ואולם מה שהוא כמו
השער אי אפשר שיהיה לא מעצם הכליות ולא מעצם המקוה. ואמר ג׳אלינוס כי הוא ראה   20
אנשים קרה להם שהשתינו השיער הזה וקצתן היה ארכו כחצי זרוע מפני שהם אכלו מאכלים
מולידים ליחה עבה. וזאת הליחה העבה כאשר פעל בה החום עד שישרפה וינגבה בכליות

_____

3 שהיו: לו א .add   7 הגב: أسفل الصلب a   8 ויצא השתן לבדו: نفرجت بالبول وخرجت الرياح
وحدها a   9 מהר למקוה: مهرة אל המקוה א   11 ההיא: .om ד   12 יתילד: ممنا א .add ببوله a
14 זה מבואר: הנה זה כלו מבואר א   15 אמר ... ובמקוה: .om א׳ ד   16 אמר המפרש: זה מבואר:
איהי דה .om   17 בהיותו עבה: בדהה .om ‖ השער: השערות א

יתילד ממנה השיער הזה. ורפואת החולי הזה תעיד לפי ההקש האמתי בסבתו כי כאשר
מצאם החולי הזה הנה נרפאו ברפואות המדקדקות החותכות ומאמר אבקראט הנה זה יוצא
מכליותיו הודיענו המקום שיתילד בו השער הזה.

(4.77)

[214] אמר אבקראט: מי שיצא בשתנו והוא עב כמו הסובין הנה במקוה שלו גרב.

5 אמר המפרש: זה מבואר.

(4.78)

[215] אמר אבקראט: מי שהשתין דם מבלתי דבר קודם יורה זה שנבקע עורק בכליותיו.

אמר המפרש: זה מבואר.

(4.79)

[216] אמר אבקראט: מי שהיה צולל בשתנו דבר דומה לחול הנה אבן מתילד במקוה שלו.

(4.80)

[217] אמר אבקראט: מי שהשתין דם קרוש והיה בו הטפת שתן ומצאהו כאב בשפל בטנו
10 וסביב הערוה הנה מה שקרוב ממקותו כואב.

(4.81)

[218] אמר אבקראט: מי שהיה משתין דם ומוגלא וקליפות או שהיה לשתנו ריח מוסרח הנה
זה יורה שיש נגע במקותו.

(4.82)

[219] אמר אבקראט: מי שיצא באמתו מורסא הנה כאשר תתבשל ותפתח יתך חליו.

(4.83)

[220] אמר אבקראט: מי שהשתין בלילה שתן רב יורה זה שתתמעט צואתו.

15 אמר המפרש: כל אלו הפרקים מבוארים.

נשלם המאמר הרביעי מפרוש הפרקים.

---

2 אבקראט: החכם אבקראט א‎ ‏3 הודיענו: הורה א‎ ‏7 אמר המפרש: זה מבואר: א‎ om. ‏8 שהיה
צולל: שישקע א‎ ‏‖ אבן מתילד במקוה שלו: אבן יתילד לו במקוה א‎ ‏‖ שלו: قال المفسّر: هذا بيّن .add
a ‏9 אמר: עוד אמר א‎ ‏13 אמר: עוד אמר א‎ ‏14 אמר: עוד אמר א‎ ‏15 הפרקים: הם א‎ .add
16 נשלם המאמר הרביעי מפרוש הפרקים: נשלם המאמר הרביעי א ח‎ .om

המאמר החמישי מפירוש פרקי אבקראט

(5.1)

[221] אמר אבקראט: הקווץ אשר יהיה מהליברוס מאותות המות.

אמר המפרש: יקרה הקווץ משתיית הליברוס הלבן והוא המכוון בכאן אם לרוב ההרקה או
לחוזק תנועת הקיא ולעקיצת האצטו' וזה קשה להרפא.

(5.2)

[222] אמר אבקראט: הקווץ אשר יתחדש מנגע מאותות המות.   5

אמר המפרש: זה יהיה להתנפח העצבים ויעלה הכאב אל המוח וכל מה שיאמר אבקראט
מדבר שהוא מאותות המות רוצה בו גודל הסכנה ושהוא ימות ברוב.

(5.3)

[223] אמר אבקראט: כאשר יגר מן הגוף דם הרבה והתתחדש פיהוק או קווץ הנה הוא אות
רע.

אמר המפרש: זה מבואר.   10

(5.4)

[224] אמר אבקראט: כאשר התתחדש הקווץ או הפיהוק אחר הרקה מופלגת הנה הוא אות
רע.

אמר המפרש: זה מבואר.

(5.5)

[225] אמר אבקראט: כאשר קרה לשכור שיתוק פתאום הנה יתקווץ וימות אם לא שתתחדש
בו קדחת או ידבר כאשר הגיע העת שתסור בו שכרותו.   15

אמר המפרש: זה הקווץ יתחדש מפני מלוא העצבים ומדרך היין שימלא העצבים מהר כי הוא
יעמיק לדקותו וחומו והיין אם כן כאשר הרבו ממנו הנה הוא ברוב שעורו ימשוך לעצבים
קווץ אבל שהוא באיכותו ירפא ויתקן מה שהפסיד מה שהפסיד בעצבים כשיחממם וינגבם. ומי שלא יוכל

1 מפירוש פרקי אבקראט: אה om.   ‖ 3 אם: כי הוא א   5 מאותות: הוא אותות ד   6 להתנפח:
למורסא א' ‖ אבקראט: החכם אבקראט א   10 אמר המפרש: זה מבואר: אה om.   11 אמר: עוד
אמר א ‖ כאשר התתחדש: כשיקרה א ‖ מופלגת: מרובה א ‖ אות: סימן א   13 אמר המפרש: זה
מבואר: כל זה הוא מבואר א   15 בו: מעליו א   16 ומדרך: ומטבע א   17 ימשוך: ימשיך ד ‖ לעצבים:
העצבים א   18 אבל: אלא ד² ‖ ומי (= فَن): וכ- א فَتِى a

לעשות זה הנה יתחייב בהכרח שיגיע לקווץ המתחדש ממנו המות ובכח אשר אמרנו שהיין
ירפא בו הקווץ פעמים ירפאהו גם כן הקדחת והשכרות הוא נזק המתחדש בראש משתיית
היין.

(5.6)

[226] אמר אבקראט: מי שקרה לו המשיכה הנה ימות בארבעה ימים ואם עבר ארבעה ימים
5 הנה יתרפא.

אמר המפרש: המשיכה חולי חד מאד כאשר יהיה הטבע בלתי סובל טורח משיכתו כי הוא
מורכב מן הקווץ אשר יהיה לאחור והקווץ אשר יהיה לפנים ותכליתו יהיה בהקף הראשון
מהקפי ימי הנקיון.

(5.7)

[227] אמר אבקראט: מי שמצאו חולי הנופל קודם צמיחת השער סביב הערוה הנה יתחדש
10 לו העתק ואולם מי שקרה לו וכבר עברו עליו מן השנים חמישה ועשרים שנה הנה הוא ימות
והוא בו.

אמר המפרש: אמר ג'אלינוס: ירצה בהעתק תכלית החולי וזה יהיה בתיקון הליחה הקרה
המולידה לחולי הנופל והיא מליחה לבנה לחה בהעתק השנים אל היובש ובהתעמלות
ובהנהגה מנגבת עם הרפואות הנאותות. ואבקראט זכר בשער הזה השינוי אשר יהיה בסבת
15 השנים ומדת זמן צמיחת השער סביב הערוה הוא מה שבין תכלית שני השבועות ובין חמישה
ועשרים שנה.

(5.8)

[228] אמר אבקראט: מי שמצאהו חולי הצד ולא ינקה בארבעה עשר יום הנה יגיע ענינו
לעשות מוגלא.

אמר המפרש: אבקראט יקרא הרקת הליחה המולידה לחולי הצד ברקיקה נקוי.

(5.9)

[229] אמר אבקראט: רוב מה שיהיה השדפון בשנים אשר בין שמונה עשרה שנה ובין חמישה
20 ושלושים שנה.

---

1 יתחייב: יחייב א   2 ירפא: יתרפא אד² || והשכרות: הנקרא כמאר א add.¹   4 המשיכה: א¹ מתוח א
10 מי שקרה: כשקרה א || שנה: ד om. || הוא: א om.   12 תכלית: הכלות ד פי׳ שהליחה תבלה (...)
ד¹ || הקרה: الزَكِ add. a   13 לחה: א om.   14 ואבקראט: והחכם אבקראט א   15 שני השבועות:
השבוע השני א   17–18 יגיע ענינו לעשות: עניינו יגיע אל לעשות א ענינו יתהפך לעשות בח

אמר המפרש: כבר קדם כי השדפון מחליי הבחורים ובעבור שזכר חליי החזה והריאה זכר
זה גם כן.

(5.10)

[230] אמר אבקראט: מי שמצאהו אסכרא ונצל ממנו ונטתה הליחה אל ריאתו הנה הוא ימות
בשבעה ימים ואם יעבור אותם ישוב שיעשה מוגלא.

אמר המפרש: דע כי הרבו לו נסיונות אלו החליים והדומה להם בזה המין מן ההעתק ואין ספק
כי זה והדומה לו אמנם ירצה בו שהוא כן ברוב.

(5.11)

[231] אמר אבקראט: כשיהיה באדם שדפון ויהיה מה שירוק בשעול מן הרוק מוסרח כאשר
הושלך על הגחלים והיה שער הראש נושר הנה זה מאותות המות.

אמר המפרש: סרחון הריח ראיה על הפסד הליחות וחוזק עפושם ונשירות שער הראש ממה
שיחזק ראית הפסד הליחות וגם כן יורה על העדר המזון מן האברים.

(5.12)

[232] אמר אבקראט: מי שיפול שער ראשו מבעלי השדפון ואחר כן תתחדש לו שלשול הנה
הוא ימות.

אמר המרפש: שלשול אלו ראיה על חולשת הכח ולכן יורה על היות המות קרובה.

(5.13)

[233] אמר אבקראט: מי שירוק דם בקצף הנה רקיקתו אמנם היא מריאתו.

אמר המפרש: הנה הוא מבואר כי הדם אשר יצא בקצף הוא מגרם הריאה ועצמה.

(5.14)

[234] אמר אבקראט: כאשר התחדש למי שבו שדפון שלשול יורה על המות.

אמר המפרש: שלשול בעלי השדפון מורה על המות ואם זה היה עם סרחון ריח מה שירוק
ונפילת שער ראשו הנה יורה על קורבתה כמו שקדם.

_____

(5.15)

[235] אמר אבקראט: מי שהגיע בו העניין בחולי הצד לעשות מוגלא הנה אם יתנקה בארבעים יום מן היום אשר התחילה לצאת המוגלא הנה חליו ישלם ואם לא יתנקה תוך הזמן הזה הוא יפול בשדפון.

אמר המפרש: כאשר לא יצא החומר אשר נבקע והגיע בריקות החזה הנה יתעפש ויקפא וינגע 5 הריאה.

(5.16)

[236] אמר אבקראט: החום יזיק למי שהרבה להשתמש בו אלו הזקים: ירפה הבשר ויפתח העצבים ירדים השכל ויביא הגרת הדם והעלוף ויגיע לבעלי החליים האלה המות.

אמר המפרש: יאמר כי מי שהפליג בשמוש החום הנה הוא ירפה בשרו ויפתח העצבים ר״ל שיתן להם רפיון בהתיך החום לעצמו ואמרו ירדים השכל אמר ג׳אלינוס: רוצה בו חולשת 10 השכל שיסיר כחו בהתכת עצם העצבים והוא מבואר כי ימשך אחר הגרת הדם העלוף וימשך אחר העלוף המות.

(5.17)

[237] אמר אבקראט: ואולם הקור הנה יחדש הקווץ והמשיכה והשחרות והפלצות אשר יהיה עמו קדחת.

אמר המפרש: זה מבואר.

(5.18)

[238] אמר אבקראט: הקור מזיק לעצמות ולשניים ולעצבים ולמוח ולחוט השדרה ואולם 15 החום הנה הוא נאות ומועיל להם.

אמר המפרש: זה מבואר.

(5.19)

[239] אמר אבקראט: כל מקום שנתקרר הנה ראוי שיחומם אם לא שיפחדו עליו שיבקע הדם ממנו.

אמר המפרש: זה מבואר. 20

---

1 הנה: הוא א add. א ‖ 2 תוך הזמן הזה: בזה הזמן א 4 בריקות: בחלל א ‖ ויקפא: ויקרע ד
6 להשתמש: להתעסק א ‖ ויפתח: וירפה א 8 שהפליג בשמוש החום הנה הוא: שהפליג del.
לנהוג הדברים החמים א 9 בהתיך: בהתוך א ‖ אמר ג׳אלינוס: inv. א 10 שיסיר: והסרת א¹
12 והמשיכה: והמתוח א ‖ והשחרות: והשחרירות א 16 הוא: om. א 18 אם לא שיפחדו: אלא
אם יפחדו א

(5.20)

[240] אמר אבקראט: הקור עוקץ לנגעים ויקשה העור ויחדש מן הכאב מה שלא יהיה עמו
מוגלא וישחיר ויחדש הפלצות אשר יהיה עמה קדחת והקיווץ והמשיכה.

אמר המפרש: זה מבואר.

(5.21)

[241] אמר אבקראט: ופעמים ישפך על מי שבו משיכה מבלתי נגע והוא בחור בריא בשר
באמצע הקיץ מים רבים קרים ויתחדש בו התחברות מחום רב והיתה הצלתו בחום ההוא.   5

אמר המפרש: זה מבואר.

(5.22)

[242] אמר אבקראט: המים החמים יעשו המוגלא אבל לא בכל נגע וזה מן האותות
היותר גדולות לראיה על האמת והבטחון וירכך העור וירקקהו וישקיט הכאב וישבר
כח הפלצות והקיווץ והמשיכה ויתיך הכבידות אשר יקרה בראש והוא היותר טוב מכל
הדברים לשבר העצמות וכל שכן המופשטים מן העור ומן העצמות בפרט לעצמות   10
הראש וכל מה שהמיתו הקור או נגעו ולנגעים אשר יתרחבו ויתאכלו ולפי הטבעת
ולקיבה והרחם והמקוה כי הנה החום לבעלי אלו החליים מועיל ומרפא והקור מזיק להם
וממית.

אמר המפרש: העשות המוגלא אות טוב לבטוח בו בנגעים כי הוא מין מן הבישול כמו
שידעת ולא כל נגע יעשה מוגלא כי הנגעים הרעים כלם או הקשים להרפא והמתאכלים   15
לא תתילד בהם מוגלא ושאר מה שזכר מבואר כי כל אבר שיש בו עצבים ועצמות יזיקם
הקור.

(5.23)

[243] אמר אבקראט: ואולם הקר הנה ראוי שישתמשו בו באלו המקומות ר"ל במקומות
אשר יגר בהם הדם או הוא מזומן שיגר מהם ואין ראוי שישתמשו בו בעצם המקום אשר
יגר ממנו אבל סביבו ובמקום אשר יבא ממנו ובמה שהיה מן המורסות החמות והעוקצות   20

1–2 יהיה עמו מוגלא: יהיה לו קודם לכן א   2 והמשיכה: והמתוח א   4 משיכה: מתוח
א   5 התחברות: עטוף א ד¹ انعطاف a || renovatio calorem naturalem א   והיתה: ותהיה א והיה
בח   7 המים החמים יעשו: החום יעשה א || וזה: והיא ד²   7–8 מן האותות היותר גדולות: הגדול
שבאותות א כי האותות היותר גדולות ה   8 לראיה: מורות ד² המורות א || האמת והבטחון: הבטחון
א || והבטחון: ויבשל המוגלא .add א || וירקקהו: וידקדקהו אבה   9 כח: ד² בקר ד סכנת א عادنة
a || והמשיכה: והמתוח א || היותר: .om א   10 המופשטים: הערומים א || ומן העצמות: ויש העצמות
ה בח .om   11 יתרחבו: יתפשטו א   12 ולקיבה: ולקרה בח ולכלי התשמיש לזכר ולנקבה א
14 העשות: עשיית א   16 עצבים ועצמות: עצמים א

נוטה אל האדמימות ומראה הדם הטרי כי הוא אם נעשה במה שכבר נתישן בו הדם
ישחירהו ובמורסא הנקראת חמרא אם לא יהיה עמה נגע כי מה שהיה ממנה עמו נגע הוא
יזיקהו.

אמר המפרש: זה מבואר.

(5.24)

5   [244] אמר אבקראט: הדברים הקרים כמו השלג והברד מזיקים לחזה מעוררים השעול
מביאים להגרת הדם והירידה.

אמר המפרש: זה מבואר.

(5.25)

[245] אמר אבקראט: המורסות אשר יהיו בפרקים והכאבים אשר יהיו מבלתי נגע וכאבי
בעלי הנקרס ובעלי הקווץ המתחדש במקומות שיש בהם עצבים ורוב מה שדומה לאלו הנה
10   אם נשפך עליהם מים קרים הרבה ישקיטום ויכמישום ויניחו הכאב בחדשם תרדמה והתרדמה
גם כן המעט ממנה משקיטה הכאב.

אמר המפרש: השקטת הכאב באלו המקומות בהפסיקו הסבה המולידה אותו ובהרדימו
החוש.

(5.26)

[246] אמר אבקראט: המים אשר יתחממו מהר ויתקררו מהר הם יותר קלים משאר המים.

15   אמר המפרש: באר שהוא רוצה בכאן בהכבדות וקלות מהירות צאתם מן האצטומכא או
איחורם בהם.

(5.27)

[247] אמר אבקראט: מי הכריחו תאותו לשתות בלילה והיה צמאו חזק הנה אם ייש אחר
זה הוא טוב.

אמר המפרש: כשייש אחר שתית המים תבשל השינה הליחה המחייבת לצמא ולא יבוא
20   לשתות בלילה כי אם מחוזק הצמא.

2 חמרא: erisypelas ד׳   6 והירידה: והנזלים ח   9 הקווץ: הכויצה ח (...) ד הפשוח א الفسخ a
15 בכאן: om. א   16 בהם: בה א   19 תבשל השינה: יתבשל בשינה א ‖ יבוא: يَؤُذن a

(5.28)

[248] אמר אבקראט: החבוש בסמנים מושך הדם אשר יבוא מן הנשים והנה יהיו מקבלים תועלת בו במקומות רבים אחרים לולי שהוא יחדש בראש כבדות.

אמר המפרש: יאמר כי החבוש בסמנים יביא דם הנדות או דם הלידה כאשר נעצר כי זה ידקדק הדם אם היה עב או יפתח סתום אם היה שם או ירחיב פיות העורקים אם היו סתומים והנה
5   יקבלו תועלת בו גם כן בחמם המקומות הקרים או בנגב הליחות לולי היותו ממלא הראש כי כל דבר חם יגבה למעלה ויכאיב הראש.

(5.29)

[249] אמר אבקראט: ראוי שישקו למעוברת הרפואה כשיהיו הליחות בגופה מתעוררות אחר שיעברו על העובר ארבעה חדשיש ועד שיעברו עליו שבעה חדשים ויהיה הכניסו עצמו על זה מעט. ואולם מה שהיה מעט מזה או יותר הנה ראוי שיפחד ממנו.

10   אמר המפרש: אם שהוא כפל זה השער או כפלו בכונה כדי לחבר הדבור בחליי הנשים.

(5.30)

[250] אמר אבקראט: האשה ההרה אם יקיזו אותה תפיל עוברה וכל שכן אם יהיה עוברה כבר גדל.

אמר המפרש: זה מבואר.

(5.31)

[251] אמר אבקראט: כשתהיה האשה מעוברת וקרה לה קצת החליים החדים הנה זה
15   מאותות המות.

אמר המפרש: אם היה מן החליים החדים אשר עמהם קדחת הנה ימית בהפסד המזג הצריך אל שאיפת אויר רב והאיברים עמוסים ובמיעוט המזון ואם היה כמו הפלג' והקווץ הנה היא לא תסבול חוזק הכאב והמשיכה למה שתשא מהכבדות.

(5.32)

[252] אמר אבקראט: האשה כשהיא מקיאה דם ותראה דם נדותה יפסק הקיא ההוא.

20   אמר המפרש: זה מבואר.

---

1 החבוש: הקטור **בח** ‖ בסמנים: בבשמים **ה** ‖ מושך הדם: מביא דם הנדות **בהה**   3 בסמנים: בבשמים **ה**   6 יגבה **ה** יעלה **א** יגרה **בח**   7 שישקו למעוברת: שתשתה **ה**   8 אחר: בעת **ה** מעת **בח**   8–9 הכניסו עצמו על זה: التقدّم على هذا **a**   10 השער: om. **א** השער בלא כונה **א¹**   17 עמוסים: مضغوطة **a** ‖ והקווץ: והקויצה **ה**   18 והמשיכה: ורוב המשיכה **א** והמתיחה **ה**   19 ותראה: فإن بعث **a** ‖ ההוא: מפני משיכתה להפך הצד **א** add.   20 אמר המפרש: זה מבואר: om. **a**

(5.33)

[253] אמר אבקראט: כשיפסק דם הנדות הנה יציאת דם הנחירים טוב.

אמר המפרש: זה מבואר.

(5.34)

[254] אמר אבקראט: האשה המעוברת אם התמיד עליה שלשול אל יהיו בטוחים עליה שלא תפיל.

5 אמר המפרש: כשיתנועע הכח הדוחה באיברים ההם השכנים לרחם בחוזק יפחדו גם כן שיתנועע הכח הדוחה מן הרחם.

(5.35)

[255] אמר אבקראט: כשיהיה באשה חולי הרחם או קשי הלידה ויבוא אליה עיטוש הנה זה טוב.

אמר המפרש: ירצה בחולי הרחם החנק הרחם והעיטוש אות על התעוררות הטבע שיעשה
10 פעולותיו והוא גם כן סבה להשליך האיברים מה שנדבק ונסתבך בהם מן הליחות המזיקות ובזה הצד ירפא העיטוש מן הפיהוק.

(5.36)

[256] אמר אבקראט: כשיהיה דם נדות האשה משתנה במראיו ולא יהיה בעתו בואו בעתו תמיד יורה זה על היות גופה צריך לנקוי.

אמר המפרש: זה מבואר.

(5.37)

15 [257] אמר אבקראט: כשתהיה האשה הרה ויצמקו שדיה פתאום הנה תפיל.

אמר המפרש: כבר נודע שתוף השדים עם הרחם וכאשר יצמקו יורה על מיעוט המזון המגיע אליהם וכאשר ימעט גם כן המזון המגיע לרחם יפול העובר.

---

1 אמר: עוד אמר א ‖ הנה יציאת: בהגרת א ‖ טוב: כי יעלה מרעות העצר דם הנדות ד .add   2 זה
מבואר: שני אלו הפרקים הם מבוארים א   7 קשי הלידה: קשתה בלידתה א   7–8 ויבוא אליה עיטוש
הנה זה טוב: וקרה לה עיטוש זה הוא אות טוב א   9 ירצה בחולי הרחם החנק הרחם: רצונו לומר כי
האשה כשתתבטל נשימתה מחולי הרחם הנקרא החנק הרחם ומצאה עטוש הקל חליה והוא אות טוב
וסבה טובה א ‖ והעיטוש אות: כי העיטוש מורה א   10 להשליך: מן ד .add

(5.38)

[258] אמר אבקראט: כשתהיה האשה מעוברת וצמק אחד משדיה פתאום והיתה מעוברת מתאומים הנה תפיל אחד מעובריה. ואם היה צומק השד הימני תפיל הזכר ואם היה צומק השד השמאלי תפיל הנקבה.

אמר המפרש: הזכר בצד הימני על הרוב.

(5.39)

[259] אמר אבקראט: כשתהיה האשה בלתי הרה ולא ילדה ויהיה לה חלב הנה הנה דם נדותה כבר פסק.

אמר המפרש: על דרך זרות בהפסק דם הנדות ימלאו העורקים הדבקים בשדים מלוי רב ויתחדש החלב לרבוי הדם המגיע אל השד. ונראה לי כי זה לא יתאמת אם לא שיהיה גוף האשה בתכלית הנקיון ויהיה מזונה בתכלית הטוב.

(5.40)

[260] אמר אבקראט: כשיקפא לאשה בשדיה דם מורה מעניינה על בלבול השכל.

אמר המפרש: הקרוב אצלי כי הוא ראה זה פעם אחת או שתי פעמים ופסק הדין במוחלט כמו שהוא מנהגו בספרו באפידימי. וכבר זכר גאלינוס שהוא לא ראה זה מעולם והוא אמת ר"ל שזה אינו סבה מסבות בלבול השכל בשום פנים. ואולם קרה זה במקרה פעם או שתים וראה אותו אבוקראט וחשב אותו סבה.

(5.41)

[261] אמר אבקראט: אם תרצה לדעת אם האשה הרה אם לא השקה אותה כשתרצה לישן מי דבש ואם ימצאוה צירים בבטנה הנה היא הרה ואם לא ימצאוה צירים אינה הרה.

אמר המפרש: רוצה בלקחה אותו עם השינה עם המנוחה והמלוי מן המאכל ומי הדבש יוליד רוחות ויעזרהו על זה מלוי הבטן וכאשר לא ימצא הרוח מפלט לסתום הרחם דרך אותם הרוחות יתחדשו הצירים.

(5.42)

[262] אמר אבקראט: כשתהיה האשה הרה מזכר תהיה טובת מראה וכאשר תהיה הרה מנקבה יהיה מראה משתנה.

אמר המפרש: כל זה מבואר והוא ברוב.

(5.43)

[263] אמר אבקראט: כשתתחדש לאשה המעוברת המורסא אשר תקרא חומרה ברחמה הנה זה מאותות המות.

אמר המפרש: נראה מדברי גאלינוס שהוא רוצה לומר מיתת העובר וכן שאר המורסות החמות.

(5.44)

[264] אמר אבקראט: כשנתעברה האשה והיא בכחישות והרזון על ענין יוצא מן הטבע הנה היא תפיל קודם שתשמין.

אמר המפרש: יאמר שהיא כאשר נתעברה והיא בתכלית הכחישות הנה המזון המגיע אל האיברים יקחוהו האיברים כלו ולא ישאירו דבר שיזון בו העובר כשיגדל והנה היא תפיל העובר קודם שישלם גדר השומן לא בעבור שובה לטבעה בשמנות גופה.

(5.45)

[265] אמר אבקראט: כשתהיה האשה ממוצעת הגוף מפלת בחדש השני והשלישי מבלתי סבה מבוארת תיק הרחם מלא ליחה הדומה לליחה היוצאת מן הנחירים ולא תוכל להחזיק העובר לכבדותו אבל ימעד ממנו.

אמר המפרש: זה מבואר.

(5.46)

[266] אמר אבקראט: כשתהיה האשה על ענין יוצא מן הטבע בשמנות ולא תתעבר הנה הכסוי הפנימי מכסויי הבטן הנקרא החלב המכסה סותם לה פי הרחם ולא תתעבר עד שתכחיש.

אמר המפרש: לרחם צואר ארוך וקצה הצואר הוא הסמוך לקיבה ותוכו תכנס האמה יקרא פי צואר הרחם ופעמים יקרא פי הרחם ואשר יקרא פי הרחם לפי האמת הוא ראשית הצואר הסמוך לרחם והוא אשר יסתום אותו החלב מן האשה מופלגת בשומן.

7 יאמר: א om. ‖ הכחישות: הרזון ח   8 האיברים: א om.   9 קודם שישלם גדר השומן: قبل أن تثني لحيز السمن a   10 ממוצעת: מזג א2   11 תיק: ⟨...⟩ ד קרוב ב ח חללות ח   12 ימעד: ⟨...⟩ د ינתק ח ينهك   a   15 הכסוי הפנימי מכסויי הבטן הנקרא החלב המכסה: הקרום הפנימי הנקרא החלב ח   17 לקיבה: الفرج a   18 יקרא פי צואר הרחם ופעמים יקרא פי הרחם ואשר: א om.   19 לרחם: לצואר הרחם אד ‖ יסתום אותו: يَسُدُّه a

(5.47)

[267] אמר אבקראט: כשיפתח הרחם עד שיגיע אל הירך התחייב בהכרח שתצטרך אל מעשה.

אמר המפרש: רוצה במעשה מעשה היד כלומר להכניס הפתילות וכאשר נפתח במה שקרוב מחוץ הנה אז יצטרך אל הפתילות.

(5.48)

[268] אמר אבקראט: מה שיהיה מן העוברים זכר הנה הוא יותר ראוי שיהיה גדולו בימין ומה שהיה מהם נקבה בשמאל.

אמר המפרש: זה מבואר כי הצד הימני יותר חם וזכר גאלינוס כי הזרע אשר יבא מן האשה מן הצד הימני מן אחד מביציה בו עובי וחום ואשר יבוא מן הצד השמאלי דק מימי ויותר קר מן האחר ואיני יודע אם הגיע לו זה בנבואה או שהגיע אליו בהקש ואם היה שגדר וסדר זה הסדר בהקש הנה הוא הקש נפלא.

(5.49)

[269] אמר אבקראט: כשתרצה שתפיל השליא הכנס בחוטם רפואה מעטשת וסתום הנחירים והפה.

אמר המפרש: כדי שיתחדש לבטן משיכה וקושי ויעזור על נפילת השליא.

(5.50)

[270] אמר אבקראט: כשתרצה שיעצר דם הנדות שים בכל אחד משדיה כלי זכוכית מן היותר גדולים שיהיו.

אמר המפרש: זה מבואר כי הוא משיכה להפך הצד.

(5.51)

[271] אמר אבקראט: פי הרחם מן האשה המעוברת יהיה סתום.

אמר המפרש: זה מבואר.

---

1 כשיפתח הרחם עד שיגיע אל הירך: כשיפתח הרחם בירך ויעשה מוגלא עד שיגיע אל הירך د מتى
تقیّح الرحم حیث یستبطن الورك a‎ 3–4 נפתח במה שקרוב מחוץ: וכשיבא לידי טרי מה שסמוך ממנו
لחוץ א וכאשר עשה מוגלא במה שקרוב מחוץ בח تقیّح مّا یلی منه خارج a‎ 5 מה: מיא אח ‖ ומה: ומיא א
8 השמאלי: הוא א add. ‖ וייתר: והוא יותר د ‖ קר: דק וקר د‎ 9–10 ואם היה שגדר וסדר זה הסדר
בהקש: א om. ואם היה זה שסדר זה הסדר בהקש א‎ ‖ ואם היה זה הוא בהקש د‎ 10 נפלא (= عجيب BP)
عجيب غريب a‎ 11 רפואה מעטשת: מעטש א‎ 14 הנדות: المرأة a add. ‖ משדיה: משני שדיה אח

(5.52)

[272] אמר אבקראט: כשיצא החלב משדי המעוברת יורה זה על חולשת העובר וכאשר יהיו אוצרים יורה זה על שהעובר יותר בריא.

אמר המפרש: אמנם יצא החלב ויגר מן המעוברת למלוא העורקים אשר בין הרחם והשדים לרבוי ואמנם ירבה שם להמצא הדם כשיהיה העובר מעט המזון ולא ימשך מן העורקים ההם
5 כי אם מעט דבר.

(5.53)

[273] אמר אבקראט: כשיהיה ענין האשה הולך אל ההפלה הנה שדיה יצמקו ואם היה הענין בהפך זה ר״ל שיהיו שדיה קשים הנה ימצא כאב בשדים או בירכים או בעינים או בשתי ארכובותיה ולא תפיל.

אמר המפרש: צמיקת השדים ראיה על מעוט הדם כמו שזכרנו וגדלם ראיה על שווי שעורו
10 וקשים ראיה על רבוי הדם ועביו ולכן ישתדל הטבע לדחות המותר ההוא הנוסף לאבר אחר קרוב מן הרחם או מן השדים ויתחדש באבר ההוא כאב ובכלל אלו הראיות כלם בלתי אמתיות ולא שיהיו ברוב וכל אלו הפרקים והדומה להם נמשך אחר מה שקרה פעם או שתי פעמים וראה אותו כי אבקראט התחיל המלאכה.

(5.54)

[274] אמר אבקראט: כשיהיה פי הרחם קשה הנה התחייב בהכרח שיהיה סתום.

15 אמר המפרש: זה מבואר.

(5.55)

[275] אמר אבקראט: כשתקרה קדחת לאשה הרה והוחמה חמום חזק מבלתי סבה נגלית הנה לידתה תהיה בקושי וסכנה או תפיל ותהיה בסכנה.

אמר המפרש: צריך לקלות הלידה שיהיו שני הגופות יחד חזקים גוף האם וגוף הולד.

(5.56)

[276] אמר אבקראט: כשיתחדש אחר הגרת דם הנדות קוץ ועלוף הנה זה רע.

20 אמר המפרש: זה מבואר.

(5.57)

[277] אמר אבקראט: כשיהיה דם הנדות יותר נוסף ממה שראוי יקרו מזה חליים. ואם לא ירד
דם הנדות יתחדשו מזה חליים מפני הרחם.

אמר המפרש: זה מבואר.

(5.58)

[278] אמר אבקראט: כשיקרה בקצה פי הטבעת או ברחם מורסא ימשך אחריו הטפת השתן
וכן כאשר נפתחה הכוליא ימשך אחריו הטפת השתן וכשיתחדש בכבד מורסא ימשך אחר
זה פיהוק.

אמר המפרש: הטפת השתן יהיה לחולשת כח המקוה המחזיק או לחדוד השתן וחולשת הכח
תהיה להפסד המזג או ממורסא תתחדש שם וחדוד השתן תהיה למה שיתערב בו מן הליחה
העוקצת וכשתהיה מורסא באחד משני אלו האיברים הנה יזיק המקוה לשכונתו ויחלש כוחה
וכאשר יהיה החולי בכליות הנה יתחדש עקיצה בשתן ולא ימשך אחר מורסת הכבד פיהוק
אם לא שתהיה גדולה.

(5.59)

[279] אמר אבקראט: כשתהיה האשה בלתי מעוברת ותרצה לדעת אם היא יכולה להתעבר
או לא כסה אותה בבגדים ועשן ועשן תחתיה ואם ראית כי ריח העשן יעבור בגופה עד שיגיע אל
נחיריה ופיה הנה תדע כי אין סבת העדר ההריון בעבורה.

אמר המפרש: העישון יהיה בדברים טובים להם חדוד כמו הלבונה והמירא והאצטרק.

(5.60)

[280] אמר אבקראט: כשתהיה האשה המעוברת נגר דם נדותה בעונותיו הנה אי אפשר
שיהיה עוברה בריא.

אמר המפרש: אמר ג'אלינוס: ידמה שיהיה דם הנדות הנגר מן מעוברות מן העורקים אשר
בצואר הרחם כי השליא תלוייה בפיות כל העורקים אשר מבפנים בחלל הרחם ואי אפשר
שיצא מזה דבר לרקות הרחם.

---

1 אמר: עוד אמר א‎ 3 זה מבואר: שני אלו הפרקים מבוארים א‎ 4 בקצה: בקצת אה‎ 5 וכן כאשר
נפתחה הכוליא ימשך אחריו הטפת השתן om.‏ א‎ וכן כאשר נתנפחה הכוליא ימשך אחריו הטפת השתן
א‎ا וכן כאשר נפתחה השליא(?) ימשך אחריו הטפת השתן د‎ وكذلك إنْ تقيّحت الكلى تبع ذلك تقطير البول a
9-8 תתחדש שם וחדוד השתן תהיה למה שיתערב בו מן הליחה העוקצת וכשתהיה מורסא: א‎ا
15 טובים: طيّبة الرائحة a‏ 16 בעונותיו: בעונתיה א‎ בעתותיה ה‎ 18 אמר: د‎ om.‏ || דם: د‎ om.‏

(5.61)

[281] אמר אבקראט: כשלא יגר דם נדות האשה בעונותיו ולא יתחדש בה פלצות ולא קדחת
אבל יקרה לה צער ועלוף ורוע נפש דע שהיא כבר נתעברה.

אמר המפרש: זה מבואר.

(5.62)

[282] אמר אבקראט: כשיהיה רחם האשה קר קשה לא תתעבר וכשיהיה גם כן לח מאד
לא תתעבר כי לחותו יכסה הזרע ויקפיאהו ויכבהו וכשיהיה גם כן יותר נגוב ממה שראוי או
שיהיה חם שורף לא תתעבר כי יעדר המזון מן הזרע ויפסד וכאשר היה מזג הרחם שוה בין
שני הענינים תהיה האשה רבת ההולדה.

אמר המפרש: זה מבואר.

(5.63)

[283]

(5.64)

[284] אמר אבקראט: החלב לבעלי כאב הראש רע והוא גם כן למוקדחים רע ולמי שהיו
המקומות שלמטה מן החלצים ממנו עולים ובהם קרקור ולמי שבו צמא ולמי שהגובר על צואתו
המרה האדומה ולמי שהוא בקדחת חדה ולמי שיש בו שלשול מדם רב ויועיל לבעלי השדפון
כשלא יהיה בהם קדחת חזקה מאד ולבעלי הקדחת הארוכה החלושה כשלא יהיה עמה דבר
ממה שהקדמנו ספורו והיו גופותם נתכים על זולת מה שיחייבהו העלה.

אמר המפרש: החלב הוא מן הדברים אשר ימהר אליהם השינוי אם באצטו' אשר היא יותר
מדי קרה הנה יתחמץ ואם באצטו' אשר היא יותר מדי חמה הנה ישתנה אל העשון ואולם
מה שיתבשל לפי מה שראוי הנה יוליד מזון רב טוב אבל שהוא בעת בשולו פעמים יחדש
נפח במה שלמטה מן החלצים ויכאיב הראש זה פעולתו בבריאים ואולם בחולים הוא כל מה
שנזכר.

---

1 יגר: ירד אה ‖ בעונותיו: בעונותיה א בעתותיה ח   2 ועלוף (=وغشي P): وغشي a   3 אמר המפרש:
זה מבואר: א om.   4 אמר: עוד אמר א   5-4 וכשיהיה גם כן לח מאד לא תתעבר: א om. וכשיהיה גם
כן לח מאד א'   5 לחותו: הלחות א ‖ יכסה: تغمر a   6 ויפסד: א om.   8 אמר המפרש: זה מבואר:
This aphorism is missing in the Arabic and Arabic-Hebrew   9 אלו השני פרקים הם מבוארים א
translations   11 ולמי: مَن a   14 העלה: החולי א   16-15 היא יותר מדי קרה הנה יתחמץ ואם
באצטו' אשר היא: ד om.   16 הנה ישתנה: א om.   17 יחדש: יתחדש א   18 כל: על א

(5.65)

[285] אמר אבקראט: מי שנתחדש בו נגע היציאה ומצאו בסיבתו נפח אי אפשר שימצאהו
קווץ ולא שטות ואם הלך הנפח פתאום והיה הנגע מאחוריו יקרה לו קווץ או משיכה ואם היה
הנגע לפניו יקרה לו שטות או כאב חד בצד או העשות מוגלא או שלשול דם אם היה הנפח
ההוא אדום.

אמר המפרש: איני צריך לכפול כי רוב אלו המשפטים אשר יאמר אותם אבקראט קצתם הם
על הרוב או על השווי ועם האמת ימצא קצת המשפטים שהם על המעט ואולי ראה אותו פעם
ויחס הענין בו לסבה שאינו סבתו באמת.

וסברת ג׳אלינוס בזה השער שהוא רוצה בנפח המורסא וכל עובי יוצא מן הטבע ומה שהוא מן
הגוף באחריו הנה יש בו עצבים ומה שהוא ממנו לפנים הגובר עליו העורקים הדופקים וכאשר
תעלה הליחה המולידה את המורסא מן העצבים אל המוח יהיה הקווץ ואם יעלה בעורקים אל
המוח יהיה השטות ואם תהיה הליחה ההיא אל החזה תוליד הכאב בצד והרבה פעמים ימצא
בעל חולי הצד עשיית המוגלא.

(5.66)

[286] אמר אבקראט: כאשר יתחדשו יציאות גדולות משונות ואחרי כן לא יראה בהם נפח
הנה הוא רעה גדולה.

אמר המפרש: רוצה ביציאות משונות אשר יהיו בראשי הגידים או בתכליתם או מה שיהיה
מן הגידים הגובר בו העצבים ואם לא תתחדש נפח במה שהיה ענינו כן מן הנגעים לא יהיה
בטוח מהיות הליחות הנשפכות אל הנגעים יעתקו מהם אל מקום אחר יותר נכבד ממקומות
הנגעים.

(5.67)

[287] אמר אבקראט: היציאה הרפה משובחת והנאה מגונה.

אמר המפרש: יאמר ג׳אלינוס שהוא רוצה בנאה הקשה להדחות והוא הפך הרפה כי כל קשה
הנה ליחתו בלתי מבושלת.

---

1 נגע היציאה: היציאה א נגע ח יציאה בח قرحة a ‖ בסיבתו: בסיבתה א 2 ולא שטות: .om ד
3 העשות מוגלא: .om ד 5 איני צריך לכפול: צריך אני לכפול א 6-5 אשר ... המשפטים: א¹
6 ואולי: ואולם א 7 בו: א ‖ .om ד ‖ שאינו: שאינה א 8 רוצה בנפח: يرضة بنفوخ א 9-8 ומה
שהוא מן הגוף באחריו הנה יש בו עצבים: .om ד 11-10 יהיה הקווץ ואם יעלה בעורקים אל המוח:
א¹ 13 יציאות (= خراجات A): خراجات a ‖ משונות: خبيثة a 15 ביציאות משונות (الخراجات
الخبيثة AP): بالجراحات الخبيثة a 16 כן: ד .om ‖ הנגעים: א¹ היציאות א 19 היציאה הרפה: الرخوة a
الأورام الرخوة APt 20 להדחות: להראה א

(5.68)

[288] אמר אבקראט: מי שמצאו כאב באחורי ראשו ונחתך לו העורק העומד אשר במצח יקח תועלת בחתוכו.

אמר המפרש: המשיכה אשר אל חלוף הצד בצואר הוא מאחור אל פנים ומפנים אל אחור.

(5.69)

[289] אמר אבקראט: הנה הפלצות רוב מה שיתחיל בנשים משפל הגב ואחר כן יעלה בגב אל הראש והוא גם כן באנשים מתחיל מאחור יותר ממה שיתחיל מלפנים כמו שמתחיל מהזרועות והירכים וזה כי העור גם כן בקודם מן הגוף ספוגי ויורה על זה השער.

אמר המפרש: יבא מהר לגב להיותו יותר קר לרוב העצמות שם ומיעוט הבשר והנשים יותר קרות מן האנשים והביא ראיה מרפיון הקודם מצמיחת השער שם.

(5.70)

[290] אמר אבקראט: מי שקרהו הקדחת הרביעית הנה אי אפשר שיקרהו הקווץ ואם היה שקרהו הקווץ קודם הרביעית ואחר כן התחדשה הרביעית ירפא הקווץ.

אמר המפרש: סברת ג׳אלינוס כי הוא אמר שזה המין מן הקווץ הוא המתהווה ממלוא ורפואתו תהיה ביציאת הליחה היוצאת או תתבשל ובקדחת רביעית תצא בחוזק ותתבשל בחום הקדחת.

(5.71)

[291] אמר אבקראט: מי שהיה עורו נמשך כחוש קשה הנה הוא ימות מבלתי זיעה ומי שהיה עורו רפה ספוגי הנה הוא ימות עם זיעה.

אמר המפרש: רוצה במי שקרב מן המות ממי שהיה עורו בזה הענין.

(5.72)

[292] אמר אפוקרט: מי שהיה בו ירקון הנה אי אפשר שיתילדו בו הרוחות.

---

1 באחורי: אחורי ד ‖ לו: ד .om ‖ העומד: ד .om ‖ מאחור .add 3 הצד: מן המאוחר אל הקודם ד ‖ מאחור אל פנים ומפנים אל אחור: מפנים אל אחור ומאחור אל פנים א מבפנים אל האחור ומהאחור לפנים ח 6 שמתחיל מהזרועות: שמתחיל מהזרוע ד שהוא מתחיל לפעמים מן הזרועות א 8 המפרש: الوَرد a .add 10–11 אי ... הרביעית: א[12 ממלוא: ממלוי א וירפא ד .add 13 ביציאת: بِانْفِاض a ‖ תתבשל: بِنُضجه a ‖ בחוזק: الثَّافِض a .add 15 מבלתי: בלא א 16 עורו רפה ספוגי: מתחלחל עורו א עורו ספוגי ורפה א[18 בו: לו א

אמר המפרש: מסבות התילד הרוחות תמצא הליחה הלבנה הנאה במקום הולדה וזה לא יהיה
עם ירקון לתגבורת המרה האדומה.

נשלם המאמר החמישי מפרוש הפרקים.

---

1 הליחה הלבנה הנאה: الْبَلْغَم a ‖ הולדה: הולדם א   3 מפרוש הפרקים: א .om   בעזרת ה׳ מנת חלקי
וכוסי ואתחיל בעזרתו המאמר הששי ה

המאמר הששי מפירוש פרקי אבקראט

(6.1)

‏[293] אמר אבקראט: כשתתחדש הקבסה החמוצה בחולי אשר תקרא קלוח המעים אחר
הארכו ולא היתה כן קודם זה הנה היא אות טוב.

אמר המפרש: כאשר היה חולי קלוח המעים לחולשת הכח המחזיק ויצא קודם שיתבשל ואחר
כן תתחדש הקבסא החמוצה הנה זה ראיה על שהמזון חזר להשאר באצטומ׳ שעור מה שיהיה
אפשר עמו שיתחיל לשנותו קצת שנוי שעור מה שיתחמץ ושהטבע התחיל שישובו פעולותיו.

(6.2)

‏[294] אמר אבקראט: מי שהיה בנחיריו בטבע לחות נוסף והיה זרעו דק הנה בריאותו קרוב
אל החולי ומי שהיה העניין בו בהפך זה הנה גופו בריא.

אמר המפרש: דברים אלו יורו על לחות המוח ויבשות שאר האיברים ולכן שב דק זרעו.

(6.3)

‏[295] אמר אבקראט: המניעה מן המאכל בשלשול הדם הנושן אות רע והוא עם קדחת יותר
רע.

אמר המפרש: שלשול הדם כאשר היה עם חמרמרות המעיים וארך עמידתו יתוספו החפירות
בעומק האיברים וישובו נגעים בהם עפוש ותכאב האצטו׳ בשותפות וישיג בשולה הנזק
וכאשר עלה החולי לפי האצטומ׳ תפול התאוה והיה זה ראיה על שקיעת החולי ואריכות הזקו.

(6.4)

‏[296] אמר אבקראט: מה שהיה מן הנגעים נקלף והיה נושר ונופל מה שסביבו הנה הוא מסוכן.

אמר המפרש: נפילת מה שסביב הנגע מן השיער וקלפת העור ראיה על חדוד מה שישפך
אליה ולכן יתאכל מה שסביבו בסוף.

(6.5)

‏[297] אמר אבקראט: ראוי שישתכל מן הכאבים אשר יקרו בצלעות ופני החזה וזולת אלו
משאר האיברים גודל חלופם.

---

1 מפירוש פרקי אבקראט: **אה** .om   5 להשאר: להתעכב **א** ‖ מה: **ד** .om   7 בטבע: טבע **ד**
‏10‏–‏11 והוא עם קדחת יותר רע: ואם יהיה עם קדחת הוא יותר רע **א** ושם קדחת יותר רע **ח** והוא עם
קדחת **בח**   14 שקיעת: مَكَّن a ‖ ואריכות: وامتداد a   15 נקלף: **אדבח** .om ‖ והיה נושר ונופל מה
שסביבו: יהיה נושר נופל מה שסיביבו **א** והיה שערו נופל מה שבסביבות **ה** יהיה השער נושר וקלוף העור
בח ‖ מסוכן: خبيث a   19 גודל: וגודל **ד**

אמר המפרש: ר״ל שלא יספיק לו ידיעת המקום הכואב לבד מבלתי שיעיין בגודל החולי או
חולשתו ושיקח ראיה על זה מחוזק הכאב ומה שימצא עמו מן העקיצה והחדוד והמשיכה
והדומה לזה מחלוף המקרים וחוזקתם הנמשכים לכאב האבר ההוא.

(6.6)

[298] אמר אבקראט: החליים אשר יהיו במקוה ובכליות קשים להרפא בזקנים.

5   אמר המפרש: זה מבואר.

(6.7)

[299] אמר אבקראט: מה שהיה מן כאבים אשר יקרו בבטן במקום יותר עליון הוא יותר קל
ומה שלא היה מהם כן הוא יותר חזק.

אמר המפרש: אמר ג׳אלינוס שהוא רוצה בעליון מה שסמוך לנראה מן הבטן על הכסוי
המשוך על המעים והאצטומכא ואמרו מה שלא היה מהם כן רוצה בו מה שהיה מהם במעים
10   והאצטומכא.

(6.8)

[300] אמר אבקראט: מה שיקרה מן הנגעים בגופות בעלי השקוי אינו נקל להרפא.

אמר המפרש: הנגעים לא יחתימו עד שיתנגבו נגוב שלם ולא יקל זה במזג בעלי השקוי.

(6.9)

[301] אמר אבקראט: הגרב הרחב אי אפשר שיהיה עמו חכוך.

אמר המפרש: הגרב והנגעים שימשכו ברחב ולא יהיה להם נפח ראיה על היות החומר קר
15   ולכן לא יחדש חכוך לקור החומר.

(6.10)

[302] אמר אבקראט: מי שהיה בו כאב הראש ודפיקה חזקה בראשו ויצא מנחיריו או מאזניו
מוגלא או מים הנה חליו יתך בזה.

אמר המפרש: זה מבואר.

---

1 הכואב: לו ד‏ .add   6 יותר: אה‏ .om   7 הוא: הנה הוא א‏   9 המשוך על: המושך למעלה מן
א‏ ‖ מהם: א‏ .om   12 יחתימו: יתרפאו א‏ יסתמו בח‏   16 כאב הראש: وجع شديد في رأسه a ‖ ודפיקה
חזקה בראשו: דפיקה חזקה א‏ ووجع شديد في رأسه a

(6.11)

[303] אמר אבקראט: בעלי הוסואס מן המרה השחורה ובעלי מורסת הראש כאשר יתחדש בהם הטחורים היה זה אות טוב בהם.

אמר המפרש: הוסואס אשר מהמרה השחורה הוא ערבוב השכל המתהוה מן המרה השחורה והוא אשר שמו בלשון יון מאלנכוניא ומורסת הראש הנקראת ברסאם היא מורסא חמה בקרום המוח וכבר באר באר כי כאשר נטה החומר אל הפך הצד ובה בהפתח פיות העורקים יתוקן העניין.

(6.12)

[304] אמר אבקראט: מי שנתרפא מטחורים נושנים עד שהבריא ואחר כן לא ירד מהם אחת לא יהיה בטוח מהתחדש בו שקוי או שדפון.

אמר המפרש: כי הוא כאשר לא ירד מהם אחד מה שירוק ממנו הדם העכור ישוב הדם ההוא וירבה על הכבד ויכבה חומו בריבויו ויתחדש השקוי או ישליחהו בעורקים אחרים ויבקע עורק בריאה ויתחדש ממנו השדפון ר״ל כי פעמים יתחדשו שני אלו החליים ופעמים יתחדש מזה זולתם.

(6.13)

[305] אמר אבקראט: כאשר קרה לאדם פיהוק ויתחדש בו עטוש ינוח פיהוקו.

אמר המפרש: רוב מה שיהיה הפיהוק ממלוא והוא אשר יתרפא בעיטוש בחסר הלחויות בתנועת העיטוש המזעזע.

(6.14)

[306] אמר אבקראט: כשיהיה באדם שקוי וילכו המים ממנו בעורקיו אל בטנו ויהיה זה התכת חליו.

אמר המפרש: זה מבואר כי הנה יעשה הטבע באותם המימות מה שיעשה בנקיונות החליים החדים החומר המחליא.

(6.15)

[307] אמר אבקראט: כשיהיה באדם שלשול ארוך והתחדש בו קיא מעצמו יפסק בו שלשולו.

אמר המפרש: זה מבואר כי הטבע משך החומר בהפך הצד.

---

1 הוסואס: השעמום א‎ 1‏‎–4 כאשר ... הנקראת ברסאם: א‎¹ 7 ירד: הניח א يَرُك a ירד: יניח 9
א עזב ח يَرُك a 10‏‎–9 הדם ההוא וירבה: om. ד‏ 10 ויכבה חומו בריבויו: וירבה חומו ובריבויו
ד 14 ממלוא: ממלוי אבהח‏ ‖ הלחויות: הליחות אבהח‏ 15 בתנועת: בתנועות ד‏ ‖ המזעזע: المزعزع
18 הנה: הוא דח‏ ‖ בנקיונות: בגבולי ח a

(6.16)

[308] אמר אבקראט: מי שקרהו חולי הצד או חולי הריאה והתחדש בו שלשול הנה זה אות רע.

אמר המפרש: אמנם יהיה השלשול אות רע בשני אלו המינים כשיהיה החולי גדול מאד עד שיתרכך הטבע מחולשת הכח.

(6.17)

[309] אמר אבקראט: כשיהיה באדם לפלוף הוא קצידה ויקרה לו שלשול הנה זה טוב.　　　5

אמר המפרש: זה מבואר.

(6.18)

[310] אמר אבקראט: כשיתחדש במקוה קריעה או במוח או בלב או בכליות או בקצת המעים הדקים או באצטומ' או בכבד הנה הוא ממית.

אמר המפרש: אמר ג'אלינוס: אבקראט יעשה ממית מה שימית בהכרח ומה שימית על הרוב. והנה ראיתי איש מצאוהו במוחו חבורות גדולות עמוקות ונרפאו אבל זה בזרות.　　　10

(6.19)

[311] אמר אבקראט: כאשר נחתך עצם או אליל או עצב או המקום הדק מן הלחי או קצה הגיד לא יצמח ולא יתחבר.

אמר המפרש: לא יצמח ר"ל לא יתחדש כמוהו בנגע עמוק ואם היה בקיעה לא יתחבר כי הם איברים יבשים ויתרחקו גם כן בבקוע והחיתוך ריחוק גדול.

(6.20)

[312] אמר אבקראט: כאשר ישפך דם אל מקום פנוי בהפך הענין הטבעי לא יהיה בטוח　　　15 מעשות מוגלא.

אמר המפרש: רוצה באמרו מהעשות המוגלא שישתנה ויפסד צורת הדם ממנו.

---

3 המינים: الرَضِين a　　5 לפלוף הוא קצידה: לפלוף הוא קצירה ח רמד ה　　9 מה שימית בהכרח ומה שימית על הרוב: מה שימית בהכרח ומה שימית על הרוב ד מה שממית בהכרח א יומה ממית על הרוב א מה שימית על הרוב ומה שימית בהכרח ה מה שימית על הרוב בח　　10 ונרפאו: ונתרפא א　　11 הדק: אי הרך א　　12 הגיד: הערלה א　　17 מהעשות המוגלא: יבא לידי מוגלא א שלא יעשה מוגלא בח בעשות מוגלא ה ‖ שישתנה: כי ישתנה א

(6.21)

[313] אמר אבקראט: מי מצאהו שטות והתחדש בו הרחבת העורקים הנקראים דליות או טחורים יותך ממנו שטותו.

אמר המפרש: זה מבואר לנטית החומר בהפך הצד ובתנאי שיהיו הליחות ההם המולידות הסכלות הם אשר נטו אל השוקים וכבר ידעת כי משפטיו אינם כלליים.

(6.22)

[314] אמר אבקראט: הכאבים אשר ירדו מהגב אל המרפקים יתיכם הקזת העורק. 5

אמר המפרש: כאשר היה סבת הכאבים ההם ליחות ונטו אצל המרפק והורקו מן המקום אשר נטו אליו יועיל זה בלא ספק.

(6.23)

[315] אמר אבקראט: מי שהתמיד בו הפחד ורוע הנפש זמן ארוך הנה חליו ממרה שחורה.

אמר המפרש: כשיקרה לאדם פחד ורוע נפש מבלתי סבה נגלית הנה סבת זה מדרך המלנכונייה ואע״פ שלא יהיו המקרים ההם תמידיים וכאשר היה התחלת אלו המקרים מסבה 10 נגלית כמו כעס או חרון אף או פחד ואחר כן האריכו והתמיד עמידתם הנה התמדתם יורה על המלנכונייה.

(6.24)

[316]

(6.25)

[317] אמר אבקראט: העתק המורסא הנק׳ חמרה מחוץ אל פנים אינו טוב אבל העתקו מבפנים לחוץ הוא טוב. 15

אמר המפרש: זכר מורסת החמרה דרך משל והוא הדין בכל מורסא וכל ליחה שתצא מבפנים אל חוץ שהוא אות טוב וכשיהיה העניין בהפך הנה הוא אות רע כי הוא ראיה על חולשת הטבע.

1 מצאהו: ימצאהו אה 3 החומר: המים דה הליחות בח 4 הסכלות: והשטות א ‖ משפטיו:
משפטיה ד 5 המרפקים: הפרקים (המפרקים א²) הנקראים קובטי א המפרקים בהח 6 המרפק:
המפרק אבה 9–8 ורוע ... פחד: א¹ 8 זמן ארוך: מבלתי זמן ד זמן ה 11 אף: ד This 13 om. ד
16–17 aphorism is missing in the Hebrew MSS and in the Arabic MSS ABC מבפנים אל חוץ: א²
מחוץ אל פנים אד

(6.26)

[318] אמר אבקראט: מי שקרה לו בקדחת השורפת רעש הנה ערבוב שכלו יתיכהו ממנו.

אמר המפרש: כבר ביאר ג'אלינוס בלבול המאמר בשער הזה וזה כי חומר הקדחת השורפת
בעורקים ואם יעתק החומר לעצבים יתחדש הרעש וכאשר נשקע במוח יתערבב השכל והוא
יותר סכנה מן הקדחת השורפת ואין בדמיון זה יאמר אם נתכה הקדחת אבל הענין אשר
התחדש בו יותר חזק הסכנה ויותר רע.

(6.27)

[319] אמר אבקראט: מי שנכוה או נבקע מן הנפוחים או המשוקים ויגר ממנו מן החומר או
מן המים שעור רב פתאום הנה הוא ימות בלא ספק.

אמר המפרש: הנפוחים יקרא כל מי שהיה בו מוגלא במקום הפנוי אשר בין החזה והריאה
ויצטרך אל הכויה בעל החולי הזה כדי שיתנגב הלחות ההוא כאשר יגע מיציאתו ברקיקה וכן
בעלי השקוי המימי יבוקעו וזכר כי ההרקה הזאת פתאום ממיתה והנה יראה גם כן בשאר
האיברים כשהתחדש באחד מהם מורסא גדולה והורקה המוגלא ממנו פתאום הוא סכנה
כי הנה יקרה לבעליו מיד העילוף ונפילת הכח עוד שהוא אחר זה ישאר בחולשה יקשה
להשיבה.

(6.28)

[320] אמר אבקראט: הסריסים לא יקרה להם הנקרס ולא הקרחות.

אמר המפרש: כי הם כנשים וכמו שלא יקרה הקרחות לנשים ללחות מזגם כן לא יקרה לאלו
וימעט נפילת הנקרס בהם כמו שיבאר.

(6.29)

[321] אמר אבקראט: האשה לא ימצאה הנקרס אם לא שפסק דם נדותה.

אמר המפרש: כבר נתן הסבה במעוט היות הנקרס בנשים וזה להרקת מותריהן בדם הנדות.

(6.30)

[322] אמר אבקראט: הנער לא ימצאהו הנקרס קודם שיתחיל להיות נזקק עם האשה.

אמר המפרש: אמר ג'אליאנוס כי בעשית המשגל להולדת הנקרס הוא ארטיטיקא כח גדול
מאד ולא באר סבה זאת. והקרוב אצלי כי סבת זה היות הרגלים מעטי הבשר ויש בהם הרבה

---

1 ממנו: מעט אה   2 בלבול: ד .om   4 אבל הענין: מפני שהענין א لكون الأمّ a   6 הנפוחים:
المتقيّحين a ‖ החומר: المدّة a   8 הנפוחים: المتقيّحين a   10 יבוקעו: יפתחו בטנם א   11 גדולה: فتقيّح
א   12 עוד: עד א   add. a   15 לנשים: בנשים א

עצבים ומיתרים והם יוצאים לאויר. וכאשר הזיק המשגל בעצבים בכלל בעבור הרקת רוחו
והקרו אותו יהיה נזק זה בעצבי הרגלים יותר חזק. ואנחנו נראה תמיד כי כאשר יתקררו
הרגלים ילך הקושי וזה ראיה על היות קצת שיתוף ביניהם מצד העצבים.

(6.31)

[323] אמר אבקראט: כאיבי העינים יתיכו אותם שתית היין החי או המרחץ והרטיה או הקזת
העורק או שתית המשלשל. 5

אמר המפרש: כבר באר ג׳אלינוס אופן ערבוב זה השער והיותו הולך על זולת דרך הלימוד
המועיל במלאכת הרפואה וזכר שאם היו החמרים חדים והיה הגוף נקי יועיל המרחץ וינוח
הכאב וכאשר נפסק גם כן הגרת החומר עם הנקיון מן הגוף תועיל הרטיה במים החמים
וכאשר היו עורקי העין מלאות כבר דבק בהם דם עב מבלתי שיהיה בגוף כלו מלוא והיתה
העין נגובה הנה שתית היין תתיך המורסא ההיא ותריקנה ותבדילה מן העורקים אשר נדבקה 10
בהם.

וזכר ג׳אלינוס כי אילו המינים השלשה מן הרפואה סכנה גדולה מאד אם לא ימצא בהם מקומם
באמת ואולם ההקזה אם היה המלאו מדם או הרקת הליחה הגוברת בשלשול הוא ענין מבואר
אמתי והוא הנעשה תמיד.

(6.32)

[324] אמר אבקראט: העלג יקרה להם בפרט שלשול ארוך. 15

אמר המפרש: רוב מה שיהיה העלגות בעבור לחות רב ורכות ולכן יהיה העלגות לנערים
ללחותם ורכותם ועם המזג הזה יתרכך הטבע על הרוב.

(6.33)

[325] אמר אבקראט: בעלי הגיהוק החמוץ אי אפשר שימצא להם חולי הצד.

אמר המפרש: רוב מה שיתילד חולי הצד הוא מליחה דקה ילך אל המכסה אשר על הצלעות
מבפנים ויתדבק בה ובעלי הגיהוק החמוץ מעט שתתילד בהם זאת הליחה. 20

(6.34)

[326] אמר אבקראט: הגבח לא יקרה לו מן העורקים אשר יתרחבו הנקראים דליות דבר רב
ומה שיתחדש בו מן הגבחים מן הדליות ישוב שער ראשו ויצמח.

_____

1 רוחו: כחו א   2 והקרו: והריקו אה וَتَبرِيدِه a   3 ילך: א¹ פחית (= יפחות) א   6 זולת: ד .om
8 הנקיון מן הגוף: נקיון הגוף אבהח   9 שיהיה בגוף כלו מלוא: שיהיה הגוף כלו מלא אה   10 היין: החי
א .add ‖ המורסא: الدم ‖ ותבדילה: وَيُزِّعُه a   19 דקה: حادّ a .add   21 הגבח: الصلع a   22 מן
הדליות: ד .om

אמר המפרש: יאמר ג׳אלינוס: רוצה בכאן הקרחות וכאשר נעתקה הליחה ההיא הרעה למטה
יתחדש הדליות ויצמח השער.

(6.35)

[327] אמר אבקראט: כשיתחדש בבעל השקוי שעול הוא רע.

אמר המפרש: ר״ל כאשר היתה סבת השעול השקוי וזה בשירבה הליחות המימי עד שיגיע
בקנה הריאה ויהיה כבר הגיע על שיתאמת הלחות ההוא.

(6.36)

[328] אמר אבקראט: הקזת העורק יתיד עוצר השתן וראוי שיחתכו העורקים הפנימיים.

אמר המפרש: תקן ג׳אלינוס זה השער שאמר פעמים יתיד עוצר השתן וזה כאשר היה סבתו
מורסא מדם עם רבוי הדם והנשאר מן השער אמר שהוא נוסף במאמר אבקראט והראוי
שיהיה ההקזה אז בארכובה.

(6.37)

[329] אמר אבקראט: כשתראה המורסא בגרגרת מחוץ במי שקרה לו האסכרא יהיה אות
טוב.

אמר המפרש: באר הוא כי הטוב העתק החולי מן האברים הפנימיים לחיצוניים.

(6.38)

[330] אמר אבקראט: כשיתחדש באדם סרטן נסתר הנה טוב שלא יתרפא שאם ירפא ימות
ואם לא ירפא ישאר זמן ארוך.

אמר המפרש: ר״ל בנסתר אשר יהיה בעומק הגוף ולא יהיה נראה או יהיה נגלה ולא יהיה נגע
ור״ל בעזיבת הרפואה מין החתוך או הכויה לא ההשקטה.

---

1 רוצה: כי רצה לומר א יאמר א || אמר בח || הקרחות: בעלי הנתק א add. א 3 הוא
רע: יהיה זה סימן רע עליו א كان دليل رديئا a 4 כאשר היתה: כי בהיות א || בשירבה ד
4–5 עד שיגיע בקנה הריאה: עד שיתעלג בקנה הריאה بدحح إلى أَنْ تَبلغ قصبة الرئة a 5 ויהיה כבר
הגיע על שיתאמת: ויהיה כבר הגיע עד שהשיגו (שיגבר עליו אי) אה ויהיה כבר הגיע שיתאמת בח فيكون
قد أَشفى على أَنْ تَحنقه a 6 יתיד: יתיר אי 8 השער: הפרק א 9 בארכובה: בעורק הארכובה א
בעורק התיכון באורך הארכובה ח في مأبض الركبة a בכל מקום יאמר אבוק׳ שהם למעלה מן הכבד מן
העורק שתחת הארכובה ומן העורקים שהם הנגלים הנקרא כעב (נ״א מאבץ אי) א add. א 12 באר הוא
כי הטוב: באר כי הוא הטוב א באר כי הוא טוב ח 13–405.14 טוב ... הליחה ההיא: om. ד

(6.39)

[331] אמר אבקראט: הקוץ יהיה מן המלוי או מן ההרקה וכן הפיהוק.

אמר המפרש: זה מבואר הסבה.

(6.40)

[332] אמר אבקראט: מי שקרה לו כאב במה שלמטה מן החלצים בלא מורסא ואחר כן התחדש בו קדחת יתך הכאב ההוא ממנו.

אמר המפרש: כשיהיה הכאב ההוא בסבת רוח או סתום תתיכהו הקדחת וכאילו הוא יאמר שתתיכהו וכבר רדפתי משפטי זה האיש כי משפטיו רובם וגדוליהם חסרי התנאים או על דרך זרות וקצתם נאמרים בלי עיון כי הם נפלו במקרה וחשב בעבור כי השאר הדבור יתבאר במקרה שאחד מהם סבה לאחר. כן יאמר מי שלא יתעקש ואולם מי שיתעקש יאמר מה שירצה.

(6.41)

[333] אמר אבקראט: כשיהיה מקום מן הגוף כבר עשה מוגלא ולא התבאר העשותו מוגלא הנה שלא יתבאר מפני עובי החומר או המקום.

אמר המפרש: באר הוא כי מפני עובי החומר או עובי המקום יקשה ידיעת החומר.

(6.42)

[334] אמר אבקראט: כשיהיה באדם ירקון ויהיה בכבדו קשי אות רע.

(6.43)

[335] אמר אבקראט: כשימצא בעל הטחול שלשול דם וארך בו יתחדש בו שקוי או קלוח המעים וימות.

אמר המפרש: בעל הטחול הוא אשר בטחול שלו קושי נושן וכשיתחדש שלשול דם או דרך העתק הליחות העבות ההם אשר ממרה שחורה אשר היו מסובכות בגרם הטחול יקבל תועלת בזה כמו שיבאר אחר זה ואם ארך השלשול ההוא ועבר השיעור ישחית כחות המעים בלכת

---

2 זה: كلّ هذا a   5 ההוא: א .om   6–5 וכאילו הוא יאמר שתתיכהו: בחח .om فكأنّه يقول قد تحلّه الحمى
a   6 רדפתי: זכרתי לך a اطّردت كبي א² .add || האיש: הלכו על דרך זו א .add   7 נאמרים בלי עיון:
وهم a   8–7 כי השאר הדבור יתבאר במקרה: אי ח .om لأنّ الشیئین المقترنین بالإتّفاق a   10 העשותו
מוגלא: מוגלתו א   12–11 עובי החומר או המקום. אמר המפרש: באר הוא כי מפני: אי   13 אמר
אבקראט: כשיהיה באדם ירקון ויהיה בכבדו קשי אות רע: בח .om אמר אבקראט: בהיות הכבד במי
שבו ירקון קשה זה סימן רע לו א || רע: قال المفسّر: هذا بين a .add   17 מסובכות: סבה א מסבבות ח

אלו הליחות הרעות בהם ויתחדש קלוח המעים ויכבה החום הטבעי ובעבור שתוף המעים עם הכבד יחלש הכבד ויתחדש השקוי.

(6.44)

[336] אמר אבקראט: מי שהתחדש בו (מן) הטפת השתן הקולון הידוע באילאוס הנה הוא ימות בשבעה ימים אם לא שיתחדש בו קדחת ויגר ממנו שתן רב.

אמר המפרש: כבר ספק ג׳אלינוס בזה השער והביא סברות רחוקות לאמת מאמר גלוי ההפסד   5 מפעולת הבטלים.

(6.45)

[337] אמר אבקראט: כאשר עבר על הנגע שנה או זמן יותר גדול מזה יתחייב בהכרח שיצאו ממנו עצמות ושיהיה מקום הנגע אחר החתמו עמוק.

אמר המפרש: רוב מה שיארך זמן הנגע מפני ריעוע שהשיג העצם וכשיצא העצם הנפסד   יתרפא וישאר המקום עמוק.   10

(6.46)

[338] אמר אבקראט: מי שמצאו חטוטרת ושעול קודם שיצמח שער הערוה זה ימות.

אמר המפרש: כשהתחדש חטוטרת מבלתי סבה מתחלה הנה היא ממורסא קשה וכאשר חייב זה צרות על הריאה בעבור העתק השנים ובזמן הגידול בתוספת הריאה ולא יהיה אפשר שיתרחב המקום הפנוי מן החזה ולא יקבל כלו הגידול בעבור חטוטרת וסבתה ולכן יחנק   וימות.   15

(6.47)

[339] אמר אבקראט: מי שיצטרך אל ההקזה ושתיית הרפואה המשלשלת הנה ראוי שישתה הרפואה ויקיז באביב.

אמר המפרש: זה מבואר למי שיצטרך אליו על צד השמירה כמו שיעשו הבריאים תמיד.

---

1 בהם: עליהם א ‖ ויתחדש: מזה א add. ‖ 3 הקולון: הקולונג׳ ח ‖ באילאוס הנה הוא add. a מنه וتفسيره المستعاذ
5 ספק: פסק א ‖ והביא: وتكلّف a 6 הבטלים: הבטל א البطّالين 7 על הנגע: על המכה בח ‖ מזה:
והיא נגרת מוגלא א add. ח add. ‖ 9 מפני: א¹ ‖ ריעוע: א¹ آفة a 11 חטוטרת: מג׳ניש ח add. מגיניש ב add.
من ربو a add. 12 מתחלה: פועלת א מתחלת א¹ באד a 13 העתק השנים: שובו כקשת א הנתק השנים
ב التقويس a ‖ ובזמן הגידול: בזמן גדול ב ובזמן ח ‖ בתוספת הריאה: تزيد الرئة a 17 הרפואה: א om.

(6.48)

[340] אמר אבקראט: כשיתחדש בבעל הטחול שלשול דם הנה זה טוב.

אמר המפרש: כבר קדם ביאורו.

(6.49)

[341] אמר אבקראט: מי שהיה מן החוליים מדרך הנקרס והיה עמו מורסא חמה הנה מורסתו
תנוח בארבעים יום.

5   אמר המפרש: כבר קדם על איזה צד נותן אילו הגדרים.

(6.50)

[342] אמר אבקראט: מי שהתתחדש במוחו חתוך הנה אי אפשר שלא התחדש בו קדחת וקיא
מרה אדומה.

אמר המפרש: כשיתנפח המוח בעבור החתוך בהכרח ימשך אחר זה קדחת וקיא המרה
האדומה בעבור שתוף המוח עם האצטו'.

(6.51)

10   [343] אמר אבקראט: מי שהתתחדש בו והוא בריא כאב פתאום בראשו ונשתתק מיד וקרה לו
כמו גסוס הנה הוא ימות בשבעה ימים אם לא התחדש בו קדחת.

אמר המפרש: הגסוס אות חזק השתוק וכבר ידעת שהוא ממית אם לא התחדש קדחת כי
פעמים תתיך אותם הליחות העבות או הרוח העבה.

(6.52)

[344] אמר אבקראט: הנה ראוי שיעיין בעת השינה ואם יראה כלום מלובן העין והעפעף נדבק
15   ולא יהיה זה אחר שלשול או שתיית רפואה משלשלת הנה הוא אות רע ממית מאד.

אמר המפרש: אמנם יתבאר הלובן כאשר לא ידביק העפעף והיות העפעף בלתי נדבק אמנם
הוא בעבור היובש והוא מהיר לבוא בגבינים ליבשותם בטבע או בעבור הכח חולשת הכח כמו
שיחלש בחולים על סתום הפה.

10 והוא בריא כאב פתאום בראשו: כאב פתאום בראשו והוא בריא א   11 גסוס: כאב גסוס א
12 התחדש: בו א   .add א   14 שיעיין: باطن العين .add a || השינה: בחליים החדים א   .add || יראה: לא א
.add || והעפעף נדבק: והעפעף אינו נדבק בטוב א   15 יהיה זה אחר: יהיה אחר זה אחר בח || שתיית:
שתייתו א || אות: .om א   17 בגבינים: בגביני העינים א   18 בחולים על סתום הפה: בחולים החלושים
שאינם יכולים לסתום הפה א בחוליים החלושים על סתום הפה ח في المرضى المدنفين عن إنطباق الفم a

(6.53)

[345] אמר אבקראט: מה שהיה מערבוב השכל עם שחוק הוא טוב ומה שהיה עם יגון ואנחה הנה יותר סכנה.

אמר המפרש: אין ממיני השטות דבר טוב והיותר רע מהם מה שהיה עמו הקדמה להלחם וחטיפה והוא השטות והיותר מעט ברוע מה שהיה עם שחוק ושמחה בלתי נהוג כמו שותה היין ואשר עמו יגון ופחד ומחשבה ועיון הוא ממוצע וכל זה מחולי במוח או בעבור השתתפו לאבר אחר ואשר יהיה מחום לבד מבלתי ליחה הוא דומה לערבוב אשר יהיה משתית היין ואשר יהיה מן המרה השחורה יהיה עמו יגון ופחד וכאשר הוסיף שריפה ונטה אל השחורה נטה הערבוב אל השטות.

(6.54)

[346] אמר אבקראט: נשימת הבכי בחליים החדים אשר תהיה עמהם קדחת אות רע.

אמר המפרש: רוצה שתהיה נשימת החולה תפסק ותשוב כנשימת מי שבוכה מן הדין וזה יהיה אם לחולשת הכח מלמשוך הנשימה או מיובש כלי הנשימה וקשים עד שלא יוכל הכח שישטחם או מענין קרוב מן הקווץ וכל זה בחליים החדים רע.

(6.55)

[347] אמר אבקראט: חליי הנקרס יתנועעו באביב ובחורף על הרוב.

אמר המפרש: באביב להגרת הליחות ותוספתם להתכת קפיאתם הסתוית ובחורף למה שקדם מאכילת פירות הקיץ.

(6.56)

[348] אמר אבקראט: החליים אשר ממרה שחורה יפחד מהם שיביאו אל השתוק או אל הפלג או אל הקווץ או אל השטות או אל העורון.

אמר המפרש: אמר ג'אלינוס: השתוק והפלג והקווץ והעורון יהיו מן הליחה הלבנה ומן הליחה השחורה ואולם השטות לא יקרה כי אם משריפת האדומה עד שתשוב שחורה.

---

1 מה: מי אה ‖ טוב: أَسْلَم a 3–4 הקדמה להלחם וחטיפה: إِقْدَام وَتَهَجُّم a 4 והיותר מעט: והפחות א ‖ ושמחה: וששון א add. a 5 במוח: أَوَّلِيَّة a ‖ add. a ‖ השתתפו: השתתפותו א השתתפות ה 6 מחום לבד: בעבור חמימות א ‖ לערבוב: הדעת א add. a ‖ אשר יהיה: המתהווה א 7 השחורה: الصَّفْرَاء a 10 מי שבוכה מן הדין: مِنْ خَنِقِه البُكَاء a 11 מלמשוך הנשימה: عَن اسْتِيفَاء التَّنَفُّس a 12 שישטחם: להתפשט א 13 חליי: חלי א חולי ה ‖ הנקרס: הנקראץ בח ‖ יתנועעו: יתנועע אה 16 שיביאו: או שיבואו א 18 אמר ג'אלינוס: om. בח

(6.57)

[349] אמר אבקראט: והשתוק והפלג יתחדשו בפרט במי שיהיו שנותיו במה שבין הארבעים שנה עד הששים שנה.

אמר המפרש: סברת ג'אלינוס בזה השער עד שיהיה מאמר אמתי אמר: רוצה השתוק והפלג אשר יתחדשו מן המרה השחורה כי המרה השחורה תגבר על בעלי השנים ההם. ואולם לפי הסברא האמתית הנה התחדש אלו השנים מן המרה השחורה הוא בדרך זרות גדול ורוב התחדשם ברוב יהיה מן הליחה הלבנה ומן הששים שנה עד סוף החיים.

(6.58)

[350] אמר אבקראט: כשיצא לחוץ החלב הנה הוא בלא ספק יתעפש.

אמר המפרש: זה מבואר.

(6.59)

[351] אמר אבקראט: מי שהיה בו כאב גיד הנשה ותקע יריכו ואחר תשוב הנה התחדש בה לחות כדמות הליחה היוצאת מן הנחירים.

אמר המפרש: בעבור הליחה ההיא המדובקת יובללו המיתרים ויקל להוקע כף הירך.

(6.60)

[352] אמר אבקראט: מי שקרהו כאב הירך זמן גדול והיתה ירכו נוקעת הנה כל רגלו תצמוק וישוב חגר אם לא יכוה.

אמר המפרש: התנגב הליחה ההיא המדובקת בכויה וכאשר לא יתנגב הליחה ההיא בכויה יתחדש החגרות ולא ילך הרגל כמנהגו ויצמק.

נשלם המאמר הששי מפרקי אבקראט.

---

1 בפרט: בלבד א¹ ‖ במה שבין: בן בח   3 סברת: דברי א   4 כי המרה השחורה תגבר: הגוברת
א   5 התחדש: יתחדשו בח תתחדש ח ‖ אלו השנים: אלו השני חליים א   6 התחדשם: התחדש בח
תתחדש ח ‖ ומן הששים שנה עד סוף החיים: ומן השנים בסוף החיים בחה   7 החלב: המכסה א² ‪.add‬
9 ותקע: ונשמט א ‖ בה: בירכו א בו ח   11 המדובקת: الخاطئة a ‖ יובללו: א¹ יתבטלו א ‖ המיתרים:
הנותרים בח המותרים ח ‖ להוקע: להשמט א   12 כל: א² ‪.om‬ ח   13 וישוב חגר: ויקצר ויעות וישוב
חגר א וישוב ויקצר וימות חגר ח   14 ההיא: ‪starts again‬ ד   15 ילך: تغني a ‖ ויצמק: ‪.om‬ א
16 נשלם המאמר הששי מפרקי אבקראט: נשלם המאמר הששי מפירוש הפרקים בח ח ‪.om‬

המאמר השביעי מפירוש פרקי אבקראט

(7.1)

[353] אמר אבקראט: כשיתקררו הקצוות בחליים החדים אות רע.

אמר המפרש: זה אצלי ראיה על חולשת החום הטבעי והיותו בלתי מגיע אל הקצוות עם היות
החולי חד ר״ל חם כי אבקראט יקרא חליים חדים החליים אשר תהיה הקדחת בהם דבקה
5 והקצוות הם קצה החוטם והאזנים והכפיים והרגלים.

(7.2)

[354] אמר אבקראט: כשיהיה בעצם חולי והיה מראה הבשר עליו חשוך הנה הוא אות רע.

אמר המפרש: המראה הזה נמשך אחר כבוי החום הטבעי.

(7.3)

[355] אמר אבקראט: הפיהוק ואדמימות העינים אחר הקיא אות רע.

אמר המפרש: כאשר לא יסתלק הקיווץ אחר הקיא הנה זה ראיה שסבתו אם מורסא בראש
10 העצבי ר״ל המוח ואם מורסא באצטומ׳ ואדמימות העינים נמשך אחר שתי המורסות האלה.

(7.4)

[356] אמר אבקראט: כשיתחדש עם הזיעה פלצות אין זה אות טוב.

אמר המפרש: כבר אמר אבקראט כי מקרי הנקיון כשלא יתחדש מהם נקיון יורה על מות או
קשי נקיון כי הטבע נבוך.

(7.5)

[357] אמר אבקראט: כשיתחדש אחר השטות שלשול דם או שקוי או בהלה הנה הוא אות
15 טוב.

אמר המפרש: אולם השקוי והשלשול ירפאו בהעתק החומר ואולם המבוכה כי המקרים
כאשר נוספו והתחזקו התעורר הטבע והתנועע לדחות כל מה שיזיק בדרך הנקיון כן סברת
ג׳אלינוס.

_____

1 מפירוש פרקי אבקראט: א .om ‖ 2 כשיתקררו: קור בח ‖ בחליים: מחליים ד ‖ 3 מגיע: ﺗﻨﺸﺮ a
9 שסבתו: על כי סבתו א ‖ 10 העצבי: העצב אה ‖ 12 אבקראט: החכם אבקראט א ‖ 13 נבוך (=)
ﺗﺤﺎﺭ‎: כלומר הטבע יחלש ויכבה א ﺗﺤﻮﺭ a ‖ 16 המבוכה: והבהלה א׳ .add ‖ 17 התעורר: أرهقت a

(7.6)

[358] אמר אבקראט: סור התאוה בחולי הנושן והצואה הפשוטה אות רע.

אמר המפרש: רוצה בצואה הפשוטה אשר לא יתערב עמה דבר מן הלחות המימי אבל יצא
החולי אשר בגוף לבד בין שהיה ממיני המרה האדומה או ממיני השחורה הנה זה יורה על
שהלחות הטבעי כלו כבר נשרף מחום הקדחת.

(7.7)

5 [359] אמר אבקראט: כשיתחדש מרוב שתיה רתת וערבוב שכל הנה זה רע.

אמר המפרש: התחבר הרתת עם הערבוב מעט שיקרה כי אם בקצת מרבים השכרות ויכבה
החום הטבעי ויתחדש הרתת וימלא המוח מדם חם ואיד חם ויתערבב השכל.

(7.8)

[360] אמר אבקראט: כאשר נפתחה היציאה לפנים יתחדש מזה נפילת כח וקיא והתכת נפש.

אמר המפרש: זה מבואר וירצה ביציאה המורסא הנקראת דבילה ור״ל לפנים אל האצטומכא.

(7.9)

10 [361] אמר אבקראט: כשיתחדש מהגרת הדם ערבוב השכל או קווץ הנה זה אות רע.

אמר המפרש: ערבוב השכל אחר ההרקה יהיה לצער המוח בתנועותיו ויהיה תמיד חלוש
ואבקראט יקרא ערבוב השכל החלוש הדיאן.

(7.10)

[362] אמר אבקראט: כשיתחדש מהקולון החזק קיא ופיהוק וערבוב שכל וקווץ הנה זה אות
מגונה.

15 אמר המפרש: זה מבואר.

(7.11)

[363] אמר אבקראט: כשיתחדש מחולי הצד חולי הריאה הנה זה אות רע.

אמר המפרש: כשלא יספיק אל הליחה המחדשת לחולי הצד מקומה תשפיע ממנו קצת אל
הריאה ואולם חולי הריאה אי אפשר שימשך אחריו חולי הצד.

---

5 שתיה: שתית היין **אבח** ‖ רע: دليل رديء a   6 הערבוב: ערבוב השכל **אבח** ‖ ויכבה: וירבה **א**
7 ואיד חם: **א**ⁱ   8 והתכת: והתרת **א**   9 לפנים: הגוף **א** .add   11 לצער: להצטער **א** لاضطراب
a   13 מהקולון: מקולונג **א** ‖ מהקולון החזק: عن القولنج المستعاذ منه a

(7.12)

[364] אמר אבקראט: ומחולי הריאה מורסת הראש.

(7.13)

[365] אמר אבקראט: ומהשריפה החזקה הקווץ והמשיכה.

(7.14)

[366] אמר אבקראט: ומההכאה על הראש הבהלה וערבוב השכל רע.

(7.15)

[367] אמר אבקראט: ומרקיקת הדם רקיקת המוגלא.

(7.16)

[368] אמר אבקראט: ומרקיקת המוגלא השדפון וההגרה וכאשר נעצר הרוק ימות בעל   5
החולי.

(7.17)

[369] אמר אבקראט: וממורסת הכבד הפיפוק.

(7.18)

[370] אמר אבקראט: ומהיקיצה הקיווץ וערבוב השכל.

אמר המפרש: כל זה מבואר ועניגו שהוא כאשר גדלו אלו החליים ונושנו פעמים יתחדש מהם
כך וכך כמו שמורסת הכבד כאשר גדלה והזיקה בפי האצטומכה יתחדש הפיהוק וכבר הודיע   10
כי הקיווץ וערבוב השכל פעמים יתחדשו מן היובש והיובש נמשך אחר רוב ההרקה והתנועות
הנפשיות והיקיצה.

(7.19)

[371] אמר אבקראט: ומגלוי העצם המורסא הנקראת חומרה.

אמר המפרש: באר ג׳אלינוס כי גלוי העצם לא יתחדש ממנו זאת המורסא כי אם בדרך זרות
והוא גם כן זכר כל מה שאפשר שימשך דבר אחר דבר ואפילו על המעט.   15

(7.20)

[372] אמר אבקראט: ומהמורסא אשר יקרא אלחומרא העפוש והנפח.

אמר המפרש: זה מבואר לפי מה שקדם פעמים רבות שעניינו פעמים יתחדש.

(7.21)

[373] אמר אבקראט: ומהדפיקה החזקה בנגעים יציאת הדם.

אמר המפרש: זה מבואר כי לחוזק הכאב יתנועעו העורקים תנועה חזקה לדחות המזיק.

(7.22)

[374] אמר אבקראט: ומהכאב הנושן במה שסמוך לאצטו' העשות המוגלא.

אמר המפרש: הכאב הנושן אמנם יהיה ממנו המורסא והמורסא ההיא תעשה מוגלא.

(7.23)

[375] אמר אבקראט: ומהצואה הפשוטה שלשול הדם.

אמר המפרש: רוצה שתהיה הצואה ליחה מן הליחות לבד פעמים יחדש אכול ונגע במעים.

(7.24)

[376] אמר אבקראט: ומחתוך העצם ערבוב השכל אם נגע הפנוי מן הראש.

אמר המפרש: יאמר כי כאשר נחתך עצם הראש עד שיגיע החתך למקום הפנוי המחזיק למוח יתחדש ערבוב השכל.

(7.25)

[377] אמר אבקראט: הקווץ משתית משקה משלשל ממית.

אמר המפרש: זה מבואר.

(7.26)

[378] אמר אבקראט: קור הקצוות מהכאב החזק במה שסמוך אל האצטו' רע.

אמר המפרש: זה מבואר.

2–4 זה ... אמר המפרש: ח om. ‖ 2 רבות: ד om. ‖ פעמים יתחדש: שיתחדש כך וכך א 6 אמנם:
א om. ‖ ההיא: א om. 8 פעמים יחדש: אז יתחדש א ‖ 9 נגע הפנוי: יגיע למקום הפנוי א יהיה הנגע
הפנוי בח יגע הפנוי ח 10 עד שיגיע החתך: עד שהחתוך יהיה מגיע א ‖ המחזיק למוח: המקיף למוח
א الحاوي للدماغ a 14 רע: הנה זה הוא רע א

(7.27)

[379] אמר אבקראט: כשיתחדש במעוברת פונץ יהיה סבה שתפיל.

אמר המפרש: זה מבואר.

(7.28)

[380] אמר אבקראט: כאשר נחתך דבר מן העצם או מן האליל לא ישלם.

אמר המפרש: כבר הורה ג'אלינוס שהוא כפול.

(7.29)

[381] אמר אבקראט: כשיתחדש במי שגבר עליו הליחה הלבנה שלשול חזק יתך ממנו בו　5
חליו.

אמר המפרש: הליחה הלבנה הוא השקוי הבשרי. אמר המחבר: כבר ראיתי זה שתי פעמים.

(7.30)

[382] אמר אבקראט: מי שיהיה בו שלשול והיה במה שיוצא בשלשול קצף פעמים שיהיה
סבת שלשולו דבר שיורד מראשו.

אמר המפרש: סבת הדבר שיש בו קצף התערב האויר בו ערוב חזק ופעמעם יהיה הלחות　10
ההוא היורד מן הראש או מאיברים אחרים או יתילד באצטומכא והמעים.

(7.31)

[383] אמר אבקראט: מי שהיה בו קדחת והיה צולל בשתנו שמרים דומים לסלת הגריס הנה
זה יורה על שחליו ארוך.

אמר המפרש: הליחות אשר יראה זה מהם רחוקים מן הבשול ולכן זכר אבקראט כי אלו ימותו
ברוב ומי שנצל מהם יארך חליו כמו שזכר הנה.　15

(7.32)

[384] אמר אבקראט: כשיהיה הגובר על השמרים אשר בשתן המרה האדומה והיה העליון
ממנו דק יורה שהחולי חד.

---

3 האליל: התנוך א ‖ ישלם: יתדבק א ימלט בח يﻨﻢ a   5 שלשול: שקוי ד   8–9 קצף פעמים שיהיה
סבת שלשולו דבר שיורד מראשו: שזה מליחה יורדת מן הראש ד   10 סבת הדבר: הקצוף פעמים
שיהיה סבת הדבר ד   11 אחרים: om. בדחח ‖ או: אשר א   16 הגובר: om. ד

אמר המפרש: זה מבואר ורצה באמרו דק שיהיה עליון השמרים דק ושיהיה תמונתו כדמות אם הבטנים.

(7.33)

[385] אמר אבקראט: מי שהיה השתנו משובש יורה כי בגופו צער חזק.

אמר המפרש: ר״ל מתחלף החלקים וזה ראיה על חלוף פועל הטבע בליחות.

(7.34)

[386] אמר אבקראט: מי שיהיה על שתנו אבעבועות מורה שחליו בכליות ויורה עליו   5
באריכות.

אמר המפרש: כי הוא מורה על רוח עב בתוך ליחות מדובקות ולכן יורה עליו באריכות.

(7.35)

[387] אמר אבקראט: מי שתראה על שתנו שומן כלו יורהו בכליתו חולי חד.

אמר המפרש: כשיהיה השומן יבא בפעם אחת הנה הוא ראיה שהוא מהתכת שומן הכליות
וזה ענין אמרו כלו ואולם אשר יבא מהתכת שאר האיברים הנה יבא מעט מעט.   10

(7.36)

[388] אמר אבקראט: מי שהיה בכליתו חולי וקרה לו אלו המקרים שקדם זכרם והתחדש בו
כאב בגיד הגב הנה אם היה הכאב במקומות היוצאים יפחד מיציאת תבא בו מחוץ ואם היה
הכאב ההוא במקומות הנכנסים הנה יותר קרוב שתהיה המורסא הנק׳ דבילה מבפנים.

אמר המפרש: זה מבואר.

(7.37)

[389] אמר אבקראט: מי שהקיא דם מבלתי קדחת הוא בטוח וראוי שיתרפא בעליו בדברים   15
הקובצים והדם אשר יקיאו אותו עם קדחת רע.

אמר המפרש: ר״ל שהוא אם לא תהיה שם מורסא באצטומ׳ שהקדחת נמשכת אחריו בהכרח
והיה הדם הזה בעבור עורק שנפתח או חבורה התחדשה עתה הנה אפשר שיתרפא מהר
בדברים הקובצים.

(7.38)

[390] אמר אבקראט: היָרידות אשר ירדו אל החלל העליון יעשה מוגלא בעשרים יום.

אמר המפרש: החלל העליון הפנוי מן החזה אשר בו הריאה ויום עשרים הוא יום נקיון כי הוא סוף השבוע השלישי ואמר כי זה היותר רחוק שאפשר שנתבשל בו הירידה.

(7.39)

[391] אמר אבקראט: מי שהשתין דם נקרש והיה בו הטפת השתן ומצאהו כאב בצדי הטבור ושפל הבטן יורה זה על מה שסביב מקומתו כואב.

5

אמר המפרש: נכפל ענינו.

(7.40)

[392] אמר אבקראט: מי שנעדר מלשונו פתאום כחה ורפה אבר מאיבריו הנה החולי ממרה שחורה.

אמר המפרש: כבר הודה ג'אלינוס שהוא בלתי מתחייב שיהיה זה מן המרה השחורה בלא ספק.

10

(7.41)

[393] אמר אבקראט: כשיתחדש בישישים בסבת הרקת שלשול או קיא)או(פיהוק אין זה ראיה טובה.

אמר המפרש: הפיהוק אחר ההרקות רע כי הוא נמשך אחר יובש ולזקנים יותר רע ליבשות מזגם.

(7.42)

[394] אמר אבקראט: מי שמצאהו קדחת שאינה ממרה אדומה והוצק על ראשו מים חמים הרבה תתך בו קדחתו.

15

אמר המפרש: ג'אלינוס ישתדל שיסבור בזה השער ויאמר כי כונתו באמרו קדחת שאינה ממרה אדומה אינה קדחת עפוש אבל קצת מיני קדחת יום ואין ספק כי המרחץ בהם מועיל ובו תתך הקדחת.

---

3 השלישי: א .om   4 נקרש: נקשר **אבה** קרוש **ה** ‖ הטבור: = السرة ACP الشرح ‖ P lt S, fol. 148 a
5 ושפל: ושפול **ד** ‖ על מה שסביב: על כי מסביב **ה**   11 בישישים: בזקן **א** ‖ בסבת: סבת **ד**
13 ולזקנים: וקיא הזקנים **בדח**   14 מזגם: بالسنّ .add. a   15 והוצק: והורק **א** ‖ חמים: חיים **א**
17 ג'אלינוס ישתדל שיסבור: אם תוכל שים בו **א** ‖ קדחת: כי קדחת **א** וכי קדחת **ה**   18 אדומה: והורק
על ראשו מים הרבה תתך בו **א** .add ‖ מיני: ממיני **א** ‖ המרחץ: א .om

(7.43)

[395] אמר אבקראט: האשה לא תהיה בעלת שתי ימינים.

אמר המפרש: אמר ג'אלינוס כי סבתו הוא חולשת איבריה וגידיה כי כל בעל שני ימנים הנה
(מ)עלתו חוזק העצבים.

(7.44)

[396] אמר אבקראט: מי שנכוה מאשר נעשת בו מוגלא ויצאה ממנו ליחה נקיה לבנה הנה
הוא בטוח ואם תצא ממנו ליחה עכורה סרוחה הנה הוא ימות.   5

אמר המפרש: הנעשה בו מוגלא הוא אשר תקובץ ליחה רבה בין החזה שלו ובין ריאתו והוא
שהיה מנהג הראשונים לכוותו להוציא הליחה ההיא.

(7.45)

[397] אמר אבקראט: מי שהיה בכבדו מוגלא ונכוה ויצא ממנו ליחה נקיה לבנה הנה הוא
יהיה בבטח וזה כי הליחה ההיא בו במכסה הכבד ואם יצא ממנו בדמיון שמרי השמן
ימות.   10

אמר המפרש: כשתהיה המוגלא במכסה וגרם הכבד הוא בטוח ואפשר לו הבריאות.

(7.46)

[398] אמר אבקראט: כשיהיה בעינים כאב השקו בעליו יין חי ואחר כן הכניסוהו במרחץ
וצוקו עליו מים חמים הרבה ואחר כן הקיזו אותו.

אמר המפרש: אמר ג'אלינוס כי השער הזה אינו לאבקראט ובכלל הוא טעות לגמרי אמרו מי
שאמרו.   15

(7.47)

[399] אמר אבקראט: כשיתחדש לבעל השקוי שעול לא יהיה בטוח.

אמר המפרש: כבר קדם ענינו.

2 אמר ג'אלינוס: א om. ‖ איבריה (= أعضائها A): أعضائها a 3 (מ)עלתו: ד om. ‖ سببه a om. ‖ העצבים:
העצבון א 4 שנכוה: أو بطّ (except for BCP) a add. 5-4 הנה הוא בטוח: ימלט א يَسلم a
7 הראשונים: האנשים ד 9 בו: אח om. ‖ השמן: השתן אבהה 13-12 הכניסוהו במרחץ וצוקו:
הכניסהו במרחץ ויצוק ה 14 אמר ג'אלינוס: ג'אלינוס יאמר א ‖ מי: מה ד

(7.48)

[400] אמר אבקראט: הטפת השתן ועצירתו תתיכם שתיית היין וההקזה וראוי שיחתכו העורקים הפנימיים.

אמר המפרש: זה המאמר נגלה ההפסד אבל ג׳אלינוס השתדל שיוציא לתחלת הפרק הזה פנים של יושר ואמר כשיהיה סבת זה מקור או מסיתום מתחדש מדם עב מבלתי מלוא בגוף תהיה שתיית היין הרבה מועילה מזה ואולם אמרו בזה השער שיחתוך העורקים 5 הנכנסים וכן במאמר אשר נאמר בו זה הנה כבר ביאר ג׳אלינוס כי הוא אינו אמת ואינו דעת אבקראט.

(7.49)

[401] אמר אבקראט: כאשר נראית המורסא והחמרה בקודם מן החזה במי שקרהו האסכרא יהיה זה אות טוב כי החולי כבר נטה לחוץ.

אמר המפרש: זה מבואר. 10

(7.50)

[402] אמר אבקראט: מי שמצאהו במוחו החולי הנקרא אספדלסמוס הנה הוא ימות בשלשה ימים ואם עבר זה הנה יתרפא.

אמר המפרש: זה החולי הפסד עצם המוח ואין רפואה לו כאשר נשלם ואמנם ר״ל שהוא התחלת זה החולי ואם עבר הג׳ ימים ולא מת הנה הוא ראיה שלא נשלם ושהטבע נתחזק ונתקן. 15

(7.51)

[403] אמר אבקראט: העיטוש יהיה בראש כאשר נתחמם המוח ונרטב המקום הפנוי בראש וירד האויר אשר בו ונשמע לו קול כי עברו ותנועתו יהיה במקום צר.

אמר המפרש: פעמים יהיה העטוש כאשר יתחמם המוח ויתלחלח המקום הפנוי אשר בו וימשוך הלחות ההוא איד ופעמים יעלה עם השעול רוח מלמטה וכאשר תהיה במעברי הנחירים תהיה סבה להתחדש העיטוש ומעברי החוטם יצאו אל שני מקומות הפה 20 והמוח והנקב אשר יצא אל הפה ינקה ברוח אשר תעלה מלמטה. ואולם המעברים אשר יצאו אל המוח הנה ינקו ברוח אשר תרד ממנו. ואמרו המקום הפנוי ר״ל בטני המוח.

(7.52)

[404] אמר אבקראט: מי שהיה בו כאב חזק בכבדו והתחדשה בו קדחת יתך הכאב ההוא
ממנו.

אמר המפרש: כאב חזק בכבד מבלתי קדחת אמנם יהיה מרוח עב ולכן כשתתחדש הקדחת
יתך הרוח ההוא.

(7.53)

[405] אמר אבקראט: מי שהוצרך שיוציאו מעורקיו דם ראוי שיפתחו לו העורק באביב.   5

אמר המפרש: זה מן הפרקים אשר נכפלו.

(7.54)

[406] אמר אבקראט: מי שתהיה נבוכה בו הליחה הלבנה במה שבין האצטו' והמסך והתחדש
בו כאב כשלא יהיה לה מעבר לאחד מן החללים הנה הליחה ההיא כשתלך בעורקים אל
המקוה יתך ממנו חליו.

אמר המפרש: הנה אמרו כי זה אינו לאבקראט ואמר ג'אלינוס שהוא בלתי נמנע שתמנע   10
הליחה הזאת לעורקים בדיות כי הטבע תעשה תחבולה לדקדק החמרים ולהוציאם בכל דרך
שיוכל ואפילו בדרך רחוק כמו שיוציא המוגלא המתקבצת במה שבין הריאה והחזה ובכלל
הוא מאמר שיקרה מעט ומעט התועלת מאד.

(7.55)

[407] אמר אבקראט: כשנמלא הכבד ממים ואחר כן יצאו המים ההם אל המסך אשר בפנים
ימלא בטנו ממים וימות.   15

אמר המפרש: פעמים יתחדשו נפחים רבים בכבד ואמרו כי מי שנמלא בטנו ממים ימות זה
על הרוב.

(7.56)

[408] אמר אבקראט: הסער והאשתרילאר והפלצות ירפאהו היין כאשר נמזג אחד שוה
באחד שוה.

---

3 כשתתחדש הקדחת: כשיתחדש בקדחת ד   5 שיוציאו: שהוציאו ד להוציא א   7 מי שתהיה
נבוכה בו (= مِن تَحيّر فِيه): מי שנבוכה בו ד מי שהיה בו נבוכה בח מי שתהיה בו ה مِن تَحيّر فِيه a   8 כאב:
ר״ל ד .add   11 לעורקים: העורקים ד ‖ בדיות: בכלות א בביות בח באמת ה   12 בדרך רחוק (בדרך
דחוק?): بعد ودقّ a ‖ ובכלל: הנה ד .add   16 זה: הוא ד .add   18 הסער והאשתרילאר והפלצות:
הצער והלאר (והאשתרילאר א') והפלצות א הפיהוק והאסטניצות ח הסער והאשתרילייר והפלצות ח
19–18 הסער ... באחד שוה: המצוק והפלצות הוא בדלאר והסמור והאשתריניקלארי יבריא(הו) היין אם
ימזג חלק בחלק שוה ב

אמר המפרש: רוב הסער מלחות מזקת בפי האצטומכא ושתיית היין המקבל המזג כמו שאמר
ירפא מכל זה לרחצו העורקים ותקנו הליחות.

(7.57)

[409] אמר אבקראט: מי שיצא שחין דק באמתו כשיתנפח ויפתח יכלה כאבו.

אמר המפרש: זה מן הכפולים.

(7.58)

[410] אמר אבקראט: מי שיזדעזע מוחו הנה הוא ימצאהו מיד שתוק.

אמר המפרש: אמנם יהיה זעזוע המוח או מוח חוט השדרה בנפילה או הדומה לו.

(7.59a–b)
[411]

(7.60)

[412] אמר אבקראט: מי שהיה בשרו לח הנה ראוי שירעיב עצמו כי הרעב ינגף הגופות.

אמר המפרש: זה מבואר.

(7.61)

[413] אמר אבקראט: כשיתחדש בגוף כלו שנויים ויתקרר קור חזק ואחר כך יתחמם ויהיה לו
מראה אחר ואחר כן ישתנה וישוב אל זולתו יורה על אריכות החולי.

אמר המפרש: זה מן הכפולים.

(7.62)

[414] אמר אבקראט: הזיעה הרבה אשר תגר תמיד תהיה חמה או קרה יורה על שהוא ראוי
שיוציא מן הגוף לחות אמנם בחזק מלמעלה ואמנם בחלוש מלמטה.

---

1 רוב הסער מלחות מזקת בפי האצטומכא: רוב המצ[..] ב ‖ המקבל: המקביל א القليل a ‖ המקבל
המזג כמו שאמר: מזג כמו שזכר ב   3 שחין דק: צמח קטן הנקרא בתר ב ‖ באמתו: הנה הוא
ב ‖ כשיתנפח: تقيّحت emendation editor a انفحت A انفتحت CP   6 בנפילה: בשתוק ד
add. ב
This aphorism is missing in the Arabic and Hebrew MSS, as it is a repitition of aphorisms 7
4.34-35   8 לח: רטוב ב ‖ שירעיב עצמו: שיתרעב א שירעב ב ‖ ינגף הגופות: מנגף הגופים ב
12-10 אמר ... הכפולים: בחח om.   10 ויהיה: ויבא א   12 מן הכפולים: נכפל א   13 אשר תגר:
היוצאת ב ‖ תהיה חמה או קרה: בין שתהיה חמה בין קרה ב   14 שיוציא: שיצא ב ‖ אמנם בחזק
מלמעלה ואמנם: אם בחזק מלמעלה ואם ב

אמר המפרש: אמרו כי הלחות תורק מן החזק בקיא ומן החלוש בשלשול לא יעשה כן תמיד. וכבר ידעת דרכו וכבר ספק ג׳אלינוס בזה הפרק אם הוא לאבקראט או לזולתו.

תם ונשלם תהלה לאל בורא עולם.

---

1 אמרו כי הלחות תורק: מאמרו שהלחות יהיה מורק ב‖ 2 ‖ יעשה כן תמיד: יהיה זב[..] ב דרכו וכבר ספק ג׳אלינוס: דרך אבוקרט ומנהגו וגאלינוס מסופק ב 3 תם ונשלם תהלה לאל בורא עולם: נשלם המאמר השביעי תמו ונשלמו פרקי אבוקרט ח נשלם המאמר הז׳ מפי׳ הפרקים ולוית חן הם לראש וענקי׳ כסף הבאורי׳ אמרים מדבש מתוקי׳ תהלה לאל גדול מעל שמי׳ חסדו ועד שחקים תם תם ח נשלם המאמר השבעי מפי׳ הפרקי׳ לוית חן הם לראש וענקים והם מחושקי׳ כסף הבאורים אמרים מדבש מתוקים תהלה לאל הגדול מעל שמים חסדו ועד שחקים ב א״א: מי שנעזבה צואתו עד שתנוח ולא תנוע וראית למעלה כמו הגרידה זה אם הוא מועט יהיה חליו מועט ואם יהיה הרבה חליו יהיה הרבה. עוד א״א: זה יצטרך לשלשל בטנו לא תנקה בטנו ותתן לו מזון כל מה שיזסיף ממנו יוסיף הזק. עוד א״א: בקדחת אשר לא תוסיף ממנה הרקיקה הנוטה לשחרות הדומה לדם והמוסרחת והיא כמו הדיו כלן רעות ואם נפתחה מאד היא טובה וכן הענין במי שיצא מן הבטן ומן השלפוחית וכל אשר יהיה יוצא ונפסקה יציאתו מבלתי היות הגוף נקי זה הוא רע. עוד א״א: צאת הגוף מן טבעו צאת הגוף מן הבטן ובמה שיורק מן הבשר או מזולתו מן הגוף אם יהיה מעט (יהיה החולי מעט) אם יהיה הרבה יהיה החולי הרבה (ואם יהיה הרבה) מאד ויזרה על מות והצדקה לנפשו תציל ממות נפשו. א״ה: כל אלו הפרקים הם מבוארים אינם צריכים לפירוש. והנה נשלמה כתיבת הז׳ מאמרים מפרקי אבוק׳ ופירושם והעתיקם מלשון הגרי אל לשון עברי החכם השוע הנכבד והנעלה החכם ר׳ משה בן החכם הפילוסוף אבי המעתיקים הה״ר שמואל בן החכם הה״ר יהודה אבן תבון. בריך רחמנא דסייען מריש ועד כען. בעזר האל נשלם יום שני יד׳ לחדש אייר שנת הרמ״ג ליצירה מכתב שמואל הצעיר אלעזר פרנס א

Commentary on Hippocrates' Aphorisms: Second Hebrew Translation (Zeraḥyah Ḥen)

[1] אמר משה בן עביד אלה הישראלי הקרטבי זצ״ל איני חושב ששום אחד מן החכמים אשר
חיברו הספרים חבר ספר מאחד ממיני החכמות והוא יהיה מכוין שלא יובנו דברי ספרו עד
שיהיה צריך לפירוש כי אילו כיון זה כיון זה שום חכם ממחברי הספרים היה מבטל בלא ספק תכלית
כוונת ספרו אשר חבר כי המחבר לא יחבר ספרו שהוא יבין ספרו לבדו אבל יחברהו כדי
שיבינו בו אחרים כי אילו כיון זה היה ספרו אשר חבר בלתי מובן אלא בספר אחר הנה בטל
זה תכלית ספרו.

[2] והסבות אשר הביא לאחרונים לפרש ספרי הקדמונים ולבאר אותם הן לפי דעתי ארבע
סבות. הסבה הראשונה: שלימות חכמת המחבר כי הוא בעבור שכלו הטוב ידבר בעניינים
עמוקים נסתרים רחוקים מהשיג במאמר קצר ויהיה זה אצלו מבואר אינו צריך לתוספת.
וכאשר יחשוב הבא אחריו להבין אותם העניינים מאותו המאמר הקצר יקשה זה עליו מאד
ויצטרך המפרש אל אריכות דברים נוספים במאמר עד אשר יובן העניין אשר כיון אותו המחבר
הראשון.

[3] והסבה השנית שעזב הקדמות הספר והוא שהמחבר חבר ספרו והיה סומך שהמעיין
קדמה לו ידיעה באותן ההקדמות הפלוניות וכאשר יחשוב להבין אותו הספר מי שאין לו
חכמה באותן ההקדמות לא יבין בו שום דבר ויצטרך המפרש להביא אותן ההקדמות והבנתם
או שיעירנו על הספרים אשר התבארו בהם אותן ההקדמות וישירנו בהן ולפי זאת הסבה כמו
כן יפרש המפרש עלות מה שלא זכר המחבר עלתו.

[4] והסבה השלישית הכרעת המאמר כי רוב המאמרים בכל לשון יהיה סובל פירוש ואיפשר
שיובן מאותו המאמר עניינים משתנים אבל קצתם הם זו הפך זו אבל סותרים זה את זה. ויפול
השינוי בין המעיינים באותו המאמר ויבארהו אדם אחד אחד פירוש אחד ויאמר מה שרצה בו
המחבר אל זה העניין. ויבארהו אדם אחר פירוש אחר ויצטרך המפרש לאותו המאמר אל
הכרעת אחד מהפירושים ולהביא על אמתתו ראייה ולהיות פוסל מה שאומר זולתו.

[5] והסבה הרביעית הספקות הנכנסות על המחבר או המאמר המוכפל או מה שלא יהיה
בו תועלת כלל ויצטרך המפרש לעורר עליהם ויביא ראייה בביטולם או שיהיה אותו הדבר
בלתי מועיל או מוכפל. וזה אינו נקרא פירוש באמת אבל תשובות והערות. אבל נהוג אצל בני
אדם שיראו הספר ואם זה מה שנא׳ בו רובו הוא נכון ישר תמנה ההערה על אותם המקומות

---

4 כי המחבר לא יחבר ספרו שהוא יבין ספרו לבדו: זⁱ   8 חכמת: فضيلة a   10 יחשוב: رام a
11 אריכות דברים: بسط a   21 אל זה העניין: إلّا هذا المعنى a

המועטים מכל הפירוש ויאמר חשב המחבר במאמרו כך והאמת הוא כך וזה יצטרך לזכרו או
זה הכפלת המאמר בו ויבאר זה כלו. אבל אם היה מה שאמר באותו הספר רובו טעות יהיה
נקרא החיבור האחרון אשר יגלה אותן הטעיות תשובות לא פירוש. ואם זכר בספר התשובה
שום דבר מן המאמרים האמתיים אשר נזכרו בחבור הראשון נאמר אמנם אמרו כך הוא אמת.

5   [6] וכל מה שפירוש מספרי ארסטו' אמנם התבאר פירוש לפי הסבה הראשונה והשלישית
לפי הנראה לנו. וכל מה שהתבאר מספרי הלימודים אמנם התבאר לפי הסבה השנית. והנה
נתפרשו קצת מאמרים לימודיים לפי הסבה הרביעית כמו כן. כי זה הספר הנקרא אל מגסטי
עם גדולת מחברו נכנסו לו בספרו ספקות התעוררו עליהם קהל מן הספרדיים וחברו ספרים
בזה. וכל מה שפורש או שיפורש מספרי בקראט הוא לפי הסבה הראשונה והשלישית
10   והרביעית רובה וקצת מאמריו הם מפורשים לפי הסבה השנית.

[7] אלא שגאלינוס לא יורה זה ולא ירצה בשום פנים שיהיה בדברי אבוקרט ספק אבל יפרש
בו מה שלא יסבול פירושו וישים פירוש המאמר מה שלא יורה אותו המאמר בשום פנים על
שום דבר ממנו כמו שתראהו שעשה בפירושו לספר הליחות ואע"פ שהיה ספק על גאלינוס
אם הוא לאבוקרט או לזולתו והביאו לזה מה שהוא אותו הספר מבולבל בעניינים והיותם
15   דומים חיבורי בעלי הקימייא או בא מהם. ויותר ראוי אצלי להקרא ספר הבלבול אבל מפני
שייחוסו מפורסם שהוא לאבוקרט פרשו זה הפירוש מופלא. וכל מה שאמרו גאלנוס באותו
הפירוש כולו הוא מאמר אמיתי לפי מלאכת הרפואות אבל לא יורה שום דבר מאותו הפירוש
על שום דבר מן העניין המפורש ואינו נקרא זה פירוש על האמת כי הפירוש הוא להוציא
באותו המאמר בכח לפי ההבנה אל הפועל עד שאתה כשתשוב ותשתכל המאמר המפורש
20   אחר שהשיבנת אותו מן הפירוש תראה אותו המאמר מורה על מה שהשיבנת אותו מן הפירוש.
זהו אצלי הנקרא באמת פירוש לא שיביא האדם מאמרים אמתיים ויאמר זה פירוש מאמר
האומר כך כמו שעשה גאלנוס בקצת מאמרי בקראט. וכמו כן אותם שיולידו תולדת מדברי
חכם ויקראו זה פירוש. אין זה אצלי פירוש אבל חיבור אחר כרוב פירושי אקלידס ללגרזי כי
אני איני קורא זה כולו פירוש.

25   [8] וכן תמצא גאלנוס כמו כן בבארו לספרי אבוקרט שיבאר המאמר הפך המובן בו כמו
שעשה בספר השבועות באמרו בקראט שהארץ תקיף במים. פירש זה המאמר גאלנוס
במאמרו אפשר שירצה לומר שהמים מקיפים באדמה. כל זה עד שלא יאמר שאבוקרט היה
טועה או נכנס עליו ספק בזה הדבר. וכשינוצח בעניין ומצא מאמר מבואר הטעות ולא ימצא
תחבולה יאמר זה מיוחס לאבוקרט ונכנס במאמרו או הוא מאמר אבוקרט הפלוני לא אבוקרט
30   המפורסם כמו שעשה בפירושו לטבע האדם. וכל זה מרוב תאווה לאבוקרט ואע"פ שהיה
אבוקרט מן הגדולים שברופאים ומנכבדיהם בלא ספק אין התאווה מדה טובה אע"פ שזה
בחוק אדם נכבד.

---

[9] וידוע כי כל ספר שפורש או יפורש אין כל מה שבו יצטרך אל פירוש רק עכ"פ יהיה בו
דבר מבואר אינו צריך לבאר. אבל כוונת המפרשים בפירושם כדרך המחברים בחיבוריהם
כי יש מחברים שיכוונו לקצר ולא יחמוד בעניין עד שאם יהיה לו לדבר דבריו המכוונים
במאה דבר לא היה דבר מדברם במאה דבר ודבר. ויש מהם שיכוין להאריך ולהרבות ולהגדיל
5   הספר ולהרבות מספר חלקיו ואע"פ שיהיה כל זה מעט עניין. כך המפרשים יש מהם שמפרש
מה שצריך לפרש בקיצור גדול ויעזוב זולת זה ויש מהם שיאריך ויבאר מה שאין צריך לבאר
או צריך לבאר ביותר ממה שראוי.

[10] והייתי חושב כי גאלנוס היה מן המאריכים כמו שנראה ברוב חיבוריו עד שראיתיו כלומר
גאלנוס יאמר בתחילת פירושו לספר החזקים לאפלטון דבר זה לשונו אמר: ראיתי קצת מן
10   המפרשים שפירשו זה המאמר שאמר אבוקרט והוא זה: כשיגיע החולי לעמידתו באותו זמן
ראוי שתהיה ההנהגה בתכלית האחרון מן הדקדוק. ופרשו זה המאמר ביותר ממאה ספרים
כל אחד מהם היה בפני עצמו ספר בלא עניין ולא סבה.

[11] אמר משה: כשראיתי זה המאמר לגאלנוס קיבלתי התנצלותו בחיבוריו ובפירושיו וידעתי
שהוא קצר בהם הרבה לפי אותם המפרשים שהיו באותם הזמנים. אבל יש בהם מהאריכות לא
15   ירחיק זה אלא מתאוה. ואני אמנם אדבר עם מי שהוא נפשי מהתאוות ויכון לאמת בכל דבר.
וזכר גאלנוס במאמר השישי מתחבולת הבריאות כי חבריו האריכו לדבר באותם המאמרים.

[12] ואני בראותי ספר הפרקים לאבוקרט שהוא מועיל יותר משאר ספריו עלה בדעתי לבארו
כי הם פרקים ראוי שכל רופא יהיה זוכר אותם אבל ראיתי מי שאינו רופא שהיה זוכר אותם
כזכור הנער הקטון מה שכתוב בלוח.

20   [13] ואלו הפרקים פירקי אבוקרט יש מהם פרקים מסופקים יצטרכו אל פירוש ויש מהם
מבוארים בפני עצמם ויש מה כפולים ויש מה שאין מועילים במלאכת הרפואות ומה ספק
גמור. אבל גאלנוס כמו שידעת לא ירצה זה ויפרש כמו שירצה. אבל אני אבאר אותם על דרך
ההודאה כי אני לא אפרש אלא מה שהוא צריך לביאור ואהיה נמשך בזה אחר כוונת גאלנוס
אלא בקצת פרקים כי אני זוכר מה שעלה בדעתי לפרש בו ומייחסו לי. אבל כל פירוש שאני
25   זוכרו סתם הוא מאמר גאלנוס כלומ' ענייניו כי אני לא אהיה חושש במלותיו כמו שעשיתי
בספריו אשר קצרתי אותם. אבל היתה כוונתי בזה הפירוש לקצר לבד למען יהיה נקל לזכור
ענייני אלו הפרקים הצריכים אל פירוש ואכוון למעט מדברים בעניין זה בכל יכולתי אלא בפרק
הראשון שאני אאריך בו מעט לא שזה על דרך הפירוש האמיתי לאותו הפרק אבל אועיל קצת
תועלת שמצאתי לי בו בין שאבקרט מכוין לו או לא יכוין זה כמו שאני מתחיל לפרש.

———————
3 יחמוד: يحلّ a   4 דבר: مثلا   8 כמו שנראה ברוב: كأكثر a   add. a   11 ופירושו: ופירושו ז فإنّه فسّر
a   15 מתאוה: متعصّب a ‖ מהתאוות: عن الأهواء a   16 מתחבולת: מתועלת זט נ"א מתחבולת זיטי
a   18–19 שהיה זוכר אותם כזכור הנער הקטון מה שכתוב בלוח: يحفظونها للصبيان في المكتب حتّى أنّ فصولا
كثيرة منها يحفظها من ليس بطيب حفظ الصغر من المكتب a   23 ההודאה: الإنصاف a   26 אותם:
בהם זט

המאמר הראשון

(1.1)

[14] אמר אבוקרט: הזמן קצר והמלאכה ארוכה והעת צר והנסיון פחד והדין קשה וראוי לך
שלא תהיה מקצר לעשות מה שראוי זולתי מה שיפעל החולה ומשרתיו גם כן והדברים אשר
מבחוץ.

אמר המפרש: ידוע שהקצר והארוך ממאמר המצטרף ואם ירצה לומר באמרו החיים קצרים   5
בהקישך אל מלאכת הרפואות אמרו והמלאכה ארוכה כפל לשון אין בו צורך ואין הפרש
בין זה ובין אמרך ראובן יותר קצר משמעון ושמעון יותר ארוך מראובן. ואם אפוקרט רצה
לומר שחיי האיש האחד קצרים בהקישו לעשות אי זו חכמה שתהיה מן החכמות ומלאכת
הרפואות ארוכה בהקישה אל שאר המלאכות זאת ההכפלה מועילה כאילו הוא אומר כמה
רחוק שלימות האדם בזאת המלאכה. זה כלו לאהוב על המשתדל בה.   10

[15] אבל היות מלאכת הרפואות ארוכה יותר משאר המלאכות העיוניות והמלאכיות
זה מבואר כי היא לא תתום ותגיע תכליתה אלא בחלקים הרבה לא יספיקו חיי האדם
להקיף באותם החלקים כלם על השלימות. וכבר זכר אבונצר אלפרבי כי החלקים אשר
בידיעתם תתום מלאכת הרפואות הם שבעה חלקים. החלק הראשון מה שצריך לרופא
לדעת מקום המלאכה והם מיני גוף האדם וזהו לדעת חכמת הנתוח ולדעת מזג כל אבר ואבר מן   15
האברים בכלל ולדעת פעולתו ותועלתו ועניין עצמותו בקושי ובחלקות ובדחיקות ובספוגות
וצורת כל אבר ואבר מהם ומקומות האברים הפנימים והנראים ודבקות קצתם בקצתם.
וזה השיעור אי אפשר לרופא שיסכל שום דבר ממנו ויש בו מן האריכות מה שאינו
נעלם.

[16] והחלק השני לדעת מה שישיג הגוף מעניין הבריאות בכלל לכל הגוף ומיני אבר ואבר.   20

והחלק השלישי לדעת מיני מיני החליים וסבתם והמקרים הנמשכים אחריהם הכל בכלל או באבר
אבר מאיברי הגוף.

והחלק הרביעי לדעת סדרי הראיות והם איך יוקחו מאותם המקרים המשיגים לגוף סימנים
מורים על מין ומין ממיני הבריאות ועל כל מין ומין ממיני החולי בין שיהיה זה בגוף כולו או באי
זה אבר מאיבריו ואיך יבדיל בין חולי לחולי אחר כיון שנתדמו רוב הסימנים.   25

1 הראשון: ל om.‏ כ״ה פרקים ז add.‏ 2 הזמן קצר: החים קצרים זיט ²לי‏ ‖ פחד: נ״א מסופק זי מסופק
ט²לי‏ ‖ והדין: והקץ ל והדין לי‏ 3 שלא תהיה מקצר לעשות: أن لا تقتصر على توخّي فعل a‏ 5 באמרו:
במאמרו זט לעשות: استكال a‏ 8 כמה: הוא ל add.‏ 9 לאהוב: لِيحضَ a‏ 15 מקום: מקומות
זט موضوع a‏ לדעת: לי‏ 20 הגוף: الموضوع a‏ הבריאות: وهو معرفة أنواع الصحّة add. a‏ 25 אבר:
שיהיה זט add.

והחלק החמישי סדרי הנהגת בריאות הגוף בכלל ובריאות כל אבר מאיבריו בכל שנה מן
השנים ובכל פרק מפרקי השנה ולפי מדינה ומדינה עד שיתמיד כל גוף וכל אבר על בריאותו
המיוחד לו.

והחלק השישי לדעת הסדרים הכוללים אשר תנהג בהם החולים עד שובם לבריאותם אשר
נעדר מהם אם שיהיה כל הגוף או אבר מאיבריו.

והחלק השביעי לדעת הכלים אשר בהם יעשה הרופא מלאכתו עד שיעמיד הבריאות הנמצא
באדם או להשיבה אם נעדרה והוא לדעת מזון האדם ורפואתו לפי שינוי מיניהם פשוטיהם
ומורכביהם והקישורים והמשיחות והטיבולים מזה הכת וכן הכלים אשר יחתוך בהם והמזלגים
אשר יתלה בהם ושאר הכלים אשר הם נעשים בחבלות ובחליי העין כלם מזה הכת. ובכלל זה
החלק מן המלאכה הוא לדעת צורת כל צמח וכל מקור שיהיה במלאכת הרפואות כי
אתה אם לא תדע אלא שמותיהם לא באת בהם עד התכלית וכמו כן תצטרך לדעת שמותיהם
המשתנים בהשתנות המקומות עד שיודע בכל המקומות אי זה שם יבקש.

[17] וידוע כי ידיעת אילו החלקים השבעה כולם ושמירתם הוא מן הספרים המונחים לכל חלק
מהם לא יגיעו בו יגיעו אל תכלית פעולת הרופא ולא יגיע לאותו היודע שלימות המלאכה עד שישא ויתן
עם האנשים בזמן בריאותם ועניין חליים וייגיע לו קניין בהכרת הסימנים המורים על החולי איך
הם מורים ושידע בקלות עניין עניין זה האיש ועניין מזג כל אבר מאיבריו ועניין עצם איבריו וכן
יודע בנקלה באורך מעשיו עם האנשים ובאותם הצורות הרשומות בדעתו איך ישמש אותם
הכלים כלומר המזונות והרפואות ושאר הכלים וזה צריך אל זמן ארוך מאד.

[18] הנה התבאר לך כי ידיעת אותם החלקים בכלל ושמירת אותם הסדרים עד שלא יחסר
מהן שום דבר צריך לזמן ארוך מאד וכן לישא וליתן עם בני אדם עד שירגיל בהנהגת הבריאות
איש אחר איש ובהנהגת רפואת חולי וחולי מכל אדם ואדם ובשימוש אותם הכלים שימוש כל
אחד ואחד מהם באנשים כלומר להרכיב פעם ולהפריד פעם ולבחור זו הרפואה או זה המזון
על רפואה אחרת ממינה. כל זה צריך אל זמן ארוך מאד. אם כן אמת אמר כי זאת המלאכה
יותר ארוכה מכל מלאכה למי שירצה להיות בה שלם. ואמר גאלנוס בפירושו מספר טימאוס
אמר: אי אפשר לאדם שיהיה חכם במלאכת הרפואות בעצמה.

[19] אמר המחבר: ואם תרצה להורות על האמת תהיה יודע שכל מי שאינו שלם במלאכת
הרפואות יזיק יותר ממה שהוא מועיל כי היות האדם בריא או חולה בלתי מתנהג בעצת רופא
כלל הוא טוב לו יותר מהיותו מתנהג בעצת רופא שיהיה טועה בו ולפי קוצר הרופא יהיה
טעותו ואם מצאה ידו די רפואתו יהיה במקרה. ובעבור זה פתח זה הנכבד ספרו שהאדם

---

5 או אבר מאיבריו: أو إلى ذلك العضو الذي إعتلّ a   6 בהם: ל .om   7 נעדרה: **ט'** הופקדה ז**'ט**
8 והמשיחות: والتقميط a ‖ יחתוך בהם: يبطّ بها ويقطع اللحم a ‖ והמזלגים: والصنّارات a   15 עם: ז**'ט**
.om   16 מאיבריו: في أيّ نوع هو من أنواع الصحة أو أنواع المرض وكذلك حال فعل كلّ عضو من أعضاء
هذا الشخص a .add   22 באנשים: ז**'ט'**   25 בעצמה: بأسرها a

צריך להיות שלם במלאכה באמרו החיים קצרים והמלאכה ארוכה והעת צר והנסיון פחד
והדין קשה. אמנם אמרו שהנסיון פחד זה מבואר אבל אני מוסיף בו ביאור.

[20] ואמרו והעת צר נ״ל שירצה לומר בו שזמן החולי יהיה צר מאד לפי הנסיון כי אתה אם לא
תדע הדברים כולם אשר התאמתו בנסיון אבל עתידים עדיין שיהיו מנוסים בזה החולה אם כן
העת ייצר בענין זה אע״פ שיש בעתידות הנסיון בזה החולה פחד ויכון המאמר כולו להשקיף
על השלמות במלאכה עד שיהיה כל מה שניסה ברוב השנים קרוב בזיכרונך.

[21] והדין קשה: נראה לי שירצה לומר בו תכלית החולי בחולים אם יהיה למות או להצלה או
שיתחדש שנוי מן השנוים. ובכלל הקדמת הידיעה במה שעתיד להיות כי זה הוא קשה מאד
במלאכת הרפואות מפני הגרת החומר ומיעוט קיומו על ענין אחד. וכבר ידעת כי העניינים
הטבעיים כלם הולכים אחר הרוב אינם מתמידים וכמה פעמ׳ יהיו הסימנים בתכלית הריעות
וינצל החולה וכמה פעמ׳ יתבשר האדם בסימנים טובים ולא יאמת מה שהורה עליהם זה. ועל
כן יצטרך להרגל ארוך בענין הסימנים בכל אחת ואחת מהם ואז נוכל לדון במה שיתחדש
בעין טוב יהיה קרוב מן האמת. ויהיה זה המאמר כמו כן להעירך שתהיה דורש תמיד על
המלאכה.

[22] אבל פני הפחד בניסיון לפי מה שאספר. דע כי כל גשם טבעי יש בו שני מינים מהמקרים:
מקרים ישיגוהו מצד חומר שלו ומקרים ישיגוהו מצד צורתו. המשל בזה האדם ישיגהו
הבריאות והחולי והשינה והיקיצה מצד חומרו כלומ׳ מצד היותו בעל חיים. וישיגהו שיחשוב
ויתייעץ ויפלא וישחק כל זה מצד צורתו. ואלו המקרים המשיגים לגוף מצד צורתו הם הנקראים
סגולות כי הם יחוד באותו המין לבדו. כן כל צמח וכל מקור וכל אבר מאיברי בעלי חיים ימצאו
לו שני אלו המינים מן המקרים.

[23] ויהיה נמשך לכל מקרה מהם פעולה אחת בגופותינו. כי הפעולות אשר תפעלם הרפואה
בגופותינו מצד החומר הוא שתחמם או שתקרר או שתיבש או שתלחלח. ואלו הם אשר
יקראום הרופאים הכוחות הראשונות ויאמרו שזאת הרפואה תחמם בטבעה או תקרר וכן
יאמרו כמו כן תפעל באיכותו וכן הפעולות הנמשכות לאלו הכוחות הראשונות והם אשר
יקראום הרופאים הכוחות השניות כמו שתהיה הרפואה תקשה או תחליק או תרפה או תקבץ
ושאר מה שזכרנו כולם תעשה הרפואה מצד החומר.

[24] כפעולות אשר תעשה הרפואה בגופותינו מצד צורתה המינית והיא אשר יקראוה
הרופאים הסגולות. וגאלנוס ידבר בעבור זה המין מן הפעולות והוא שיאמר: פועל בכל עצמותו
הענין שהוא יש לו פעולה יפעל אותה מצד צורתו המינית אשר בה התעצם אותו הגוף והיה זה
לא שהיא פעולה נמשכת אחר איכותו ויקראום כמו כן הכוחות השלישיות והם כמו שלשול

1 פחד: מסופק זט ל׳   5 אע״פ שיש בעתידות: مع ما في استئناف a ‖ ויכון: ויכון זט ‖ להשקיף: ז׳ט
לאהוב זט׳ في الحضّ a   6 קרוב: حاضرا a   7 בחולים: .om.a   10 כלם: רוביים זטל׳   .add   12 בענין:
مباشرة a   19 כן: כי זט   25 תקבץ: يكثّف a   27 כפעולות: والأفعال a

הרפואה המשלשלת או הרפואה המקיאה או שתיית סם ממית או מצילה ממי ששתה סם
המות או למי שנשך אחד מבעלי הסמים. כל אלו הפעולות הם נמשכות לצורה לא לחומר.

[25] והמזון כמו כן מזה המין כלומ׳ היות זה המין מן הצמחים יזון המין הפלו׳ מן הבעלי חיים
ואין זה שב לאיכות הראשונים המופשטים ולא כמו כן למה שיהיה בעבורו מן הקושי והחלקות
5 והדחיקות והאספוגות אבל זה פעולה בכל העצמות כמו שאמ׳ גאלנוס. הסתכל איך נהיה
נזונים בדברים הם קרובים מטבע העצים ויעשה בהם מקור וישנה אותן כמו הערמונים היבשים
והגלנד היבשים והכרוביות היבשות ולא ישוב מקור בשום קליפת פנים קליפת גרעיני הענבים ולא
קליפת התפוחים ודומיהם אלא שכמו שהם נכנסים בגוף כך הם יוצאים כי אין בעצמותם דבר
שמקבל ממקור שום מעשה בשום פנים.

10 [26] וכבר באר גאלנוס איך נקח ראייה על טבעי הרפואות ופעולותיהם באיכותם מטעמם
בספרו המפורסם ברפואות הנפרדות. אמנם הכרת מה שתעשהו הרפואה מצד צורתה
המינית והיא אשר יאמר שהיא תעשה בכל עצמותה אין לנו ראייה בשום פנים שנקח ממנה
בעניין זאת הפעולה ואין לנו דרך אחרת שבו נוכל לדעת זה אלא הנסיון. וכמה רפואה מרה
מוסרחת בתכלית הסרחון והיא רפואה מועילה וימצא העשב אשר יהיה טעמו וריחו כשאר
15 טעמי המזונות וריחם שיהיה סם המות אבל ימצאו עשבים יחשב בהם שהם ממיני המזונות
אלא שהוא מדברי לבד לא פרדסי ויהיה סם המות. הנה התבאר לך פחד הנסיון כמה הוא גדול
ורוב הצורך אליו עם זה כי כל המזונות אין אתה יודע כוחותיהם מצד היותם מזון אלא בנסיון.
וכן רוב הרפואות אין אתה יודע פעולתם אלא בנסיון על כן ראוי לך שלא תהיה מקדים בנסיון
ושתזכור כל מה שניסוהו זולתך.

20 [27] ודע ששם רפואה תהיה פעולתה נמשכת אחר החומר שלה הוא הנראה
המבואר ופעולתה הנמשכת אחר צורתה לא ישוער בה ישוער אשר לא יתואר אליהם
יחוד ולא סגולה בפעולה. ושם רפואות שיהיה פעולתם נמשכים אחר צורתם נגלה
מאד כרוב המשלשלים והסמים והמצילים ולא יעשו מעשה בגופותינו מצד החימום והקירור
אלא מעשה מועט או מפני מיעוט מה שנאכל מהם ואם יהיו חמים או קרים או מפני שאין
25 להם איכות מתגבר נראה כי אין ספק כי שתי הפעולות בהכרח כלומ׳ הנמשך אחר
החומר והנמשך אחר הצורה. ועל כן תהיה רפואה מיוחדת באצטומכא ורפואה מיוחדת בכבד
ורפואה מיוחדת בטחול ורפואה מיוחדת בלב ורפואה מיוחדת במות. ומצד הצורה המינית
כמו כן ישתנו מיני הרפואה ואע״פ שתהיה טבעם אחד כי אם תשתכל תמצא רפואות הרבה
במדרגה אחד בעצמם מן החמימות והיובש על דרך משל ולכל רפואה מהם פעולות בלתי
30 פעולות הרפואה האחרת. וזה כלו אמנם מצאהו הנסיון ברוב הזמנים.

_____

1 מצילה: מציל זט   4 לאיכות הראשונים המופשטים: لمجرّد الكيفيّات الأوّل a   5 הסתכל: הסתכל זט
6 מקור: זי מזון זטי מعدنا a   7 והכרוביות: والخروب a ‖ מקור: זי מזון זטי מعدنا   9 ממקור: זי ממזון
זטי من مَعدنا a   11 הכרת: לדעת זטילי   13 הנסיון: בנסיון: זי ששם: זי שיש זט²   21 צורתה:
خفيّ جداً حتّى a add.   23 בגופותינו: טי בפעולותינו טל add. a   24 מועט: جداً טל   25 נראה: נגלה ז
26 ועל כן תהיה: ومن أجل الفعل التابع للصورة صارت a

[28] ולרוב מעלת אבקרט אמר בזה הפרק אשר פתח בו וצוה שלא יהיה הרופא קצר מעשות
מה שראוי לבד ויעמוד כי זה בלתי מספיק בהגיע הבריאות לחולה אבל תשלם התכלית
ויתרפא כשיהיה החולה כמו כן וכל מי שהוא אצלו יפעל בחולה מה שראוי לעשות וידחה
המונעים כולם אשר מבחוץ המונעים החולה שלא יתרפא וכאילו יצוה בזה הפרק שהרופא
יהיה לו יכולת להנהיג החולים ושתקל מלאכת הרפואות עליהם כשתיית הרפואה המרה
והקרישטירי והחיתוך והכוייה וזולתה ושידבר לחולים ומי שסביביו וישמרהו וישמרהו שלא יחטא
בעצמו וישים מי שסביביו יעמדו בהנהגתו כמו שראוי בזמן היותם חוץ ממנו ולא יהיה עמו.
וכן יסיר המונעים אשר מבחוץ אשר כל מה שיהיה אפשר לו לפי איש ואיש. המשל בזה כמו שיהיה
החולה עני והוא במקום שיוסיף על חליו ואין לו יכולת לעמוד במקום אחר וכן יתקן לו המזון
או הרפואה כל זמן שלא יהיה לו אלו ודומיהם מהדברים היוצאים ממה שהרופא חייב לעשות
מצד מלאכתו אבל הם הכרחיים בהגעת התכלית אשר יחשוב הרופא להגיעו בזה החולה.
אבל שיצוה לבד מה שראוי לעשות וילך לדרכו לא טוב לעשות כי לא יגיע מזה הכוונה
המכוונת.

(1.2)

[29] אמר בקראט: אם יהיה מה שיריק מן הגוף בהיות לו התרת הבטן והקיא אשר יהיו מרובים
מן המין אשר ראוי שינוקה ממנו הגוף יועילנו זה ויקל שאתו ואם זה לא יהיה כן יהיה העניין בהפך
וכן הרקת העורקים כי אלו הורקו מן המין הראוי להריק ממנו יועילנו זה ויוקל שאתו ואם
לא יהיה כן העניין יהיה הפך. וראוי שיראה כמו כן בזמן ההוה מזמני השנה ובמקום ובשנים
ובחליים אם הם ראויים להריק אם לא.

אמר המפרש: אמרו וכן הרקת הגידים ירצה לומ' בהגרת השתן והזיעה והגרת דם ופתיחת
פיות הגידים ויהיה זה המותר כולו מרובה. אמר גאלנוס כי אמרו בהרקת הגידים ההרקה
אשר תהיה עם הרפואה ועל כן יהיה הפרק האחרון מזה המאמר אצלו מוכפל עד שיצטרך לו
פירוש. ואחר כן זכר כשתחשוב להריק המין אשר הוא ראוי כשתהיה לך סימן גובר ראוי כמו
כן שתשים חלק לזמני השנה והמקום והשנים וטבע אותו החולי ותנהיג העניין לפי מה שהוא.
כי אם תריק הקולורא בזמן הקור או במקומות הקרים או בשני הזקנים או בחליים הקרים יהיה
קשה ולא יסבול. וכן הרקת הליחה הלבנה בקיץ או במקומות החמים או בנערים או מן החליים
החמים הוא קשה ולא יסבול.

(1.3)

[30] אמר בקראט: שומן הגוף המופלג לבעלי הטורח פחד בהיותם מגיעים בו לתכלית
האחרון כי אי אפשר שיעמדו על עניינם ולא ינוחו ומפני היותם בלתי נחים בלא העתק אי

---

1 ולרוב מעלת: عظم فضيلة أخلاق a   4 החולה: المرض a   5 המרה: החדה והמרה זט   6 לחולים:
לחולה זט   7 כמו שראוי בזמן היותם חוץ ממנו ולא יהיה עמו: في حال غيبة الطبيب a   9 אחר: فينقله
هو من موضع إلى موضع a add.   14 מרובים: برضون ز² طوعا a   15 כן: זה ז   16 הרקת: ל⁵ העדר ל
17 כן: זה ל   20 המותר (= المختار): الفصل a ‖ אמר: פי׳ לפי כוונת גלי׳ בזה הפרק הוא לפי איכות
הליחות ובפרק הבא אחר זה הוא לפי יתרון הכמות וחסרונו ט¹ add.   27 המופלג: ז¹ נ״א המרובה ז

אפשר שיוסיפו תיקון ונשארו מטים אל ענין יותר רע ועל כן ראוי שיפחות שמנות הגוף בלתי איחור כדי שישוב הגוף ויתחיל לקבל המזון ולא יגיע מהרקתו התכלית האחרון כי זה סכנה אבל בשיעור סבול טבע הגוף אשר יבוקש הרקתו וכמו כן כל הרקה שתגיע בה אל התכלית האחרון הוא פחד וכל מזון שיהיה כמו כן עד התכלית האחרון הוא כמו כן פחד.

5

אמר המפרש: ירצה לומר בבעלי הטורח המתאבקים ודומיהם מאותם שעושים הטורח המרובה כמו מלאכתם כי הגידים שיתמלאו יותר מן הראוי אינם מובטחים מלהבקע או שיתחזק החמימות הטבעי בהם ויתכבה וימותו על כן ראוי שיהיה בגידים הרקה לקבל מה שיגיע אליו מן המזון.

(1.4)

[31] אמר בקראט: ההנהגה הדקה בתכלית בכל החליים הארוכים אין ספק שהיא סכנה

10

ובחליים החדים כשלא יסבלה החולה וההנהגה אשר תגיע בקצה האחרון מן הדקות היא קשה ורעה.

אמר המפרש: ההנהגה אשר בתכלית האחרון מן הדקות הוא שיעזוב המזון מכל וכל. וההנהגה אשר בתכלית הדקות אלא שהוא אינו בתכלית הקצה הוא שיאכל מן מי הדבש ודומהו. וההנהגה הדקה אשר אינה בתכלית הוא הפארי של שעורים ודומה לו.

15

(1.5)

[32] אמר בקראט: בהנהגה הדקה יחטיאו החולים על עצמם חטאה מבוארת שהיזקה גדול עליהם כי כל מה שיהיה ממנו יותר גדול ממה שיהיה מן המזון אשר בו עובי מועט. ומקודם זה תהיה ההנהגה הגמורה בדקות בבריאים כמו כן פחד כי סבלם מה שיקרה מטעותם ומשגגתם פחות. ועל כן היתה ההנהגה הגמורה בדקות ברוב העניינים יותר גדול פחד מן ההנהגה שהיא יותר גסה מעט.

20

אמר המפרש: זה מבואר נגלה.

(1.6)

[33] אמר בקראט: ההנהגה היותר טובה בחליים אשר בתכלית הקצוי היא ההנהגה אשר בתכלית הקצוי.

אמר המפרש: החליים אשר בתכלית הקצוי הם החליים החדים מאד.

1 שיפחות: ל' שימנע ל   8 שיתחזק: تُختنق a   12 ורעה: لَا مَحَالَة add. a   17 כי כל מה שיהיה ממנו יותר גדול ממה שיהיה מן המזון אשר בו עובי מועט: ז' שכל חולי כשיהיה יותר גדול יעשה יותר גדול בדיקדוק ממה שיעשה מן המסעדים הגסים ז   18 ומשגגתם: في التدبير الغليظ add. a

(1.7)

[34] אמר בקראט: ובהיות החולי חד מאד והכאבים אשר בתכלית האחרון הקצוי
יבואו בו תחילה וראוי בהכרח שיעשה בו ההנהגה אשר בתכלית האחרון מן הדקות.
ואם לא יהיה כן ויהיה העניין הפך אבל יהיה סובל מן ההנהגה מה שהוא יותר עב
מזה יהיה ראוי שתהיה הירידה לפי רפיון החולי וחסרונו על התכלית הקצוי וכשהפליג
5   החולי לבוא עד תכונתו הוא ראוי בהכרח שיעשה ההנהגה אשר היא בתכלית הקצוי מן
הדקות.

אמר המפרש: הכאבים אשר בתכלית הקצוי הם הכאבים הגדולים כלומ' עונות הקדחת
והמקרים והוא עמידת החולי כי אין העמידה דבר אחר אלא החלק הראשון שבחלקי החולי
ובמקרים והבן אמרו תחילה הד' ימים הראשונים או אחריהם מעט.

(1.8)

[35] אמר בקראט: כשיגיע החולי עד קצו הא' ראוי כמו כן שתראה כח החולה ותדע אם יהיה
10   מתקיים עד זמן עמידת החולי ותראה אי זו משתי דברים אם כח החולה יחלש קודם תכלית
החולי ולא ישאר על זה המזון או החולי יחלש קודם ותנוח ההזק.

אמר המפרש: וזה מפני גודל המקרים באותו הזמן ומפני שיתבשל החולי כי אין
ראוי להטריד הטבע לבשל לבשל מזון חדש שיאכל וישיב מלבשל הליחות המולידות החולי
15   אחר היות הטבע בא עליהם בכוחו כלו אבל נשאר לה המעט עד שתשלם הנצחון
עליהם.

(1.9)

[36] אמר בקראט: וראוי לך שתשקול כח החולה.

אמר המפרש: זה מבואר.

(1.10)

[37] אמר בקראט: ואותם יבואם קץ חלים תחילה ראוי שינהגו בהנהגה הדקה תחילה ואותם
20   שיתאחר קץ חלים ראוי שתושם הנהגתם בהתחלת חלים יותר עבה ומעט מעט יחסר מעביו

---

1 חד: חס ל   2 יבואו: ל¹ יבואנו ל   3 ויהיה העניין הפך: .om a   4–6 וכשהפליג החולי לבוא
עד תכונתו הוא ראוי בהכרח שיעשה ההנהגה אשר היא בתכלית הקצוי מן הדקות: .om a   5 תכונתו:
עמידתו ל¹   8 והמקרים: وجميع الأعراض a ‖ הראשון: הגדול זט והרע²ט .add أعظم a   10 קצו הא':
קצו העמידה זט העמידה ל¹ منتهاه a   10–12 ראוי ... ההזק: فعند ذلك يجب ضرورة أن يستعمل التدبير
الذي هو في الغاية القصوى من اللطافة a   14 שיאכל וישיב מלבשל: توردہ عليه عن إنضاج a   15 בא
עליהם: مكبّة عليها a   17 החולה: فتعلم إن كانت تثبت إلى وقت منتهى المرض وتنظر أقوة المريض تخور قبل
غاية المرض ولا تبقى على ذلك الغذاء أم المرض يخور قبل وتسكن عاديته .add a   19 יבואם: יבואם זט
20–19 ואותם שיתאחר: ואותם שיתמהר ל   20 מעט: ממנו ל

עד קרוב קץ החולי ובזמן קצו שיעור מה שישאר החולה עליו. וראוי שתמנע מן המזון בזמן
עמידת החולי כי התוספת בו הוא היזק.

אמר המפרש: זה מבואר.

(1.11)

[38] אמר בקראט: ובהיות לקדחת הקפה תמנע לו מן המזון בזמן העונות.

5   אמר המפרש: זה מבואר.

(1.12)

[39] אמר בקראט: שיורה על עונות הקדחת ומדרגת החליים בעצמם וזמני השנה ותוספת
ההקפות קצתם על קצתם בין שתהיה עונותיה בכל יום או יום ויום לא או ברוב זה מן הזמן
והדברים כמו כן אשר יתראו עדיין. ומשל זה מה שיהיה נראה בבעלי חולי הצד כי אם נראתה
הרקיקה מתחילת החולי יהיה החולי קצר. ואם התאחרה הראותה יהיה החולי ארוך. והשתן
10   והריעי והזיעה כשיתראו יורונו על בחראן טוב. וכן ריעותו ואורך החולי וקיצורו.

אמר המפרש: מטבע החולי בעצמו תוכל לדעת אם קצו מהר או מאוחר כי חולי הצד וחולי
הריאה והשרסאם חליים חדים והחנק והשלשול הנקרא היצה והקוץץ הם חליים חדים מאד
וההדרקון והשעמום ורקיקה היוצאת מן הגוף והטיציש היא חבלת הריאה הם חליים ארוכים
ועונות הקדחת יהיו שלישיות ברוב בחליי הצד והשרסאם. ומי שבהם יהיה צמח בעל טרי
15   באצטומכתו או בכבדו או במי שבו קדחת טיציש עונות אלו יהיו בכל יום וכל שכן בלילה.
ועונות הקדחת יהיו ברוב במי שחליו בטחול ובכלל מן המרה השחורה יום אחד ושני ימים לא.
וכן זמני השנה כי קדחת הרביעית הבאה בקיץ תהיה קצרה ברוב העניינים והבאה בימי החורף
תהיה ארוכה ברוב. וכל שכן כשתהיה סמוכה בקור.

ותוספת העונות יורה על תוספת החולי ובקרוב מעמידתו ותודע תוספת העונה השנית על
20   העונה הראשונה משלשה דברים האחד זמן עונת הקדחת והאחר אורך העונה והאחר גדלה
כלומ' חיזוקה.

(1.13)

[40] אמר בקראט: הזקנים יותר סובלים הצום משאר בני האדם ומאחריהם הכהול והבחורים
מעט הם סובלים לרעב ואותם שלא יסבלו הצום יותר מאלו כולם הם הנערים הקטנים ומי
שיהיה מהם יותר בעל תאוה למזון הוא פחות סובל הרעב.

---

1 שישאר: قوّة‎ .add a   6 ומדרגת: ومرتبته ونظامه‎ a   11 לדעת: העונה שלו זטי‎ .add   12 והשרסאם:
ליתרגיאס ט‎²   14 בחליי: ברוב חליי ל‎ ‖ צמח: .om ל   18 כשתהיה: כשהיא זט   19 החולי: החולה
ל   22 הכהול: בין מ' שנה ‹...› ל‎ⁱ

אמר המפרש: אשר זכר אותו בזה הפרק כבר זכר סבתו בפרק אשר אחריו כי כל מה
שיהיה החום הטבעי יותר יהיה צריך אל מזון יותר והניתך מגופות הנערים בעבור לחותם
הוא יותר וזה אשר זכר מסבול הזקנים לרעב אמר גאלנוס שהוא הזקן שלא הגיע לגבול
הכלה. אבל הזקנים אשר הם בתכלית הזקנה לא יסבלו לעמוד מן המזון רק הם צריכים לאכול
מעט מעט פעם אחר פעם להתקרב חומם מן הכיבוי ועל כן צריכים לדבר שיאריכנו מעט
מעט.

(1.14)

[41] אמר אבקראט: מה שיהיה מן הגופות בגידול החום הטבעי בהם בתכלית הריבוי וצריך
ליוקדת יותר ממה שצריכים אליו שאר הגופות ואם לא יאכלו כצריך יתך גופם ויחסר. אבל
הזקנים חמימותם מועטת ומפני זה לא יצטרכו יקידה אלא הדבר המועט כי חומם תכבה מרוב
ימיהם ומפני זה כמו כן לא תהיה הקדחת בזקנים חדה כמו שהיא באותם שהם בגידול כי גופם
של הזקנים קר.

אמר המפרש: אמר גאלנוס: העצם אשר בו החמימות בילדים יותר שיעור וזה העניין הוא אשר
יאמר בעבורו תמיד כי החמימות נוסף בכמות כמו שבאר בספר המזג.

(1.15)

[42] אמר בקראט: הגופות בקור וביומי ניסן הם בטבע יותר חמים מכל שאר הזמנים והשינה
תאריך יותר על כן ראוי בשתי אילו הזמנים שיקח מן המזון יותר כי החום היסודי בגופות
בשתי אילו העיתים הוא הרבה ועל כן יצטרך אל יותר מזו והראיה על זה עניין השנים ובעלי
ההתאבקות.

אמר המפרש: וראייה על זה השנים והמתאבקים כי הנערים מפני היות החמימות הטבעי יותר
בהם יצטרכו מן המזון אל מה שהוא יותר והמתאבקים כמו כן מפני היות חומם היסודי תגדל
בריבוי טרחם יוכלו לאכול מן המזון יותר.

(1.16)

[43] אמר אבקראט: המזון הלח הוא ניאות לכל המוקדחים כל שכן לנערים ומי שהרגיל לאכול
מזון לח.

אמר המפרש: זה מבואר והוא משל יוקח ממנו הסדר הכולל והוא שכל חולי ינוגד בהפכו.

8 ליוקדת: ז' רוב המזון זט' ‖ הגופות: من الغذاء add. a ‖ 9 יקידה: מזון ז' ‖ 13 החמימות: הוא זט .add
15 על כן ראוי בשתי אילו הזמנים שיקח מן המזון יותר: ל .om ‖ 16 יותר: ל' מעט ל הרבה זט (= كثير
A) ‖ 18 והמתאבקים: قال جالينوس (except for B) add. a ‖ 20 בריבוי: בעבור ל

(1.17)

[44] אמר בקראט: וראוי שיותן לקצת מהחולים בפעם אחת וקצתם בב׳ פעמים ויושם מה
שיותן להם פחות או יותר וקצתם מעט מעט וראוי גם כן שיותן לעת ההוה מזמני השנה חלקו
מזה והמנהג והשנים.

אמר המפרש: בתתו הסדר בכמות המזון תחילה ואחר כן באיכותו לקח שיתן במקום זה הסדר
בצורת קחתו אותו והעיקר בזה לדעת כח החולה והתחלי ויתן חלקו לשנים ולמנהג ולמזג האויר
המיוחד כי הכח החזק ראוי לו לאכול מן המזון בבת אחת והכח החלוש צריך שיאכל בעליו
מאכלו מעט מעט וחסרון הגוף וכחשו ראוי שיותן לו מזון מרובה ומילויו צריך למזון מועט. אם
כן יבוא מזה כי אם יהיה הכח חלוש והגוף בעניין החסרון יותן לו מזונו מעט מעט בפעמים
מעטים זה אם יהיה הכח חזק והכימוסים יהיו הרבה. אבל אם יהיה הכח חזק והגוף בחסרון
או ענין הפסד ליחות ראוי שיאכיל החולה מזון הרבה ופעמים רבות כי ענין גופו יצטרך אל
מזון מרובה וכוחו חזק יספיק לבשלו. ואם מנעו עונות הקדחת ולא ימצא זמנים הרבה למזון
תתן לו בפעמים מועטים.

כן הראיה לפי הכח והחולי. אבל העת והשנים והמנהג ודומהו על זה המשל. הקייץ יהיה ראוי
בו להאכיל לפעמים רבות ומעט בכל פעם ופעם ובימות הגשמים ראוי להרבות המזון ולמעט
הפעמים אבל אמצע הזמן הנקרא וַיר ובערבי אלרַבִיע כשיתקרב מן הקיץ ראוי שיפרנס במזון
מועט בין שעות ארוכים כי זה העת אפשר שיהיו הגופות בו מלאים כי הכימוסים אשר היו
נקפאים בימי הקור יתכו ויזובו. אבל החורף מי שלא ירגיש בו חמימות יצטרך אל תוספת זה
אחר זה ממזון טוב בעבור הפסד הכימוסין באותו עת. אבל המנהגים והשנים ענינם מבואר.

(1.18)

[45] אמר בקראט: המזון הוא קשה לסבול אותו יותר בזמן הקייץ ובזמן החורף ובימי הקור
הוא יותר נקל לסובלו ואחריו בימי הַוִר.

אמר המפרש: אמר גאלנוס: מאמרו בזה הפרק הוא בחולים ומאמרו המוקדם הוא בבריאים.

(1.19)

[46] אמר בקראט: בהיות עונות הקדחת דבקות להקפה אין ראוי בזמניה שיותן לחולה שום
דבר ולא יביאנו לקחת שום דבר אבל ראוי שיפחות מן התוספת מקודם זמני ההפרדה.

אמר המפרש: אמר גאלנוס: ירצה באמרו מקודם זמני ההפרדה קודם זמני העונות ובהיות זה
העת ראוי בו לפחות החמרים כדי שלא תגדל הקדחת וכל שכן מהוסיף בה שום דבר במזון.

---

4 לקח: התחיל לֹ‎ ‖ הסדר: תחילה ואחרי כן זט add. ‖ 9 וזה: وكذلك a ‏ 13 הקייץ: בימות החמה
לֹ‎ ‏ 15 מן: זט om. ‏ 17 בימי: בימות זט ‖ מי שלא ירגיש בו חמימות: فَن يحم فيه a ‏ 21 הוא בחולים
ומאמרו המוקדם הוא בבריאים: הוא בבריאים ומאמרו המוקדם הוא בחולים זט ‏ 23 יביאנו לקחת:
‏يضطر إلى a (emendation editor) ‏ 25 בה: זט om.

(1.20)

[47] אמר בקראט: הגופות אשר יבואם האלבחרן או שכבר באם הבחראן השלם אין ראוי
שיעירם בשום דבר ולא יחדש בהם שום חידוש לא ברפואה משלשלת ולא בזולתה מן הדברים
המעוררים אלא תניחנו.

אמר המפרש: אמרו יבואם האלבחראן ירצה לומר בו שסיבותיו נזדמנו ונראו הסימנים
שלו והוא מוכן להיות. ואמרו לא בזולתו מן הדברים המעוררים כמו ההקאה והזיעה   5
והבאת הוסת והשתן והחפיפה. והתנה שיהיה הבחראן שלם אבל האלבחראן המחוסר
טוב להשלים על חסרונו ויוציא מה שנשאר מן הליחה המחליאה במשלשל. ואמר גאלנוס
כי הבחראן השלם הוא מה שקיבץ ששה ענינים: הראשון שיקדימנו בישול. והשני שיהיה
מיומי הבחראן. והשלישי שיהיה בהרקת שום דבר שיצא מן הגוף לא בצמה. והרביעי
שיהיה הדבר המורק הוא הדבר המזיק לבד אשר היה סבת החולי. והחמישי שתהיה   10
הרקתו על היושר והממצוע מן הצד שיהיה החולי. הששי שיהיה עם מנוחה וקלות מן
הגוף.

ואמר גאלנוס כי אם יפחות אחת מאילו אינו בחראן אמיתי ושלם.

אמר המפרש: ראוי לך שתשאל במקום זה ותאמר איך יריק הליחה המחליאה בעצמו
וביום הבחראן וביושר ולא יהיה סוף המנוחה והנחת כי גאלנוס יתנה תנאי ששי והוא   15
שיהיה עם מנוחה ונחת רוח ראיה שהגיעו התנאים החמשה ולא יהיה מנוחה תשובה על זה
שאפשר זה כשההרקה תהיה מרובה ושתהיה מן המין הראוי להוציא עם שאר התנאים כי
כשיתרבה ולא יבוא בסופו מנוחה אבל חולשה ומורך הגוף ואיפשר שיתעלפה עילוף חזק.
ודע זה.

(1.21)

[48] אמר בקראט: הדברים הראוים להריק ראוי שיורקו מן המקומות אשר הם אליהם יותר   20
נוטות לאיברים אשר הם טובים להריק.

אמר המפרש: גאלנוס אמר שהדברים שראוים להריק הם הליחות המולידות לחליים אשר
בא בהם הבחראן שאינו שלם. והמקומות אשר הם טובים להריק הם המעיים והאצטומ׳
והשלפוחית והרחם והעור ועם זה כמו כן האובלי והנחירים כשאנו רוצים להריק המוח. וראוי
לרופא שיתמיד לראות הטיית הטבע לאי זו צד היא כי אם מצא שהיא נוטה לצד טוב שצריך   25
להריק מה שיריק יזמן לו מה שצריך אליו ועזרהו. ואם ראה העניין הפך מזה וראה תנועתה
תנועה מזיקה מנעה והעתיק אותה ומשוך אותה אל הפך הצד אשר נטה לצדו. ואני אמשול
לך משל כי אם תהיה בכבד כימוסים שיחדשו חולי הצדדים אשר טובים להטות להם הן שני

---

3 אלא: אבל זט   7 מה שנשאר: זט .om   9 שום דבר: בֵּין .add a   14 בעצמו: بعد النضج .add a
18 ולא יבוא בסופו מנוחה: لا يعقّبه خفّ ولا تكون معه راحة a   25 שיתמיד לראות: أن يتفقّده بتعرّف
a   28 הצדדים: המקומות זיט׳

צדדים האחד הוא צד האצטו' ובהיות ההטייה לאותו הצד תריק בשלשול שהוא יותר טוב
מהריקו בקיא והצד האחר צד הכליות והשלפוחית אבל הטיית אותם הכימוסין אל צד החזה
והריאה והלב אינו טוב.

(1.22)

[49] אמר בקראט: אמנם ראוי לך שתעשה הרפואה והתנועה אחר שההחולי יהיה מבושל אבל
כל זמן היותו נא ובתחלת החולי אין ראוי שיעשה זה אלא אם יהיה החולי צריך ואי אפשר ברוב   5
החליים שיהיה החולה צריך.

אמר המפרש: אמרו הרפואה ירצה בה המשלשל. והחולי אשר התעורר הוא שיהיו הכימוסים
צערו החולה והזיקו בחום שהיה לו חזק והגרה מאבר אל אבר בהתחלת החולי ויצערהו ויחדש
לו צרה והמיה ולא יניחהו לנוח אבל יתנועעו ויזובו מאבר לאבר וזה רחוק מהיותו אבל ברוב
העניין יהיו הכימוסים נחים וקיימים באבר אחד ובאותו האבר יהיה בישולו בכל זמן החולי כלו   10
עד שיפחות.

(1.23)

[50] אמר אבקראט: ואין ראוי שנקח ראייה על השיעור הראוי להריק מן הגוף מריבויו אבל
ראוי שישתדל בהרקה כל זמן שהדבר הראוי להריק הוא אשר יורק והחולה יסבול לו בקלות
ונחת ובמקום הראוי ותהיה ההרקה עד שיתעלף אבל ראוי שיעשה זה בהיות החולה סובל
אותו.   15

אמר המפרש: גאלנוס אמר: אם היה הדבר הגובר הוא אשר הריק גוף החולה יקל בהכרח
ממה שהיה בו הריק עם הדבר היוצא מהטבע דבר טבעי החולה יתרפה עכ"פ וכוחו יחלש
וירגיש בכובד וסערה והמיה וראוי שתהיה ההרקה עד זמן שיתחדש בעבור העילוף במורסות
החדות שהם בתכלית הגודל ובקדחות השורפות מאד והכאבים החזקים מאד ויקדים על זה
השיעור מן ההרקה בהיות הכח חזק. והנה ניסינו זה פעמים רבות בלא מספר ומצאנוהו יועיל   20
תועלת חזקה ולא נדע בכאבים החזקים מאד רפואה יותר חזקה ויותר מופלגת מן ההרקה
עד שיקרה העילוף אחר שתשמור ותדע אם ראוי שנקיז גיד או נעשה השלשול עד שיקרה
העילוף.

(1.24)

[51] אמר אבקראט: יצטרך בחליים החדים לעת רחוק לעשות הרפואה המשלשלת בתחילה
וראוי שתפעל זה אחר שתקדים ותנהיג העניין כראוי.   25

----

4 אמנם: ל .om   5 שיעשה: זט .om ‖ 5 שיעשה: זט .om   6 צריך (= محتاجا): محتاجا a   6 צריך (= محتاج): محتاجا a   8 חזק: היזק זט   9 רחוק מהיותו: أقلّ ما يكون a   10 בכל: כל ל   13 שישתדל: أن يستغني a   18 בעבור: عنه a   22–23 אחר שתשמור ותדע אם ראוי שנקיז גיד או נעשה השלשול עד שיקרה העילוף: ל .om

אמר המפרש: באר לנו שהוא לא יתיר השלשול בתחילת החוליים אלא בקצת חליים חדים
המעוררים כמו שזכר זה קודם ועם כל זה ראוי הוא שיעשה זה בשמירה רבה ואחר הכנת
הגוף כל מה שאפשר ואחר ידיעת רקיקות הליחה.

אמר גאלנוס: הפחד לעשות הרפואה המשלשלת על זולתי הראוי בחליים חדים יש לפחד
עליו כי הרפואה המשלשלת כלה חמה ויבשה והקדחת באשר היא קדחת אינה צריכה לדבר
מחמם ומיבש אלא תצטרך להפך זה כלומ' דבר שיקרר וילחלח אבל יעשהו בעבור הכימוס
הפועל לה. על כן ראוי להיות התועלת בהרקת הכימוס אשר בעבורו התחדש החולי יותר מן
ההיזק אשר יבוא לגופות באותו העניין בעבור הרפואה המשלשלת אבל יהיה התועלת יותר
כשיריק הכימוס המזיק כלו בלא היזק. ראוי שישמור תחילה אם גוף החולה מזומן מוכן לזה
השלשול. כי אשר היה תחילת חליים ממלוי הנק׳ תוכם בערבי ובלע״ז אמפונמינטו או ממזון
יתר ויסקום וגס ואשר יהיו מבני אדם מתחת צלעותיהם בהמשכה או בניפוח או חום חזק מאד
או שיהיה שם בקצת הקרבים עם כל זה מורסא אין כל גוף אחד מהם מוכן לשלשול. ראוי שלא
יהיה שום דבר מזה נמצא ושיהיו הכימוסים בגוף החולה יותר טובים ממה שאפשר שיהיו
מקלות מרותצת כלומ׳ שיהיו הכימוסים שבגוף החולה רקיקים ולא יהיה בהם שום דבקות
ושיהיו המהלכים אשר יהיה עובר בהם השלשול רחבים פתוחים אין בהם שום סתימה. נעשה
אנו אלה העניינים ונקדים ונזמן הגוף בזה העניין כשאנו רוצים לשלשלו.

(1.25)

[52] אמר בקראט: אם הורק הגוף מן המין אשר ראוי שינוקה ממנו יועיל זה ויסבלנו בקלות
ואם היה העניין הפך יהיה זה קשה.

אמר המפרש: זה הפרק אצלי אינו כפול למה שכלל בו הפרק השני כי אותו הפרק מדבר במה
שיהיה מורק מעצמו מרובה וזה הפרק מדבר במה שאנו מריקים ברפואה. ומפני ששם גאלנוס
הפרק השני יכלול שני העניינים כלם הוצרך לתת סבה להכפלת הפרק.

נשלם המאמר הראשון מפרקי אבקראט.

2 כמו: כמה זט 4 הפחד: הספק ל׳ 5–4 יש לפחד עליו: הוא דבר גדול ל׳ 6 בעבור: لكان
a ‖ הכימוס: הליחה ל׳ 10 תוכם: תוכום ל ‖ אמפונמינטו: אמפוניטו זט 11 ויסקום: ויסקוסו זט
12 שם: זט om. ‖ בקצת: באחד ל׳ 13 ושיהיו: וכשיהיו זט 14 דבקות: من النوع الذي ينبغي أن ينقى
منه نفع ذلك واحتمل بسهولة فإن كان الأمر على ضدّ ذلك add. a (إلى قوله B) 18 היה העניין הפך יהיה
זה קשה: יהיה העניין הפך זה יהיה העניין קשה זט 20 מעצמו מרובה: מעצמו מֵרוּבָה ז מעצמו מֵרוּבָה
ט طوعا a 21 הוצרך: التجأ a

המאמר השיני

(2.1)

[53] אמר אבקראט: בהיות השינה בחולי מן החליים מחדש כאב זה מסימני המות ובהיות השינה מועילה אין זה מסימני המות.

אמר המפרש: ירצה לומ' באמרו כאב הזיק ויש שם חליים ושעות מן החולי שיזיק בהם השינה
ועל כן ראוי שיצוה החולה בהם בתעורה כי אם היה אז ישן היה מזיק. ושם זמנים שיועיל 5
בהם השינה כי אם היה ישן החולה בהם ונתחדש לו בה הזיק אותו סימן מות כי במקום
שקוינו התועלת בא ההזק. וזה אמנם יהיה נהוג בהיות לחות הגוף רעות מאד ואונסות לחום
היסודי. אבל החליים אשר תזיק השינה לעולם יהיה בהתחלת מורסות האיברים הפנימיים
ובהגרת החמרים להאצטומ' או בהתחלת עונת הקדחת וכל שכן בהיות עמה קרירות או
פלצות. והשעות אשר יועיל בהם השינה הוא אחר כלות התחלת העונה והמורסא וכל שכן 10
בעת העמידה. והיותר מועיל ממה שיוכל להיות השינה שהיא נעשת בזמן הירידה כי אם תזיק
בזה העת הוא סימן מות ואע״פ שהשינה תועיל כמו שידעת מתועלת השינה בזה העת לא
יוסיף לנו בסימן שום דבר.

(2.2)

[54] אמר בקראט: כשיהיה לשום אדם בלבול הדעת בחליו ויניחנו השינה זה סימן טוב.

אמר המפרש: זה יורה על שהחמימות היסודי נצח הכימוסים ואנסם. 15

(2.3)

[55] אמר בקראט: השינה והתעורה כששום אחד מהם יעבור השיעור הראוי זה סימן רע.

אמר המפרש: זה מבואר.

(2.4)

[56] אמר בקראט: לא השובע ולא הרעב ולא זולתם מכל העניינים טוב כשיעברו השיעור הטבעי.

אמר המפרש: זה מבואר. 20

(2.5)

[57] אמר בקראט: העיפות שלא יודע לו סבה הוא מורה על החולי.

---

4 ושעות: وأوقات a   6 אותו סימן: فتلك علامة a   10 והשעות: والأوقات a   15 ואנסם: والحلیشם
זט   16 הראוי: القصد a

אמר המפרש: זה יורה שהשליחות התעוררו על המנהג הטבעי ובעבור זה נחלו האיברים או מריעות איכותם או מכמותם ועל כן הוא מורה על החולי.

(2.6)

[58] אמר בקראט: מי שיכאב לו שום דבר מגופו ולא ירגיש בכאבו ברוב ענייניו שכלו מבולבל.

אמר המפרש: ירצה באמרו במקום זה סבת הכאב כמו שיהיה בחולה מורסה חמה או ריציפלא או חבלה או ריצוץ בשר והדומה לזה ויהיה בלתי מרגיש בו דעתו של זה מבולבל.

5

(2.7)

[59] אמר בקראט: הגופות אשר יקבלו הרזון בזמן ארוך ראוי שתהיה תשובתם עם המזון אל השמנות בזמן ארוך והגופות אשר יקחם הרזון בזמן מועט ישובו לשמנותם נקל.

אמר המפרש: זה בעבור כי הגופות אשר יקחם הרזון בזמן מועט אמנם נתחדש להם זה הכחש והרזון מהרקת הלחויות לא מהתכת האיברים הנקפאים. אבל הגופות אשר נכחשו ונרזו בזמן ארוך הותך מהם הבשר ושב רקיק ונתכו שאר האיברים אשר בהם יהיה העיכול והתפשט המזון בגוף ותולדת הדם ולא יוכל לבשל מן המזון השיעור אשר יצטרך אליו הגוף ועל כן ראוי שישוב אל השמנות בנחת ובזמן ארוך.

10

(2.8)

[60] אמר בקראט: הנקי מן החולי בקחתו מן המזון ולא יתחזק זה יורה על שהוא יסבול מן המזון יותר ממה שהוא סובל ובהיות זה שהוא לא יבואנו ממנו זה יורה על שגופו צריך אל הרקה.

15

אמר המפרש: כבר באר הסבה בפרק אשר הורנו בו כי הגוף שאינו נקי כל אשר תזונהו תוסיף עליו היזק.

(2.9)

[61] אמר בקראט: כל גוף שאתה רוצה לנקותו ראוי שתשים מה שאתה רוצה להוציאו ממנו יצא בנקלה.

אמר המפרש: יהיה זה בשתפתח ותרחיב כל דרכיו ותחתוך ותדקדק ותתיך הלחויות אשר בהם אם היה להם שום דבר מן העובי והדבקות.

20

---

1 על המנהג: على غير مجراها a (except for B)   4 באמרו: بالوجع a ‖ ריציפלא: حمرة a   5 ריצוץ בשר: والفسخ والشدخ a   7 נקל: **ל** om.   10 ונתכו: ونهكت a   פفي زمان يسير a   11 המזון: הרזון **זט**   12 בנחת ובזמן ארוך: في زمان طويل a   13 הנקי (= النقي): الناقه a ‖ יסבול: يكقح **ל**י יקח **זט**י
18 לנקותו: בנקיותו **זט**

(2.10)

[62] אמר בקראט: הגוף שאינו נקי כל מה שתוסיף במזונו הוספת בו מדון.

אמר המפרש: זה מבואר הסבה וכל שכן בהיות האצטומ׳ מליאה מכימוסים רעים ובזמן זה
יקרה בה אשר זכר אבוקרט שיקרה לנקי והוא שלא יוכל לקחת מן המזון.

(2.11)

[63] אמר בקראט: למלאות הגוף משתייה הוא יותר נקל ממלוא אותו ממזון.

אמר המפרש: רצה בזה הדברים הלחים והשתיות הלחות אשר לגופותינו בהם מזון כי המזון
הלח וכל שכן בהיותו בטבעו חם הוא יותר במהירות ובנקל מזון לגוף.

(2.12)

[64] אמר בקראט: ההשאריות הנשארות מן החולי אחר הבחראן ממנהגם שיביאו חזרת
החולי.

אמר המפרש: ברוב יתעפשו אותם ההשאריות בהאריך הימים ויולידו קדחת כי כל לחות
זר שמטבע הגוף המקיף אותו אין ראוי שיזון אותו ולא יכלה ענינו אלא לעיפוש ברוב.
ובהיות עם זה המקום אשר הוא מתקבץ בו חמימות ישוב לעיפוש מהרה וביותר חזק ממה
שאפשר.

(2.13)

[65] אמר בקראט: מי שיבואנו הבחראן יקשה חליו בלילה אשר קודם עונת הקדחת אשר
יבוא בו האלבחראן ובלילה האחרת יהיה זה יותר נקל.

אמר המפרש: בהבדיל הטבע הדבר הרע מן הטוב והכנתו לדחות ולהוציא יתחדש מזה סערה.
וראוי בהכרח בזמן הסערה שהחולה יצטער ויקשה עליו חליו וממנהג בני אדם שיישנו בלילה
וכשימנע אותה הסערה מהשינה יתבאר סער החולה וקושי חליו ביאור נגלה. ויוכל להיות זה
ביום בהיות האלבחראן מוכן להיות בלילה הבאה אחריו ואמרו שזה יהיה יותר נקל כי רוב
האלבחראן יכלה בטובה.

(2.14)

[66] אמר בקראט: בהגרת הבטן יועיל בשינוי המראים שיתראו בצואה כל זמן שזה השינוי
לא יהיה נוטה אל מינים רעים.

---

1 מדון: شرّا a‎ 2 מכימוסים: מליחות ל‎¹ 3 לנקי: للنقي (=):للناقه a‎ 10 אלא: ז‎¹ יבוא זט‎¹ 14 בו: ל
‎.om ‖ האחרת: الّتي بعدها a‎ 15 בהבדיל: בבחור ל‎¹ 19 יכלה: סופו זט‎²ל‎¹ 20 בהגרת: בהתרת
זט

אמר המפרש: כי רוב המראים והצבעים יורו על מינים רבים מהכימוסיס. והמינים הרעים הם
שיהיה בהם שום דבר מסימני התכות הגוף והיא היציאה הדשנה או מסימני העיפוש והיא
ריעות הריח.

(2.15)

[67] אמר בקראט: כשיתרעם אדם מן הגרון או שיצא בגוף בתור או צמחים ראוי שתעיין
תמיד מה שיצא מן הגוף כי הוא אם היה הגובר עליו המרות יהיה הגוף עם זה חולה. ואם יהיה 5
מה שיצא מן הגוף דומה למה שיצא מגוף הבריאים היה בטוח והקדים לזון הגוף.

אמר המפרש: אמר גאלנוס: הגרון כמו כן יקבל הכימוסיס היורדים מן המוח והבתור והצמחים
אמנם יהיו בהתחמם הדם בעבור המרות הצטריני על כן ראוי שתראה תמיד אם דחה הטבע
כל המותרות אל אותם האיברים אשר נתבטלו ותדע אם יהיה מה שיצא מבטנו כמו אותו
שיצא מהגוף מהבריא כי אין במזונו אז פחד. ואע״פ שלא התנקה הגוף מן הליחות לגמרי 10
ומשך היותר גובר על מה שיצא מן הגוף מן המרות ואז ראוי שינוקה ותריק קודם שיתפרנס
כי הגוף שאינו נקי כל אשר תוסיף במזונו תוסיף עליו רעה.

(2.16)

[68] אמר בקראט: בהיות האדם רעב אין ראוי שיטרח.

אמר המפרש: עם מעט מן המזון הוא ראוי שתעזוב הטורח וסיבת ענין זה מבוארת.

(2.17)

[69] אמר בקראט: כשתכניס בגוף מזון חוץ מן הראוי הטבעי יותר מדאי זה יחדש חליים ויורה 15
זה על שיתרפא.

אמר המפרש: נראה לי כי כוונתו בזה הפרק שיגיד כי בהיותו המזון הנכנס בגוף יוצא חוץ
מן הטבע יציאה מרובה בין שתהיה זאת היציאה בכמות או באיכות תחדש חולי וסוף מה
שיתחדש מן החולי לפי צאתו אם יצא יציאה גדולה יחדש חולי גדול ואם היתה יציאת המחליא
יציאה מועטת ויורה על זה היציאה במה שיראה מבריאותו כי אם תהיה היציאה מועטת 20
יתרפא מהרה.

1 על: استفراغ add. a ‖ מהכימוסיס: מליחות ל׳ 4 בתור: بُور a 5-4 שתעיין תמיד: أن ينظر
ويتفقّد a 9 נתבטלו: ז׳ הוזקו זט׳ اعتلّت a ‖ ותדע: ذلك add. a ‖ מבטנו (من البطن): من البدن a
11 ומשך: وجدت a 13 האדם: באדם זט 15 חוץ מן הראוי הטבעי יותר מדאי: خارج عن الطبيعة كثير
a 16-15 ויורה זה על שיתרפא: ويدلّ على ذلك بروءه a (= ויורה על זה רפואתו) 18 וסוף: ومبلغ a
19 ואם היתה: واع״ف שתהיה זטל׳ 20 מועטת: كان المرض يسيرا add. a ‖ על זה היציאה: على مقدار
خروجه a (except for B)

(2.18)

[70] אמר בקראט: מה שיהיה מן העניינים מפרנס מהר פתאום יציאתו כמו כן תהיה פתאום.

אמר המפרש: תכלית העניינים כלם אשר יפרנסו מהרה ובבת אחת הוא היין ועניין מהרה הוא אחר שיקחנו בזמן מועט. ואמרו בבת אחת שיהיה אחר שיתחיל להתפרנס שיקבל הגוף מזונו כלו בבת אחת.

(2.19)

[71] אמר בקראט: להקדים הגזר דין בחליים החדים על מות או על בריאות אינך בו על תכלית הבטחון.

אמר המפרש: אמר גאלנוס: הקדחת בחולי החד תהיה קדחת תמידית דבקה ברוב כי המעט מהחליים החדים יהיה מבלתי קדחת כמו הפלג.

(2.20)

[72] אמר בקראט: מי שיהיה בטנו בבחרותו רפה כשיהיה זקן יהיה בטנו יבש ומי שיהיה בבחרותו יבש כשיזקין יהיה בטנו לח.

אמר המפרש: כשתבקש על האמת תדע שזה העניין בלתי מקויים אם כן הוא פסק דין)ו(שקר בלא ספק. והאמת אצלי כי אבקראט ראה שני אנשים או שלשה שעניינם כן ושמו כפסק דין גמור כמו שהיה מנהגו ברוב ספר פידימיאי כי בקרות עניין אחד על שני אנשים או על שלשה ישוב אצלו הגזירה דין על המין. זהו אצלי מדת ההוראה. ואם אינך רוצה זה ותבחר להשים לזה המאמר שאינו אמיתי פנים אמתיים ותתנה לך תנאים ותדון ברצונך לך אל מה שזכר בו גאלנוס בזה הפרק.

(2.21)

[73] אמר בקראט: שתית היין יסיר הרעב.

אמר המפרש: רצונו לומר ברעב התאוה הכלביית כי שתית היינות אשר בהם חימום חזק ירפא זה הרעב. כי התאווה הכלבית אמנם תהיה או מקרירות מזג האצטומ' לבד או מכימוס חמוץ שנשתבכה בעצם האצטומ' והיין ירפא שני העניינים כלם.

---

3 שיתחיל להתפרנס: שיתפרנס ל שיתפרנס (שיתחיל ט׳) להתפרנס ט　 4 כלו: ولا يجذبه قليلا قليلا add. a　 5 הגזר דין: הפסק דין זטל׳　 8 הפלג: ס״א השתוק אפופליסאה ז׳ט׳　 10 יבש: البطن add. a
14 אצלו: לו ל ‖ מדת ההוראה: الإنصاف a　 14–15 להשים לזה: לומר בזה זטל׳　 15 ותדון ברצונך: وتفرض له فرضات a　 18 רצונו לומר ברעב התאוה הכלבית: يريد بالشراب النبيذ وهذا الجوع يريد به الشهوة الكلبية a　 20 שנשתבכה בעצם האצטומ': قد تشرّبه جرمها a ‖ והיין: الذي وصفنا add. a

(2.22)

[74] אמר בקראט: מה שיהיה מן החליים מתחדש מן המילוי רפואתו תהיה בהרקה ומה שממנו מתחדש מן ההרקה רפואתו תהיה במילוי ורפואת שאר החליים תהיה בהפך.

אמר המפרש: זה מבואר נגלה.

(2.23)

[75] אמר בקראט: כי הבחראן בחליים החדים יבוא בי״ד ימים.

אמר המפרש: אמ׳ גאלנוס: לא יעבור שום מן החליים אשר תנועתם תנועה חדה ומהירות דבק   5
זה הזמן ויוכל להיות הבחראן בהרבה חליים חדים בי״א ימים וביום התשיעי וביום השביעי
ובחמישי ולפעמים יבואו ביום ו׳ אבל אינו טוב בחליים אשר יבוא בהם הבחראן השלם. אמנם
החליים אשר יבוא בהם הבחראן השלם בי״ד או לפניו ממנהג בקראט שיקראם חליים חדים
במאמר מוחלט. אבל החליים אשר יהיה בהם בחראן מחוסר באחד מימי הבחראן אשר
יסופרו עד מ׳ יום)ו(יאמר בהם החליים החדים אשר יבוא הבחראן שלהם במ׳ יום.   10

(2.24)

[76] אמר בקראט: היום הרביעי יורה על היום השביעי ותחילת השבוע השני הוא היום השמיני
והמורה בי״ד הוא היום הי״א כי הוא הרביעי מן השבוע השנית. והיום הי״ז כמו כן יום הראות
כי הוא היום הרביעי מיום הי״ד והיום הז׳ מן היום הי״א.

אמר המפרש: אמר גאלנוס: הי״ז ⟨...⟩ כי יום העשרים הוא יום בחראן והוא סוף השבוע   15
השלישי.

(2.25)

[77] אמר בקראט: קדחת הרביעית הבאה בקיץ ברוב היא קצרה והבאה בימי החורף היא
ארוכה וכל שכן אם היא סמוכה בימות הגשמים.

אמר המפרש: אין הקדחת הרביעית לבד תהיה קצרה אבל שאר החליים כי הכימוסים יזובו
ויתפשטו בגוף כלו ויתכו ויבוא מזה שלא יאריך שום מן החליים הבאים בקיץ. ובקראט שם   20
דבריו ביותר ארוך מן החליים ושמו משל. ובימות הגשמים יקרה הפך זה כלומר שיעמדו
הכימוסים בעומק הגוף כאילו יתקשו וישאר הכח על כחו ולא החליים יבואו לתכליתם כיון
היות הכימוסים המולידים לקדחת נשארים ולא החולים ימותו כי כחם יהיה נשאר ולא יהיה
נתך.

---

3 מבואר נגלה (بيّن واضح B): واضح a   5 תנועה חדה: حركة حدة a   6 הזמן: الحدّ a   7 יבואו: יבוא זט
بعضهم add. a ‖ בחליים אשר יבוא בהם הבחראן השלם: om. a   10 יסופרו (= يعد): يعدّ a   14 (...): بعد
منذربالعشرين a   18 תהיה: في الصيف add. a   19 ויבוא: فيجب a   21 הכח: החולי זט׳

(2.26)

[78] אמר בקראט: להיות הקדחת אחר הקיווץ יותר טוב מהיות הקיווץ אחר הקדחת.

אמר המפרש: הקיווץ הוא בא ממלוי ומהרקה כי כשיקרה הקיווץ מן המלוי אמנם יתמלאו
העצבים מן הכימוס ויסקוזו הקר אשר ממנו מזונו ויחדש הקדחת אחר זה הקיווץ כי הרבה
פעמ׳ יתחמם אותו הכימוס ויתיכנו וידקדקנו ויתירנו הקדחת. וכשיקרה לאדם קדחת שורפת
ונתייבש גופו כלו ושם יהיה עצב יקרה לו הקיווץ מפני היבשות והחולי הוא חזק וגדול.

(2.27)

[79] אמר בקראט: אין ראוי לקבל ראיה בקלות שיימצא החולה הפך ההקש ואל יפחידוך
ענינים קשים מתחדשים על זולתי ההקש כי רוב מה שיקרה מזה אינו קיים ולא עומד ולא
יאריך זמנו.

אמר המפרש: כשיתחדש חולי חזק ואחר כן יקל פתאום מבלתי התקדם בישול ולא הרקה
לא תסמוך על זה כי הליחות נבהלו ונכבו ופחתה תנועותיהם לא דבר אחר. וכן אם התקדם
הבישול המבואר ואחר כן קרה לו נפש רעה ובלבול דעת ודומהו לא יפחידך זה כי הוא לא
יעמוד. והרבה פעמ׳ יורה על בחראן טוב.

(2.28)

[80] אמר בקראט: מי שהיתה לו קדחת בלתי קשה מאד אם גופו נשאר על עניינו ולא יחסר
ממנו שום דבר או שיהיה נתך יותר ממה שראוי הוא רע כי הראשון יורה באורך החולי והשני
יורה על חולשת הכח.

אמר המפרש: כחש הגוף לעולם הוא סימן רע ויורה על חולשת הכח בין שתהיה חזקה מאד
או שלא תהיה חלושה מאד.

(2.29)

[81] אמר בקראט: כל זמן שיהיה החולי בהתחלתו אם תראה בדעתך להניע שום דבר תניעהו
כי הוא בהגיע החולי אל עמידתו ראוי שינוח החולה ויעמוד.

אמר המפרש: סבה זו בפרק אשר יבוא אחריו ומה שאמר אם ראית שתניע שום דבר תניעהו
ירצה בו ההקזה לבד ואפשר שיעשה כמו כן השלשול. ואין ראוי שיעשה אחת משתי אילו
בזמן עמידת החולי כי בשול החולי באותו זמן הוא והכח הנפשי יהיה בזמן העמידה ברוב

---

5 ושם יהיה עצב יקרה לו: وعصبه ثمّ عرض له a ‖ והחולי הוא חזק וגדול: והחולי הזה חזק וקשה זט
فالآفة في ذلك عظيمة a   6 לקבל ראיה: أن يعتّر a   9 יקל: يعمود זטל׳ יפסוק זٟ²ט²   10 נבהלו: تبلّدت
a ‖ ונכבו: ל om. ‖ ופחתה: ונגרعו זטל׳   11 נפש (= نفس): نَفَس a   13 קשה: ضعيفة a   16 בין
שתהיה חזקה מאד: سواء كانت الحمّى ليست بالضعيفة جدّا a   17 או שלא תהיה חלושה: أو كانت حمّى
قويّة جدّا a

העניין הוא פני. והטוב שבעזר כדי להיות הבשול יותר מהיר הוא שיעשה ההרקה בתחילת החולי עד שיתמעט החומר שלו. ובעת העמידה הכח החיוני והכח הטבעי נשארים בכחותיהם.

אמר המפרש: הנה הקדים לך שאין ראוי שתשתלשל בהתחלה אלא בחליים המתעוררים ועל כן אמר במקום זה אם ראית שתניע שום דבר תניע.

(2.30)

5 [82] אמר בקראט: כי כל הדברים בתחילת החולי ובסופו יותר חלושים ובעמידתו יותר חזקים.

אמר המפרש: ירצה לומ' באמרו הדברים המקרים כי הם בהתחלת החולי ובסופו יותר חלושים כלומר עונות הקדחת והתעורה והצמא והכאב. אבל העניין אשר יהיה ממנו אלו המקרים והוא החולי ראוי בהכרח שיהיו בעת העמידה יותר טוב בהיות החולה מן החולים אשר יתרפאו.

(2.31)

[83] אמר בקראט: בהיות הנקי מן החולי ייטב לו מן המזון ולא יוסיף גופו שום דבר זה רע.

10 אמר המפרש: זה מבואר והנה הקדים עניין זה.

(2.32)

[84] אמר בקראט: כי ברוב העניינים כל מי שעניינו רעה וייטב לו המזון בתחילה ולא יוסיף גופו שום דבר יבוא עניינו לבסוף שלא ייטב לו המזון. אבל מי שלא ייטב לו בתחלה לקחת המזון ותהיה לו מניעה חזקה ואחר כן ייטב לו עניינו יהיה יותר טוב.

אמר המפרש: המאמר במקום זה הוא בנקי ומבואר הוא כי בעבור רוע מזגו ותאותו חזקה 15 והוא יאכל בתוספת הליחות או שיחזק רוע המזג ובטל התאווה. ובהיות תחלה לא יתאוה מפני שהטבע עסוק בבישול ואחר שיתחיל להתאות ידע כי ליחותיו נתבשלו וילך עניינו אל התיקון.

(2.33)

[85] אמר בקראט: בריאות השכל בכל חולי סימן טוב וכן הניעור תאוה למזון והפך זה סימן רע.

20 אמר המפרש: זה מבואר והנה בארנו סבה זאת בפרקים שחברנו אותם.

1 פנוי: قد كلّت a 6 ובסופו: ובסופם זט 7 והכאב: والكرب add. a 8–7 והוא החולי ראוי בהכרח שיהיו (= שיהיה): وهي المرض فيجب ضرورة أن يكون a 9 ייטב לו מן המזון: יוסיף במזון זט 11 כל: כז זט 13–12 שלא ייטב לו בתחלה לקחת המזון ותהיה לו מניעה חזקה: يمتنع عليه في أوّل أمره النيل من الطعام امتناعا شديدا a 14 בנקי: الناقه a ‖ מזגו: أوبقيّة الأخلاط لم تغتذ أعضاؤه a add. a 15 בתוספת: فتزداد a 18 הניעור תאוה: الهشاشة a

(2.34)

[86] אמר בקראט: בהיות הזמן ניאות לטבע החולי ושניו וטבעו והעת ההווה מזמני השנה פחדו פחות מפחד החולי כשיהיה בלתי נאות לאחד מאילו הסגולות.

אמר המפרש: זה מבואר. כי אם לא יהיה ניאות הוא ראיה על יציאה מרובה מהמיצוע באותו האיש.

(2.35)

[87] אמר בקראט: היותר טוב בכל חולי הוא שיהיה מה שסמוך לטבור ולעצם שלערוה לו 5 עובי וכשיהיה רקיק מאד נכאה זה רע ובהיות זה כמו כן השלשול בזה פחד.

אמר המפרש: המוֹתֶן במה שבין הערוה והטבור יהיו חלקי הבטן שלשה המקומות אשר תחת החלצים וסמוך לטבור והמותן ובהיות אותם המקומות יותר עבים הוא יותר טוב. ובהיותם כחושים העניין יותר רע וזה כי הוא סימן רע. ושהוא יורה על חולשת אותם האיברים אשר נכאו ונתכו. אמנם הוא סבה רעה כי עיכול המזון באצטומ׳ ותולדת הדם בכבד לא יהיו בזה 10 העניין לפי מה שראוי כי שתי אלו האיברים כלם יועיל להם שמה שיכסם יהיה עב ושמן בחממם אותם.

(2.36)

[88] אמר בקראט: מי שגופו בריא ותשלשל ברפואה או בקיא ימהר אליהם העילוף וכן מי שיתפרנס במזון רע.

אמר המפרש: וכן מי שהיה מתפרנס במזון רע כי הוא יוקא או ישולשל ימהר בו העילוף 15 כי בגופותם ליחה רעה וכשיעשה בו הרפואה מעט מעשה התבאר ריעותו ונתגלה. זאת היא טענת גאלנוס. ואשר נראה לי כסבת עניין זה כי אשר יתמיד המזון הרע דמו דם רע מאד נפסד האיכות וכשימשוך המשלשל בכוחו המושך ינוע כל דם שבו ויחשוב לטהר ממנו כל הפסדותיו והן הרבה מאד ומתאחדים אבל הם מוצק חיי זה האיש הנפסד ההנהגה ויחדש העילוף בהכרח בכח המשיכה וריבוי מה שיחשוב למושכו והוא מעורב מתאחד. 20

(2.37)

[89] אמר בקראט: מי שגופו בריא לעשות הרפואה המשלשלת כי הוא עניין קשה.

אמר המפרש: הבריאים כשעושים הקיא או השלשול יקרה להם גלגול הראש ועקיצה ויקשה עליהם מה שיצא מגופם ובעבור זה ימהר עליהם העילוף כי הרפואה תתקדם

1 החולי: المريض a ‖ וטבעו: وطبعته a ‖ חזיו ‏**ט**   6 נכאה: منهوكا a   8 והמותן: ولمותن ‏**ט** ‖ הוא: فالحال a   9 כחושים: أهزل a ‖ רע: وسبب ردىء add. a   10 נכאו: انتكت a   11 יועילו: יועיל ‏**ט**   18 המשלשל: המזון ‏**ט**   19 מוצק: مركب a   22 ועקיצה: a   23 תתקדם: תתחזק ‏**זטל׳** يتوق a

למשוך הכימוס הניאות לה וכשלא תמצאנו תמשוך הדם והבשר ותבחר מהם להסיר מהם
מה שבהם ממה שניאות לה.

(2.38)

[90] אמר בקראט: מה שיהיה מן המזון והיין יותר ע(ר\)ב מעט אלא שהוא יותר מוטעם וערב
ראוי שיבחרנו על מה שיהיה יותר טוב ממנו.

5   אמר המפרש: זה מבואר כי עיכול היותר מוטעם וערב הוא יותר טוב.

(2.39)

[91] אמר בקראט: בני הארבעים הנקרא בערבי כהול ברוב יהיו חולים יותר מעט מהבחורים
אלא שמה שיקרה להם מן החליים הארוכים ברוב ימותו בהם.

אמר המפרש: הכהול מפני שהם מונעים עצמם מן ההנהגה הטובה יותר מהבחורים והכח
בגופות הכהול חלוש לא יוכל להתבשל החולי מהר והחליים הארוכים כלם קרים ועל כן הם
10   חייבים מיתה.

(2.40)

[92] אמר בקראט: מה שיקרה מן הנזל והפסד הקול לזקן הכלה לא יבואו לידי בישול.

אמר המפרש: אין אילו החליים לבדם יקרה כך לזקן אלא שאר מה שיקרה מן הליחות הקרות.

(2.41)

[93] אמר בקראט: מי שיקרה לו פעמים רבות עילוף חזק מבלתי סבה נגלית ימות פתאום.

אמר המפרש: מי שיקרה לו העילוף באילו התנאים השלשה והוא שיהיה מבלתי סבה נראית
15   וחזק ופעמים רבות אמנם יקרה לו זה מפני חולשת הכח החיונית.

(2.42)

[94] אמר בקראט: השתוק אם יהיה חזק אי אפשר שיתרפא בעליו ואם הוא חלוש אינו נקל
להתרפא.

אמר המפרש: כל שיתוק אמנם יהיה כשלא יהיה הרוח הנפשיי הולך אל מה שהוא זולתי
הראש משאר הגוף. או תהיה הסבה מסוג המורסה שנתחדשה במוח או שבטני המוח נתמלאו

---

1 ותבחר מהם: واستكرههما a   3 מוטעם: ראוי לⁱ   7 בהם: מהם ל וهي بهم a   8 מונעים: לⁱ
מונעים עצמם מן ההנהגה أضبط لأنفسهم في التدبير a   11 והפסד הקול: البحوحة a ‖ הכלה: זיטⁱ הכלוח
זט   14 העילוף: ט² השיתוק טל ‖ נראית: נגלית זט   16 השתוק: אפופליסיאה טיזⁱ   18 אמנם: ל
‖ יהיה: ל om. ‖ הרוח: הכח זט   19 שנתחדשה: ל om.

מליחות פליאומטיקו. ואם השתוק נעדרה ממנו תנועת החזה זה יותר גדול ממה שאפשר
וכשיתנפש ביותר חזק ממה שיהיה מן ההדחקה שיתוקו חזק כמו כן אלא שהוא יותר חסר מן
השני ובהיותו מתנפש נפוש דבק לסדר שיתוקו חלוש. ואם אתה נתת עצמך בעניינו לכל מה
שראוי לעשות אפשר לך שתרפאנו.

(2.43)

5   [95] אמר בקראט: אותם שיחנקו ויבואו אל העילוף ולא יגיעו עד שערי מות לא ימלט מהם
מי שנתראה בפיו קצף.

אמר המפרש: וזכר גאלנוס כי קצת מי שנחנק ונראה בו הקצף ניצלו וזה לעיתים רחוקות.

(2.44)

[96] אמר בקראט: מי שיהיה גופו עב מאד בטבע המות ימהר אליו יותר מהיותו ממהר אל
הכחוש.

10   אמר המפרש: עלה זו מבוארת מפני צרות הגידים ורחבותם כמו שבאר בספר המזג. ואמר
גאלנוס שיהיה הגוף יפה בשר ממוצע עד שלא יהיה עב ולא כחוש הוא יותר משובח ואפשר
שיחיה ימים רבים ויזקין מאד.

(2.45)

[97] אמר בקראט: בעל הוציאו הנק׳ צָרְע בערבי בהיותו חדש רפואתו תהיה בהיותו נעתק
בשנים והמקום וההנהגה.

15   אמר המפרש: האלצרע והשיתוק הכימוס המוליד להם הוא קר וכשיהיה נעתק בשנים ובמקום
ובהנהגה אל החמימות והיובש ונעתק כמו כן מהנהגה הרעה אשר הולידה זאת הליחה להפך
זאת ההנהגה אפשר שיתרפא.

(2.46)

[98] אמר בקראט: בהיות שני כאבים יחד ואינם במקום אחד החזק שבהן יעלים האחר.

אמר המפרש: כשהטבע ישים מגמת פניו לצד האבר אשר בו הכאב היותר חזק יפחית הרגש
20   המקום האחר ולא ירגיש במה שבו ממה שהוא כואב.

---

2 ביותר: ניפוש יותר זט ‖ כן: ومتى كان تنفّسه من غير مجاهدة واستكراه إلّا أنّه يختلف غير لازم لنظام واحد
فسكتته قوّة أيضا add. a (except for B)   3-2 من الثاني: ز׳ مهراشون זט׳   3 נתת עצמך: تأتيت a
4 לך: ל om.   7 שנחנק: خنق أو اختنق a   13 הוציאו הנק׳ צָרְע: איפילינסיאה ז׳ ט׳ ‖ תהיה: خاصّة
add. a (except for B)   15 האלצרע והשיתוק: האיפילינסיאה והאפופליסיאה זט׳ ‖ קר: غليظ   18 בהיות: بإنسان add. a (except for B) ‖ יעלים: יעביר זטל׳   19 הכאב: החולי הכאב זט החולי ל׳

(2.47)

[99] אמר בקראט: בזמן תולדת הטרי יתילד הכאב והקדחת יותר מאשר יקרו אחר תולדתם.

אמר המפרש: כי באותו זמן יתמשך מקום המורסא יותר ויתחזק הכאב ותטה החמימות לצד הליחה ויבשלנה ויתפשט יותר ויתחזק הקדחת.

(2.48)

[100] אמר בקראט: בכל תנועה שינוע הגוף וימצא בה הגוף מנוחה בהתחלת העייפות ימנענו מהתחדש בו העייפות.

אמר המפרש: זה מבואר.

(2.49)

[101] אמר בקראט: מי שהרגיל לטרוח אם היה חלוש הגוף או זקן הוא יותר סובל אותו הטורח שהרגיל ממי שלא הרגילו ואע״פ שהוא חזק ונער.

אמר המפרש: זה מבואר.

(2.50)

[102] אמר בקראט: מה שהרגיל האדם שנים רבות ואע״פ שיהיה טוב לו שלא היה מרגיל אותו הזיקו הוא פחות על כן ראוי שיהיה נעתק האדם אל אשר לא יהיה מרגילו.

אמר המפרש: הקדים הקדמה אמיתית וחייב הראוי בה ובעבור מה שיתחייב מהתמדת הבריאות שישוב האדם ממנהג אל מנהג ובמדרגה.

אמר גאלנוס: היותר טוב לכל אחד מבני אדם שירגיל לסבול עצמו לנסות כל דבר כדי שלא ימצאנו בזמן ההכרח דבר שלא היה רגיל בו והיה מביא עצמו להזק גדול אמנם יהיה זה כשלא יהיה האדם נשאר על מה שהיה רגיל בו תמיד אבל יטריח עצמו בקצת הזמנים לעשות הפכו.

(2.51)

[103] אמר בקראט: לעשות המרובה פתאום והוא ממה שימלא הגוף או שיריקנו או שיחממנו או שינועענו במין אחד מן התנועה אי זה מן שיהיה הוא פחד. וכל אשר יהיה מרובה הוא מנגד לטבע אבל מה שיהיה מעט מעט הוא בטוח כשתרצה להעתיק מדבר אל דבר זולתו וכשתרצה זולתי זה אינו בטוח.

אמר המפרש: זה מבואר.

---

2 יתמשך: האבר ל .add   4 שינוע: שיתנועע זט   10–11 ואע״פ שיהיה טוב לו שלא היה מרגיל אותו: وإن كان أضرّ مما لم يعتده a   13 הבריאות: في جميع الحالات a .add   14 שירגיל לסבול עצמו: أن يحمل نفسه a   17 ממה: ז׳ כמו זט׳ ‖ שיחממנו: أو يبرده a .add   20 אינו בטוח: om. a

(2.52)

[104] אמר בקראט: אם אתה עושה כל מה שראוי לעשות כמו שראוי ולא היה מה שראוי להיות לא תהיה נעתק אל דבר אחר משאתה בו כל זמן שאתה רואה העניין קיים עומד מתחלתו.

אמר המפרש: זה פרק בכללו סדר גדול מסדרי הרפואה ולא בא גאלנוס בו לסוף ביאורו הראוי לו. ועניין זה כי כשיורוך הסימנים שאתה על דרך משל ראוי לך לחמם והתמדת החימום ולא יתרפא החולה אין ראוי לך שתהיה נעתק אל הקירור אבל תתמיד לחמם כל זמן שאתה רואה הדברים המורים בעשיית החימום קיימים והוא עניין אמרו כל זמן שתראהו מתחלת העניין קיים. זה העניין אמרו כלומ' שלא יהיה נעתק ממין ההנהגה אבל ראוי בהכרח שתהיה נעתק מרפואה מחממת אל רפואה אחרת מחממת ותתהפך ברפואה הנפרדת והמורכבת אשר היא כלה מחממת כי כשהגוף יאסוף לו רפואה אחת תמיד יתמעט מעשהו בו. ועוד בהשתנות מיני הרפואות אשר איכותם אחת נאות גדול מאד למזג גוף וגוף ולמזג אבר ואבר ולמקרי כל חולי וחולי. זה שורש גדול מסודות הרפואה וזה העניין בעצמו ינהיג מה שיריק בו הליחה המחליאה או בהתכה או בדקות או בישול או עבות חומר או לקבצו יתמיד לעולם מין ההנהגה אשר עליו תורה הסימנים הקיימים וְשַׁנֵּה במיני הרפואות אשר הם כלם מכת אחד והבן זה.

(2.53)

[105] אמר בקראט: מי שהיה בטנו לח ורפה כל זמן היותו בחור הוא יותר בריא ממי שבטנו יבש ואחרי כן יהיה סוף עניינו בזמן הזקנה עד שישוב יותר רע כי בטנו יהיה יבש כשיזיקין לפי הרוב.

אמר המפרש: כבר הקדים זה הדעת ברפיון הבטן ויבשותו בשני הבחורים והזקנים. וגאלנוס יחשוב לתת עלת זה וכבר אמרתי מה שבסברתי וחלקות הבטן לעולם בכל השנים מסבת התמדת הבריאות וכל יובש בטבע רע לבריאים ולחולים.

(2.54)

[106] אמר בקראט: גודל הגוף בזמן הארבעים שנה אינו דחוק אבל הוא נאהב אבל בזמן הזקנה יכבד ויקשה לשאת אותו ויהיה יותר רע מהבטן אשר הוא יותר חסר ממנו.

אמר המפרש: גאלנוס יאמר שירצה במאמרו הנה גודל הגוף ארכו עד שלא תהיה זאת הגזרה ספק גמור.

נשלם המאמר השיני מפרקי אבקראט.

---

4 בכללו: בכלל זט يَتَضمّن a ‖ סדר: קאנון ליט² קאנון סדר ז 5 לו: בו זט 10 יאסוף לו: أَلِف a

11 הרפואות: הרפואה זט ‖ גדול: לי טוב ל טוב גדול זט ‖ ולמזג: ומזגי זט 14 הרפואות: والأغذية

22 בזמן הארבעים: في الشبيبة a add. a 23 מהבטן: מהקטן זט

من البدن a 24 ארכו: ז² גבהו זט² 25 ספק: وهم a 26 מפרקי אבקראט: זט om.

המאמר השלישי

(3.1)

[107] אמר בקראט: התהפך זמני השנה הוא עניין שמוליד החליים בייחוד ובזמן אחד מהם
השינוי המרובה בקור או בחום וכן בשאר העניינים על זה ההקש.

אמר המפרש: ירצה לומר שנוי טבעי הפרקים כמו שיהיה פרק הקור חם או פרק הקייץ קר. וכן
השתנות הזמן האחד ממזגו בהיותו חזק ואע״פ שהנשאר מן הפרקים לא ישתנה יוליד חליים.   5

(3.2)

[108] אמר בקראט: כי יש מן הטבעים שיהיה עניינו בקייץ יותר טוב ובקור יותר רע. ויש מהם
שיהיה עניינו בזמן הקור יותר טוב ובקייץ יותר רע.

אמר המפרש: ירצה לומ׳ באמרו מן הטבעים ממזגי האנשים וזה מבואר כי בזמן הקור ייטבו
ענייני המוקדחים ובימי הקייץ ייטבו עניני המקוררים ולפי זה תקיש בנשארים.

(3.3)

[109] אמר בקראט: כל אחד ואחד מן החליים עניינו בדבר בלתי דבר יותר טוב ויותר רע ושנים   10
מה שאצל זמני השנה והמקומות ומיני ההנהגה.

אמר המפרש: כשתכתוב מילותיו יתבאר לך ביאור נגלה וכן יכתבו כל אחד מן החליים עניינו
בשנים בלתי שנים או בעיר בלתי עיר או בזמן מן השנים בלתי זמן או בהנהגה בלתי הנהגה
הוא יותר טוב ויותר רע. המשל בזה כי בעל החולי הקר בזמן הבחרות ובזמן הקייץ ובעיר החם
ובהנהגה החמה החמה הוא יותר טוב ובהפכי אילו הוא יותר רע. ובכלל כי עניין ההפך אצל ההפך   15
הוא יותר מתוקן והמשל היוצא מהשווי באותה השנה יותר רע. אבל בעל שנים ממוצעי המזג
ההנהגה המיושרת והזמן המיושר או העיר המיושר יותר נאות לו כי בעל זה המזג לבדו הוא
אשר יתוקן עניינו בדומהו. אבל בעלי המזג העובר לשווי במדינות ובזמנים ומיני ההנהגה הפכם
יהיה להם יותר נאות.

(3.4)

[110] אמר בקראט: בהיות ביום אחד מזמני השנה פעם חמימות ופעם קרירות יביא חידוש   20
חליים דומים לחוליי החורף.

אמר המפרש: זה מבואר.

---

1 השלישי: ל״א פרקים **זט** add. ‏   2 ובזמן: וכן כשיהיה בזמן **זט**׳   9 המוקדחים: בעלי החמימות
זטל׳ ‏ || ‏ ובימי הקייץ ייטבו עניני המקוררים: **ל**׳   12 כשתכתוב: إذا رتّب a ‏ || ‏ יכתבו: يرتّب a
16 מתוקן: טוב **זטל**׳ ‏ || ‏ מהשווי: عند المثل الخارج عن الاعتدال add. a (except for B)   18 העובר
לשווי: المجاوز للاعتدال a ‏ || ‏ במדינות ובזמנים: بالمدينة والهزمنة **זט** فالبلدان والأوقات a ‏ || ‏ הפכם: והפכם
ל   20 יביא: فتوقّع a   22 מבואר: כי יולידו ליחות שונות ויעשו חליים בלתי מסודרים **זט** add.

(3.5)

[111] אמר בקראט: הרוח הנק' ג'נוב בערבי יעשה כובד בשמיעה וסנוירים וכובד בראש ועצלה וריפיון ובהתחזק זה הרוח יקרה לחולים אילו המקרים. אבל רוח צפוני הנק' אלשמאל בערבי יחדש שעול וכאב הגרון ויבשות הבטנים ועוצר השתן והפלצות וכאב הצלעות והחזה. ובהתגבר זה הרוח וכוחו ראוי שיביא אילו המקרים בחולים.

אמר המפרש: רוח האלגנוב חם ולח ועל כן תבלבל החושים ותלחלח התחלת העצבים ויחדש העצלה ועוצר התנועה ורוח האלשמאל קרה ויבשה על כן תעבה הגרון והחזה ותיבש הבטן ותעבה הדרכים ותחדש מה שזכר.

(3.6)

[112] אמר בקראט: בהיות הקייץ דומה באלרביע בקדחת זיעה מרובה.

אמר המפרש: ראוי בהיות הקייץ יבש חזק היובש שיפנה ויתיר הלחות ובהיותו דומה באלרביע שימשוך הלחות בחמימותו אל צד העור ואי אפשר שיתיכנה על דרך האד בעבור לחותו ומפני כי זה הלחות בזמן בחראן חליים מורקים פתאום יהיה בעבורו זיעה מרובה.

(3.7)

[113] אמר בקראט: בהעצר המטר יתחדשו קדחות חדות ואם תתרבה זאת העצירה בשנה כלה ואחר כן נתחדש באויר יבש ראוי שתבוא ברוב העניינים ודומיהם.

אמר המפרש: מבואר הוא כי בהעדר המטר יתייבשו הליחות ויתעבו ויהיו הקדחות פחות במספר ואיכות יותר חם.

(3.8)

[114] אמר בקראט: בהיות זמני השנה הולכים אחר סדרם ויהיה בכל עת ממנה מה שראוי להיות יהיה מה שיתחדש מן החליים סדר טוב וקיום ובחראן טוב ובהיות זמני השנה בלתי מסודרים יהיה מה שיתחדש בהם מן החליים בלתי מסודר ובחראן מגונה.

אמר המפרש: זה מבואר.

---

1 הרוח: הדרומי .add ז דרומי .add ט‏ ‏ ‏ 2 ובהתחזק זה הרוח: فعند قوّة هذه الريح وغلبتها a ‏ ‏|| צפוני: דרום ל ‏ ‏ 3 הבטנים: הבטן זט ‏ ‏ ‏ 6 על כן תעבה: فتخشّن a ‏ ‏ ‏ בחולים: في الأمراض a ‏ ‏ 4 שיביא: أن يتوقّع a ‏ ‏|| בחולים: في الأمراض a ‏ ‏ 9 שיפנה: أن تهي a ‏ ‏ 10 ואי אפשר: ט' ואפשר זט ‏ ‏ 14 שתבוא ברוב העניינים: أن يتوقّع في أكثر الحالات هذه الأمراض a ‏ ‏ 15 ויתעבו: وتحتدّ a ‏ ‏ 16 יותר חם: وأحدّ a

(3.9)

[115] אמר בקראט: כי בחורף יהיו החליים יותר מחודדים ויותר ממיתים ברוב אמנם האלרביע הוא יותר בריא משאר הזמנים ופחות מות.

אמר המפרש: האלרביע ממוצע והחורף בתכלית השנוי.

(3.10)

[116] אמר בקראט: החורף לבעלי הטיציש רע.

5 אמר המפרש: מפני היותו קר ויבש משתנה במזגו והוא יזיק לנחלאים מאד.

(3.11)

[117] אמר בקראט: אמנם בזמני השנה אני אומר כי כשיהיה האוירנו במטר מועט ורוחו שמאלי והיה הויר בעל מטר והרוח רוח האלגנוב ראוי בהכרח שיתחדש בקייץ קדחות חדות וחולי העינים הנק׳ רמד ודם שותת ורוב מה שיקרה שלשול הדם לנשים ולבעלי הטבעים הלחים.

10 אמר המפרש: זה מבואר אחר דעת שרשי המלאכה.

(3.12)

[118] אמר בקראט: ובהיות זמן האוירנו ינשבו בו רוחות האלגנוב בעלי מטר חם ויהיה זמן הויר במעט מטר וינשב בו רוח שמאלי הנשים אשר תלדנה נגד הויר תהיינה מפילות במעט סבה. ואותם שתלדנה יהיו בניהם חלושי התנועה שדופים ונחלאים עד שהיא תמות מיד או תשאר נחלאה וכלה כל ימי חייהם. אבל שאר בני אדם יקרה להם שלשול הדם וחולי העין הנק׳
15 רמד היבש אבל הכהול יקרה להם מן הנזל מה שיסור מהרה.

(3.13)

[119] אמר בקראט: אם יהיה הקיץ במטר מועט ברוח שמאלי ויהיה החורף מטרי גנובי יקרה בימות הגשמים כאב ראש ושעול וקוריצא וקטרא ויקרה לקצת בני אדם חולי הטיציש.

(3.14)

[120] אמר בקראט: אם יהיה הקייץ שמאלי יבש יהיה נאות למי שיהיה טבעו לח ורפה ולנשים אבל בשאר בני אדם יקרה להם רמד יבש וקדחות חדות וקטארה ארוכים ומהם מי שיקרה
20 להם השעמום הקורה מן המרה השחורה.

1 בחורף: בתקופת תשרי ז²ט² ‖ האלרביע: לטיץ ויר זט add. ויר בלעז ל¹ 4 החורף: תקופת תשרי ז²ט²
5 לנחלאים: لأصحاب السلّ a 6 במטר מועט: במעט מטר זט 7–16 ראוי ... הקיץ: om. ט 8 ודם
שותת: דיסינטיריאה ז 12 תלדנה: תהרנה זל¹ 13 שדופים: דלים ל¹ ‖ שדופים ונחלאים: مسقامة a
16 הקיץ: ל¹ הציף ל 17 ראש: شديد وسعال وبحوحة add. a 18 ורפה: om. a

(3.15)

[121] אמר בקראט: כי מן ענייני האויר בשנה בכלל מעט המטר יותר בריא מן השנה שהיא מרובת המטר ופחות מיתה.

(3.16)

[122] אמר בקראט: אמנם החליים המתחדשים בהתרבות מטר ברוב העניינים הם קדחות ארוכים והתרת הבטן ועיפושים וויציאו ותרדימה ואישקויינצ'יאה. אבל החוליים המתחדשים במעט מטר הם טיצ'יש ורמד וכאב הפרקים והגרת טיפות השתן.

אמר המפרש: כל מה שהנהיג בקראט באילו החמישה פרקים מהיות החליים הפלוניים מתחדשים במין הפלוני מבני אדם בהיות האויר כן אין זה נמצא ברוב בשום פנים ולכן אין ראוי שתתן סיבותיו לפי מה שידוע בפילוסופיה אבל גאלנוס ירצה לתת סבה לכל זה ובכלל שאע"פ שמלאכת הרפואה היא יוצאת מידיעת טבעי הפרקים והאישים וסבות החוליים ושהלחות חומר העיפוש והחמימות פועל בה יקל לתת סבות לכל מה שזכר שהוא קורה.

(3.17)

[123] אמר בקראט: אמנם ענייני האויר בכל יום ויום מה שיהיה רוח שמאלי הוא מקבץ הגופות ומחזיק אותם ומטיב תנועותיהם ויעשה מראיהם יפה ויזקק השמע וינגב הבטן ויחדש בעינים עקיצה. ואם יהיה בצדדי החזה כאב מתקדם יעוררהו ויוסיף בו. ומה שיהיה גנובי יתיר הגופות וירפם וילחלחם ויחדש כובד בראש ובשמע וסיתום ובעיניים ובגוף כולו קושי תנועה ורפיון הבטן.

אמר המפרש: ידוע כי רוח שמאלי קר ויבש ושהגנוב חם ולח וכל זה מבואר.

(3.18)

[124] אמר בקראט: אמנם בזמני השנה בזמן הויר ותחלת הקיץ יהיו הנערים וסמוך להם בשנים בעניין טוב ובריאות שלם. ובשארית הקיץ וקצה החורף יהיו הזקנים יותר בטובה בעניינים מן הילדים. ובשארית החורף ובימות הגשמים יהיה הממוצע ביניהם בשנים יותר בעניין טוב.

אמר המפרש: הנה קדם לנו סבה זאת בפרק אשר שנינו בו הרכבת מילותיו.

---

5 השתן: واختلاف الدم add. a   6 שהנהיג: ذكره a ‖ הפלוניים: ל' הפנימיים ל' במעט מטר הם
טיצ'יש ורמד וכאב ל add. ‖   9 שאע"פ שמלאכת הרפואה היא יוצאת: أنّ مع ما تأصّل في الصناعة
الطبّيّة a ‖ הרפואה: הרפואות זט ‖ יוצאת: זט נודעת זט²   10 סבות: סבה זט   12 האויר: הרוח
ל'   13 יפה: ל om.   14 מתקדם: ישן זט²ל'   15 וסיתום (= وسددا): وسدرا a   20 יותר: ל om.
22 קדם: הקדים זט

(3.19)

[125] אמר בקראט: והחליים כלם יתחדשו בזמני השנה כלם אלא שקצתם לפעמים הוא יותר טוב שיתעוררו ויתחדשו.

אמר המפרש: זה מבואר.

(3.20)

[126] אמר אבקראט: יקרה בזמן אלרביע השעמום המלנקוניקו והשטות והויציאו והגרת הדם והחנק והקטרא והרוקיצא והשעול והחולה אשר יתפלץ בו העור ובוהק ובהרת והבתור והמרובים אשר יתחבלו והצמחים וכאבי הפרקים.

אמר המפרש: זה הפרק מבאר למה שקדם בפרק אשר לפניו כי הוא זכר בפרק שקדם שיתחדש כל מין ממיני החוליים בכל פרק מפרקי השנה אבל קצת החליים בקצת הפרקים יותר טוב והוא שיתחדש ברוב באותו הפרק. והשלים זה העניין בשאמר כי הוא מתחדש בזמן הויר שהוא היותר ממוצע שבפרקים חליים מלנקונקי כשעמום המלנקונקו והשטות וחליים פליאומטיקי כמו הויציאו והקטרא והפסד הקול והשעול וחליים קולייריקי כמו הבתור אשר יתנגע בו העור והצמחים וחליים בעלי דם כהגרת הדם והחנק אבל החליים המיוחדים בזמן האלרביע הן הנמשכים אחר התכת הליחות והגרתם לחוצה והטבע יתנועע לדחותם בקוה. וכן הפרק אשר אחר זה בנוי על שבארנו מהיות החליים מתחדשים בהפך טבע הפרק.

(3.21)

[127] אמר בוקראט: אבל בקייץ יקרו קצת מאלו החליים וקדחות תמדיות ושורפות וקדחות שלישיות וקיא ושלשול וחולי העיניים וכאב האזנים ונגעים בפה ועיפוש בחבלות.

(3.22)

[128] אמר בקראט: אבל בזמן החורף יקרו חולי הקיץ ברוב וקדחות רבעיות ומעורבות וטחול והדרוקן וטיציש ורבוי שתן ושלשול הדם והמעדת המעיים וכאב הירך והחנק והמין מן השעול הנקרא רבו ובלעז נקרא רֵימְפָלִי והקולון החזן והוא חולי המעי שנקרא כך ונקרא בלשון יון אליאוס. והויציאו בערבי אלצרע והשטות והשעמום המלאנקונקו.

אמר המפרש: כל זה מבואר ממה שהקדמנו.

4 והויציאו: אסויסיאו זט פי׳ חולי שמדבר החולה בינו לבין עצמו זיטי׳   5 והרוקיצא: והרוקיציאה זט
والبحوحة a ‖ והחולה: والعلّة a ‖ יתפלץ: يَسمر لi يَتقشّر a ‖ ובוהק ובהרת: والقوابي والبهق a   7 מבאר:
מבואר זט   8 השנה: ל om.   13 בקוה (=بقوّة): بقنه זק   14 בנוי: مبنية זק موكنة לi ‖ מתחדשים:
בטבע ל add.   16 שלישיות: كثيرة add. a ‖ בחבלות (= في القروح a) في الفروج emendation editor
وحصف a add.   18 ורבוי שתן: وتقطير البول a

(3.23)

[129] אמר בקראט: אמנם בזמן הקור יקרה חולי הצד וחולי הריאה והקטרא והשעול
והרוקיצא וכאבי הצדדים ועצם הנק' קוטן והכאב שבראש והסתום והשיתוק.

אמר המפרש: זה בנוי כמו כן לפי מה שקדם כי יתחדש בזמן הקור חוליים מיוחדים בו ברוב
כמו הקטרא והרוקיצא והשתוק וחליים אין מטבעו כחולי הצד.

(3.24)

[130] אמר בקראט: אמנם בשנים יקרו אלו החליים אמנם הילדים הקטנים בזמן הולדם
יקרה להם חולי הפה הנקרא קלאע והקיא והשעול והתעורה והפחד ומורסת הטיבור ולחות
האזנים.

אמר המפרש: יקרה להם החולי הנק' קלאע מפני חלקות איבריהם ומה שבחלב מן הניקיון.
ויקרה להם הקיא בעבור רבוי מה שינקו וחולשת הכח העוצר בהם בעבור חוזק הלחות.
והשעול יקרה להם מפני לחות הריאה. ורוב מה שיזוב ממוחם בעבור חוזק לחותם בריאה
והיא הסבה בלחות האזנים. ומורסת הטבור מפני שהוא קרוב מהחיתוך והפחד שיקרה להם
הוא מפני רוב השינה בעבור הפסד עכול האצטומ' באד המוח ויתחדשו בו דמיונות מפחידים.
ואמנם התעורה לא ידע גאלנוס סבתה אבל אמר כי העניין המיוחד בילדים רבוי השינה וזה
אמת. אבל הרבה פעמים יקרה להם התעורה והבכי כל הלילה וסבה זו רבוי הרגשם בעבור
חלקות גופם וכחותם כולם חלושה בלתי נאחזת ומעט דבר מכאב יעירם משנתם. ומעט שיהיה
נעדר מהם רוע עיכול וצער מפני האצטומ' לריבוי ינקתם ויעוררם אותו הכאב וייקצו ולא ישנו
ואם יוסיף מעט יבכו וזה מפורסם תמיד.

(3.25)

[131] אמר בקראט: כשיתקרב הנער שיצמחו להם השינים יקרה להם חיכוך בשנים וקדחות
וקוץ ושלשול כל שכן אם יצמחו להם השינים והשמן מן הילדים והנערים ולמי שיהיה בטנו
עצור.

אמר המפרש: זה כלו מפני היות השניים חותכים ונוקבים בשר החנכים ויתרחבו החורים ויהיה
נמשך אחר זה הכאב והקוץ ובעבור שהזמן לא יתעכל בטוב בעבור החולי והתעורה יתחדש
השלשול וברוב יקרה הקוץ לשמנים ולעצורי הבטן מפני רוב מותרי גופותם.

2 והרוקיצא: והרוקיציאה **זק** ‖ והסתום: (= والسدد): والسدر a ‖ 4 והרוקיצא: והרוקיציאה **זק**
11 האוזנים: لأنّ فضول الدماغ تندفع للأذنين (except for AB) add. a ‖ 12 באד: يتبخّر a ‖ 13 בילדים:
ל om. ‖ 15 נאחזת: מתונקנת **זטי**לי ‖ ומעט: הם **זט** add. ‖ 18 הנער: הילד **זטי**לי ‖ בשינים: في اللثة a
19 השינים: הטוחנות **זטי** add. ‖ 21 החורים: הנקבים **זטלי** ‖ 22 בעבור החולי: للألم a

(3.26)

[132] אמר בקראט: וכשיעבור הנער אלו השנים יקרה לו מורסת הגרון והכנס חליית העורף
והרבו והחול והתולעים הגדולים והתולעים הקטנים והתלולים בלע"ז פורי בדגש הריש
והחזירים ושאר הצמחים.

אמר המפרש: מאחר שיצמחו השינים עד י"ג שנה יאכלו הנערים המזונות המרובות
וירבה תאותם למזון וישימו מזון על מזון ותרבה תנועתם אחר המזון וכל זאת ההנהגה   5
מפסידה המזון ומרבה הליחות וגופותם עם זה לח ואיבריהם רפים והוא ראוי להיות כל
מה שזכר כי כשיתמרסם המושקולי של הגרון ימשוך החוליה מן העורף בעבור חלקות
הקישורים.

(3.27)

[133] אמר בקראט: אמנם מי שיעבור אלו השנים ויתקרב שיצמח בו השיער בעצם הערוה
יקרה לו הרבה מאלו החליים וקדחות יותר ארוכים והגרת דם מהנחירים.   10

אמר המפרש: באלו השנים יתרבה הדם וירוץ בהם ועל כן יתחדש להם הגרת דם מנחיריהם
בחלייהם.

(3.28)

[134] אמר בקראט: ורוב מה שיקרה לנערים מן החליים יבוא בקצתם הבחראן במ' ימים
ובקצתם בז' חודשים ובקצתם בז' שנים ובקצתן כשיצמח השיער בערוה. אבל מה שיהיה
נשאר מן החליים ולא יהיה נתך בזמן צמיחת השיער או בנקבות בזמן שיגר מהם הוסת מטבעם   15
שיאריכו וישארו עם האדם כל זמן שהוא נשאר.

אמר המפרש: ירצה לומר מן החליים הארוכים מהם.

(3.29)

[135] אמר בקראט: אמנם הבחורים יקרה להם רקיקת הדם והטיציש והקדחות החדות
והוציאו ושאר החליים אלא שרוב מה שיקרה להם הוא מה שזכרנו.

אמר המפרש: כבר ביאר גאלנוס כי אין פנים להיות הוציאו בבחורים אבל הוא מחוליי   20
הנערים.

---

2 והתלולים בלע"ז פורי בדגש הריש: والثَّوَاليل المُتعلّقة a   5 תאותם למזון: شَرِبهم a   6 המזון: لِلهضم
a   15 החליים: החולים זט   16 וישארו עם האדם כל זמן שהוא נשאר: om. a   20 הוציאו: خاصّ
add. a (except for BP)

(3.30)

[136] אמר בקראט: אבל מי שעבר אלו השנים יקרה לו האלרבו וחולי הצד וחולי הריאה והקדחת אשר יהיה עמה התעורה והקדחת אשר יהיה עמה בלבול הדעת והקדחת השורפת והשלשול הנק׳ היצה ובלע׳ אינישטיאון והשלשול הארוך ופונטי במעיים והמעדת המעיים ופתיחת פיות הגידים מתחת.

אמר המפרש: ידוע שאלו השנים והם שני הכהול הליחה השחורה נראית בו ברוב ועל כן   5
המיוחד בהם הוא בלבול הדעת והתעורה בקדחת ופתיחת פיות העורקים. אבל שאר מה
שסופר אינו מיוחד באלו השנים ואינו כן.

(3.31)

[137] אמר בקראט: אמנם הזקנים יקרה להם רוע הניפוש והנזל אשר עמו השעול וטיפות
השתן ועוצר השתן וכאבי הפרקים וכאבי הכליות והגלגול בראש והשתוק והחבלות הרעות
וחיכוך הגוף והתעורה וחלקות הבטן ולחות העיניים והאף ואפילת הראות וכובד השמיעה.   10

אמר המפרש: סבות אלו כלם מבוארים למה שנודע מעניין מזג הזקנים.

נשלם המאמר השלישי מפרקי אבקרט.

---

1 האלרבו: אזמא זⁱ‎טⁱ   2 והקדחת אשר יהיה עמה התעורה: זט .om   4 ופתיחת (= وانفتاح MSS):‎
وانتفاخ a   6 ופתיחת: (= وانفتاح MSS) وانتفاخ   emendation editor   7 השנים: وجالينوس يزعم أنّه‎
أعطى أسباب خصيصة بهذه السنّ a. add   10 הראות: والزرقة a. add   12 מפרקי אבקרט: זט .om

המאמר הרביעי

(4.1)

[138] אמר אבקרט: ראוי שתשקה האשה ההרה הרפואה בהיות הליחות בגופן מתעוררות
מיום שיעבור על העובר ד׳ חודשים ועד שיעברו עליה ז׳ חודשים ויהיה ההקדם על זה פחות
אבל מי שיהיה פחות מזה או יותר ממנו ראוי שתשתמור בעובר.

אמר המפרש: זה מבואר כי בתחלתו הוא חלוש ויהיה נקל להפילו וכן בסופו יהיה כבד וגדול   5
ויעזור על נפילתו הכובד שלו.

(4.2)

[139] אמר בקראט: אמנם ראוי שישקה מן הרפואה מה שיריק מן הגוף המין אשר כשיריקהו
מעצמו יועיל הרקתו אבל מה שתהיה הרקתו על הפך זה ראוי שתפסיקהו.

אמר המפרש: זה מבואר.

(4.3)

[140] אמר בקראט: אם הורק הגוף מן המין אשר ראוי לנקות ממנו יועיל זה ונקל הוא לסובלו   10
ואם היה העניין הפך זה הוא קשה.

אמר המפרש: הודיענו בזה על שזה יהיה סימן נדע בו איך נוכל לדעת מההרקה בקלות הסבל
או בקשיו.

(4.4)

[141] אמר בקראט: ראוי לעשות ההרקה בקיץ ברפואת הקיא ממעלה יותר ובזמן האיזורנו
מלמטה.   15

אמר המפרש: הגובר בקיץ המרה האדומה ובעבור תנועת הליחות מלמעלה על כן יבחר
להריק בקיא ובזמן האיזירנו יהיה הפך.

(4.5)

[142] אמר בקראט: אחר עלות כוכב הכלב ובזמן היותו עולה וקודם יקשה להריק הגוף
ברפואה.

---

4 מי: מה זט   12–13 איך נוכל לדעת מההרקה בקלות הסבל או בקשיו: هل أصبنا في الحدس أو أخطأنا
أعني سهولة احتمال الاستفراغ أو عسره a   16 ובעבור תנועת הליחות: ألجّوا الأخلاط متحرّكة a ‖ כן: ל
om.

אמר המפרש: זה הזמן הוא בימות החמה חזק יותר משאר ימות הקיץ והכחות חלושות מאד וחמימות האויר ימנע משיכת המזון ולא יגיע ממנו אלא חולשה וסער.

(4.6)

[143] אמר בקראט: מי שהוא רזה הגוף ויהיה הקיא נקל לעשות לו תשים הרקתך ברפואה ממעלה והשמר מעשות זה בזמן הקור.

אמר המפרש: עניין הכחוש תמיד כעניין רוב בני אדם בקיץ והנה הקדים לך המניעה מעשות   5
הקיא בזמן הקור.

(4.7)

[144] אמר בקראט: אמנם מי שיקשה עליו הקיא ויהיה בשרו ממוצע בין הדלות והשומן תשים הרקתו ברפואה מתחת והשמר מעשות זה בקיץ.

אמר המפרש: זה מבואר.

(4.8)

[145] אמר בקראט: אמנם בעלי הטיציש כשתריקם עם הרפואה השמר מהריק אותם   10
ממעלה.

אמר המפרש: כלומר המוכנים לטיציש והם הצרים בחזיהם ריאתם כמו כן צרה בסמפונות ולא תמשוך להם החמרים.

(4.9)

[146] אמר בקראט: אמנם מי שגובר עליו המרה השחורה ראוי שתריקהו ממטה עם רפואה יותר עבה אחר שתתחבר שני ההפכים אל היקש אחד.   15

אמר המפרש: אמרו ברפואה יותר עבה ירצה לומר בו יותר חזקה כי הקולורא צפה למעלה והמרה השחורה תשקע למטה וההקש האחד הוא אשר יעשה בזה לבחור אחד משני צדדים לאחת משתי הליחות כי אנו נריק כל ליחה ממקומו הקרוב לצאתו.

(4.10)

[147] אמר בקראט: ראוי לעשות רפואת ההרקה בחליים החדים מאד כשיהיו הליחות מתעוררות מיום ראשון לחלייו כי האיחור בכמו אילו החליים הוא רע.   20

---

2 המזון: الدواء a   3 לו: אילו ל   7 שיקשה עליו הקיא: שיקרה עליו ל   17 משני צדדים: משני טל
צדדים ז משני דרכים ז corr. الضّدين a

אמר המפרש: זה מבואר ויש לפחד מעזוב אלו הליחות הנגרות ממקום למקום בלתי נחות
שמא ינוחו באבר מעולה ועל כן תמהר להריקם קודם החליש הכח או שינוחו באבר המעולה.

(4.11)

[148] אמר בקראט: מי שיהיה בו עקיצה וכאב סביב הטבור וכאב בבטן תמיד לא יסור לא
ברפואה משלשלת ולא בזולתה עניינו ילך אל ההדרוקן היבש.

אמר המפרש: כשלא יהיה סר זה בשום רפואה הוא ראיה על רוע מזג שגבר על אותם האיברים   5
ונתאחז בהם ויתחדש ההדרקון התופי הוא אשר קראו ההדרוקן היבש שהוא נוכח ההדרוקן
אשר בו המים כמי הנאד ויתילד מקרירות נוסף.

(4.12)

[149] אמר בקראט: מי שיש בו המעדת המעים בזמן הקור הרקתו ברפואה ממעלה רעה.

אמר המפרש: יאמר שאפילו היה המביאו להמעדת מעים ליחה חדה ודקה צפה אשר יחייב
זה להריקו בקיא כיון שהעת איוירנו אין דרך לעשות הקיא כמו שקדם.   10

(4.13)

[150] אמר בקראט: מי שיצטרך לשתות הליברוס והיתה הרקתו ממעלה ולא

יענה בנקלה ראוי שילחלח גופו מקודם השקותו במזון יותר ובמנוחה.

אמר המפרש: זה מבואר.

(4.14)

[151] אמר בקראט: כשתשקה לשום אדם ליברוס בערבי כרבק תהיה כוונתך לנוע גופו יותר
וליישנו וחממו פחות ויורה רכיבת הספינה על שהתנועה יעיר הגופות.   15

אמר המפרש: ידוע שהליברוס מקיא ותנועת הגוף בהעתק המקומי יעזור על הקיא והורה עליו
זה ברכיבת הספינות.

(4.15)

[152] אמר אבקרט: כשתרצה שתהיה הרקת הליברוס יותר תניע הגוף ואם תרצה להשקיטו
תישן השותה אותו ולא תניעהו.

אמר המפרש: זה מבואר כפול.   20

---

3 בבטן (= في البطن): في القطن a   11 הליברוס: ל om.   12 יענה: يواتيه a   15 וחממו (= وتَسخينه):
وتَسكينه a   16 מקיא: قوّي add. a

(4.16)

[153] אמר בקראט: לשתות הליברוס פחד למי שבשרו בריא וזה שהוא יחדש קווץ.

אמר המפרש: זה מבואר

(4.17)

[154] אמר בקראט: מי שאין בו קדחת והיה בו המנע מן המזון ועקיצה בפי האצטומ' וסתימה
ומרירות בפה זה יורה על הרקתו ממעלה.

אמר המפרש: הגלגול הוא שידמה לאדם שכל מה שהוא רואה יקיף סביבו ויעדר ממנו חוש 5
הראות פתאום עד שיחשוב שהכל יתכסה מאפילה ואלו המקרים יהיו כשיהיה בפי האצטומ'
ליחות רעות ינשכוהו ועל כן ראוי כשיתראו אלו המקרים שיריקנו בקיא.

(4.18)

[155] אמר בקראט: הכאבים אשר למעלה מהמסך יורו על שההרקה ברפואה צריכה
להיות למעלה והכאבים אשר ממטה מהמסך הנק' דיאפרמה יורו על ההרקה ברפואה
ממטה. 10

אמר המפרש: לאי זה צד שיטו הליחות מאותו הצד יורקו ממעלה ברפואה מקיאה או מתחת
במשלשלת. אבל בעניין מוצק הליחות ראוי שתתמשכנה אל הפך הצד.

(4.19)

[156] אמר בקראט: מי ששתה רפואת ההרקה והריק ולא אחזו הצמא לא תפסיק ממנו
ההרקה עד שיצמא.

אמר המפרש: הצמא אחר שתות הרפואה כל זמן שלא תהיה בעבור חמימות האצטומ' או 15
יבשותה או בעבור חידוד הרפואה או מפני היות הליחה המורקת חמה יורה על ניקיון האיברים
והעדרם מאותה הליחה אשר תרצה להוציאה.

(4.20)

[157] אמר בקראט: מי שלא תהיה בו קדחת וקרה לו עקיצה וכובד בשתי הארכובות וכאב
הקוטן זה יורה על שהוא יצטרך אל הרקה ברפואה מתחת.

אמר המפרש: זה מבואר. 20

---

3 וסתימה (= وسدد): وسدر a   5 המפרש: الفؤاد فم المعدة والنخس اللذع add. a   7 שיריקנו:
שיריק בו טז   9 למעלה: ממעלה טז ‖ הנק' דיאפרמה: טז om. ‖ 11 הליחות: وتيقّنت هناك add. a
12 במשלשלת: ל om.   16–15 בעבור חמימות האצטומ' או יבשותה או: זט om.

(4.21)

[158] אמר בקראט: הצואה השחורה הדומה לדם הבאה מעצמה בין שתהיה עם קדחת
או בלא קדחת הוא מן הסימנים הרעים. וכל אשר המראים והיציאות יותר רעים יהיו אותם
הסימנים יותר רעים כי בהיות זה עם שתיית רפואה יהיו אותם סימן יותר טוב. וכל אשר יהיו
אותם המראים יותר הוא יותר רחוק מן הריעות.

(4.22)

[159] אמר בקראט: אי זה חולי שיצא בתחלתו המרה השחורה ממטה או ממעלה זה ממנו
סימן מורה על המיתה.

אמר המפרש: כל זמן היות החולי בהתחלתו אין שום דבר ממה שיצא חוץ מגוף החולה תהיה
יציאתו בתנועת הטבע אבל תהיה צאתו מקרה דבק לעניינים שבגוף יוצאים מהטבע והמרה
השחורה היא הליחה הגסה הדומה לשמרים כשתהיה שרופה ויצאה מהיות מרה שחורה
טבעית ויציאת אלו הליחות הרעות קודם הבישול יורה על נשיכתם לאיברים לחוזק ריעותם
ולא יוכלו האיברים לעצרם עד שיתבשלו.

(4.23)

[160] אמר בקראט: מי שהיה הולך ודל מחולי חם או ארוך או אשה מפלת או זולת זה ויצא
ממנו מרה שחורה או כמו דם שחור זה ימות ממחרת אותו היום.

אמר המפרש: הטבע במי שזה ענינו יהיה חלוש עד שלא יוכל לבשל ולא להבדיל ולא להריק
אלו הליחות אשר הם מן הרעות על מה שהיא עליה ולעוצם החולי ולהתרחבו ישתפך
כיון שאין דבר שיעצרנו. ואמרו או כמו דם השחור כלומר הצואה השחורה. וההפרש בין
המרה השחורה והיציאה השחורה כי המרה השחורה תהיה נתכת ועמה זריחה ונשיכה
דומה לנשיכת החומץ והאדמה תרתח ותתקלף כשיפול בה ואין מזה שום דבר ביציאה
השחורה.

(4.24)

[161] אמר בקראט: שלשול הדם בהיות התחלתו מן המרה השחורה זה סימן מות.

אמר המפרש: כשיתחיל יציאת הקולורא ותנגע המעיים ויביא הדם מכן אפשר שיתרפא
זה הפונטי. אבל אם תהיה זאת הליחה המלנקוניאה היא אשר עשתה הפונטי וגם נגעה המעיים
ואחר כן באה הדם על כל פנים יחדש במעיים דמיון הסרטן המתחדש בשטח העור.

---

2 המראים והיציאות: الألوان في البراز a ‖ 12 חם (= حارّ): حادّ a ‖ 13–14 זה ימות ממחרת אותו היום.
אמר המפרש: הטבע במי שזה ענינו יהיה חלוש: ט׳ z .om ‖ 15 ולהתרחבו: وفاقه a ‖ 17 נתכת: ניגרת
ל׳ ‖ 18 והאדמה תרתח ותתקלף: وقشر الأرض a ‖ ביציאה: بصياءة זט ‖ 21 ותנגע המעיים: فسحجت
الأمعاء أو قرّحته a ‖ 23 הדם: فلا يرء له .add a ‖ על כל פנים: لأنّ a

(4.25)

[162] אמר בקראט: יציאת הדם ממעלה על אי זה שיהיה הוא סימן רע וצאתו ממטה הוא סימן טוב כשיצא ממנו שום דבר שחור.

אמר המפרש: ירצה לומר ממעלה בקיא. אבל יהיה ממטה הוא טוב מאד כשתדחהו הטבע על דרך נקיון המותרות כמו שזה נהוג בטחורים ובתנאי שיהיה הדם מועט.

(4.26)

[163] אמר בקראט: מי שהיה בו שינוי דם ויצא ממנו דומה לחתיכות הבשר זה סימן מות. 5

אמר המפרש: כי זה ראיה על התאחז חבלת המעיים עד שתחתוך עצמותם ואי אפשר שיתדבק אותו הבשר.

(4.27)

[164] אמר בקראט: מי שיצא ממנו דם הרבה מאי זה מקום שיהיה הגרתו כי הוא בקחתו המזון יחליק בטנו ביותר מהשיעור.

אמר המפרש: מפני חולשת החום הטבעי בגופו מהרקת הדם ימעט משיכת האיברים למזון 10 ויחלש העיכול ויחליק הטבע.

(4.28)

[165] אמר בקראט: מי שיש לו שלשול מרות ואחזו חרשות יפסק ממנו אותו השינוי. ומי שיש לו חרשות ואחזו שלשול מרות סר ממנו אותו החרשות.

אמר המפרש: סבה זאת מבוארת בעבור הגרת החומר להפך הצד ומבואר הוא שהמאמר הוא בחרשות הקורה פתאום בחליים וכל שכן בסור הקרישיש. 15

(4.29)

[166] אמר בקראט: מי שאחזו בקדחת ביום הו׳ מחליו קרירות הנקרא ריגור האלבחראן שלו יהיה בצער.

אמר המפרש: כשיתחדש האלנפץ הוא ריגור בלע״ז בקדחת וכל שכן בשורפת ממנהגה שיבוא האלבחראן אחריו והנה נודע ריעות הבחראן הבא ביום השישי והוא ענין אמרו שיהיה בצער. 20

---

1 זה: ענין זט add. ‖ וצאתו: ובצאתו זט‏ 4 נקיון המותרות: הנקיון מהמותרות זט‏ 5 שינוי: נ״א דיסינטיריאה זיטי‏ 8 ממנו: في الحمّى‎ add. a‏ 9–8 בקחתו המזון: عندما ينقه فيغذى a (= הטבע‏ 11 a الطبع B): הבטן (= البطن a)‏ 14 סבה זאת: זט‏ 14 שהמאמר הוא: ל‏ .om 15–14 הסבה זט‏ 15 בסור (= مفارقة AB): مقاربة emendation editor‏ 18 האלנפץ: النافض a

(4.30)

[167] אמר בקראט: מי שהיו בקדחתו עונות באיזו שעה שיהיה עזבם לו כשיקחנו בבקר
באותה שעה בעצמה האלבחראן שלו יהיה קשה מאד.

אמר המפרש: מבואר הוא בהיות עונות הקדחת כלם באות על ענין אחד בתחלתם ובסופם
זה יורה על אורך החולי. והוא ענין אמרו בחראן שלו יהיה קשה כאילו הוא יאמר כי יקשה
שיכלו אלו הקדחות בחראן כי הבחראן אמנם יהיה לחליים החדים אבל החליים הארוכים
הם ניתכים באורך הזמן.

(4.31)

[168] אמר בקראט: בעל העייפות בקדחות ברוב יצאו צמחים בפרקיו ולצד הלחיים.

אמר המפרש: בעבור חמימות הקדחת וחמימות האיברים מבעל העייפות ידחה המותר אל
הפרקים ובעליון הגוף כי יקבלהו הבשר הרך אשר בפרקי הלחיים.

(4.32)

[169] אמר בקראט: מי שקם מחולי ונחלש ממנו מקום מגופו יתחדש לו באותו המקום צמח.

אמר המפרש: מבואר כי הנקי מחלייו אם טרח אבר מאיבריו ומצאו בו כאב הוא יצא לשם
צמח והסבה מבוארת. והנה זכר גאלנוס כי חידוש הכאב נקרא ביטול.

(4.33)

[170] אמר בקראט: ואם כמו כן הקדים והטריח אבר מן האיברים קודם שיחלה בעליו באותו
האבר יתאחז החולי.

אמר המפרש: זה מבואר זכר במקום זה הטורח שקדם לחולי עד שתהיה זאת הסבה לחולי
זכר בפרק אשר קודם הטורח אשר יהיה אחר היציאה מן החולי זכר בשלישי אשר קודם זה
הטורח אשר יהיה בעצם החולי ואמנם יפלו כמו אילו היציאות כלם בבחארין אשר אין בהם
הרקה נראית.

(4.34)

[171] אמר בקראט: מי שקרה לו קדחת ואין בגרונו נפיחה ויקרה לו חניקה פתאום זה יורה על
המות.

אמר המפרש: החנק הבא פתאום אמנם תהיה מפני סיתום הגרון והמוקדח יצטרך אל שאיפת
הרוח הקר המרובה וכשימנע האויר ימות בלא ספק. אבל התנאי הוא שלא תהיה שם נפח כי

---

1 בקדחתו: בקדחותיו ל   10 ונחלש: فكّ a   11 הנקי: الناقه a   12 ביטול: אلאل a   19 חניקה: לי
חניקת זט נפיחה ל   21 סיתום: עצירת לי עצירת סיתום זט

תוכל להיות הקדחת נמשך אחר מורסת הגרון ויהיה החנק בא מעט מעט לתוספת המורסא
ובעמידתה אפשר שיפחות כמו כן מעט מעט וינצל החולה.

(4.35)

[172] אמר בקראט: מי שאחזתו קדחת ונתעותה צווארו ויקשה עליו הבליעה עד שלא יוכל
לבלוע המזון ולא יהיה נראה בו נפח זה מסימני המות.

אמר המפרש: עוות העורף ועוצר הבליעה יהיה עם הסרת אחת מן החליות והסרתם תהיה   5
מפני מורסא ויהיה לתגבורת היובש. ואשר ירצה במקום זה הוא ההווה מתגבורת היובש כי
זה ראייה על התאחז רוע המזג באיברים ושליטת היובש.

(4.36)

[173] אמר בקראט: הזיעה משובחת במוקדחים אם תתחיל ביום השלישי או ביום החמישי
או בשביעי או בתשיעי או בי״א או בי״ד או בי״ז או בכ׳ או בכ״ד או בכ״ז או בל׳ או בל״ד או
בל״ז כי הזיעה אשר תהיה באלו הימים יהיה בו בחראן החליים אבל הזיעה שלא תהיה באלו   10
הימים יורה על חולי או על אורך מן החולי.

אמר המפרש: אין זה הדין בזיעה לבדה אבל בכל ההרקות אשר יהיה בהם הבחראן כי טבע
אלו הימים ידעתם בניסיון וכל בחראן שיהיה עם הזיעה או בזולתו מן ההרקות שהוא נמצא
בנסיון יהיה ברוב באלו הימים.

(4.37)

[174] אמר בקראט: הזיעה הקרה בהיותה עם קדחת חדה תורה על מות ובהיותה עם קדחת   15
ונחה תורה על אורך החולי.

אמר המפרש: חוזק הקדחת תכבה החמימות הטבעי ולא יתבשלו הליחות הקרות מאד אשר
בנגלה הגוף אשר מהם תצא הזיעה הקרה וסימן פגות אילו הליחות וחוזק קרירותם היות חום
הקדחת החזק לא תוכל לחמם מה שיצא ממנו.

(4.38)

[175] אמר בקראט: ובמקום שתהיה הזיעה מן הגוף יורה על שהחולי באותו המקום.   20

אמר המפרש: ועל כן תהיה הזיעה מאותו המקום לבדו אשר בו הליחה הנחבאה.

---

4 המזון: إلّا بكّ‎ a .add   9–10 או בל׳ או בל״ד או בל״ז: أو في الواحد والثلاثين أو في الرابع والثلاثين a
11 חולי: رعى لا آفة a   13 הימים: الباحوريّة‎ a .add   18 בנגלה: بشطح زט‎²   21 הנחבאה: المحتقن a

(4.39)

[176] אמר בקראט: אי זה מקום מן הגוף יהיה קר או חם באותו המקום יהיה החולי.

אמר המפרש: זה מבואר.

(4.40)

[177] אמר בקראט: ובהתחדש בגוף כלו שינוי ויהיה הגוף מתקרר פעם ואחר כן יתחמם פעם
אחרת או שישתנה מראיהו יורה על אורך החולי.

5   אמר המפרש: החולי שהוא ממינים הרבה הוא לעולם יותר ארוך מן החולי אשר הוא ממין
אחד.

(4.41)

[178] אמר בקראט: הזיעה המרובה אשר תהיה בשינה מבלתי סבה מבוארת יורה על שבעליו
יסבול על גופו מן המזון יותר ממה שיסבול. ואם יהיה זה והוא לא יקח המזון תדע כי גופו יצטרך
להריק.

10   אמר המפרש: זה מבואר.

(4.42)

[179] אמר בקראט: הזיעה המרובה אשר תגר תמיד חם או קר הקר ממנו יורה על שהחולי
יותר גדול והחם ממנו יורה על שהחולי יותר נקל.

אמר המפרש: יאמר שהזיעה אשר תהיה בשאר ימי החולי על דרך הבחראן מה שממנו יהיה
קר יהיה יותר רע כי הוא יורה על קרירות החומר.

(4.43)

15   [180] אמר בקראט: בהיות הקדחת בלתי נבדלת ואחרי כן תתחזק ותשוב קדחת שלישית
היא מיותר פחד. ואם תהיה נבדלת על איזה שיהיה תורה על שאין בה פחד.

אמר המפרש: זאת שהיא תמידית ותתחזק שלישית שהיא בעלת פחד היא מטריקוינו בערבי
שטר גב כלומ' חצייה קדחת שלישית.

(4.44)

[181] אמר בקראט: מי שמצאו קדחת ארוכה יקרה לו או צמחים או חולשה בפרקיו.

---

4 או שישתנה מראיהו: أو يتلوّن بلون ثمّ بغيره a   16 איזה: وجه add. a   17 תמידית: קונטינואה
זט² || מטריקוינו: מטריטיגו זט

אמר המפרש: או מרוב החומר או מקרירותו או מפני עובי הליחה והחומר אשר הוא עניינו
ברוב יהיה נדחה או לאבר אחד מן האיברים ויחדש צמח או למקום פנוי מהפרקים ויחדש
כאב הפרקים.

(4.45)

[182] אמר בקראט: מי שמצאו צמח או חולשה באברים אחר הקדחת יאכל מן המזון יותר
ממה שהוא סובל.

אמר המפרש: ירצה לומר אחר סור הקדחת בכלל והוא כבר נקיא.

(4.46)

[183] אמר בקראט: כשיקרה ריגור עם קדחת שאינו נבדל למי שכבר נחלש זה מסימני המות.

אמר המפרש: אמר גאלנוס שאמרו כשיקרה יורה על התמדת הריגור פעם אחר פעם כי
חידושו פעם אחר פעם. והקדחת נשאר בלתי נבדל יורה על היות הטבע תשתדל לנקות הליחה
המחליאה לא יוכל לעצרו באיברים ויוסיף הכח סער והתכה מפני היותו בלתי סובל רעות
הריגור והזדעזעה לגוף.

(4.47)

[184] אמר בקראט: בקדחת אשר לא תבדיל הרוק האדום והדומה לדם והמוסרח ואשר הוא
מסוג המרירות כלם רעות ואם פסק הפסק טוב הוא טוב. וכן העניין ביציאה ובשתן ואם יצא
מה שלא יועיל מאחד מאלו המקומות זה רע.

אמר המפרש: המאמר הכולל מן הדברים אשר יורקו יורו על עניינים רעים בגופות אשר יריקו
מהם אלא שהוא אפשר שיהיה יציאתם כיציאת המגל מן החבלות המתעפשות ולא יועיל לו
ביציאתם ואפשר שתהיה יציאתם כיציאת הטרי מחוצה יפתח יהיה בו נקיות טוב לאבר אשר
בו המחלה. והסימנים המורים עם שיציאת מה שיצא טוב הוא בישולו לבד וסבלנות הגוף
ליציאתו בנקלה וקלותו בו ועם זה טבע החולה ומאחריו העת ההווה מהשנה והמקום והשנים
וטבע החולה.

(4.48)

[185] אמר בקראט: בהיות בקדחת בלתי נבדלת נראה הגוף קר ותוכו יהיה שורף ויהיה עמו
צמא זה מסימני המות.

---

1 המפרש: طول الحمّى ‖ add. a (except for BP)‏ 4 צמח او: זט .om 6 כבר: بعد a ‖ נקיא: ناقه a
10-9 לנקות הליחה המחליאה: نفض الخلط المرض وإخراجه a 10 לעצרו באיברים: لِثبوته وتبقّيه في
الأعضاء a ‖ רעות (רדا P): رعدة a 12 הרוק: ל .om ‖ האדום: الكدم: رعدة a 13 פסק הפסק (= انقضت
انقضاء): اتفضت اتفاضا a 15 הדברים: الرديئة a add. a (except for BP) 16 המגל: الموغلا זט: המוגלא
17 מחוצה יפתח: من خراج ينفجر a 19 החולה: المرض a

אמר המפרש: אמר גאלנוס כי זה המקרה לא ימצא לעולם אלא בקצת הקדחות שאינם
נבדלות וסבתו אמר הוא שתתחדש מורסה חמה בקצת האיברים הפנימיים ויבואו הדם והרוח
אל האבר החולה מן הגוף כלו ועל כן יהיה שורף הפנימי שלגוף כלו והעור קר כמו שיקרה
בתחלת עונות הקדחת. זה מה שאומר גאלנוס וזהו הטעם שנותן בעניין זה והוא בלתי אמיתי
כי אם היה זה בהכרח היה זה המקרה ראוי בכל מורסה חמה מתחדשת באיברים הפנימיים   5
ואנו נראה תמיד בעלי חלי הצד וחלי הריאה וחולי הכבד עורותיהם חמה מאד כמו שהוא
תוך גופותם. ואשר נראה לי כי עלה זאת היא היות החמרים אשר בנראה הגוף עבה מאד
קרה מאד לא תוכל לאנוס אותו חמימות הליחה המעופשת המולידה לקדחת אשר נתעפש
בתוך הגוף. וכשנתלהב אותו הדבר המעופש ועלה החמימות נוכח שטח הגוף יבקש מאין יכול
לצאת ולהתנפש מצא מסך קר ימנע אותו החמימות מצאת אל שטח הגוף ותתהפך החמימות   10
שב בחזק גדול וישרוף תוך הגוף יותר ותתחזק הצמא ויקרה בחמימות באותו זמן כמו שיעשו
הנפחים בהזותם המים על הפחם היוקד מאד ויעשו זה כדי שיתחזק חמימות האש ויתך הברזל
וזהו טעם אמיתי וטבעי אין חולק בה.

(4.49)

[186] אמר בקראט: כשנתעותה השפה והעין או האף או המסך או שלא יראה החולה או לא
ישמע אי זה מאלו יהיה בקדחת תמידית והוא יהיה חלוש המות יהיה קרוב ממנו.   15

אמר המפרש: זה מבואר כי כשיהיו נראים אלו הסימנים עם חולשת הכח ויתקדם הקדחת
תדע שהיובש נתגבר על התחלת העצבים ועל כן יתחדש עיות וזולתו ממה שזכר.

(4.50)

[187] אמר בקראט: כשיתחדש בקדחת תמידית רוע הניפוש ובלבול בדעת זה מסימני המות.

אמר המפרש: זה מבואר כי החמימות התאחזו באיברים עד שהעצבים קבלו חולשה
המונעים לחזה והמסך ונתרועע הניפוש.   20

(4.51)

[188]

(4.52)

[189] אמר בקראט: הדמעות אשר תהיינה נגרות בקדחת או בזולתו מן החליים אם יהיה זה
עם רצון החולה אינו רחוק. ואם הוא מבלתי רצון הוא רע הרבה מאד.

---

1 אלא: ל‎ .om   3 שלגוף: טי‎ז‎² מן הגוף זט‎   9–10 יבקש מאין יכול לצאת ולהתנפש: تطلب منفسا
تتنفّس منه‎ a   10 מצאת: מצאתו זט‎   12 הפחם היוקד מאד: النار في الكور‎a ‖ חמימות האש: حرارة
باطن النار‎ a   14 המסך (= المجاب): الحجاب‎ a   17 ممה: מה ל‎   19 התאחזו: יתאחזו זט ‖ חולשה:
أيضا‎ .add   21 This aphorism is missing in all the Hebrew MSS   23 אינו רחוק: فليس ذلك بمنكر‎
add. ‖ הוא: יותר זטי‎ ‖ a

אמר המפרש: זה מבואר שהוא בעבור חולשת הכח המחזיק ואמרו הוא יותר רע יורה על
שגם הראשון הוא כמו כן רע כי רע אם בכה ברצון זה יורה על חולשת לבו ועל כן ימהר הפעלתו
למעשה הבכיה.

(4.53)

[190] אמר בקראט: מי שנתכסו שיניו מדבר ויסקוז הקדחת שלו חזקה.

אמר המפרש: אילו העניינים הויסקוז אמנם יתחדשו מחמימות חזק שעשה בלחיות   5
הפלואומטיקי עד שיבש אותם.

(4.54)

[191] אמר בקראט: מי שקרה לו בקדחת שורפת שעול יבש מרובה ואחר כן יעוררהו מעט
לא יוכל להיות לו צמא.

אמר המפרש: אמר גאלנוס: עכ״פ בשעול ואע״פ שלא ירוקק שום דבר ילחלח קנה ריאתו
במה שיהיה נמשך לה בזמן השעול ועל כן לא יצמא.   10

(4.55)

[192] אמר בקראט: כל קדחת שתהיה עם מורסת הבשר הרך אשר באינגוינלי ודומיהם היא
רעה אלא אם תהיה קדחת יום.

אמר המפרש: בהיות סבת הקדחת מורסא האנגינאליה ודומהו מן הבשר הרך תהיה קדחת
יום. אבל בהיות לקדחת סבה אחרת ונתחבר עמו כלומר האינגינליה הוא סבת התמרסם
האינגינאליה יהיה אז זה נמשך אחר צמיחת אחד מהדקים וזאת המורסה הפנימית היא סבת   15
הקדחת המתקדמת ועל כן היא בעלת פחד.

(4.56)

[193] אמר בקראט: בהיות באדם קדחת ואחזתו זיעה והקדחת לא תפסק זה סימן רע כי הוא
יורה על אורך החולי ויורה על לחות מרובה.

אמר המפרש: זה מבואר.

(4.57)

[194] אמר בקראט: מי שקרה לו קיוץ או המשכה בלע׳ טומור ואחרי כן אחזתו קדחת חליו   20
יהיה נתך ויסור.

_____

1 המחזיק: העוצר לי‎   8 לא יוכל להיות לו צמא: لا يكاد يعطش a   14 ונתחבר עמו כלומר האינגינליה
הוא סבת: واقترن معها ورم الخالبين ونحوه فهي رديئة لأنّ سبب a ‖ כלומר: מורסת זט‎ add. ‖ הוא: זט‎
om.   15 מהדקים: الأحشاء a   17 כי: לו ז‎

אמר המפרש: הקיווץ שלשה מינים: אשר מאחור והקיווץ שהוא מפנים והטומור ולא תראה
שהאברים יתקווצו בו כי הם יתמשכו אל אחור ואל פנים המשכה שווה וכל מיני הקיווץ יהיה או
ממילוי האיברים העצביים או מהרקתם. אמנם אם יהיה נמשכת אחר הקיווץ קדחת שורפת
ראוי שתהיה מן היובש ומה שיהיה הקיווץ מתחדש יתחדש בתחילה ופתאום ראוי שיהיה מן
5   המילוי וכשיתחדש אחריו קדחת תתיך קצת מלחויות מותריות ובשלה קצת לחותיה.

(4.58)

[195] אמר בקראט: כשיהיה באדם קדחת שורפת וקרה לו הריגור הנק' בערבי אל נפיץ' בו
תתך קדחתו.

אמר המפרש: כשהקולורא תתנועע לצאת תחדש ריגור ויחדש קיא קוליריקו והתרת הבטן
למען שיצא אותו המותר המוליד לקדחת וכשינקו גידיו תתך קדחתו.

(4.59)

10   [196] אמר בקראט: הקדחת השלישית ברוב תהיה נתכת בשבעה עונות.

אמר המפרש: אמר גאלנוס: הנה מצאנו הבחראן ברביעית ומצאנוהו שהוא לפי מנין ההקפות
לא לפי מספר הֵ‍ימים. מזה שהז' בשלישית יבוא ביום השלשה עשר מתחלתה ובאותו היום
ברוב הימים יהיה בזמן החולי וכלותו מבלתי חכות בו הי''ד ומאמר בקראט במקום זה הוא
בשלישית הפשוטה.

(4.60)

15   [197] אמר בקראט: מי שמצאו בקדחת באזניו חרשות ונגר מנחיריו דם או הותר בטנו סר
חולייו מעליו.

אמר המפרש: הנה קדמה עלת ענין זה.

(4.61)

[198] אמר בקראט: אם לא תהיה סר הקדחת מהמוקדח ביום מימי האחדים מטבעה לשוב.

אמר המפרש: גאלנוס יאמר כי זה טעות סופר ובמאמר בקראט הוא ביום מימי הבחראן בין
20   שיהיה זה זוג או נפרד.

---

1 מינים: הן זט‏ .add   4 ומה שיהיה הקיווץ מתחדש יתחדש: وما كان من التشنّج يحدث a   5 לחותיה
‏(= رطوبتها‏P): برودتها a   8 ויחדש: ويتبعه a   10 בשבעה: בשלשה ל ‏|| עונות: הקפות לי‏   11 מצאנו:
رصدنا وتفقّدنا a ‏|| ברביעית: والغبّ‏ .add a   12 שהז': ולغבّ‏ .add. זט‏ ‏|| עונות זט‏ .add‏   ‏|| שהז' בשלישית:
‏السابع في الغبّ‏ a   13 הימים ‏(= الأيّام‏ BP): الأمر a ‏|| ויהיה בזמן ‏(בחראן‏ ט‏ .add): يكون بحران
المرض a   15 בקדחת: الحادّة‏ .add a

(4.62)

[199] אמר בקראט: כשיקרה האיקטריציאה בקדחת קודם יום ז' הוא סימן רע.

אמר המפרש: יקרה האיקטריציאה על דרך הבחראן ולא יהיה בחראן באיקטריציאה קודם יום השביעי אבל סבתו חלי מחליי הכבד ועל כן תהיה סימן רע.

(4.63)

[200] אמר בקראט: מי שמצאו בקדחתו ריגור בכל יום קדחתו תכלה בכל יום.

5 אמר המפרש: ירצה באמרו תכלה בכל יום שהקדחת תסור ממנו ותניחנו בכל יום בהרקת הליחה העושה לקרירות בתנועתה לצאת וכן העניין בשלישית ורביעית.

(4.64)

[201] אמר בקראט: כשיקרה לו האיקטריציאה בקדחת בז' או בט' או בי"ד זה טוב אלא אם יהיה הצד הימיני מתחת החלצים קשה ואם היה כן אין עניינו משובה.

אמר המפרש: סבת עניין זה מבואר ממה שקדם.

.

(4.65)

10 [202] אמר בקראט: בהיות בקדחת התלהבות חזק באצטו' ודפיקת לב ב(א)לפואד זה זה סימן רע.

אמר המפרש: אם ירצה לומר באלפואד פי האצטו' עניין אמרו דפיקה יהיה נשיכה בפי האצטומ' להסתבד בו הליחות הקוליריקי ואם ירצה לומ' שהאלפואד יהיה ימצאנו סינקופיץ שהוא דפיקת הלב להתאחז החמימות ממנו ושני אילו המקרים רעים מאד.

(4.66)

15 [203] אמר בקראט: הקווץ והכאבים הקורים בקרבים בקדחות החדות סימן רע.

אמר המפרש: הקדחת החזקה תיבש העצבים כמו האש ותמשכם ועל אילו הפנים יתחדש הקווץ הממית ואפשר שיקרה בגופות כמו כן כאב מזה העניין בעצמו כלומר מחוזק ההתלהבות והיובש.

(4.67)

[204] אמר בקראט: הפחד והקווץ הקורים בקדחת בעת השינה הוא מהסימנים הרעים.

אמר המפרש: בהיות הגוף מלא מליחות בזמן השינה יתמלא ראשו ויכבד המוח. ואם תהיה הליחה הגוברת נוטה אל המרה השחורה יקרה לו פחד ואם לא יהיה כן יקרה ממנו הכאב והקווץ. אמר גאלנוס שהוא ראה פעמים רבות בחליים ממיתים הפחד והכאב והקווץ יתחדש מהשינה וידמה זה שיהיה קורה בלכת הליחה המזיקה בזמן השינה למוח.

(4.68)

5   [205] אמר בקראט: בהיות האויר ישתנה ברוצו בגוף זה רע כי יורה על הקווץ.

אמר המפרש: ירצה לומ׳ באויר אויר הניפוש כשיעצרנו שום דבר בדרכיו עד שיהיה נחתך בעניין הכנסו או צאתו או בהם יחד.

(4.69)

[206] אמר בקראט: מי שיהיה שתנו עב דומה בדם ואין גופו נקי מקדחת כשישתין שתן מרובה ורקיקה יועילנו. ורוב מה שישתין זה השתן מי שישקע בשתנו מתחלת חליו או אחר מכן מעט
10   שמרים.

אמר המפרש: העניין ההולך ברוב במוקדחים הוא שיהיה בתחלת החולי מועט וכל אשר יתקרב הסוף יתעבה עצמותו. וספר אפוקרט בעניין זה הבא לפעמים רחוקים והוא שיהיה השתן דומה לדומן ומעט בתחילת החולי וסבת מיעוטו כי הוא לא יעבור אל הכליות אלא בטורח וכשהשורקה הליחה הרעה ונתבשלה מה שיהיה נשאר ממנו יריק מן השתן בזמן זה מה
15   שהוא יותר רקיק והרבה.

(4.70)

[207] אמר בקראט: מי שהשתין שתן עכור דומה לשתן הבהמות יש בו כאב ראש מיד או עתיד להתחדש בו.

אמר המפרש: אמנם יהיה השתן כך כשהחמימות יעשה בחומר ארוך ומרובה ומה שיהיה מן החמרים על זה התאר ביחוד כשתעשה בו החמימות היוצא יתיילדו ממנו הרוחות עד שיתעבו
20   כמו השעווה והזפת והרשינה היא הקלפוניאה. והרוחות העבים עם החמימות וימהר לעלות אל הראש ויעשה כאב הראש. ואפשר שיהיה עם העכור ואפשר שיהיה קודם ואפשר שיהיה אחריו.

(4.71)

[208] אמר בקראט: מי שיבואנו הבחראן ביום השביעי יתראה בשתנו ביום ד׳ ענן אדום ושאר הסימנים יהיו על זה ההקש.

_____

7 בהם: בשניהם זט (= a) فيما ‖ a   8 בדם: بالعبيط a يسيرا add. a   9 מה: מי זט   11 שיהיה: البول add.
a ‖ מועט: رقيقا a   14 וכשהשורקה: أكثر ذلك add. a   18 ארוך: غليظة a   21 ואפשר שיהיה עם
העכור: وترى الصداع ربّما كان مع البول المتثوّر a

אמר המפרש: היום הרביעי מורה על מה שעתיד להיות ביום השביעי וכל סימן בעל שיעור
יתראו בו שיורה על הבישול יורה שבחראן עתיד להיות בשביעי. אבל העמוד הלבן יותר ראוי
שיורה על זה ויותר ראוי ממנו הוא הענן הלבן הנתלה באמצע השתן. ובהיות החולה בעל
תנועה ממהרת יהיה שינוי המראה לבדו ושינוי העצמות הוראה מספקת על הבחראן שיהיה
ביום השביעי. ואמר גאלנוס כי בקראט זכר העמוד האדום אשר היא יותר חלושה למען הבין
עניין שאר הסימנים אשר הם יותר חזקים כי יורו על שהבחראן מוכן. וכן הסימנים אשר יהיו
נראים בימי ההראות ביציאה או ברקיקה על זה ההקש.

(4.72)

[209] אמר בקראט: בהיות השתן בהיר ולבן הוא רע וכל שכן בבעלי הקדחת אשר עם מורסת
המוח.

אמר המפרש: זה השתן בתכלית הרוחק מהבישול ויורה על אורך החולי ויורה עם זה כי תנועת
המרה האדומה למעלה נוכח הראש.

(4.73)

[210] אמר בקראט: מי שהיה בו במקומות אשר מתחת הצלעות רוחות גוברות ואחר כן
נתחדש בו כאב בסוף גבו למטה בטנו ישתלשל אלא אם ישולחו ממנו רוחות הרבה או ישתין
שתן מרובה וזה בקדחות.

אמר המפרש: כשהרוח יורד עם הלחות הראוי ונח והגיע למטה יפחות הנפח וירד אל מה
שסמוך למטה מהגב וימשך האברים אשר שם ויחדש הכאב. ואפשר רתחה אותה הלחות
בעורקים ויצאה השתן ויצאו הרוחות לבדם. ואפשר שיצאו יחד הרוח והלחות מן המעים
ויחליקו הבטן. ואפשר כי שניהם יעברו יחד אל העורקים ויעברו מהרה אל השלפוחית והלחות
והרוח. ובמי שיש בו קדחת ביחוד תהיה בוטח באלו הסימנים ותדע שהטבע חשב לדחות
הדבר המזיק ויוציאנו בשתן או בציאה.

(4.74)

[211] אמר בקראט: מי שיצא צמח באחד מפרקיו יוכל להנצל מאותו הצמח בשתן הרבה ועב
שישתין כמו שיתחיל ביום הד' במי שיש בו קדחת עם עייפות שאם יצא דם מנחיריו יסור חליו
בעבור זה מהרה.

אמר המפרש: זה מבואר.

---

2 העמוד: الغمامة a   3 החולה: المرض a   5 העמוד: الغمامة a   6 מוכן: مز مع a   7 ההראות:
ההראה ז ההראות ט الإنذار a   12 רוחות גוברות: عالية فيها قرقرة a   15 הראוי ונח: الموجبة للقراق
a ‖ יפחות הנפח וירד: يخطّ الانتفاخ a   16 רתחה: تأدّت a   19 בוטח: بتوخ זט   21 מי שיצא: من
يتوقع له أن يخرج به a ‖ ועב: أيضا a .add

(4.75)

[212] אמר בקראט: מי שהיה משתין דם וטרי זה יורה על שהחבלה בכליותיו או בשלפוחיתו.

אמר המפרש: זה מבואר.

(4.76)

[213] אמר בקראט: מי שהיה בשתנו חתיכות בשר קטנות או כמו השערות והשתן עב זה יוצא
מכליותיו.

אמר המפרש: אמנם חתיכות הבשר הקטנות הם מעצם הכליות ממש אבל מה שהוא כמו   5
השערות אי אפשר שיהיה לא מעצם הכליות ולא מעצם השלפוחית. ואמר גאלנוס שהוא ראה
מי שהשתין זה השיער והיה ארכו כמו חצי זרוע מפני שהם היו עושים מאכלים שהיו מולידים
ליחה גסה. וזאת הליחה העבה כשתתעשה בה החמימות עד שתשרפנה בכליות יתיילד ממנה
זה השיער. ורפואת זה החולי יורה על בריאות ההקש בסבתו כי אותם שקרה להם זה החולי
אמנם נתרפאו ברפואה המחתכת. אם כן מאמר כי זה יצא מכליותיו הודיענו מקום שזה השער   10
נולד בו.

(4.77)

[214] אמר בקראט: מי שיצא בשתנו והוא עב כמו סובין שלפוחיתו מלאה גרב.

(4.78)

[215] אמר בקראט: מי שהשתין דם מבלתי דבר קודם זה יורה על שגיד נסדק בכליותיו.

(4.79)

[216] אמר בקראט: מי שישתין דם עב והיו בו טיפות שתן עם כאב בתחתית בטנו ועצם ערותו
יורה כי יש כאב בסמוך לשלפוחיתו.   15

(4.80)

[217] אמר בקראט: מי שישקע בשתנו כמו החצץ החול נולד בשלפוחיתו.

אמר המפרש: זה כלו מבואר.

---

3 בשתנו: وهو غليظ add. a ‖ والشتن עב: om. a ‖ والشتن عب: 5 مה: מי ל 8 שתשרפנה: وتجفّفه add. a (except
for BP) 10 ברפואה המחתכת: بالأدوية الملطّفة المقطّعة a ‖ מאמר: أبقراط add. a 14–17 אמר
בקראט ... בשלפוחיתו: Aphorisms 4.79–80 feature the other way around in the Arabic and the
other Hebrew translations. 16 החצץ: الرمل a

(4.81)

‏[218] אמר בקראט: מי שהיה משתין דם וטרי וקליפות או שיהיה לשתנו ריח רע זה יורה על‏
‏שהחבלה בשלפוחיתו.‏

(4.82)

‏[219] אמר בקראט: מי שיצאה בתור בקצה האמה שלו כשתפתח יסור חליו.‏

(4.83)

‏[220] אמר בקראט: מי שישתין בלילה שתן הרבה יורה זה כי צאתו תמעט.‏

5   ‏אמר המפרש: זה מבואר. וכן שאר הפרקים מבוארים.‏

‏נשלם המאמר הרביעי מפרקי אבקרט.‏

‏3 שלו: ל .om ‖ כשתפתח (= انفتحت AC): تقيّحت وانفجرت a   6 מפרקי אבקרט: זט .om‏

המאמר החמישי

(5.1)

[221] אמר בקראט: הקווץ אשר יהיה בא מאכילת הליברוס הוא מסימני המות.

אמר המפרש: יקרה הקווץ משתיית הליברוס הלבן והוא המכוון במקום זה או לריבוי ההרקה
או לחוזק תנועת הקיא ומפני נשיכתו באצטומ׳ וזה תקשה רפואתו.

(5.2)

5   [222] אמר בקראט: הקווץ אשר יהיה מתחדש מצמח הוא מסימני המות.

אמר המפרש: זה אם יהיה לו מורסה ויעלה הכאב עד המוח וכל מה שאמ׳ אבקרט שהוא
מסימני המות ירצה לומר בו שהוא סכנה גדולה ושהוא ברוב ענין איבוד.

(5.3)

[223] אמר בקראט: כשיגר מן הגוף דם מרובה ויבוא לו שנגלוניצו או קיווץ זה סימן רע.

(5.4)

[224] אמר בקראט: כשיקרה הקווץ או השנגלנצו אחר הרקה מרובה הוא סימן רע.

10   אמר המפרש: כל זה מבואר.

(5.5)

[225] אמר בקראט: כשיקרה בשיכור השיתוק פתאום זה יתקווץ וימות אלא אם יתחדש בו
קדחת או שידבר מיד שיסור מעליו יינו.

אמר המפרש: זה הקווץ יקרה מפני מילוי העצבים ומטבע היין שימלא העצבים מהרה כי הוא
שוקע מפני דקדוקו וחומו. והיין כשיתרבה האדם ממנו בריבוי התלהבו יחדש בעצבים קווץ
15   אלא שהוא באיכותו ירפא ויתקן מה שיפסיד בעצבים אחר שיחממם ויבשם. וכשאינו יכול
לעשות זה יהיה ראוי בהכרח שישיג הקווץ המתחדש ממנו המות. ובכח אשר אמרנו כי היין
ירפא הקווץ ירפא כמו כן הקדחת והחולי הנק׳ כמאר הוא ההזק המתחדש בראש משתיית
היין.

---

2 מאכילת (من شرب A): من ‖ a   הליברוס: הלבן ל .add   6 מורסה: العصب   add. a (except for P)
8 רע: قال المفسر: هذا بين add. a   11 השיתוק: חולי השיתוק זט   14 התלהבו: جمه a   17 כמאר:
שכרות לז²טײ²

(5.6)

[226] אמר בקראט: מי שקרה לו ההמשכה הוא ימות בארבעה ימים ואם יעבור הד׳ ימים יתרפא.

אמר המפרש: ההמשכה הוא חולי מחודד אחר שהטבע לא יסבול המשכתו כי הוא מורכב מהקווץ אשר יהיה מאחור והקווץ אשר יהיה מלפנים כי סופו יהיה בתחלת ההקפה מהקפות
5 ימי הבחראן.

(5.7)

[227] אמר בקראט: מי שמצאו הוציאו הנק׳ בערבי אלצרע קודם צמוח השיער בבית הערוה יתחדש לו העתק. אבל מי שקרה לו ועברו עליו מן השנים כ״ה שנה ימות בו.

אמר המפרש: אמר גאלנוס: ירצה באמרו העתק סוף החולי וזה יהיה בתיקון הליחה הקרה הויסקוזה המולידה לויציאו והוא פליאומטיקו לח בהעתק השנים אל היובש ועם הטורח
10 וההנהגה המדקדקת עם הרפואה הנ!אותה. ובקראט זכר בזה הפרק השינוי אשר יהיה בעבור השנים וזמן צמיחת השיער בערוה בין כלות השבועים ובין כ״ה שנה.

(5.8)

[228] אמר בקראט: מי שקרה לו חולי הצד ולא ינקה בי״ד ימים ענינו יבא לידי מוגלא.

אמר המפרש: בקראט יקרא הרקת הליחה המולידה לחולי הצד עם הרקיקה נקיון.

(5.9)

[229] אמר בקראט: רוב מה שיהיה בו הטיציש הוא בשנים שהן בין י״ח שנים ובין ל״ה שנה.

15 אמר המפרש: הנה התקדם שהטיציש מחולי הבחרות ובזכור בקראט חליי החזה והריאה זכר זה כמו כן.

(5.10)

[230] אמר בקראט: מי שמצאתו החנק ונמלט ממנו ונטה המותר אל ריאתו זה ימות עד ו׳ ימים ואם עברם יבוא העניין לידי המוגלא.

אמר המפרש: בלא ספק שרבים נסו אלו החליים ודומיהם בזה הצד מן ההעתק ובאלו ודומיהם
20 ירצה לומ׳ בהם שהם ברוב.

---

1 ההמשכה: טֵיאטַאנו ז2ט9 3 מחודד: جدّا add. a ‖ יסבול: تعب add. a 10 המדקדקת: المجفّف a
17 עד ו׳: في سبعة a 19 שרבים נסו אלו החליים: أنّه كثرت له تجربة هذه الأمراض a ‖ ובאלו: ولا ريب أنّ هذا a

(5.11)

[231] אמר בקראט: בהיות בשום אדם הטיציש ויהיה מה שירקקנו עם השעול דבר מאוס בריחו כשיושם על הגחלים ויהיה שיער ראשו נמרט זה מסימני המות.

אמר המפרש: סרחון הריח יורה על הפסד הליחות וחזק עיפושם ומריטת שערות הראש ראיה על הפסד הלחות וכן יורה זה על העדר האברים למזון.

(5.12)

[232] אמר בקראט: מי שנפלו שערות ראשו מבעלי הטיציש ואחר כן נתחדש בו שלשול זה ימות.

אמר המרפש: שינוי אלו סימן על חולשת הכח זה יורה על מות קרוב.

(5.13)

[233] אמר בקראט: מי שרקק דם דומה לקצף אמנם הוא בא מריאתו.

אמר המפרש: מבואר הוא כי מי שירוקק דם קצפו הוא מעצם הריאה ממש.

(5.14)

[234] אמר בקראט: בעל הטיציש כשיתחדש בו שלשול יורה זה שהוא ימות מזה.

אמר המפרש: שלשול בעלי הטיציש יורה על המות ואם זה יהיה זה עם סרחון ריח ממה שהוא מרוקק וימרט ראשו יורה זה על שהמיתה קרובה כמו שקדם זה.

(5.15)

[235] אמר בקראט: מי שבא עניינו מבעלי חולי הצד עד המוגלא אם ינקה ממנו עד מ' יום מיום שהתחיל לרוקק חליו יבוא לקץ רפואה ואם לא ינקה לזה הזמן יבוא לידי טיציש.

אמר המפרש: אם לא יצא החומר אשר פתח והגיע בחלל החזה יתעפש ותתחדד ותנגע הריאה.

(5.16)

[236] אמר בקראט: החום יזיק למי שירבה לעשותו זה ההזק: ירפה הבשר ויפתח העצבים ויבלבל הדעת ויביא הגרת הדם והעילוף וישיג בעלי אלו המות.

אמר המפרש: יאמר כי מי שהרבה בעשיית הקדחת ירפה בשרו ויפתח העצבים כלומ' יחליקם וירפם בהתיך החמימות לעצמותם ויבלבל הדעת. אמר גאלנוס: ירצה לומר בו חולשת השכל ויסור כוחו בהתכת עצם העצבים ומבואר הוא שיהיה נמשך אחר הגרת הדם לעילוף ואחר העילוף תהיה המות.

(5.17)

[237] אמר בקראט: אמנם הקר יתחדש הקווץ וההמשכה והשחרות וריגור שיהיה עם הקדחת.

אמר המפרש: זה מבואר.

(5.18)

[238] אמר בקראט: הקור מזיק לעצמות ולשיניים ולעצבים ולמוח ולחוט השדרה אבל החם טוב להם מאד.

אמר המפרש: זה מבואר.

(5.19)

[239] אמר בקראט: כל מקום שנתקרר ראוי לחממו אלא אם יהיה פחד מהגרת הדם.

אמר המפרש: זה מבואר.

(5.20)

[240] אמר בקראט: הקר נושך החבלות ויקשה העור ויחדש מהכאב מה שלא היה לו קודם לכן ישחיר ויחדש הריגור שבא עם הקדחת והקיווץ וההמשכה.

אמר המפרש: זה מבואר.

(5.21)

[241] אמר בקראט: מי שיש בו המשכה מבלתי חבלה והוא נער ויפה בשר ובחצי הקייץ ישפוך מים קרים על גופו יעשה לו טובה אשר יחזיר חמימות מרובה אל תוך גופו ואפשר שינצל מחולייו באותו החמימות.

אמר המפרש: זה מבואר.

---

1 ויפתח (= وِيفتح): وِيفنخ a 3 לעילוף: الغَشي a = העילוף 13–14 קודם לכן: تقييح a 17 על גופו: كَثيرٍ a ‖ יעשה לו טובה אשר יחזיר חמימות مرובה אל תוך גופו: وأحدث فيه انعطاف من حرارة كثيرة

a

(5.22)

[242] אמר בקראט: החם מביא המוגלא אבל לא בכל מוגלא וזה כי רוב הסימנים מורים על
הבטחון והאמונה ויבשל המוגלא ויחליק העור ויפחות היזק הקרירות הנק׳ נאפץ והקיווץ
וההמשכה ויתיר הכבידות הקורה בראש והוא מן היותר נאות לשברון העצמות וכל שכן
לאצטומ׳ ולעצמות הראש ולכל מה שהמיתו הקרירות או חבל אותו ולחבלות המתפשטות
והמתאכלות ולפי הטבעת ולחבלות שברחם ולשלפוחית כי החמימות לבעלי אילו החליים
5 מועיל ומרפא והקור להם מזיק וממית.

אמר המפרש: המוגלא סימן טוב ומשובח בחבלות כי הוא מין מן הבישול כמו שידעת. ואין כל
חבלה בא לידי מוגלא כי כל החבלות הפרדולינט כלם או הקשים להתרפאות לא יתיל בהם
מוגלא. ושאר מה שזכר מבואר כי כל אבר בעל עצבים כמו כן יזיק להם הקרירות.

(5.23)

10 [243] אמר בקראט: אמנם הקר ראוי שיעשה באילו המקומות כלומר במקומות אשר ירוץ
בהם הדם. ואין ראוי לעשות במקום זה במקום עצמו אשר יהיה נגר אבל תעשהו סביבו ומן
המקום הבא. ויועיל הקר במורסות החדות והנושכות והנוטות אל האודם ולמראה הדם הלח
שאם יעשהו בדבר שכבר נתישן בו הדם ישחר אותו ובמורסא הנקרא רציפלא כל זמן שלא
נתחבלה כי אותה שכבר באה לידי חבלה יזיק הקר.

15 אמר המפרש: זה מבואר.

(5.24)

[244] אמר בקראט: כי הדברים הקרים כמו השלג והכפור יזיק לחזה מעוררים לשעול מושכין
להגרת הדם ולקטרא.

אמר המפרש: זה מבואר.

(5.25)

[245] אמר בקראט: המורסות אשר יהיו בפרקים והכאבים אשר יהיו מבלתי חבלה וכאבי
20 (בעלי) הפודגרא ובעלי ההפסד הבא במקומות העצביים ורוב מה שהוא דומה לזה כי כשיוצק
עליהם מים קרים והרבה יחממם ויכחידם וישקיט הכאב במה שיתחדש מן הביטול והביטול
כמו כן המעט ממנו משכך הכאב.

אמר המפרש: ישכך הכאב בכמו אלו המקומות בהפסיקו הסבה המולידה לו או בבטלו החוש.

---

2 ויבשל המוגלא: om. a ‖ העור: ويرقّقه ويسكّن الوجع add. a ‖ ויפחות היזק הקרירות: ويكسر عادية
النافض a 4 לאצטומ׳: المعرّى منها a 5 הטבעת: والفرج add. a 9–8 כי כל החבלות הפרדולינט
כלם או הקשים להתרפאות לא יתיל בהם מוגלא: טי ז om. a (except for
P) 11 הדם: أو هو مزمع بأن يجري منها a הבא: منه a add. a (except for P) ‖ החדות: الحارّة:
20 a ההפסד: الفسخ a 21 יחממם (= سخّنها) يحممها a ‖ ויכחידם: سكّنها a ‖ ويضمرها a

(5.26)

[246] אמר בקראט: והמים אשר יחממו הרבה ויתקררו הרבה אלו הם היותר קלים שבבמימות.

אמר המפרש: מבואר הוא שהוא ירצה במקום זה בכובד ובקלות מהירות צאתו מן האצטומ' או איחורו בה.

(5.27)

[247] אמר בקראט: מי שהביאתו תאותו לשתות בלילה ויהיה צמאו חזק זה אם יישן אחר זה הוא טוב.

אמר המפרש: כשיישן אחר שתות המים יבשל השינה הליחה המביאה לשינה ולא תורה על שתייתו בלילה אלא מחוזק הצמא.

(5.28)

[248] אמר בקראט: המשיחה עם הבשמים ימשוך דם הבא מן הנשים ויועיל במקומות אחרים הרבה אלא שהוא יחדש בראש כובד.

אמר המפרש: יאמר כי המריחה עם הבשמים ישלחו דם הווסת או יתירו ההריון כשתמנע כי זה ירקק הדם אם הוא עב או שיפתח סיתומה אם היא לשם או שירחיב פיות העורקים אם נאספו. ויועילו כמו כן לחמם המקומות הקרים או ליבש הלחות אלא שהם ממלאים הראש כי כל דבר חם יעלה למעלה ויכאיב הראש.

(5.29)

[249] אמר בקראט: ראוי שתשקה הרפואה להרות כשיהיו הליחות בגופן נעורות מאחר עבור על העובר ד' חדשים ועד הגיעה לז' חדשים ויהיה ההקדם על זה פחות. אבל מה שהיה פחות מזה או יותר גדול ממנו ראוי להזהר עליו.

אמר המפרש: זה הפרק אפשר שנכפל עליו שלא מדעתו או ששנהו בכוונה להדביק המאמר בחליי הנשים.

(5.30)

[250] אמר בקראט: האשה ההרה אם תקיז דם תהיה מפלת וכל שכן אם יהיה הוולד גדול.

אמר המפרש: זה מבואר.

---

1 הרבה: سريعا a ‖ הרבה: سريعا a   6 לשינה: לצמא זⁿ²ט² = للعطش a   8 הבשמים: לⁱ התבלין ל
10 יתירו ההריון: دم النفاس a   12 נאספו: انضمّت a   15 פחות: קטון לⁱ מעט זט²

(5.31)

[251] אמר בקראט: אם תהיה האשה הרה וקרה לה קצת מן החליים החדים זה מסימני המות.

אמר המפרש: אם יהיה מן החליים החדים אשר עמהם קדחת ימיתו ברוע המזג הצריך לשאוף אויר מרובה והאיברים דחוקים ובמיעוט המזון. ואם יהיה כמו הפלג והקוץ והאשה ההרה אינה סובלת חוזק הכאב או ההמשכה בעבור שהיא סובלת הכובד.

(5.32)

5 [252] אמר בקראט: האשה כשתקיא דם והווסת שלה יבוא עליה יפסק הקיא.

אמר המפרש: זה מבואר.

(5.33)

[253] אמר בקראט: כשיפסק הווסת בהגרת הדם מהאף זה טוב.

אמר המפרש: זה מבואר.

(5.34)

[254] אמר בקראט: האשה ההרה כשבטנה יהיה משלשל אינה בטוחה מהיותה מפלת.

10 אמר המפרש: כשהכח הדוחה תתנועע באותם האיברים השכנים לרחם בכח יש לפחד גם כן שמא תתנועע כח הרחם הדוחה.

(5.35)

[255] אמר בקראט: כשתהיה ברחם חולי או שתעצור האשה מלדת וימצאנה עיטוש זה הוא טוב.

אמר המפרש: ירצה לומר בחולי הרחם חניקת הרחם והעיטוש יורה על הערת הטבע שיפעל 15 פעולתו והוא כמו כן סבה לנקות האיברים ממה שדבק בהם ונשתבד מן הליחות המזיקות ובזה הצד ינקה העיטוש השוונגלוצו.

(5.36)

[256] אמר בקראט: בהיות וסת האשה משתנה במראהו ולא יהיה בא בזמנו תמיד יורה זה על שגופה תצטרך לנקות.

אמר המפרש: זה מבואר.

7 בהגרת הדם מהאף: فالرعاف a   11 הרחם הדוחה: **זט** inv.

(5.37)

[257] אמר בקראט: בהיות האשה הרה ושדיה יהיו נסתרות פתאום זאת תהיה מפלת.

אמר המפרש: הנה נודעה שתוף השדיים לרחם וכשנסתרו יורה זה על מיעוט משיכתם למזון הבא אליהם ובהתמעט המזון המגיע לרחם כמו כן תפיל האשה העובר.

(5.38)

[258] אמר בקראט: בהיות האשה הרה ואחת משדיה החבאו ונסתרו ותהיה הרה תאומים היא תפיל אחד מעובריה. ואם השד הימני יהיה נסתר תפיל הזכר ואם השמאלי תפיל העובר הנקבה.

5

אמר המפרש: והזכר בצד הימני ברוב.

(5.39)

[259] אמר בקראט: בהיות האשה בלתי הרה ולא ילדה ותהיה לה חלב יסתלק וסתה.

אמר המפרש: בעיתים רחוקות בהעצר וסת האשה יתמלאו העורקים הדבקים בשדיים מילוי יתר ויתחדש החלב בעבור ריבוי הדם המגיע אל השדיים. ונראה לי שזה לא יהיה אמת אלא אם יהיה גוף האשה בתכלית הנקיון ויהיה מזונה בתכלית היושר.

10

(5.40)

[260] אמר בקראט: אם נקפא הדם בשדיה יורה זה מעניינה על שטות.

אמר המפרש: היותר קרוב אצלי שאבקראט ראה זה העניין פעם או פעמיים והתיר הפסק דין כמנהגו בספרו ספר איפידימיאה.

וזכר גאלנוס שהוא לא ראה זה והוא האמת כלומר שאין זה סבה מן סבות השטות בשום פנים. אבל קרה זה במקרה פעם או פעמיים וראהו בקראט וחשבו סבה.

15

(5.41)

[261] אמר בקראט: אם תרצה לדעת אם האשה הרה או אינה הרה תשקנה כשתרצה לישן מי הדבש ואם מצאה עקיצה בבטנה היא הרה ואם לא מצאה עקיצה אינה הרה.

אמר המפרש: ירצה לומר באמרו כשתרצה לישן בזמן המנוחה ומילוי מהמזון ומי הדבש הוא יוליד רוחות ויעזרנו על זה מילוי הבטן וכשהרוחות לא ימצא דרך לצאת מפני דוחק הרחם יחדש עקיצה.

20

---

1 נסתרות: فضمر a   2 וכשנסתרו: فإذا ضمرتا a ‖ מיעוט משיכתם למזון: قلّة الغذاء a   4 החבאו
ונסתרו: فضمر a   5 נסתר: الضامر a   13 והתיר הפסק דין: فأطلق القضيّة a   14 בספרו ספר: בספר
זט   20 הרחם: لطريق تلك الرياح add. a

(5.42)

[262] אמר בקראט: בהיות האשה הרה מזכר יהיה מראה יפה ובהיותה הרה מנקבה יהיה מראה פלידו.

אמר המפרש: כל זה מבואר והוא הולך אחר הרוב.

(5.43)

[263] אמר בקראט: כשתתחדש באשה ההרה המורסה הנקראת ריציפלא ברחמה זה מסימני 5 המות.

אמר המפרש: נראה לי מדברי גאלנוס שהוא ירצה לומר מות הוולד וכן שאר המורסות החמות.

(5.44)

[264] אמר בקראט: כשהאשה תהיה הרה והיא מן הכחש והרזון על עניין יוצא מן הטבע היא תהיה מפלת קודם שתשמין.

אמר המפרש: יאמר שהיא כשתהיה הרה והיא בתכלית מן הרזון המזון המגיע לאיברים יקחו 10 אותו האברים בכלל ולא יוותר ממנו שום דבר שיתפרנס העובר כשיגדל ועל כן תפיל קודם שתגיע לגבול השומן לא להיותה שבה לטבעה בהשמין גופה.

(5.45)

[265] אמר בקראט: בהיות האשה וגופה ממוצע ותפיל בחודש השיני והשלישי מבלתי סבה מבוארת תחתית רחמה מלא ליחות כמו מותרי האף ולא יוכל להחזיק על הוולד אבל יהיה נכאה מהן. 15

אמר המפרש: זה מבואר.

(5.46)

[266] אמר בקראט: בהיות האשה על עניין השומן עד שהוא דבר יוצא מהטבע לא תהר כי הקרום הפנימי מקרוס(י) הבטן אשר נקרא החלב המכסה ידחק פי הרחם ולא תוכל להרות עד שתשוב כחושה.

אמר המפרש: יש לרחם צואר ארוך וקצה אותו הצואר הוא הסמוך לערוה ובתוכו יגיע קצה 20 האמה ונקרא פי צואר הרחם ונקרא פי הרחם. והנקרא פי הרחם באמת הוא התחלת הצואר ממה שהוא סמוך לרחם והוא אשר ידחקנו החלב המכסה מהאשה השמנה מאד.

---

14 הוולד: لِفْقله add. a   15 נכאה: זʾטʾי נדחה זט يَنهَك a   20 וקצה: emendation editor וקצר(?) ט
וקצת זל   21–20 קצה האמה: emendation editor קצת האמה زטל الإحليل a

(5.47)

[267] אמר בקראט: כשהרחם יהיה נחבל ומוגלא יהיה בה במקום תחת הירך יהיה ראוי
בהכרח שתצטרך אל פתילה.

אמר המפרש: כלומר שהיא צריכה למאלכת היד ולהכניס הפתילות וכשיבוא לידי טרי מה
שסמוך ממנו לחוץ אז יצטרך אל פתילות.

(5.48)

5   [268] אמר בקראט: מה שיהיה מן העוברים זכר הראוי הוא שיהיה תולדתו בצד הימני ומה
שהוא נקבה תהיה בשמאל.

אמר המפרש: זה מבואר כי הצד הימני הוא יותר חם. וזכר גאלנוס כי הזרע הבא מן האשה מן
הצד הימני מאחת מביציה שבו עובי וחמימות ואשר יבוא מן הצד השמאלי רקיק מימיי ויותר
קר מהאחר. וזה תימה אם בא לו מזה כעין נבואה או הביאו לזה ההקש. ואם דקדק זה בהקש
10   זה הקש זר.

(5.49)

[269] אמר בקראט: אם תרצה להפיל השליה תכניס באף רפואה מעטשת ותחזיק הנחירים
והפה.

אמר המפרש: כי יחדש בבטן המשכה ויתרות ויעזור על השליה שתהיה נופלת.

(5.50)

[270] אמר בקראט: כשתרצה לעצור וסת האשה תשים בכל אחת ואחת משדיה כוס גדול
15   בין הרחם והשדיים.

אמר המפרש: זה מבואר כי הוא ימשוך להפך הצד.

(5.51)

[271] אמר בקראט: פי הרחם מן האשה ההרה יהיה סתום ומקובץ.

אמר המפרש: זה מבואר.

1 יהיה נחבל ומוגלא יהיה בה: تقيّح a   2 פתילה (= الفتل A): العمل a   9 דקדק זה בהקש: حدّد وحرّر
هذا التحرير بقياس a   11 ותחזיק: وتسهم לⁱ ותסתור זט   13 נופלת: אמר בקראט: האשה ההרה אם
יבוא לה טינזמן תפיל זטⁱ .add   14 משדיה: ר״ל תחתיהם זⁱט² .add   15 בין הרחם והשדיים: a .om
17 בקראט: כי ל .add

(5.52)

[272] אמר בקראט: בהיות החלב יוצא משדי האשה ההרה יורה זה על חולשה מהעובר. ובהיות שני השדיים אוספים חלביהן יורה שהעובר הוא בריא.

אמר המפרש: אמנם יגר וירוץ מן ההרות החלב מפני מילוי העורקים אשר בין הרחם והשדיים בהיותו הרבה אבל יתרבה שם מציאות הדם כשיהיה העובר מתפרנס מעט ולא יהיה מושך מזונו מאותם הגידים אלא מעט דבר.

(5.53)

[273] אמר בקראט: כשהאשה עתידה להפיל שני שדיה יכחשו. ואם היה העניין הפך זה כלומר אם יהיו שדיה קשים ימצאנה הכאב בשתי שדיה או בירכיה או בשתי העינים או בארכובותיה לא תפיל.

אמר המפרש: כחש השדיים יורה על מיעוט הדם כמו שזכר ועביו הוראה על שווי שעורו וקשייו הוראה על ריבוי דם ועוביו. וכן אפשר שידחה הטבע אותו המותר הנוסף לאבר אחר קרוב מן הרחם או מן השד ויחדש באותו האבר כאב. ובכלל כי אלו הסימנים בלתי אמיתיים ולא הולכים אפילו אחר הרוב. וכל אילו הפרקים ודומיהן לפי דעתי הם נמשכים אחר מה שראה בקראט פעם או פעמים כי הוא היה מתחיל המלאכה.

(5.54)

[274] אמר בקראט: בהיות פי הרחם קשה ראוי בהכרח שיהיה מקובץ.

אמר המפרש: זה מבואר.

(5.55)

[275] אמר בקראט: כשתקרה הקדחת לאשה הרה ונתחממה חימום חזק מבלתי סבה נגלית הוולד שלה יהיה קשה ויש לפחד עליו.

אמר המפרש: יצטרך בקלות הלידות שיהיו שני הגופות חזקים גוף האם וגוף העובר.

(5.56)

[276] אמר בקראט: כשיתחדש אחר הגרת הווסת קווץ והעילוף זה הוא רע.

אמר המפרש: זה מבואר.

---

2 אוספים חלביהן: مكتنزين a ‖ בריא: أصحّ a   9 שזכר: واكتنازهما دليل على اعتدال مقداره وصلاحيتهما   10–9 ועביו הוראה על שווי שעורו וקשייו הוראה על ריבוי דם ועוביו: -emen دليل على كثرة الدم add. a   dation editor   ועביו וכן אפשר שידחה הטבע שעורו וקשייו הוראה על ריבוי דם ועוביו זטל   10 וכן: ولذلك a   17 הוולד: ولادها a   19 הווסת: השתן ל ‖ והעילוף: העילוף ל

(5.57)

[277] אמר בקראט: בהיות הווסת יותר מן הראוי יקרה מזה חליים וכשלא ירד הווסת יתחדשו מזה חליים בעבור הרחם.

אמר המפרש: זה מבואר.

(5.58)

[278] אמר בקראט: כשיקרה בקצה פי הטבעת או ברחם מורסה יהיה נמשך אחר זה הטפת השתן וכן אם באו הכליות לידי מוגלה יהיה נמשך אחר זה הטפת השתן וכשיתחדש בכבד
5 מורסא יהיה נמשך אחר זה שנגלוצו.

אמר המפרש: הטפת השתן יהיה בעבור חולשת כח השלפוחית העוצר או בעבור חידוד השתן. וחולשת הכח בעבור רוע המזג או בעבור מורסה מתחדשת שם וחידוד השתן מפני שיתערב בו מן הליחה הנושכת. וכשתהיה מורסא באחת משתי אלו האיברים זה יזיק
10 לשלפוחית עם השכנות ויחלש כחה ובהיות חולי בכליות יחדש נשיכה בשתן. ולא תהיה נמשכת אחר מורסת הכבד שנגלוצו אלא אם תהיה גדולה.

(5.59)

[279] אמר בקראט: בהיות האשה בלתי הרה ותרצה לדעת אם רחמה נעצר מהריון או אינו נעצר תכסה אותה עם בגדים ואחרי כן תעשן תחתיה אם תראה כי ריח העישון יעבור בגופה עד שיגיע אל נחיריה ובה תדע כי אין ההמנע מסיבתה.

15 אמר המפרש: העישונים יהיו בדברים שיהיה להם חידוד כמו האוליבנום והמירא והאשטורג׳.

(5.60)

[280] אמר בקראט: בהיות האשה הרה ווסתה נגרת בעתה אי אפשר שיהיה העובר בריא.

אמר המפרש: אמר גאלנוס: ידמה שיהיה הווסת הניגר מן ההרות מן הגידים אשר בצואר הרחם כי השליה תלוייה בפיות כל העורקים אשר בתוך הרחם ואי אפשר שיצא שום דבר
20 לפנוי שלרחם.

---

4 בקצה פי הטבעת: في طرف الدبر a   5 וכן אם באו הכליות לידי מוגלה יהיה נמשך אחר זה הטפת השתן: טל²ו¹   8 בעבור: רוע זט .add   12 מהריון: להריון זט   13–12 או אינו נעצר: אם לאו זט 14 ובה: وفيها = a ‖ ופיה   כי אין ההמנע מסיבתה: أنّه لیس سبب تعذّر الحبل من قِبلها a   15 בדברים: طِيّبة الرائحة a .add

(5.61)

[281] אמר בקראט: כשלא יבוא וסת האשה בזמנו ולא יתחדש בה פלצות ולא קדחת אבל
יקרה לה סער ועילוף ורוע נפש תדע שהיא הרה.

אמר המפרש: זה מבואר.

(5.62)

[282] אמר בקראט: בהיות רחם האשה קרה וקשה לא תהר וכשיהיה כמו כן לח לא תהר כי
לחותה תקפיא הזרע ויכבנו. וכשיהיה כמו כן יבש יותר מן הראוי או שיהיה חם שורף לא תהר
כי הזרע יעדיר המזון ויפסד. ובהיות מזג הרחם ממוצע בין שני העניינים תהיה האשה מתרבה
בהריון.

אמר המפרש: זה מבואר.

(5.63)

[283]

(5.64)

[284] אמר בקראט: החלב לבעלי הכאב של הראש רע והוא כמו כן למוקדחין רע ולמי שיהיו   10
המקומות אשר תחת הצלעות ממנו עלוי ובהם רוחות ולמי שבו צמא ולמי שיגבר על הציאה
שלו המרות ולמי שיש לו קדחת חדה ולמי שנשתלשל דם מרובה. ויועיל לבעלי הטיציש כל
זמן שלא יהיה בהם קדחת חזקה מאד ולבעלי הקדחת הארוכה החלושה כל זמן שלא יהיה
עמה שום דבר ממה שקדמנו להגידו ויהיה גופם ניתך יותר ממה שראוי לפי החולי.

אמר המפרש: החלב הוא מן המזון אשר ימהר אליו השינוי. אמנם באצטומ׳ אשר הוא יותר   15
מחמם ישתנה אל העשן אבל אשר יתעכל לפי מה שראוי יוליד מזון מרובה וטוב אלא שבעת
העיכול יחדש נפיחה בתחת הצלעות ויחדש כאב בראש זה פעולתו בבריאים אבל בחולים
כמו שזכר.

(5.65)

[285] אמר בקראט: מי שנתחדשה בו חבלה ומצאו בסבתה ניפוח לא יוכל לאחוז בו קווץ ולא
שטות. ואם נסתרה אותה הנפיחה פתאום ואחרי כן תהיה התבלה מאחוריו יקרה לו הקווץ   20
או ההמשכה. ואם תהיה החבלה מבפנים יקרה לו שטות או כאב חד או תעשה מוגלא או
שלשול דם אם יהיה אותו השלשול אדום.

---

2 ועילוף (= وغشي P): وغشي a   5 לחותה: تغمر add. a   6 יעדיר: ז²ט² יעביר זט   This aphorism 9
מشرفة a   15 מן: ל .om   ‖ הוא: أبرد فيحمض وإمّا في المعدة التي هي add. a   19 חבלה: מבפנים ז מפנים
is missing in the Arabic and Hebrew translations   10 והוא כמו כן למוקדחין רע: עלוי   11 .om ל:
ז²ט²   20 הקווץ: שפזגנ ז²ט²   21 ההמשכה: טיטנו ז² טיטאנו ט²   ‖ חד: חם ל   ‖ מוגלא: אימפימא
ז²ט²   22 שלשול דם: דיסנטיריאה ז²ט²   ‖ השלשול: الاستفاخ a

אמר המפרש: איני צריך להכפיל שזה הפסק דין אשר יאמר אותו בקראט קצתם הולכים אחר הרוב או על השווי ולפי האמת ימצאו קצת מפסקיו הולכים אחר המיעוט. ואפשר שראה אותו פעם אחת וייחס זה לסבה שאין זה סבתה באמת.

זה הפרק לפי דעת גאלנוס שהוא ירצה לומ' בניפוח המורסה וכל עובי יוצא מן הטבע. ומה שהוא מן הגוף מאחריו הוא עצביי ומה שהוא מפנים הגובר בו הוא הגידים הדופקים. וכשתעלה הליחה המביאה למורסה מן העצבים למות יהיה הקווץ ואם יעלה בגידים אל המוח יהיה השטות ואם יגיע זאת הליחה אל החזה תוליד הכאב בצד. והרבה פעמים ימצא בעל חולי הצד המוגלא.

(5.66)

[286] אמר בקראט: כשיתחדשו צמחים גדולים ורעים ואחרי כן לא יתראה בהם שום מורסה הרעה היא גדולה מאד.

אמר המפרש: ירצה לומר בצמחים הרעים בלע"ז פררולינ"ט אותם שיולדו בקצה המושקולו או בסופו או מה שיהיה מן המושקולו הגובר עליו העצבים. וכשלא תתחדש מורסה במי שזה עניינו בצמחים לא יהיה בטוח מהיות הליחות המורקות אל הצמחים שיהיו נעתקות מהם אל מקום יותר מעולה.

(5.67)

[287] אמר בקראט: הלחות הרכות טובות והניות רעות.

אמר המפרש: יאמר גאלנוס שהוא ירצה לומר באמרו הנא הקשה הדופק שהוא הפך הרך כי כל דבר קשה ליחתו בלתי מבושלת.

(5.68)

[288] אמר בקראט: מי שמצאו כאב באחורי ראשו וחתך לו בגיד העומד אשר במצחו יועילינו חיתוכו.

אמר המפרש: המשיכה אל הפך הצד הוא מן המאוחר אל המוקדם ומן המוקדם אל המאוחר.

(5.69)

[289] אמר בקראט: הקרירות הנק' ריגור ברוב מתחיל בנשים ממטה לגב ואחר כן יעלה בנראה אל הראש. והוא כמו כן באנשים יתחיל מאחור יותר משהוא מתחיל

---

2 מפסקיו: מפרקיו זט 5 מפנים: בפנים זט 14 מעולה: من مواضع الجراحات add. a 16 הנא: הוא ל || הדופק: المدافع a 18 העומד: הזקוף זטיל' 23 בנראה (= في الظاهر a): في الظهر a || משהוא: מה שהוא ל

מפנים כמו שיתחיל משתי הזרועות והירכים. זה כי העור במקדים הגוף מתרפה ויורה על
זה השער.

אמר המפרש: הקרירות ימהר לבוא בגב מפני היותו קר מרוב העצמות שיש שם ומיעוט הבשר
והנשים יותר קרות מן האנשים והורה זה על שאחורי הראש הוא יותר רפה מפני ששם יצמח
5   השיער יותר.

(5.70)

[290] אמר בקראט: מי שקרה לו קדחת רביעית לא יוכל לקרות לו הקווץ. ואם יקרה הקווץ
קודם הקדחת הרביעית ואחר כן נתחדשה הקדחת הרביעית ישכך הקווץ.

אמר המפרש: פירש גאלנוס שהוא אמר שזה המין מן הקווץ הוא ההווה מן המילוי ורפואתו
תהיה בנקיון הליחה היוצאה או יבשלנה ובקדחת רביעית תצא בחוזק הריגור ויתבשל
10   בחמימות הקדחת.

(5.71)

[291] אמר בקראט: מי שהיה עורו מתמשך וקשה זה ימות מבלתי זיעה ומי שהיה עורו רך
ורפה זה ימות עם זיעה.

אמר המפרש: ירצה לומ׳ על מי שהוא נטוי למות והיה עניינו כמו זה.

(5.72)

[292] אמר בקראט: מי שהיה בו ירקון בלע״ז איקטיריציאה אי אפשר שיתילדו בו הרוחות.

15   אמר המפרש: מסבות תולדת הרוחות הוא מציאות הליחה הלבנה אשר במקום תולדתה זה
לא יהיה עם הירקון מרוב תגבורת המרות.

נשלם המאמר החמישי מפרקי אבקרט.

---

1 העור: أيضا‏ add. a   4 שאחורי הראש: المقدّم a   9 היוצאה (= الخارج AP): الخارج ‖ יבשלנה:
بنضجه a   11 מתמשך: قلا‏ add. a   13 נטוי למות: أشرف على الموت ‖ עניינו: جلده a   17 מפרקי
אבקרט: זט‏ om.

המאמר השישי

(6.1)

[293] אמר בקראט: כשיתחדש הרוטו החמוץ בחולי אשר יאמר לו המעדת המעים אחר האריכו ולא היה קודם לכן הוא סימן טוב.

אמר המפרש: בהיות חולי המעדת המעים בעבור חולשת הכח העוצר ויצא קודם שיתעכל ואחרי כן נתחדש הרוטו החמוץ זה ראיה על שהמזון ישאר באצטומ׳ מזמן שאפשר שיתחיל הכח לשנותו אחר שנות שיעור מה שיחמיץ ושהטבע התחיל לשוב לפעולותיו.

(6.2)

[294] אמר בקראט: מי שהיה בחוטמו בטבע לחות עודף והזרע שלו יהיה יותר רקיק בריאותו יותר קרובה אל הדלדול. ומי שיהיה בו העניין הפך זה הוא בריא בגופו.

אמר המפרש: אלו הם דברים מורים על לחות המוח ויובש שאר האיברים ועל כן יהיה הזרע שלו רקיק.

(6.3)

[295] אמר בקראט: ההמנע מן המזון בהגרת הדם שזמנו ארוך הוא סימן רע והוא עם הקדחת יותר רע.

אמר המפרש: שינוי הדם בהיותו עם שלשול המעיים הנק׳ סחג׳ פונט ויאריך יוסיף לחפור בעומק האיברים וישוב נגע בעל עיפוש והכאב באצטומ׳ עם השיתוף ויקח בה ההזק. ובעלות החולי לפי האצטומ׳ תסור תאוות המזון ממנה ויהיה זה ראייה על שהחולי נאחז והמשך ריעותו.

(6.4)

[296] אמר בקראט: מה שיהיה מן החבלות נופל מה שסביבותיה הוא סימן רע.

אמר המפרש: כשיפול מה שסביב החבלה מן השיער ויתקלף העור יורה על חידוד מה שהוא מורק לה.

(6.5)

[297] אמר בקראט: ראוי שתתחשוב בכאבים הקורים בצלעות ומוקדם החזה וזולת זה משאר האיברים כצלעות רוב שנויים.

6 אחר (= بعد): بعض a   8 הדלדול: السقم a   14 ויקח בה: فينال هضمها a   15 והמשך: وامتداد a
17 מה: مي ל   19 לה: فلذلك تأكّل ما حولها أخيرا add. a   21 כצלעות: om. a

אמר המפרש: ירצה לומ' שלא יקצר על מקום הכאב לבדו מבלתי ראותו בגודל החולי או חולשתו. והראיה על זה מחוזק הכאב ומה שימצא עמו מן העקיצה והארס וההמשכה ודומים לאלו משינוי המקרים וחזקם הנמשכים אחר לחליי אותו האבר.

(6.6)

[298] אמר בקראט: החליים אשר יהיו בכליות ובשלפוחית יקשה רפואתם בזקנים.

5   אמר המפרש: זה מבואר.

(6.7)

[299] אמר בקראט: מה שיהיה מן החליים הכאבים אשר יקרו בבטן במקום עליון ויותר יוצא הוא יותר נקל ומה שיהיה מהם בלתי כן הוא יותר רע.

אמר המפרש: יאמר גאלנוס שהוא ירצה לומר במקום יותר עליון מה שהוא סמוך בגב הבטן למעלה מהמקרום המכסה המעיים והאצטומכא ואמרו מה שממנו בלתי כן ירצה לומ' בו מה
10   שהוא במעיים ובאצטומ'.

(6.8)

[300] אמר בקראט: מה שיקרה מן הצמחים בגופות בעלי ההדרקון לא תקל רפואתו.

אמר המפרש: החבלות אינם נרפאות עד שהם מתייבשות יבשות שלימה ולא יקל זה בגופות בעלי ההדרקון.

(6.9)

[301] אמר בקראט: הבתור הרחב אי אפשר להיות עמו חיכוך.

15   אמר המפרש: בהיות החבלות והבתור יתמשכו ברוחב ולא יהיה להם גוף נראה יורה שהחומר קר ועל כן לא יחדש חיכוך בעבור קרירות החומר.

(6.10)

[302] אמר בקראט: מי שיש בו כאב ראש והכאב חזק וירד מחוטמו או מאוזנו מוגלא או מים חליו יהיה נתך בזה.

המפרש: זה מבואר.

---

1 יקצר: יספיק לⁱ   2 והארס: والدغ a   3 לחליי: لألّم a   לחלי: om. a   6 החליים: אלם a   במקום עליון ויותר
יוצא: أعلى موضعا a   8 בגב הבטן (= ظهر البطن): ظاهر البطن a   9 המכסה: הנמשך לⁱ הנמשך המכסה
זנ   12 בגופות: في مزاج a   14 הבתור: = البثور a   15 גוף נראה: شخوص a

(6.11)

[303] אמר בקראט: בעלי השעמום הבא ממרה שחורה ובעלי הברסאם כשיתחדש בהם
הטחורים יהיה סימן טוב בהם.

אמר המפרש: השעמום הבא ממרה שחורה הוא ערבוב הדעת המתהוה מן המרה השחורה
והוא שנקרא בלשון יון מלנקוניאה והברסאם מורסה חמה בקרומות המוח ומבואר הוא כי
5   כשהחומר יעשה אל הפך הצד ובא בפתיחת פיות העורקים יהיה העניין מתוקן.

(6.12)

[304] אמר בקראט: מי שנתרפא מטחורים שעמדו זמן גדול עד שיהיה בריא ולא עזב אחת
מהם אינו בטוח מהתחדש בו ההדרקון או הטיציש.

אמר המפרש: כי הוא אם לא יעזוב מהם מה שריק מהם הדם העכור ישוב אותו הדם ויתרבה
על הכבד ויכבה חומו בריבויו ויתחדש ההדרקון או ישליחנו בגידים אחרים ויחתך גיד בריאה
10   ויחדש הטיציש כלומ׳ שני אילו החליים ויתחדש מזה זולתם.

(6.13)

[305] אמר בקראט: כשיקרה לשום אדם שנגלוצו ונתחדש עמו עיטוש ינוח השנגלוצו שלו.

אמר המפרש: ברוב יהיה השונגלוצו ממילוי והוא אשר יתרפא בעיטוש מפני נקיון אותם
הלחויות בתנועת העיטוש.

(6.14)

[306] אמר בקראט: בהיות באדם ההדרקון ונגר המים ממנו בגידיו אל שלפוחיתו ויצא מפי
15   האמה מעצמו יסור חלייו בזה ויכלה.

אמר המפרש: זה מבואר כי יעשה הטבע באותו המים כמו שיעשה בבחראן החליים החדים
החומר המחליא.

(6.15)

[307] אמר בקראט: בהיות באדם שלשול ארוך ונתחדש בו קיא מעצמו יפסק בזה שלשולו.

אמר המפרש: זה מבואר כי הטבע משך החומר אל הפך הצד.

---

1 הברסאם: פירנסיאה z²ט²   5 יעשה: انصرف a   12 נקיון: استقاص a   14 שלפוחיתו: بطنه a
14–15 ויצא מפי האמה מעצמו: om. a

(6.16)

[308] אמר בקראט: מי שקרה לו חולי הצד או חולי הריאה ונתחדש בו השלשול סימן רע.

אמר המפרש: אמנם יהיה השלשול סימן רע בשני אלו החליים בהיות המחלה גדולה מאד עד שיחליק הטבע מחלשת הכח.

(6.17)

[309] אמר בקראט: בהיות באדם חלי העין הנק' רמד וקרה לו שלשול זה טוב.

5   אמר המפרש: זה מבואר.

(6.18)

[310] אמר בקראט: אם נתחדשה בשלפוחית קריעה או במוח או בלב או בכליות או בקצת המעים הדקים או באצטומ' או בכבד זה הוא ממית.

אמר המפרש: אמר גאלנוס: בקראט יעשה משל במה שימית בלא ספק ובמה שהוא ממית ברוב. וראיתי אדם שקרה במוחו חבלה גדולה ועמוקה ונתרפא אלא שזה יקרה לזמן רחוק.

(6.19)

10   [311] אמר בקראט: כשיחתוך עצם או תנוך או עצב או המקום הרך מהלחי או הערלה לא יצמח ולא יתדבק.

אמר המפרש: אמרו לא יצמח כלומ' לא יתחדש בחיתוך כמוהו בחבלה עמוקה ואם יהיה חיתוך לא יתדבק כי אלו הם איברים שאינם צומחים ליבשותם ויתרחקו בקריעה כמו כן ובחיתוך הרחקה גדולה.

(6.20)

15   [312] אמר בקראט: בהשתפך דם המקום אל פני על הפך הענין הטבעי על כל פנים יבוא לידי מוגלא.

אמר המפרש: ירצה לומר באמרו יבוא לידי מוגלא ישתנה ותפסד צורתו הדמית.

(6.21)

[313] אמר בקראט: מי שנתחדש בו שטות ונתחדש בו רוחב הגידים אשר הם נקראים הגפנים או הטחורים סר מעליו שטותו.

---

8 משל (= مثل B): قَتّال a (قَتّال B): מי (= مثل B): קריעה 13   om. a :(add. P والقطع بالشق) לי בקריעה :בחיתוך 12   a לי ‖ איברים שאינם צומחים ליבשותם: أعضاء يابسة a   15 המקום אל פני: המקום הפנוי זט إلى فضاء

a

אמר המפרש: זה מבואר שהוא מפני חזרת החומר הפך הצד ובתנאי שיהיו אותם הליחות המולידים לשטות היא אשר תטה אל השוקים. וכבר ידעת כמו כן שפסק דינו אינו כללי.

(6.22)

[314] אמר בקראט: הכאבים אשר ירדו מהגב עד הפרקים הנקראים קופְטי יתירם הקזת הגידים.

אמר המפרש: בהיות סבת אותם הכאבים ליחות ונטו לצד הגופטו והורקו מן המקום אשר נטו אליו יועילהו זה עכ״פ.

(6.23)

[315] אמר בקראט: מי שהתמיד בו הפחד ורוע נפש זמן ארוך החולי שלו מרה שחורה.

(6.24)

[316]

(6.25)

[317] אמר בקראט: העתק המורסה הנק׳ ריציפלא מחוץ אל פנימה אינו טוב אבל העתקתו מבפנים אל חוצה הוא טוב.

אמר המפרש: זוכרו מורסת הריציפלא הוא משל והוא ההקש בכל מורסה וכל חומר יוצא מבפנים אל חוצה כי הוא סימן טוב. ואם יהיה העניין בהפך הסימן הוא רע כי הוא סימן על חולשת הטבע.

(6.26)

[318] אמר בקראט: מי שקרה לו בקדחת שורפת רעש בלבול דעתו יתירה.

אמר המפרש: כבר ביאר גאלנוס מבוכת המאמר בזה הפרק כי חומר הקדחת השורפת בגידים וכשתעתק החומר בעצבים יתחדש הרעש וכשיתאחז במוח יתבלבל הדעת והוא יותר פחד מן הקדחת השורפת ואין בכמו זה יאמר אם הותרה הקדחת מפני שהעניין אשר נתחדש הוא יותר פחד ויותר רע.

(6.27)

[319] אמר בקראט: מי שהוכוה או נקרע מן הנפוחים או מבעלי ההדרקון ונגר ממנו מן המרה או מן המים הרבה פתאום זה ימות בלי ספק.

אמר המפרש: המוגלא נקראת כל מי שיש בו חומר במקום הפוני אשר בין החזה והריאה. ויצטרך אל הכויה בעל זה החולי ליבש אותו הלחות כשייעף מצאתו ברקיקה וכן בעלי ההדרקון הממיי יפתחו עצמם וזכר כי זאת ההרקה ממיתה. וכן אמר בשאר האיברים כשיתחדש באחד מהם מורסה גדולה ותבוא לידי מוגלא והורק ממנה פתאום הוא פחד כי יקרה לבעליו מיד העילוף ונפילת הכח ואחר כן ישאר בחולשה שיקשה להשיבו.

(6.28)

[320] אמר בקראט: הסריסים לא יקרה להם הפודגרא ולא יקרה להם ראש קרח.

אמר המפרש: מפני שהם כמו הנשים וכמו שלא תקרה הקרחה לנשים מפני לחות מזגם כן לא יקרה לסריסים הקרחה ומיעוט בוא להם חולי הפודגרא.

(6.29)

[321] אמר בקראט: האשה לא תקרה לה חולי הפודגרא אלא אם היה נפסק וסתה.

אמר המפרש: הנה נתן הסבה במיעוט בוא הפודגרא לנשים זה בעבור הרקת מותריהן עם הווסת.

(6.30)

[322] אמר בקראט: הנער לא יקרה לו הפודגרא עד שיתחיל בתשמיש.

אמר המפרש: אמר גלאנוס כי בעניין התשמיש בתולדת הפודגרא כח גדול מאד ולא יבאר סבה זאת. והקרוב אצלי כי סבת זה הוא היות הרגליים במעט בשר ולהם עצבים הרבה ומיתרים והם נגלים לאויר וכשירבה התשמיש ויעשה מעשה בעצבים בכלל מפני הרקת האישפיריט ומפני שהוא מתקרר בתשמיש תהיה ההזק ההזק בעצבי הרגלים יותר חזק ואנו רואים תמיד כי כשהרגליים יתקררו יפחות הקושי וזה ראיה על שתופם מצד העצבים.

(6.31)

[323] אמר בקראט: כאבי העינים יתיר אותם שתות היין שאינו מזוג או המרחץ או המישוש הנק' תכמיד בערבי או הקזת הגיד או שתית הרפואה.

---

1 הנפוחים: المتقيّحين a ‖ המרה: المدّة a 3 המוגלא: المتقيّحين a 4 מצאתו: זי מהוציאו זטילי
5 עצמם: זי בטנם זטילי ‖ ממיתה: دفعة add. a (except for BP) 10 הפודגרא: كَ تين .add. a
12 הרקת: ל .om 17 וכשירבה התשמיש ויעשה מעשה: فإذا أضرّ الجماع بالعصب a ‖ ויעשה: ויפעל זטילי

אמר המפרש: הנה באר גאלנוס מבוכת זה הפרק והיותו בלתי בא על דרך הלימוד המועיל
במלאכת הרפואות וזכר שהוא בהיות החמרים חמים ויהיה הגוף נקי יועיל המרחץ וישקיט
הכאב. ובהפסק כמו כן המשך החומר עם נקיות הגוף יועיל המישוש במים חמים ובהיות גידי
העינים מלאים נכנס בהם דם עבה מבלתי היות בגוף כלו מילוי ויהיה העין מתייבש. שתיית היין
יזיב אותו הדם ויריקהו ויוציאהו מן הגידים אשר נכנס בהם.

5

ואמר גאלנוס שאלו המינים השלשה מהרפואה יש לפחד עליהם מאד אם לא ימצא בה מקום
האמתות. אמנם ההקזה אם יהיה המילוי מדם או שיריק הליחה הגוברת עליו בשלשול הוא
ענין מבואר אמתי והוא הנעשה תמיד.

(6.32)

[324] אמר בקראט: הנערים יקרה להם שלשול ארוך.

אמר המפרש: ברוב תהיה סבת בעבור לחות מרובה וחלקות ועל כן הנערים בעבור לחותם
וחלקותם ועם זה המזג ישלשל הטבע ברוב.

10

(6.33)

[325] אמר בקראט: בעלי הרוטו החמוץ לא יוכל להיות להם חולי הצד.

אמר המפרש: רוב תולדת חולי הצד אמנם הוא מליחה חדה ורקיקה תרוץ אל הקרום אשר
מתחת הצלעות ויתדבק בהם. ובעלי הרוטו החמוץ למיעוט יהיה נולד בהם זאת הליחה.

(6.34)

[326] אמר בקראט: הקרחים לא יקרה להם מאד חולי הגפנים והם גידים מתרחבים ומי שיהיה
לו מאלו גפנים אליו יצמח שער ראשו.

15

אמר המפרש: אמר גאלנוס שהוא ירצה במקום זה באמרו הקרחים בעלי הנתק וכשזאת
החומר הרע יהיה נעתק למטה יחדש הגפנים בשוקים ויצמח השיער.

(6.35)

[327] אמר בקראט: כשיתחדש בבעלי ההדרקן שעול יהיה זה סימן רע.

אמר המפרש: ירצה לומר כי בהיות סבת השעול ההדרוקן וזה בהתרבות הלחויות המימיים
עד הגיעם עד קנה הריאה.

20

---

2 חמים: حادّة a   3 המשך (تَجَلّب): ל .om تَحَلّب a   4 נכנס בהם: قد لجج فيها a ‖ היין: الصرف .add
a (except for P)   9 הנערים יקרה להם: اللثغ يعتريهم خاصّة a   10 סבת: اللثغ .add a ‖ הנערים: يبلغ
الصبيان a   15 מאד: .om a   16 אליו יצמח: אילו יצמח זט عاد a   21 הריאה: فيكون قد أشفى على أنّ
تحنقه تلك الرطوبة .add a

(6.36)

[328] אמר בקראט: הקזת העורקים תתיר עוצר השתן וראוי שתתתוך העורקים הפנימיים.

אמר המפרש: תיקן גאלנוס זה הפרק כשאמר יתיר עוצר השתן וזה בהיות סבתו מורסא מדם וריבוי דם. והנשאר מהפרק אמר שהוא נכנס במאמר בקראט והראוי שתהיה ההקזה אז בתחת הארכובה.

(6.37)

5 [329] אמר בקראט: כשתהיה נראית המורסה בגרון במי שקרהו החנק זה משובח.

אמר המפרש: זה מבואר כי בהיות החליים נעתקים מהאברים הפנימיים לאברים הנגלים הוא יותר טוב.

(6.38)

[330] אמר בקראט: בהתחדש באדם סרטן נסתר הוא יותר טוב שלא תרפאהו כי אם תרפאהו ימות ואם לא תרפאהו יחיה זמן ארוך.

10 אמר המפרש: ירצה לומ' באמרו נסתר אשר יהיה בעומק הגוף ולא יהיה נראה או יהיה נראה ולא יהיה עמו חבלה וירצה לומר בעזבו הרפואה כמו הכויה והחיתוך לא החימום.

(6.39)

[331] אמר בקראט: הקווץ יהיה מהמילוי ומן ההרקה וכן השונגולוצו.

אמר המפרש: כל זה מבואר הסבה.

(6.40)

[332] אמר בקראט: הקורה אליו כאב מתחת חלציו מבלתי מורסה ואחר כן נתחדשה בו קדחת יתיר אותו הכאב ממנו.

15 אמר המפרש: בהיות אותו הכאב בסבת רוח או המשכה יתירינו הקדחת. וכאילו הוא יאמר שהתירהו הקדחת וכבר זכרתי לך משפטי זה האיש כי גזר דיניו רובם חסרי התנאי או זרים וקצתם ספק שהם נפלו בהזדמנות וחשב שני הדברים המחוברים עם ההזדמנות שהאחד מהם סבה לאחר כן יאמר מי שלא ילד אחר תאוותו אבל ההולך אחר תאוותו יאמר מה שירצה.

20

──────────

5 משובח: دليلا محمودا a   11 החימום (= التسخين) a   15 יתיר: יתר ל   16 המשכה (= امتداد): سدد a   17 וכבר זכרתי לך: وقد اطّردت a   18 ספק: وهم a   19 מי שלא ילד אחר תאוותו אבל ההולך אחר תאוותו: من لا يتعصّب وأمّا من يتعصّب a

(6.41)

[333] אמר בקראט: בהיות מקום מן הגוף בא לידי מוגלא ולא יתבאר מוגלתו לא יתבאר מפני עובי החומר או המקום.

אמר המפרש: מבואר הוא כי מפני עובי החומר או עובי המקום יקשה הכרת החומר.

(6.42)

[334] אמר בקראט: בהיות הכבד במי שיש בו ירקון קשה זה סימן רע.

5   אמר המפרש: זה מבואר.

(6.43)

[335] אמר בקראט: כשיקרה לבעל הטחול שלשול דם והאריך בו יתחדש בו הדרוקן או המעדת המעים וימות.

אמר המפרש: המוטחל הוא מי שיש בטחולו קושי ארוך וכשיתחדש שלשול דם על דרך העתק אותם הליחות העבות המילנקוניקי אשר היו סבה בחולי הטחול יועילנו זה כמו שיבאר עדיין.
10   ואם יאריך אותו השלשול ועבר אותו השיעור יפסיד על כוחות המעים בלכת אלו הליחות הרעות עליהם והתחדש מזה המעדת המעים ויכבה החמימות היסודי ומפני שתוף המעים הגדולים יחלש הכבד ויתחדש ההדרוקן.

(6.44)

[336] אמר בקראט: מי שהתחדש בו הטפת השתן ויהיה נמשך אחר מכן החולי הנקרא איליאוס זה ימות בשבעה ימים אלא אם נתחדש בו קדחת ויגר ממנו שתן מרובה.

15   אמר המפרש: הנה ספק גאלנוס בזה הפרק והעמיס על עצמו פירושים רחוקים לאמת מאמר נגלה הדלות מפעולת הבטלנים.

(6.45)

[337] אמר בקראט: כשיעבור על החבלה זמן והיא נגרת מוגלא ראוי בהכרח שזה התאחז בעצם ושיהיה מקום המעשה עמוק אחר היותה מתחילה להתרפאות.

---

9 היו סבה (= كانت سبب P): كانت تَشبّثَت a ‖ בחולי הטחול: في جرم الطحال a   12 הגדולים: للكبد a   13–14 מי שהתחדש בו הטפת השתן ויהיה נמשך אחר מכן החולי הנקרא איליאוס: من حدث به من تقطير البول القولنج المعروف بإيلاوس a   14 איליאוס: add. a وتفسيره المستعاذ منه   16 הדלות: السقم a ‖ הבטלנים: البطّالين a   17 זמן: حول a ‖ והיא נגרת מוגלא (= مدّة): أو مُدَّة أطول من ذلك a   17–18 התאחז בעצם: يتبيّن منها عظم a   18 המעשה: الأثر a

אמר המפרש: זמן החבלות ברוב הוא מאריך מפני חולי שהשיג העצם וכשיצא העצם הנפסד
תתרפא וישאר המקום עמוק.

(6.46)

[338] אמר בקראט: מי שמצאו גבנות מפני שעול הנק' רבו או שעול אחר קודם שיגדל זה
ימות.

אמר המפרש: כשיתחדש הגבנות מבלתי סבה מבוארת היא בעבור מורסא קשה וכשיחייב   5
זה צרות על הריאה בעבור העקמימות ובזמן הגידול תהיה הריאה נוספת ואי אפשר שיתרחב
מקומה ולא תקבל הגידול מפני הגבנות וסבתה על כן יאחזנו החנק וימות.

(6.47)

[339] אמר בקראט: מי שיצטרך אל ההקזה או שתיית הרפואה ראוי שיקח הרפואה
המשלשלת ויקיז בזמן הויר בערבי רב(י)ע.

אמר המפרש: זה מבואר למי שיצטרך זה על דרך שמירת הבריאות כמו שיעשו הבריאים   10
תמיד.

(6.48)

[340] אמר בקראט: כשיתחדש במוטחל שלשול דם הוא טוב.

אמר המפרש: זה כבר קדם ביאורו.

(6.49)

[341] אמר בקראט: מי שהיה מן החליים מדרך הפודגרא והיה עמו מורסה מורסתו תהיה
שוככת במ' ימים.   15

אמר המפרש: כבר קדם על איזה צד יותן אלו הגבולים.

(6.50)

[342] אמר בקראט: מי שהתחדש במוחו חתוך על כל פנים יתחדש בו קדחת וקיא ומרות.

אמר המפרש: כשיתמרסם המוח בעבור החיתוך בהכרח יהיה נמשך אחר זה קדחת וקיא
המרירות בעבור שיתוף המוח לאצטומ'.

---

3 אחר: om. a ‖ שיגדל: ז²טי² שיצמח זטלי קודם הבחרות טי أَنْ يَنْبُت له شعر في العانة a   7 מקומה:
فضاء الصدر a ‖ תקבל: كلّه add. a   14 מורסה: حاّر add. a ‖ מורסתו: لـ om.   16 הגבולים:
التحديدات a   17 וקיא ומרות: وقيء مرار a

(6.51)

[343] אמר בקראט: מי שנתחדש בו כאב פתאום בראשו והוא בריא ומיד אחזו חולי השתוק וקרה לו חולי הנק' גטיטא בערבי זה ימות בז' ימים אם לא תתחדש בו קדחת.

אמר המפרש: הגטיט סימן כח השתיקה וכבר ידעת שהוא דבר ממית אלא אם נתחדש בו קדחת ואפשר שיהיה נתך בה הליחה הגסה או הרוחות הגסות.

(6.52)

[344] אמר בקראט: ראוי שייגין הרופא בת העין בזמן השינה בחליים החדים. ואם התבאר שום דבר מלובן העין והעפעפים ואין זה אחר שלשול ולא שתיית רפואה משלשלת זה סימן רע מאד ומורה על מות.

אמר המפרש: אמנם יהיה נראה הלובן כל זמן שלא יסתם העפעף והעפעפים אינם נסתמים מפני היובש והיובש ימהר לעפעפים בעבור יבשותם בטבע או בעבור חולשת הכח כמו שיחלש בחולים שאינם יכולים לסתום פיהם.

(6.53)

[345] אמר בקראט: מה שיהיה מבלבול דעת עם שחוק הוא יותר בטוח ומה שיהיה עם מחשבה ושמירה הוא יותר פחד.

אמר המפרש: אין ממיני הליחות שום דבר שיהיה בלא פחד והיותר רעה היא אותה שיהיה עמה הקדם ומהירות והיא השטות. ואותה שהיא פחות רעה היא שתהיה עם שחוק ושמחה שאין זה מנהגו כמו השיכור. ואשר יהיה עמו מחשבה ועיון ורעיון הוא בינוני. וכל זה מחולי במוח או בעבור שתוף אבר אחר. ואשר יהיה בעבור חמימות מבלתי ליחה הוא דומה לערבוב הדעת המתהוה בעבור שתיית היין ואשר יהיה מן המרה האדומה יהיה עמו מחשבה ורעיון. וכשיוסיף שריפה ותטה אל המרה השחורה יטה זה הערבוב אל השטות.

(6.54)

[346] אמר בקראט: הבכי עם ניפוש בחליים החדים אשר יהיה עם קדחת הוא סימן רע.

אמר המפרש: ירצה לומ' שיהיה ניפושו נפסק וחוזר כניפוש מי שחנקו הבכי וזה יהיה או עבור חולשת הכח מהספיק הניפוש מיובש כלי הנפש וקשים עד שלא יוכל הכח להתפשט או מעניין קרוב מן הקווץ וכל זה בחוליים החדים רע.

2 בערבי: ל .om ‖ הרופא: .om a ‖ בת: זט .om ‖ בחליים החדים: .om a ‖ התבאר: נראה
זטל‪1‬‪2‬   5 הרופא: .om a   6 והעפעפים: مطبق .add a   10 בחולים: בחוליים זט   12 מחשבה ושמירה: هم وحزن a
13 הליחות (= الأخلاط): الاختلاط a ‖ שום דבר: ס"א שום בלבול דעת זט‪1‬   14 הקדם ומהירות:
ס"א הקצה ובהלה זט‪1‬ إقدام وتهجم a   15 מחשבה ועיון ורעיון: هم وحرص وفكرة a   16 במוח: أوّلة
17 מחשבה ורעיון: هم وحرص a   19 הבכי עם ניפוש: نفس البكاء a ‖ עם: רוע זט‪2‬ .add
20 ניפוש: אֲנֵילִיטוֹ בלעז זט‪1‬ .add ‖ הניפוש: أو .add a   21 להתפשט: أن تبسطها a

(6.55)

[347] אמר בקראט: חליי הפודגרא יתנועעו בזמן הויר ובחורף וזה נמצא ברוב.

אמר המפרש: בזמן הויר בעבור הגרת הליחות ותוספתם מפני התרת הקפאתם בזמן הקור
ובחורף מפני שקדם עליהם אכילת הפירות בקיץ.

(6.56)

[348] אמר בקראט: החליים המילנקוניקי יהיה עליהם פחד שמא יתירו אל השתוק והפלג או
אל הקווץ או אל השטות או אל הסנוירים.

אמר המפרש: אמר גאלנוס: השתוק והפלג והקווץ והסנווירים יהיו מן הליחה הפליאומטיקא
ומן הליחה המילנקוניקא. אבל השטות לא יקרה אלא משריפת הקולורא עד שובה מרה
שחורה.

(6.57)

[349] אמר בקראט: והשתוק והפלג יתחדשו לבד בין המ׳ שנה והששים שנה.

אמר המפרש: פירש גאלנוס זה הפרק עד שיהיה מאמר אמת. אמר: ירצה לומ׳ בו השתוק
והפלג אשר יבואו בעבור המרה השחורה כי המרה השחורה גוברת על בעלי אילו השנים.
אבל לפי האמת כי התחדש שתי אילו החליים מן המרה השחורה הוא רחוק מאד וחידושם
ברוב יהיה מן הליחה הלבנה ומן הששים עד סוף חייו.

(6.58)

[350] אמר בקראט: כשהחלב יהיה יוצא ונראה עכ״פ יתעפש.

אמר המפרש: זה מבואר.

(6.59)

[351] אמר בקראט: מי שיש בו כאב גיד הנשה ויריכו נשמט וחזר תדע כי נתחדשה בו לחות
דומה למותרי החוטם.

אמר המפרש: בעבור הלחות הדומה למותרי החוטם יתבטלו הקשרים ובנקלה יהיה נמשך
עצם הירך מהירך.

(6.60)

[352] אמר בקראט: מי שקרה לו כאב הירך זמן ארוך ויריכו נשמטת רגלו כולו יהיה נכחש
ויהיה פסח אם לא יכוה.

_____

3 בקיץ: ל‏ני בציף (= في الصيف) ל‏   4 פחד: זט om. ‖ יתירו: ثؤول a   18 יתבטלו (= تبطّل): بطّل a

אמר המפרש: אותם הלחויות יתייבשו בכויה וכשלא יתייבשו אותן הלחויות בכויה יתחדש
הפסחות ולא יתפרנס הרגל לפי מנהגו ויכחש.

נשלם המאמר השישי מפרקי אבוקרט.

---

1 הלחויות: الخاطية‎ a .add   3 מפרקי אבוקרט: זט‎ .om

<h1 style="text-align:center">המאמר השביעי</h1>

(7.1)

[353] אמר בקראט: קרירות הקצוות בחליים החדים הוא סימן רע.

אמר המפרש: זה אצלי ראייה על חולשת החמימות הטבעי והיותו בלתי מתפשט אל הקצוות
עם היות החולי מחודד כלומ׳ חם כי אבקרט יקרא חליים חדים החליים שיהא בהם הקדחת
תמיד. והקצוות הם קצה האף והאזנים והכפיים והרגלים.

(7.2)

[354] אמר בקראט: בהיות בעצם חולי ויהיה מראה הבשר בעבורו שחור זה הוא רע.

אמר המפרש: זה מראה נמשך אחר כבות החמימות היסודי.

(7.3)

[355] אמר בקראט: חדוש השנגלוצו ואודם העיניים אחר הקיא סימן רע.

אמר המפרש: כשלא יסתלק הקווץ אחר הקיא זה סימן כי סבתו או מורסא בהתחלת העצבים
כלומ׳ המוח או מורסה באצטומ׳ ואודם העיניים נמשך אחר שתי אילו המורסות.

(7.4)

[356] אמר בקראט: בהתחדש בעבור הזיעה סימור בלעז פְלוֹרִגְ אין זה סימן טוב.

אמר המפרש: כבר אמר בקראט כי מקרי הבחראן כשלא יתחדש מהם בחראן יורה על המות
כי הטבע יחלש ויכבה.

(7.5)

[357] אמר בקראט: בהתחדש מהשטות שלשול דם או הדרוקן או חיכוך זה סימן רע.

אמר המפרש: אמנם ההדרוקן והשלשול יתרפאו בהעתקת החומר. אבל החיכוך המקרים
כשיהיו נוספים ומתחזקים יניעם הטבע לדחות כל מה שהוא מזיק על דרך הבחראן כן יפרש
גאלנוס.

---

1 השביעי: ס״ד פרקים זט .add   2 הקצוות: הקצות ל לעז זטרימימיטי לּ   4 עם: עד זט   6 שחור:
كدا a   11 אמר ... טוב: ט׳ ‖ בלעז פְלוֹרִגְ: זט   12–13 אמר ... om. זט   12 המות: أو عسر
بحران add. a   13 יחלש ויכבה: تخور a   14 חיכוך (= حكّة): حيرة a ‖ רע: טוב ט׳ محمود a   15 החיכוך
(= الحكّة): חזוק זט׳ الحيرة a

(7.6)

[358] אמר בקראט: בסור תאות המזון בחולי הארוך והציאה הפשוטה סימן רע.

אמר המפרש: ירצה לומ' באמרו הציאה הפשוטה אשר לא יתערב עמה שום דבר מן הלחות
המימיי אבל יצא החולי אשר בגוף לבד בין שיהיה ממיני הקולורא או ממיני המרה השחורה
כי זה יורה על שהלחות הטבעי כלו נשרף מחום הקדחת.

(7.7)

5   [359] אמר בקראט: כשיתחדש מרבוי היין סמור ובלבול דעת זה רע.

אמר המפרש: התקבץ הסימור עם בלבול הדעת לא יקרה אלא לעיתים רחוקות אלא במי
שיתרבה בשכרות והחמימות הטבעי יהיה מתכבה ויתחדש הסימור וימלא המוח דם חם
ויתבלבל הדעת.

(7.8)

[360] אמר בקראט: כשיהיה פותח בפנים לגוף צמח יתחדש מזה נפילת הכח וקיא והתכת
10   נפש.

אמר המפרש: זה מבואר. וירצה לומר בצמח מורסה הנקראת דובילא וירצה לומר בפנים לגוף
אל האצטומ'.

(7.9)

[361] אמר בקראט: כשיתחדש בעבור הגרת הדם בלבול הדעת או קווץ זה סימן רע.

אמר המפרש: בלבול הדעת אחר ההרקה יהיה בעבור הצטער המוח בתנועותיו ויהיה לעולם
15   חלוש ובקראט יקרא לבלבול הדעת החלוש הזיה.

(7.10)

[362] אמר בקראט: כשיתחדש בעבור החולי הנק' קולנג' קיא ופואק הוא שונגלוצו ובלבול
דעת הוא סימן רע.

אמר המפרש: זה מבואר.

(7.11)

[363] אמר בקראט: כשיתחדש בעבור חולי הצד חולי הריאה הוא סימן רע.

_____

7 מתכבה: emendation editor מתרבה **זטל** فتطفأ a ‖ חם: أو بخارا حارّا add. a   9 וקיא: בקיא **ל**
11 בצמח מורסה הנקראת דובילא וירצה לומר: **ז** .om   14 בעבור הצטער: لاضطراب a   16 קולנג':
פי' איפוקונדריאה **זؐ²ט²** المستعاذ منه add. a

אמר המפרש: כשלא תביל הליחה המחדשת לחולי הצד מקומו ישפע ממנו שום דבר אל הריאה אבל חולי הריאה אי אפשר שיהיה נמשך אחריה חולי הצד.

(7.12)

[364] אמר בקראט: ובעבור חולי הריאה הברסאם.

(7.13)

[365] אמר בקראט: ובעבור השריפה החזקה הסתימה.

(7.14)

[366] אמר בקראט: ובעבור ההכאה על הראש הבהלה ובלבול הדעת רע.   5

(7.15)

[367] אמר בקראט: ובעבור רקיקת הדם רקיקת המוגלא.

(7.16)

[368] אמר בקראט: ובעבור המוגלא הטיציש וההגרה וכשתהיה הרקיקה נעצרת ימות בעל החולי.

(7.17)

[369] אמר בקראט: ובעבור מורסת הכבד יהיה השונגלוצו.

(7.18)

[370] אמר בקראט: ובעבור התעורה הקיווץ ובלבול הדעת.   10

אמר המפרש: אלו כלם מבוארים. ועניינם שהם כשיתחזקו ויקחו גבול גדולה יתחדש מהם כך כמו שמורסת הכבד כשיגדל ויזיק בפי האצטומ' יתחדש השנגלוצו. והנה הוא ידוע שהקיווץ ובלבול הדעת מתחדש בעבור היובש והיובש עם ריבוי ההרקה והתנועות הנפשיות והתעורה.

(7.19)

[371] אמר בקראט: ובעבור הגלות העצם המורסה הנקראת רציפלא.   15

אמר המפרש: באר גאלנוס כי הגלות העצם לא יהיה ממנו זאת המורסה אלא לזמן רחוק כי הוא גם כן זכר כל מה שאפשר שיהיה נמשך ואפילו במיעוט.

---

3 הברסאם: פי׳ פירניסיאה זיט² ‏   4 הסתימה: التَّشَنّج والتَّمَدّد a ‏   7 המוגלא: نفث المدّة a   11 ויקחו
גבול גדולה: وثاقت a   12 כך: كذا وكذا a

(7.20)

[372] אמר בקראט: ובעבור הרציפלא העיפוש והמוגלא.

אמר המפרש: זה מבואר לפי מה שקדם פעמים רבות שעניינו שיתחדש כך וכך.

(7.21)

[373] אמר בקראט: ומהדפיקה החזקה בחבלות הגרת הדם.

אמר המפרש: זה מבואר כי מחוזק הכאב יתנועעו הגידים תנועה חזקה לדחות הדבר המזיק.

(7.22)

5 [374] אמר בקראט: ובעבור הכאב אשר זמנו ארוך והוא סמוך לאצטומ׳ המוגלא.

אמר המפרש: הכאב הארוך יהיה בעבורו המורסה ואותה המורסה עתידה לבוא לידי מוגלא.

(7.23)

[375] אמר בקראט: ומהיציאה היחידה עירוב הדם.

אמר המפרש: כלומ׳ שתהיה הצאיה ליחה מן הליחות לבד אז יתחדש איכול וחבלה במעיים.

(7.24)

[376] אמר בקראט: ומחיתוך העצם בלבול הדעת אם יגיע למקום הפנוי.

10 אמר המפרש: יאמר כשיחתך עצם הראש עד שהחיתוך יהיה מגיע למקום פנוי המקיף במוח יחדש בלבול הדעת.

(7.25)

[377] אמר בקראט: הקיווץ משתיית הרפואה הוא ממית.

אמר המפרש: זה מבואר.

(7.26)

[378] אמר בקראט: קרירות הקצוות בעבור הכאב החזק סמוך לאצטו׳ הוא סימן רע.

15 אמר המפרש: זה מבואר.

_____

2 שיתחדש כך וכך: قد يحدث a   7 היחידה: الصرف a ‖ עירוב: اختلاف a

(7.27)

[379] אמר בקראט: כשיתחדש באשה ההרה שלשול מעיים הנק' בערבי זחיר תהיה סבה
להיותה מפלת.

אמר המפרש: זה מבואר.

(7.28)

[380] אמר בקראט: כשיהיה שום דבר נחתך מן העצם או מן התנוך לא יתדבק.

5   אמר המפרש: גאלנוס הורה שזה הפרק כפול.

(7.29)

[381] אמר בקראט: כשנתחדש במי שגבר בו ליחה לבנה שלשול חזק יתר ממנו חולייו.

אמר המפרש: הליחה הלבנה היא ההדרוקן הבשרי. אמר המחבר: כבר ראיתי זה שני פעמים.

(7.30)

[382] אמר בקראט: מי שיהיה בו שלשול ויהיה מה שיצא כמו קצף יהיה סבת שלשולו דבר
שירד מראשו.

10   אמר המפרש: סבת הדבר הדומה לקצף הוא עירוב האויר עירוב חזק. ותהיה אותו הלחות מן
הראש או מאיברים אחרים שיתיל באצטומ' ובמעיים.

(7.31)

[383] אמר בקראט: מי שהיה בו קדחת וישקע בשתנו דבר דומה לגרישים זה יורה כי חלייו
יאריך.

אמר המפרש: הליחות אשר נראה מהם זה הם רחוקים מהבישול ועל כן אמר בקראט שאלו
15   ימותו ברוב ומי שימלט מהם יאריך חלייו כמו שזכר הנה.

(7.32)

[384] אמר בקראט: בהיות הגובר על השמר אשר בשתן המרות ויהיה עליונו רקיק יורה על
שהחולי מחודד.

אמר המפרש: זה מבואר. ירצה באמרו רקיק שיהיה עליון השתן רקיק ויהיה דמותו כמו פיניי.

─────────────

5 הורה: אמר זט   10 הלחות: المنحدرة add. a   12 לגרישים: بالسويق الجريش a

(7.33)

[385] אמר בקראט: מי שיהיה שתנו מפוזר יורה על שבגופו סערה חזקה.

אמר המפרש: כלומ' משתנה החלקים זה ראייה על שינוי פעולת הטבע בליחות.

(7.34)

[386] אמר בקראט: מי שיהיה למעלה בשתן גרעינים יורה על שחלייו בכליות ויורה על אורך חולי.

5   אמר המפרש: כי זה יורה על רוח עב בתוך הליחות דבק ועל כן יורה על אריכות.

(7.35)

[387] אמר בקראט: מי שיראה למעלה שומן הרבה יורה על שיש בכליותיו חולי חם.

אמר המפרש: כשיהיה השומן בא בבת אחת זה יורה על שהוא התכת שומן הכליות וזהו עניין אמרו בבת אחת. אבל אותו שיבוא מהתכת שאר האיברים יבוא מעט מעט.

(7.36)

[388] אמר בקראט: מי שיהיה חולי בכליותיו וקרו לו או המקרים אשר קדמו והתחדש
10   בו כאב במושקלי קשים. אם יהיה אותו הכאב במקומות היוצאים יורה על צמח יוצא בו מבחוץ. ואם היה אותו הכאב במקומות הפנימיים יותר קרוב הוא שתצא הצמח הנק' דבילה מבפנים.

אמר המפרש: זה מבואר.

(7.37)

[389] אמר בקראט: הדם אשר יקיא מבלתי קדחת אין בו פחד וראוי שירופא בעליו עם
15   הדברים העוצרים והדם המוקא עם הקדחת הוא סימן רע.

אמר המפרש: ירצה לומ' כי כשלא תהיה שם מורסא באצטומ' אשר הקדחת נמשך אחריו בהכרח ויהיה קיא זה הדם מגיד שנקרע או חבלה נתחדשה וראוי שתתרפא מהרה בדברים העוצרים.

(7.38)

[390] אמר בקראט: הנזילות היורדות אל התוך העליון יבואו לידי מגל בעשרים יום.

---

3 גרעינים: عنب a   6 למעלה: بوله add. a   ‖ הרבה: z²טיל בבת אחת ל' جملة a   ‖ חם: حادّة a
10 קשים (= صلبة): صلبه a   15 סימן רע: رديء a   17 וראוי: فيمكن a

אמר המפרש: התוך העליון הוא המקום הפנוי שבחזה אשר בו הריאה ויום העשרים הוא יום הבחראן כי הוא בסוף השבוע השלישי. ואני אומר שזה הזמן הוא יותר רחוק ממה שאפשר שנתבשלו בו הנזילות.

(7.39)

[391] אמר בקראט: מי שישתין דם ויהיה בו הטפת השתן ומצאו כאב בצידי הטבור ועצם הערוה יורה זה על שסמוך לשלפוחית יש כאב. 5

אמר המפרש: זה כפל ענין.

(7.40)

[392] אמר בקראט: כשיהיה נעדר הלשון מכוחו פתאום או שהתרפה אבר מאבריו החולי הוא מלנקוניקו.

אמר המפרש: הנה הורה גאלנוס שאינו מוכרח שיהיה זה בעבור הליחה השחורה עכ״פ.

(7.41)

[393] אמר בקראט: כשיתחדש בזקן בסיבת הרקת שלשול בטן או קיא שנגלוצו אין זה סימן 10 טוב.

אמר המפרש: השנגלוצו אחר ההרקות הוא רע כי הוא נמשך אחר היובש ובזקנים הוא יותר רע מפני יובש מזג שנותם.

(7.42)

[394] אמר בקראט: מי שמצאו קדחת שאינו בא מן המרות והורקו על ראשו מים הרבה חמים יסור מעליו קדחתו. 15

אמר המפרש: גאלנוס יאמר כי כוונתו באמרו קדחתו שאינה מן המרות אינו קדחת עיפוש אבל קצת ממיני קדחת יום ואין ספק שהחימום בה מועיל ובו יתר הקדחת.

(7.43)

[395] אמר בקראט: האשה לא תהיה בעלת שני ימינים.

אמר המפרש: אמר גאלנוס כי סבת זה הוא חולשת העצבים שלה והמושקולי כי כל בעל שני
ימינים אמנם סבתו כח העצבים. זה נמצא בנ״א: אמר המפרש: יזכור סבת בעל שני הימינים
ויאמר כי האשה חלושה בחמימות בלא ספק ולא יגיע מן החמימות עד שישתוה הימין לשמאל
והוא מאריך באותו המאמר.

(7.44)

[396] אמר בקראט: מי שהוכוה או נפתח מבעלי המוגלא ויצא טרי נקי לבן זה ימלט ואם יצאה   5
ממנו טרי דומה לדומן מוסרח ימות.

אמר המפרש: בעלי המוגלא הם אותם אשר יתקבץ בין חזיהם וריאתם מוגלא והם אשר היה
מנהג הקדמונים לכוות אותם ולהוציא אותה המוגלא משם.

(7.45)

[397] אמר בקראט: מי שהיתה מוגלא בכבדו ויכוה ויצאה ממנו מוגלא נקייה ולבנה זה ימלט.
כי אותו הטרי בקרום הכבד ואם יצאה ממנו כמו שמרי השמן ימות.   10

אמר המפרש: בהיות הטרי בקרום ועצם הכבד יהיה בריא אפשר שיתרפא.

(7.46)

[398] אמר בקראט: כשיהיה בעינים.

אמר המפרש: גאלנוס יאמר שזה הפרק הוא מזוייף על אבוקרט. סוף דבר שהוא טעות גמור
ואמרו מה שאמרו.

(7.47)

[399] אמר בקראט: כשיתחדש בבעל ההדרוקן שעול אין בו תקוה.   15

אמר המפרש: כבר קדם עניין זה.

(7.48)

[400] אמר בקראט: הטפת השתן ועיצורו יתיר אותו שתיית היין וההקזה וראו שתחתוך
הגידים הפנימיים.

2-4 זה ... המאמר (= هذا وجد في نسخة أخرى قال المفسّر): يذكر علّة ذا اليمينين ويقال إنّ المرأة ضعيفة الحرارة
بلا شكّ ولا يصل حرها إلى حيز يساوي اليمين الشمال وتبسط القول في ذلك add. P يذكر علّة ذا اليمينين ويقال
إنّ المرأة قليلة (ضعيفة B¹) الحرارة بلا شكّ ولا يصل حرها إلّا حيز يساوي اليمين الشمال وتبسط القول في ذلك
add. B   10 השמן: השتن זל   12 בעינים: וجع add. B وجع فاسق صاحبه شرابا صرفا ثم أدخله الحمّام
وصبّ عليه ماءا حارّا كثيرا ثمّ أفصده add. a   15 תקוה: תקנה זט

אמר המפרש: זה המאמר הפסדו מבואר נגלה. אבל גאלנוס רצה להוציא לתחלת זה
הפרק תיקון ואמר כשיהיה סבת זה קרירות או סיתום מתחדש מדם עב ממזון שמלא
הגוף יהיה שתית היין המרובה יועיל מזה. אבל אמרו בזה הפרק וראוי שתחתוך הגידים
הפנימים וכן במאמר אשר קודם אלו כבר ביאר גאלנוס שזה בלתי אמת ולא הוא דעת
5 בקראט.

(7.49)

[401] אמר בקראט: כשתהיה המורסא והריציפלא נראית במוקדם החזה במי שקרה לו החנק
בלע״ז אישקינגנציאה יהיה סימן טוב כי החולי הוא נוטה אל חוצה.

אמר המפרש: זה מבואר.

(7.50)

[402] אמר בקראט: מי שקרהו במות החולי הנקרא סקקילוס זה ימות בג׳ ימים ואם יעברם
10 יתרפא.

אמר המפרש: זה החולי הוא הפסד עצם המוח ועל כל פנים כשיהיה גמור אין לו רפואה. וירצה
לומ׳ כשיתחיל זה החולי ויעבור ג׳ ימים ולא ימות אינו גמור ושהטבע יתחזק ויקבל תיקון.

(7.51)

[403] אמר בקראט: העיטוש יהיה מן הראש כשיתחמם המוח ויתלחלח המקום הפנוי אשר
בראש וירד האויר אשר בו וישמע לו קול כי עברו וצאתו יהיה במקום צר.

15 אמר המפרש: יהיה העיטוש בהתחמם המוח ויתלחלח המקום הפנוי ויתך אותו הלחות אד.
ולפעמי״ יעלה עם השעול רוח ממטה ובהגיעו בדרכי החוטם תהיה סבה להתחדש העיטוש.
ודרכי האף יעברו אל שני מקומות הפה והמוח כי הנקב אשר יעבור בפה ינקה ברוח העולה
ממטה. אבל הדרכים העוברים אל המוח ינקה ברוחות אשר ירדו ממנו. ואמרו המקום הפנוי
ירצה בו בטני המוח.

(7.52)

[404] אמר בקראט: מי שיש לו כאב חזק בכבדו ויתחדש בו קדחת יתר אותו הכאב ממנו.
20

אמר המפרש: כאב חזק בכבד בלתי קדחת אמנם יהיה מרוח גס ועל כן כשנתחדש הקדחת
נתך אותו הרוח.

---

1 רצה: تَكَلَّف a ‖ לתחלת: בתחלת ל 2 ממזון (= من غذاء): من غيرة a 7 אישקינגנציאה: אשכננציאה
ל 9 סקקילוס: سفاقيلوس a 11 ועל כל פנים: om. a ‖ add. a فذلك دليل أنَّه 12 ימות: فذلك دليل أنَّه ‖ ויקבל תיקון:
ויקבל המזון ל فأصلحت a

(7.53)

[405] אמר בקראט: מי שנצטרך להוציא דם מגידיו ראוי שתחתוך לו הגיד בזמן הויר הנק׳ בערבי רביע.

אמר המפרש: זה הפרק מן הפרקים אשר נכפלו.

(7.54)

[406] אמר בקראט: מי שהקפיא בו ליחה לבנה בין האצטומ׳ והמסך המבדיל והתחדש בו כאב אם יהיה בלא מעבר ולא אל אחד משני המקומות הפנויים אותה הליחה הלבנה כשתהיה נגרת בגידים אל השלפוחית יסור ממנו כאב.

אמר המפרש: כבר נאמר שזה הפרק אינו לאבקראט ואמר גאלנוס שלא יהיה נמנע מעבור זאת הליחה בגידים באומֶמֶינְטו כי הטבע יתחבל לדקדק החמרים ולהוציאם בכל דרך שיוכל כמו שיוציא המרה המתקבצת כמו בין הריאה והחזה. ובכלל הוא מאמר שהוא מעט התועלת.

(7.55)

[407] אמר בקראט: מי שנתמלא כבדו מים ואחר כן יצא אותו המים אל הקרום הפנימי יתמלא בטנו ממים וימות.

אמר המפרש: יתחדשו אלו האבעבועות מאד בכבד ומאמרו שמי שנתמלא בטנו מים ימות ברוב.

(7.56)

[408] אמר בקראט: הסערה וְהַאֲלַר והסימור ירפאנו היין כשיהיה מזוג מעט.

אמר המפרש: רוב הסערה היא מלחות מזיק בפי האצטומ׳ ושתות היין מזוג מעט כמו שזכר ירפא מכל זה מפני שהוא מרחץ הגידים ומתקן הליחות.

(7.57)

[409] אמר בקראט: מי שיצאה בַּתְרָה בראש האמה שלו כשתפתח יסור כאבו.

אמר המפרש: זה מן המוכפלים.

---

8 באומֶמֶינְטו: بالرشح a ‖ יתחבל: ישתדל ט‎²   8–9 בכל דרך שיוכל: ولو بعد ودقّ a   13 מאד: emen-dation editor‏ מאז זבל كثيرا a   14 ברוב: ذلك على الأكثر a   15 מעט: واحد سواء بواحد سواء a

(7.58)

[410] אמר בקראט: מי שנזדעזע מוחו יקרה לו שיתוק מיד.

אמר המפרש: אמנם יהיה זעזוע המוח או חוט השדרה בנפילה או דומה לה.

(7.59a–b)

[411]

(7.60)

[412] אמר בקראט: מי שהיה בשרו לח ראוי שיתרעב כי הרעב ייבש הגוף.

5   אמר המפרש: זה מבואר.

(7.61)

[413] אמר בקראט: בהתחדש בגוף כלו שינוי ויתקרר קרירות חזק ואחר כן יתחמם ויצטבע
במראה ואחרי כן ישתנה וישוב למראה אחר יורה זה באורך החולי.

אמר המפרש: זה הפרק הוא כפול.

(7.62)

[414] אמר בקראט: הזיעה המרובה אשר תהיה ניגרת בין שתהיה חמה או קרה יורה על שהוא
10   ראוי שיצא מן הגוף לחות בחזק ממעלה ובחלוש מתחת.

אמר המפרש: מאמרו שהלחות יהיה מורק מן החזק בקיא ומן החלוש בשלשול לא יהיה זה
תמיד. וכבר ידעת דרך בקראט ומנהגו וגאלנוס היה מסופק בזה הפרק אם הוא לאבקרט או
לזולתו.

(7.68)

[415] אמר בקראט: מי שנעגבה צואתו עד שתנוח ולא תניעה וראית למעלה כמו הגרידה זה
15   אם הוא מועט יהיה חליו חליו מועט ואם יהיה הרבה יהיה חליו הרבה. וזה יצטרך לשלשל בטנו כי
אם לא תנקה גופו ותתן לו מזון כל מה שיוסיף ממנו יוסיף הזק.

(7.70)

[416] אמר בקראט: בקדחת אשר לא יסור ממנה הרקיקה הנוטה לשחרות הדומה לדם
והמוסרחת והוא כמו הדיו כלם רעות כלם ואם נפתחה מאד היא טובה. וכן העניין במה שיצא
מן הבטן והשלפוחית וכל אשר יצא ונפסקה יציאתו מבלתי היות הגוף נקי זה הוא רע.

This aphorism is missing in the Arabic and Hebrew MSS, as it is a repetition of aphorisms 4.34–   3
Aphorisms 7.68, 70, and 81 are missing in the Arabic MSS and the other Hebrew 512.5–14   35
translations (except for א, see Appendix 2)

(7.81)

[417] אמר בקראט: צאת מטבעו כמו שיצא במה שיורק מהבטן ובמה שיורק מן הבשר או
מזולתו מן הגוף אם יהיה מעט יהיה החולי מעט ואם יהיה הרבה יהיה החולי הרבה (ואם יהיה
הרבה) מאד ויורה על מות.

אמר: כל אילו הפרקים מבוארים אינם צריכים לפירוש.

5   נשלם המאמר השביעי ובהשלמתו ישלם ספר פרקי אבקרט תהלה לשם ית׳ ויתברך.

_____

4 לפירוש: ומי שאינו יודע אין די לו בביאור ‹...›: **ל** .add   5 ובהשלמתו ... ויתברך: ונשלם ספר הפרקים
לאפוקרט עם הפירוש שפירש בהם כבוד רבינו משה בן ה״ר מיימון ז״ל **ט** העתקת זרחיה בן יצחק מן
העיר וורזילונה זצ״ל **ל** .add ונשלם ספר הפרקים לאפוקרט עם הפירוש שפירש בהם כבוד רבינו משה
בן ה״ר מיימון ז״ל בריך רחמנא דסייען ז נשלמו אילו הפרקים עם האמפוריזימי על ידי מרדכי בכ״ר בנימין
ויכ״י אספילו זלה״ה וכתבתיו לכבוד מורי הנכבד והיקר ר׳ משה דודי בכ״ר מרדכי כבתוי״א (ושלמתים
ז‹²›) בליל ו׳ ב׳ בשבט שנת חמשת אלפי׳ ומאה לבריאת עולם. ה׳ שזיכני לכותבם ולהשלימם הוא יזכהו
להגות בו ולכלותו (כחפצו הטוב ז‹²›) עם שאר חפציו הוא וזרעו וזרע זרעו עד סוף כל הדורות אמן ואמן
סלה ועד. וחלקי המחוקק יהיה ספון עם מצדיקי הרבים ככוכבים לעולם ועד. חזק הכותב ואמיץ כל
הקורא בו ז .add

Commentary on Hippocrates' Aphorisms: Third Hebrew Translation (Anonymous)

[1] אמר השר משה בן עבד האלהי׳ הקרטובי הישראלי לא אחשוב אחד מן החכמים אשר
חברו ספרים חבר ספר במין ממיני החכמות והוא יכוון שלא יובן מה שיכללהו ספרו עד
שיפורש. ואלו כיון כן אחד ממציעי הספרים היה כבר בטל תכלית חבור ספרו כי המחבר
לא יחבר חבורו להבין עצמו מה שיכללהו החיבור ההוא. ואמנם יחבר מה שיחבר להבין זה
5 לזולתו. וכאשר היה מה שחברו לא יובן אלא בחבור אחר אחר כבר נתבטל תכלית חבורו.

[2] ואמנם הסבות המביאות לאחרונים לפרש ספרי הקדמונים ולפרשם הוא אצלי אחד
מארבע סבות: הראשונה מהם שלמות חשיבות המחבר כי הוא לטוב שכלו ידבר בענינים
עמוקים רחקו ההבנה במאמר קצר ויהיה זה אצלו מבואר לא יצטרך לתוספת. וכאשר השתדל
המתאחר אחריו להבין אלו הענינים מזה המאמר הקצר יקשה עליו מאד ויצטרך המפרש
10 להציע תוספת מלות במאמר עד שיובן הענין אשר כיונו המחבר.

[3] והסבה השנית: דילוג הקדמת הספר וזה כי המחבר כבר יחבר ספרו בהשענו על היות
המעיין בו כבר קדמה לו ידיעת הקדמת הפלוניים. וכאשר השתדל להבין זה הספר מי שאין לו
ידיעה באלו ההקדמות לא יובן לו דבר ויצטרך אל המפרש שיציע אותם ההקדמות ויבארם לו
(או) שיעורר על הספר אשר נתבארו בו אלו ההקדמות וירמוז עליהם. וכפי זאת הסבה גם כן
15 יבאר המפרש עלות אחר לא יזכור המחבר עלתו.

[4] והסבה השלישית: הכרעת המאמר. וזה כי רוב המאמרים בכל לשון יסבול הביאורים ויתכן
שיובן מזה המאמר ענינים המתחלפים אבל קצתם מתהפכים אבל סותרים ויפול המחלוקת
בין המעיינים בזה המאמר ויבארהו איש אחד (...) ביאור אחר ויצטרך המפרש לזה המאמר
להכריע אחד מן הבאורים ולהורות על אמתתו ולזייף זולתו.

20 [5] והסבה הרביעית: השגגות הנופלות למחבר או המאמר המוחזר או מה שאין תועלת בו
כלל ויצטרך המפרש שיעורר עליו ויורה על בטולו או (על) היות אותו המאמר בלתי מועיל או
שהוא מוחזר. וזה לא יקרא פירוש באמת אבל יקרא תשובות והערות. אבל כבר נהג המנהג
אצל בני אדם בעיינו בספר ואם זה מה היה מה שנאמר בו רובו אמת ימנה ההערה על אלו המקומות
המועטים מכלל הפירוש ויאמר שגג המחבר באמרו כן והאמת כך הוא או זה לא יצטרך
25 לזוכרו או זה הוא חזרת דברים ויבאר זה כלו. ואמנם אם זה מה היה מה שנאמר בזה הספר רובו

1 השר: السيّد العالم الفاضل الإمام a ‖ הישראלי: قدّس الله نفسه (except for B) a add.   7 מהם: והם צ
8 רחקו: emendation editor בחכו MSS خفيّة بعيدة a ‖ במאמר: ממאמר צ   9 המתאחר: = المتأخّر
10 a המחבר: الأوّل   15 עלות: add. a   עלול ק עליו צ emendation editor   17 ענינים המתחלפים:
ענין המתחלף צ   18 (...): ويقول ما أراد به المؤلّف إلّا هذا المعنى ويتأوّله شخص آخر a

טעיות אז יקרא המחבר האחרון אשר גלה אלו הטעיות משיב לא מפרש. וכאשר זכר בספר
התשובות דבר מן המאמרי' האמתיים אשר נזכרו בחבור הראשון ואמר אמנם אמרו כך הוא
אמת.

[6] וכל מה שנתפרש מספרי אריסטו אמנם נתפרשו כפי הסבה הראשונה והשלשית במה
שנראה לנו. וכל מה שנתפרש מספרי הלימודיות אמנם נתפרשו כפי הסבה השנית. וכבר 5
יפורשו קצת מאמרים למודיים כפי הסבה הרביעית ג״כ כי זה ספר אלמגסטי עם גדולת מחברו
כבר נפלו לו בספרו שגגות העירו עליהם רבים מן האנדלוסיים וכבר חברו בזה. וכל מה
שנתפרש או יפורש מן ספרי אבוקרט הוא כפי הסבה השלישית והרביעית והראשונה רובם
וקצת מאמריו יפורשו כפי הסבה השנית.

[7] אלא שג׳אלינו' ימאן זה ולא יראה בשום פנים שיש בדברי אבוקרט שום שגגה אבל 10
יבאר מה שלא יסבול הביאור וישים פירוש המאמר מה שלא יורה זה המאמר עליו על דבר
ממנו. כמו שתראהו עושה בפירושו לספר הליחות נסתפק ג׳אלינו' בספר הליחות האם הוא
לאבוקרט או לזולתו והביאו לזה בו מתערובת ענינים והיותו דומה לחיבורי בעלי הכימיא או
פחות מזה. והראוי שבשמות אצלי שיקרא ספר התערובות. אבל להיותו מיוחס מפורסם
לאבוקרט פרשו זה הפירוש הנפלא. וכל מאמר המפורש על דבר מן הפירוש ולא יקרא זה 15
פירוש לפי האמת כי הפירוש הוא הוצאת מה שיש במאמר ההוא בכח אצל המבין אל הפעל
עד שאתה כשתחזור ותתבונן המאמר המפורש אחר שהבנתו מן הפירוש. זהו אשר יקרא
פירוש על האמת כי שיבא אדם במאמרים אמתיים ויאמר זהו פירוש מאמר האומר כך כמו
שיעשה ג׳אלינו' בקצת מאמרי אבוקרט. וכמו כן אלו אשר יולידו תולדות מדברי איש ויקראו
זה פירוש. לא יראה זה אצלי פירוש אבל חבור אחר כרוב פירושי אקלידאס לספר הנירוזי ואני 20
לא אקרא לזה פירוש.

[8] וכן נמצא ג׳אלינוס ג״כ בפירושו לספרי אבוקרט כבר יפרש המאמר בהפך הבנתו עד
שישים המאמר ההוא מיושר כמו שעשה בספר השביעי כשיאמר אבוקרט כי הארץ תקיף את
המים. ופירש ג׳אלינו' זה המאמר כשיאמר רצונו באמרו זה כי המים יקיפו בארץ כל כדי שלו
יאמר כי אבוקרט שגג או טעה בזה המאמר. וכאשר היה מנוצח בענין ומצא מאמר מבואר 25
הטעות ולא היה לו בו תחבולה אמר: זה מיוחס לאבקרט והכניסוהו במאמרו או הוא מאמר
אבוקרט הפלוני לא אבוקרט. וכל זה להפך אחר זכות ואע״פ שהיה אבוקרט מגדולי חשובי
הרופאים בלא ספק אך הנה רדיפת הזכות בדברי שקר אינו חשיבות ואפילו היה זה בחק
החשוב.

---

12 הליחות: وإن كان قد .add .a   15 וכל: ما قاله جالينوس في ذلك الشرح هو كلّه كلام صحيح بحسب صناعة
الطبّ لكن لا يدلّ ذلك .add .a   16 המבין (= الفاهم): الفهم   17 הפירוש: رأيت ذلك الكلام دالًّا
على ما فهمته من الشرح .add .a   18 פירוש מאמר: פירוש על האמת ממאמר צ   20 לספר הנירוזי:
לספר הנירוזי צ للنيريزي a   23 השביעי: الأسابيع a   27 אבוקרט: كما فعل في شرحه لطبيعة الإنسان
.add || להפך אחר זכות: تعصّب لأبقراط a   28 רדיפת הזכות בדברי שקר: التعصّب a

[9] וידוע כי כל ספר מפורש או שיפורש אין כל מה שבו צריך אל פירוש אבל על כל פנים
יש בו מאמר מבואר לא יצטרך לפירוש. אכן כונות המפרשים בפירושיהם כדרך המחברים
בחבוריהם מי שיכוין הקצור שלא יאריך בענין עד שאילו היה אפשר לו הדבור במה שרוצה
לחברו במאה דבורים על דרך משל לא יעשהו מאה ואחד דבורים. ויש מי שכונתו ההארכה
והרבוי ולהגדיל תמונת הספר ולהרבות מספר חלקיו ואף אם יקבץ זה כלו ענינים מעטים. כן   5
המפרשים מהם מי שיפרש הדבר הצריך לפירוש בקצור מה שיתכן לו ויניח מה שזולת זה.
ומהם מי שיאריך מה שאין צריך לפרש או מה שצריך אל פירוש ביותר ממה שצריך.

[10] וכבר חשבתי כי ג'אלינוס מן המאריכים בפירושיו מאד כרוב חיבוריו עד שראיתיו
לגלינו' יאמר בתחלת פירושו לספר הנימוסים לאפלטון דבר זה לשונו אמר: כבר ראיתי קצת
המפרשים פירשו זה המאמר ממאמרי אבוקרט והוא זה: וכאשר הגיע החולי לתכליתו אז צריך   10
שיהיה ההנהגה בקצה האחרון מן הדקות וכי הוא פי' זה ביותר ממאה קלפים בלא ענין וללא
סבה.

[11] אמר משה: כאשר ראיתי זה הדבור לג'אלינו' זכיתיו בחיבוריו ופירושיו וידעתי כי
כבר קיצר בם הרבה בהצטרפות אלו המחברים האחרים אנשי הדורות הם להיותם בענין
ההארכה מה שלא יכחיש זה המודה באמת. ואני אמנם אספר עם מי שיסיר התאוות ויכוין   15
אל האמת בכל דבר. וכבר זכר ג'אלינו' במאמרו הששי הספר הנקרא תחבולת הבריאות כי
חביריו האריכו דברים במאמרים ההם.

[12] וכאשר ראיתי ספר הפרקים לאבוקרט הטוב שבספריו והמועיל ראיתי לפרשו כי הם
פרקים יצטרך ליודעם כל רופא אבל טובי הרופאים ראיתים ילמדו לנערים בבית הספר עד
שפרקים רבים מהם ידעום מי שאינו רופא הרגיל מקטנותו בבית המדרש.   20

[13] ואלו פרקי אבוקרט מהם פרקים מסופקים יצטרכו אל פירוש ומהם מבוארים בעצמם
ומהם מוחזרים ומהם מה שאין בו תועלת במלאכת הרפואה ומהם טעות גמור. אכן ג'אלינו'
כמו שידעת מיאן זה הדבר ופירש כמו שרצה. אמנם אני אפרשהו על דרך היושר וזה שאני
לא אפרש אלא מה שצריך לפירוש ואמשך בזה לכונת ג'אלינו' חוץ מקצת פרקים שאזכיר מה
שנפל לי בו מיוחס אלי. ואמנם כל פירוש שאזכור סתם הוא דבר גאלינוס ר"ל כונתו כאשר   25
אני לא אשגיח לצמצם מלת לשונו ממש כמו כמו שעשיתי בשלישיתי בספר המבחרים. ואמנם היתה כונתי
בזה הפירוש הקיצור לבד להקל שמירת עניני אלו הפרקים הצריכים לפירוש. ואשתדל למעט
הדבור בזה בכל כחי חוץ מהפרק הראשון שאני מאריך בו מעט לא שזה הוא על דרך הפירוש
האמיתי לזה הפרק אבל להזכיר קצת תועלות שנתבארו לי בו או היתה זו כונת אבקרט או
שלו כיון בם.   30

3 שלא יאריך בענין: الذي لا يحلّ بالمعنى a   7 שיאריך: وشرح: מה: emendation editor: || add. a מי
MSS מا a   8 כרוב: ברוב ק كَأكثر a   16 בכל: emendation editor: כלא MSS في كلّ a   19 טובי
הרופאים: غير الأطبّاء a   20 ידעום ... הרגיל מקטנותו: يحفظها ... הרגיל מקטנותו a   26 בספר המבחרים:
في المختصرات a

⟨המאמר הראשון⟩

(1.1)

[14] אמר אבוקרט: החיים קצרים והמלאכה ארוכה והעת צר והנסיון סכנה והמשפט קשה.
וכבר צריך לך שלא תכוין על הזהרת פעולת מה שצריך לבד זולת שתזהיר מה שצריך שיעשהו
החולה ומי שלפניו כמו כן והדברים אשר מחוץ.

פירוש: ידוע כי הקצר והארוך הם ממאמר המצטרף. ואם רצה באמרו החיים קצרים 5
כהצטרף אל מלאכת הרפואה היה אמרו והמלאכה ארוכה חזרת דברים אין צורך לו.
ואין הפרש בין זה ובין אמרך יותר קצר מחיים וחיים יותר ארוך מיוסף. ואם היה
ר"ל כי חיי איש מן האנשים קצרים בהצטרפות אל שלימות אי זה חכמה היתה מן
החכמות ומלאכת הרפואה ארוכה בהצטרפות אל שאר המלאכות היה אז זה חזרת
דברים מועיל כאלו יאמר ומה רחוק שלימות האדם בזאת החכמה זה כלו לזרז וליסר 10
עליה.

[15] ואמנם היות מלאכת הרפואה ארוכה משאר המלאכות העיוניות והמלאכתיות זה
מבואר כי היא לא תושג ותגיע תכליתה אלא בחלקים רבים לא יספיק חיי איש איש מבני
האדם להקיף החלקים ההם כלם על השלימות התמימות. וכבר זכר אבונצר אלפרבי
כי החלקים אשר תושג בידיעתם מלאכת הרפואה שבעה חלקים. הראשון: מה שיתלה 15
ברופא מידיעת נושא מלאכתו והוא גוף האדם וזהו ידיעת חכמת הנתוח וידיעת מזג כל
אבר מהאברים על הכלל וידיעת פעולתו ותועלתו (ו)ענין עצמותו בקושי והרכות והמקשיי
והספוגיי וצורת כל אבר מהם ומקומות האברים הפנימיים והחיצוניים וחיבורי האיברים
קצתם בקצת. וזה השיעור לא יתכן שיסכל הרופא מהם מאומה ויש בו מהאורך מה שלא
יעלם. 20

[16] החלק השני: ידיעת מה שיפגע לנושא מענין הבריאות והוא ידיעת מיני הבריאות בכללם
בכל הגוף ומיני ⟨בריאות⟩ אבר אבר.

החלק השלישי: ידיעת מיני החליים וסבותם והמקרים הנמשכים להם בגוף על הכלל או באבר
אבר מאברי הגוף.

החלק הרביעי: ידיעת דרכי ההוראות והוא איך ילקחו מאלו המקרים הפוגעים למונח ראיות 25
יורו בהם על אי זה מין מין ממיני החולי יהיה זה בגוף כלו או באי זה אבר מאבריו ואיך יבדיל בין חולי
לחולי אחר שידמה לו ברוב הראיות.

---

3 תכוין על הזהרת פעולת מה שצריך: تقتصر على توخّي فعل ما ينبغي a ‖ זולת שתזהיר מה שצריך
שיעשהו: دون أن يكون ما يفعله a   10–11 לזרז וליסר עליה: ليحضّ على الدأب عليها a   16 ברופא:
הרופא MSS emendation editor   26 ממיני: الصحّة وعلى نوع نوع من أنواع .add a

החלק החמישי: דרכי הנהגת בריאות הגוף על הכלל ובריאות כל אבר מאיבריו בכל שנה
מהשנים ובכל פרק מפרקי השנה וכפי עיר ועיר עד שיתמיד כל הגוף וכל אבר על בריאותו
אשר תיחדהו.

החלק הששי: ידיעת הדרכים הכוללים אשר ינהגו בהם החולים עד שתשוב הבריאות אל הגוף
כלו או אל זה אבר הנכשל.

החלק השביעי: ידיעת הכלים אשר בהם יעשה הרופא עד שתתמיד הבריאות שנמצאת או
תושב הבריאות הנחסרה כמו מזונות האדם ורפואת סממניו לפי חלוף מיניהם ופשוטיהם
ומורכביהם והדחיקה והקשירה והנטילה מזה המין. וכן המלקחים הכלים שיאחז בהם ויחתוך
הבשר המזלגות והחחים שיתלה בהם ושאר הכלים אשר ישתמשו בפצעים ובתחלואי העין
כלם מזה המין. ובכלל זה החלק מן המלאכה ידיעת צורת כל צמח וכל מחצב שישמש במלאכת
הרפואה שאתה אם לו תדע מהם זולת שמותם לא תגיע אל התכלית. וכמו כן צריך לידע
שמותם המתחלפים לפי חלוף המקומות עד שידע בכל עיר לבקשו בשמו.

[17] וידוע כי ידיעת זה החלק השביעי כלו ושמירתם מן הספרים המוצעים לכל חלק מהם
לא יגיע אליו תכלית פעולת הרופא ולא ישיג לזה החכם השלם במלאכה עד שישמש את
האנשים בענין בריאותם וענין חוליהם ויגיע אצלו קנין בהכרת הראיות אשר יורו בהם איך
יורה וידע בקלות ענין מזג זה האיש וענין מזג כל אבר מאיבריו ואי זה מין הוא ממיני הבריאות
או מיני החולי וכן ענין כל אבר מאיברי האיש וענין עצם איבריו. וכן ידע בקלות לאורך שמושו
את האנשים ובצורה ההיא הנרשמת בשכלו איך ישתמש בכלים ההם ר"ל המזונות והסמנים
ושאר הכלים. זה צריך אל זמן ארוך מאד.

[18] וכן שמוש האנשים עד שירגילו בהנהגת הבריאות איש אחר איש ובתשמישי אלו הכלים
תשמיש פרטי ר"ל פרטיהם ונפרדיהם פעם והרכבת קצתם עם קצת פעם ולבחור איש הסם
או המזון על איש אחר ממינו כל זה צריך אל זמן ארוך מאד. ובאמת נאמר כי זאת המלאכה
ארוכה מכל המלאכות למי שיכוין השלימות בו. ואמר ג'אלינ' בפירוש לספר טימאוס: אי
אפשר לו לאדם שידע מלאכת הרפואה בכללה.

[19] אמר המחבר: ולפי האמת דע כי כל בלתי שלם בה כי הוא יזיק יותר ממה שהועיל כי
היות האיש בריא או חולה שלא יתנהג בעצת רופא כלל הוא טוב לו מאשר יתנהג בעצת רופא

5 הנכשל: الذي إعتلّ a		7 כמו: وهي معرفة a || ורפואת סממניו: وأدويته a		8 והדחיקה: emen-
dation editor והרחיקה MSS والشدّ a || המלקחים הכלים שיאחז בהם: وكذلك الآلات التي يبطّ بها a
9 המזלגות והחחים: والصنّارات a		13 החלק השביעי כלו: الأجزاء السبعة كلّها a (= החלקים השבעה
כלם)		14 תכלית פעולת הרופא: פי'(?) emendation editor פעולת תכלית הרופא ק פירו' פעולת
תכלית הרופא צ		17 שמושו: مباشرة a		19 מאד: فقد بان لك أنّ معرفة تلك الأجزاء على العموم وحفظ
تلك القوانين حتّى لا يشذّ عنه منها شيء يحتاج إلى زمان طويل جدّا add. a		20 שירגילו: يرتاض (= שירגיל)
a || איש: وفي تدبير شفاء مرض شخص بعد شخص add. a

שיטעה עליו. ולפי שיעור קוצר ידיעת כל איש יהיה טעותו ואם נפל ממנו האמת זהו במקרה.
ומפני זה פתח זה החסיד ספרו להזהיר על השלימות בזאת המלאכה באמרו: החיים קצרים
והמלאכה ארוכה והעת קצר והנסיון סכנה והמשפט קשה. אמנם הנסיון היות סכנה זה מבואר
ועוד אוסיף בו ביאור.

[20] ואומרו: והעת צר יראה לי שרוצה בזה עת החולי יצר מאד מן הנסיון שאתה כשלא
תדע העניינים כולם שנתבחנו כבר בנסיון אבל תרצה מכאן ואילך שתתנסה עניינים בזה החולה
או העת יצר מזה להתלמד הנסיון בזה החולה מה שיש בו מן הסכנה. ויהיה המאמר כלו
להזהיר על השלמות במלאכה עד שיהיה כל מה שנתנסו על אורך השנים שעברו מוכנים
בזכרונך.

[21] אמנם אמרו: והגזירה קשה יראה לי שרוצה בזה הגזירה על ענין החולה הינצל או יאבד או
שיתחדש שנוי מן השנויים ובכלל הקדמת הידיעה במה שיהיה כי זה יקשה במלאכת הרפואה
מאד לשפיכת החומר ומיעוט קיומו על ענין אחד. וכבר ידעת כי העניינים הטבעיים כולם
מאודיים לא תמידיים וכמה פעמים תהיה הראיה בתכלית הרוע וינצל החולה וכמה פעמים
תתבשר בטוב הראיות ולא יבא מה שהורה עליו. ולזה צריך אל הרגל ארוך בשמושי הראיות
הפרטיות ואז תוכל לגזור מה שיתחדש בדקדוק טוב קרוב אל האמת. ויהיה זה המאמר גם כן
הזהרה על ההתמדה בהשגת זאת המלאכה.

[22] ואמנם אופני הסכנה בנסיון הוא כמו שאגיד לך. דע כי כל גשם טבעי ימצא בו שני מינים
מן המקרים: מקרים יגיעוהו מצד חמרו ומקרים ישיגוהו מצד צורתו. דמיון זה האדם: הנה
יפגענהו זה הבריאות או החולי והשינה והיקיצה מצד חמרו מצד שהוא בעל חיים ויפגענהו
שיחשוב ויצייר ויתמה ויצחוק מצד צורתו. ואלו המקרים הפוגעים לגשם מצד צורתו הם אשר
יקראו סגולות כי הם מיוחדים בזה המין לבדו. כן כל צמח וכל מחצב וכל איבר מאיברי ב"ח
ימצאו לו אלו שני מינים מן המקרים.

[23] וימשך לכל מקרה מהם פועל אחד בגופינו. והפועל שיפעלהו הסם בגופינו מצד חומרו
הוא שיחמם או יקרר או ירטיב או ייבש. ואלו אשר יקראו הרופאים הכחות הראשונות ויאמרו
כי זה הסם יחמם בטבעו או יקרר וכן יאמרו גם כן יפעל באיכות. וכמו כן הפעולות הנמשכים
לאלו הכחות השניות כמו שהסם יקשה או ירכך או יסתים או יעבה ושאר מה שמנו כלם יפעלם
הסם מצד.

---

7 או העת: فالوقت a ‖ להתלמד הנסיון: مع ما في استئناف التجربة a   10 ענין החולה (= حال المريض):
ميل المرض a (emendation editor)   12 לשפיכת: لسيلان a   مال المرض ABC   13 מאודיים: أكثر
a   פעמים: تهيه الرؤية צ .add   15 בדקדוק: بحدس a   16 בהשגת: بالشغاحة צ في ملازمة a
20 ויצייר: ويروي a   23 הסם: emendation editor الدواء a החם MSS   26 הכחות: الأول وهي التي
يسميها الأطباء القوى .add a   27 הסם: بגופינו צ .add ‖ מצד: مادته. والأفعال التي يفعلها الدواء في أبداننا
من جهة .add a

[24] צורתו הם אשר יקראו הרופאים הסגולים. וג'אלינו יבאר בעבור זה המין מן הפעולות
כשיאמר יפעל בכלל עצמותו הענין כי הוא פעל יפעלהו מצד צורתו המיניית אשר בה נתעצם
זה הגשם והיה זה שהוא פעל נמשך לאיכות ויקראום גם כן הכחות השלישיות והם כמו שלשל
הסמנים המשלשלים או מקיאים או היותם הורגים או מצילים משתיית סם המות או מעיקצת
אחד מבעלי הארס. כל אלו הפעולות נמשכות לצורה לא לחמר.   5

[25] והמזונות ג״כ הם מזה המין רצוני היות זה המין מן הצמח יזוננו המין הפלוני מב״ח אין
זה חוזר לפשיטות האיכויות הראשונות ולא גם כן למה שיתחייב בעבורם מן הקושי והרכות
והמקשי הספוגי אבל זה פעל בכללות העצם כמו שאמר ג'אלינו'. התבונן איך תזון בדברים
הם קרובים מטבע העצים ותפעל בהם קיבתינו ותיכם כמו הערמונים והכרשינים והחירובים
היבשים ולא תתיך קיבתינו בשום פנים גרעיני הענבים ולא קליפות התפוחים וכיוצא   10
בהם אלא כמו שירד אל הגוף כן יצא כי אין בעצמותם שיקבלו מקיבתינו רושם בשום פנים.

[26] וכבר ביאר גאלינוס איך נקח ראיה על טבעי הסמנים ופעולתם)מן הטבעיות(הנמשכים
לאיכויותיהם מן טעמיהם בספרו הידוע בסמנים הנפרדים. אמנם ידיעת מה שיעשה הסם מצד
צורתו המיניית והם אשר יאמר כי יפעלו בכללות עצמותו אין אצלינו ראיה בשום פנים יורה
בה על אלו הפעולות ואין לידיעת זה דרך אחר בשום פנים זולת הנסיון. וכמה סם מר מסריח   15
בתכלית הסרחון והוא סם מועיל. וכבר ימצא צמח שיהיה טעמו וריחו כשאר טעמי המזונות
וריחם והוא סם הורג. וכבר יתבאר לך סכנת הנסיון מן הטעמים וחוזק הצורך אליהם עם זה
כי כל מזון לא יודע כחם מצד שהם מזון אלא בנסיון וצריך לך שלא תקדם ותתחיל בנסיון
והסתפק לשמור כל מה שבחנו בלעדיך.

[27] ודע כי יש סמים יהיה פעולתם בגופינו הנמשך לחמרם והוא נגלה מבואר ופעולתם   20
הנמשך לצורתם נעלם מאד עד שלא ישוער בו כרובי הסמים אשר לא יתואר בהם סגולה ולא
ייוחד בפעל. ויש סמנים יהיה פעולתם בגופינו הנמשך לצורתם גלוי מאד כסמנים המשלשלים
והארסים והמצילים ולא ירשמו בגופינו מצד שיחממו או יקררו אלא רושם מעט מזער או
מפני שאין להם איכות גובר בגלוי. ואי אפשר שלא ימצאו שני הפעולות בהכרח ר״ל הנמשך
לחמר והנמשך לצורה. ומפני הפועל הרביעי אשר לצורה היו סמנים מיוחדים לאצטומ' וסמנים   25
מיוחדים לכבד וסמנים מיוחדים לטחול וסמנים מיוחדים ללב וסמנים מיוחדים למות. ומפני
הצורה המיניית גם כן נתחלפו פעולות הסממנים ואף אם היה טבעיהם אחד. אתה כשתתבונן
תמצא סמנים רבים במדרגה אחת בעצמה מן החום והיובש על דרך משל ולכל סם מהם
פעולות בלתי פעולות הסם האחר. וזה כלו אמנם הוציאהו הנסיון לפי אורך הזמן.

---

1 צורתו: النوعية (= ותחיכם add. a   9 ותתיכם (= وتحلّها): وتحيلها a ‖ והכרשינים: والبلّوط a   10 תתיך (= تَحلّ):
تَحيل a   11 רושם: emendation editor أثرا MSS אשם a   17 הורג: بل قد يوجد نبات يظنّ أنّه من
أنواع الأغذية إلّا أنّه برّي فقط لا بستاني وهو سمّ قاتل .add. a ‖ מן הטעמים: ما أعظمه a   18 כחם:
emendation editor בהם MSS قواها a ‖ בנסיון: وكذلك معظم الأدوية ما علمت أفعالها إلّا بالتجربة .add.
a   19 והסתפק: والستفقوت ‎ק ‖ והסתפקות ואן تستظهر a   23 מזער: إمّا من قبل نزارة ما يتناول منها وإن كانت حارّة
أو باردة .add. a   25 הרביעי (= الرابع): التابع a ‖ סמנים: אחחים(!) ‎ק .add. ‎צ אחרים ‎ק .add.

[28] ולגודל חשיבות המדות של אבוקרט צוה בזה הפרק אשר פתח בו שלא יתכוין הרופא על
שיעשה מה שצריך לבד ויעמוד כי זה בלתי מספיק בהגעת הבריאות לחולה. ואמנם להשלים
התכלית צוה בשיהיה החולה החולה גם כן וכל מי שלפניו לעשות לחולה מה שראוי לעשותו ויסיר
המונעים כולם אשר מחוץ אשר ימנעו הסרת החולי. וכאלו צוה בזה הפרק שיהיה הרופא
עליהם משער בהנהגת החולה ויקל עשיית הרפואה עליהם כשתיית הסמנים המרים ועצירת
תשומת כלי וכריתת הברזל והכויה והדומה להם שיספר לחולה ולמי שאצלו ויזהירנו שלא
יחטא על עצמו. וישים למי שלפניו שישתדלו בהנהגתו כמו שצריך בחק טובי הרופאים. וכן
יסיר המונעים אשר מחוץ מה שאפשר לו כפי איש ואיש. דמיון זה אם יהיה החולה עני והוא
במקום יוסיף בחליו ואין יכולת לו על מקום אחר יעתיקנו הוא ממקום למקום. וכן יכין לו
המזון והסמנים כשלא יהיו זה עמו. ואלו והדומה לאלו הם הדברים אשר מחוץ ודאי יתחייב
הרופא מצד מלאכתו להיותה הכרחית בהגעת התכלית שישתדל הרופא להגיעה לזה החולה.
אמנם שיספר לבד מה שצריך לעשותו ברוח פיו ולא יעשה זה הוא לא תגיע מזה התכלית
המכוונת.

(1.2)

[29] אמר אבוקרט: אם היה מה שיורק מן הגוף עם גרישת הבטן והקיא אשר תהיינה נאותות
מן המין אשר צריך שינוקה הגוף ממנו יועיל זה ויקל סובלו ואם לא היה כן הנה הענין להפך.
וכן הרקת העורקים שאם הוא הורק מן המין שצריך שיורק ממנו יועיל זה ויקל סובלו ואם
לא יהיה כן יהיה הענין בהפך. וראוי ג״כ שיעיין בעת ההו(ה)י'(ה מעתות השנה ובעיר ובשנים
ובתחלואים האם ראוי להריק מה שזממת להריקו.

אמר המפרש: אמרו וכן הרקת העורקים ר״ל הזלת השתן או הזיעה או דם הנידות או פיתוח
פיות העורקים ויהיה הפרק הזה כלו במה שהביא בו מצורך. אמנם ג׳אלינו׳ שאמר: ירצה
בהזלת העורקים ההרקה אשר תהיה בסמנים יהיה אם כן הפרק האחרון מזה המאמר לפי
דעתי מיותר וחזרת דברים עד שצריך לו ביאור. אחר כן זכר שכאשר זממת להריק המין
אשר יצטרך כשנתבורר לך אותות תגבורתו אז צריך כן שתשים מגמתך לעתות השנה
והעיר והשנים וטבע זה החולי והנהג הדבר במשפטו. כי אם תריק המרה הכרכומית בסתיו
או במקומות הקרים או בשנות הזקנה יקשה ולא יסבול. וכן הרקת הליחה הלבנה בקיץ או
במקומות החמים או מן הבחורים או בתחלואים החמים יקשה ולא יסבלנו.

(1.3)

[30] אמר אבוקרט: שומן הגוף המופלג לבעלי העמל סכנה כשהפליגו ממנו בקצה אחרון וזה
כי לא יתכן שיעמדו על ענין ולא יתקיימו וכאשר לא יתקיימו על ענין זה אי אפשר שיוסיפו

---

1 יתכוין (= يَقتَصد): يَقتَصر a   3 צוה: وَيُبرئ a   4 הסרת: شفاء a   5 משער: قدرة a   5–6 ועצירת
תשומת כלי: والحقَن a   7 שישתדלו: يَقومون a ‖ טובי: غِيبة a   10–11 אשר מחוץ ודאי יתחייב הרופא:
الخارجة عمّا يلزم الطبيب a   14 גרישת הבטן: اسطلاق البطن a ‖ נאותות: طوعا a   19 דם הנידות:
النزف a   20 במה שהביא בו מצורך: فيما يأتي طوعا a   22 דעתי: عنده a   24 במשפטו: بحسبه a
25 הזקנה: أو في الأمراض الباردة add. a   28 ולא יתקיימו וכאשר לא יתקיימו על ענין: צ om.

טובה ונשארים כן שיטו אל ענין יותר רע ולזה יצטרך שיחסר שומן הגוף בלי איחור עד שישוב
הגוף ויתחיל לקבל המזון ולא יפליג בהרקה על הקצה האחרון כי זה סכנה אבל כפי שיעור
סבל טבע הגוף אשר יכוין להריקו. וכן כל הרקה יפליג בה עד הקצה האחרון הוא סכנה וכל
הזנה ג״כ היא אצלינו בקצה האחרון סכנה גמורה.

אמר המפרש: ירצה בבעלי התנועה הטרחנים ודומיהם ממי שלקח התנועה המתמדת לו   5
לאומנות וזה כי העורקים כשיתמלאו יותר מזה שראוי לא תאמין שלא יכוסה או יחנק החום
היסודי בהם ויכבה וימותו והוא צריך שיהיה בעורקים ריקות כדי שיקבל מה שיבא אליהם מן
המזון.

(1.4)

[31] אמר אבוקראט: ההנהגה המופלגת בכל החליים הישנים בלי ספק סכנה ובחליים החדים
ג״כ כשלא יסבלו וההנהגה המופלגת עד קצה התכלית מן הדקות הוא בהם קשה מר ורע בלי   10
ספק.

אמר המפרש: ההנהגה אשר בקצה התכלית מן הדקות הוא הנחת המאכל לגמרי וההנהגה
הדקה שאינה בתכלית הוא כמו תבשיל שעורים ודומיהם.

(1.5)

[32] אמר אבוקראט: בהנהגה הדקה כבר יחטאו החולים על עצמם חטא גדול הנזק עליהם.
וזה כי כל מה שיהיה מהם יותר נזק יהיה ביותר דק והוא מה שיהיה ממנו במזון שיש לו עובי   15
מעט. ובעבור זה היתה ההנהגה המופלגת בדקות בבריאים גם כן סכנה כי מה שיקרה להם
מן החטא בהנהגה העבה יקל סבלם ולזה היתה ההנהגה המופלגת בדקות ברוב הענינים יותר
סכנה מההנהגה שהיא יותר עבה.

אמר המפרש: זה נגלה מבואר.

(1.6)

[33] אמר אבוקראט: הטוב שבהנהגות בחליים אשר בקצה התכלית ההנהגה אשר בקצה   20
התכליתי.

אמר המפרש: החוליים אשר בקצה התכליתי הם החליים החדים מאד.

---

4 אצלינו בקצה האחרון: عند الغاية القصوى a ‖ גמורה: om. a   5 המתמדת: العنيفة a   6 יכוסה:
تصدع a   9 המופלגת: في اللطافة add. a   10 בהם: om. a ‖ מר ורע: مذموم a   12 וההנהגה: الذي
هو في الغاية من اللطافة إلّا أنّه ليس في أقصاها هو تناول ماء الشعير ونحوه والتدبير add. a   15 יותר נזק יהיה
ביותר דק והוא מה שיהיה ממנו במזון: أعظم ما يكون منه في الغذاء   18 עבה: قليلا add. a

(1.7)

[34] אמר אבוקראט: וכשיהיה החולי חד מאד והיו הכאבים אשר בקצה התכלית מן הדקות וכשלא יהיה כן אמנם יסבול מן ההנהגה מה שהוא יותר עב מזה ויצטרך שיהיה ההורדה כפי רכות החולי וחסרונו מקצה התכלית. וכאשר הגיע החולי בתכליתו ועם זה צריך שיהיה ההנהגה אשר היא בקצה האחרון מן הדקות.

אמר המפרש: הכאבים אשר בקצה התכלית הם הכאבים הגדולים ר״ל תחת זמן בקדחת וכל המקרים והוא תכלית החולי כי אין התכלית דבר אחר זולת גודל חלקי החלי במקריו. תבין מאמרו בתחלה הארבעה ימים הראשונים או אחריהם מעט.

(1.8)

[35] ⟨(...)⟩ ואמרו שיעשה ההנהגה הדקה בתכלית זה לגודל המקרים בעת ההיא בעבור מה שיתבשל החולי. וזה כי אינו צריך שיתעסק הטבע בבשול המזון שירד עליו וימנענו מלבשל החולי ר״ל התערובות המולידים לחולי כאשר הטבע בעת ההיא מתעורר עליהם בכחותיו כלם ואמנם נשאר לו מעט כח עד שישלם להתגבר עליהם.

(1.9)

[36] אמר אבוקראט: וראוי שתשקול גם כן כח החולה ותדע אם תתקיים עד עת תכלית החולי ותעיין אי זה משני דברים יהיה אם כח החולה יכשל קודם תכלית החולי ולא תשאר על זאת ההזנה או החולי יכשל קודם ושוב תן לו.

אמר המפרש: זה מבואר.

(1.10)

[37] אמר אבוקרט: ואשר יבא תכלית חליים בתחלה צריך שיתנהגם בהנהגה הדקה בתחלה ואשר יתאחר תכלית חוליים ראוי שיעשה הנהגתם בתחלת חליים יותר עבה ואח״כ יחסר מעורבים מעט מעט כל אשר יקרב אל תכלית החולי ובעת התכלית כפי מה שישאר כח החולה עליו וראוי למנוע מן המזון בעת תכלית החולי כי ההוספה בו מזקת.

אמר המפרש: זה מבואר.

---

1 התכלית: تأتي فيه بدءا ويجب ضرورة أن يستعمل فيه التدبير الذي في الغاية القصوى add. a ‏3–4 וכאשר ... מן הדקות: om. a ‏5 תחת זמן: نوائب a ‏8 (...): قال أبقراط: إذا بلغ المرض منتهاه فعند ذلك يجب ضرورة أن يستعمل التدبير الذي في الغاية القصوى من اللطافة a ‏|| ואמרו שיעשה ההנהגה הדקה בתכלית זה: وذلك a ‏9 המזון: جديد add. a ‏10 החולי ר״ל: om. a ‏11 מעט :emendation editor מעיר MSS ‏14 ושוב תן לו: وتسكن عاديته a ‏18 מעורבים: من غلظه a (= מעובים)

(1.11)

[38] אמר אבוקרט: כשהיו לקדחת סבובים תמנע מהם המזון בעת עונותיהם.

אמר המפרש: זה מבואר.

(1.12)

[39] אמר אבוקרט: הנה יורה על עונות הקדחות וסדר החולי ומדרגתו החליים בעצמם
ועתות השנה ותוספת הסבובים קצתם על קצת יהיה עונתו בכל יום ויום לא או היותר
מזה הזמן. והדברים גם כן אשר יראו אחרי כן דמיון זה מה שיראה בסובלי חולי הצד הוא
כשיראה הרוק בתחלה מעת החל החולי היה החולי קצר ואם נתאחר הראותו היה החולי
ארוך. והשתן והרעי והזיעה כשנראה אחרי כן יורנו על טוב הגבול ורעתו ואורך החולי
וקצורו.

אמר המפרש: מטבע החולי עצמו תדע האם קץ(ו)ה(ו) ימהר או יאחר. כי מדוה הצד ומדוה
הריאה ומדוה הטרפש הם חליים חדים והאסכרה וכאב הקיבה וחולי הקוץ הם חליים חדים
מאד. והשקוי וחולי הדאגה וחולי מיעים והכליה והוא נגע הריאה הם חליים ישנים. ועונת
זמן הקדחת הרוב מה שיהיו במדוה הצד והטרפש חזקים. ורוב מה שיהיה במי שיש בו צמח
במרירתו או בכבדו או בקבתו או במי שיש בו הכלייה בכל יום וכל שכן בלילה. ורוב מה שיהיה
עונת זמן הקדחת במי שחלתו בטחולו מן המרה ובכלל מן המרה השחורה יום ויומם לא. וכן
עתות השנה כי הקדחת הרביעית בקיץ היא קצרה מאד העניין ובחורף ארוכה וכ״ש כשתגיע
בסתיו.

ותוספת העונות יורה על תוספת החולי וקורבת תכליתו. ויודע תוספת העונה השנית על העונה
הראשונה משלשה דברים אחד מהם עת זמן העונה והשני אורך זמן העונה והשלשי גדלו ר״ל
חזקו.

(1.13)

[40] אמר אבוקרט: הישישים היותר סובלים שבאנשים לצום ואחרי כן הזקנים והבחורים
מעט יסבלו הצום והמעט שבאנשים לסבול הצום הם הנערים. ומה שיהיה מן הנערים חזק
התאוה הוא פחות סובל לו.

אמר המפרש: אשר זכרו בזה הפרק כבר זכר עלתו בפרק שאחריו וזה כי כל מה שהיה החום
היסודי יותר צריך למזון יותר וההתוך מגופי הנערים לרטיבותם הרבה. וזה אשר זכרו מסבול

---

1 עונותיהם: فإنّ الزيادة فيه مضرّة add. a   6 הרוק: النفث   7 הגבול: المرض add. a   10 ומדוה
הטרפש: والسرسام a   11 וחולי הדאגה: والوسواس a ‖ וחולי מיעים: ومدّة الجوف a ‖ והכליה: والسلّ
a   12 והטרפש: والسرسام a ‖ חזקים: غبّا a   12–13 צמח במרירתו: خراج فيه مدّة a   15 מאד העניין:
في أكثر الأمر a   18 העונה: الحمّى a add. a   20 הזקנים: الكهول a

הישישים לצום זכר ג'אלינו' כי הוא הישיש שלא הגיע לגדר השהיה. אמנם הישישים שהם
בתכלית הזקנה לא יסבלו ההמתנה מן המאכל אבל צריכים שינתן להם מעט מעט פעם אחר
פעם לקרוב חומם היסודי להכבות וצריך אל הנהגתם מי שיגיעם מעט אחר מעט.

(1.14)

[41] אמר אבוקרט: מי שהיה מן הגופים בזמן הגדול החום היסידי בהם בתכלית מה שיהיה
מן הרבוי ויצטרך מן המזון יותר ממה שיצטרכו אליו שאר הגופים ואם לא יאכילהו מן המזון   5
כל צרכו יבלה גופו ויחסר. ואמנם הישישים החום היסודי בהם מעט ומפני זה לא יצטרכו אל
מזון אלא המעט המעט כי חומם תכבה מן ההרבה ומפני זה גם כן לא תהיה הקדחת בישישים חדה
כמו שתהיה באשר בעת הגדול וזה כי גופותם קרים.

אמר המפרש: ⟨אמר⟩ ג'אלינו': העצם אשר בו החום היסודי הוא בנערים יותר רב השיעור וזהו
העניין אשר בעבורו אמר ג'אלינו' תמיד כי החום יותר בכמות כמו שנתבאר במזגים.   10

(1.15)

[42] אמר אבוקרט: הגופים בסתיו ובאביב הם יותר חמים מכל מה שיהיה בטבע. והשינה
יותר ארוכה ממה שיהיה. ויצטרך באלו העתים שיהיה מה שינתן להם מן המזונות הרבה וזה
כי החום היסודי בגופים באלו שני הזמנים הרבה ולזה צריכים אל מזון רב. והראיה על זה השנים
והטרחניים.

אמר המפרש: אמר ג'אלינו': וכי זה בנערים למה שהיה החום היסודי בהם יותר יצטרכו לזה   15
למזונות יותר. והטרחנים גם כן כאשר היה החום היסודי יגדל בהם ברוב תנועותיהם היתה
שיעור צרכם אל המזון הרבה.

(1.16)

[43] אמר אבוקרט: המזונות הלחים יאותו לשאר המחוממים וכל שכן לנערים ומי שכבר
הנהיג המאכלים הלחים.

אמר המפרש: זהו מבואר וזה כמו שיקח מזה דרך ונתיב לזו החכמה והוא שהבריאות ישמר   20
בדומה והחולי ירופא בהפכו.

---

1 השהיה: الهرم a   3 וצריך אל הנהגתם מי שיגיעם: فتحتاج إلى متابعة ما يمدّها a   5 המזון: الوقود
a ‖ הגופים: من الغذاء add. a   9 החום היסודי: حرارة a   11 הגופים: الأجواف a ‖ ובאביב: emendation editor בואבים MSS   15 המפרש: ودليل على ذلك أمر الأسنان والصريعين add. a   18 לשאר
(= سائر C): جميع a   20 דרך ונתיב לזו החכמה: القانون العامّ a   21–20 שהבריאות ישמר בדומה
והחולי ירופא בהפכו: وهو أنّ كلّ مرض يقابل بضدّه a

(1.17)

[44] אמר אבוקרט: וצריך שיתנו לקצת החולים מזונותם בפעם אחת ולקצתם בשני פעמים
וישים מה שיתן לו מן המזון רב ומעט ולקצתם מעט וצריך גם כן שישים מגמתו אל העת
ההווה מעתות השנה והמנהג והשנים.

אמר המפרש: כאשר נתן הדרך בכמות המזון תחלה אחרי כן באיכותו התחיל עתה לתת
הדרך בצורת ההגעה אליו. והעקר בזה התבוננות כח החולה והתבוננות החולי. וישים מגמתו   5
גם כן אל השנים והמנהג ומזג האויר. וזה כי הכח החזקה ראוי לה הגעת המזון בפעם אחת
והחלושה ראוי לה הגעתו מעט מעט. וחסר הגוף הכחוש ראוי לו שיגיעו לו מזון הרבה ומלא
הגוף ראוי לו מיעוט המזון. ויתחייב מזה כשתהיה הכח חלושה והגוף כחוש שינתן לו מאכליו
מעט ופעמים רבות וכשתהיה הכח חלושה והגוף אינו כחוש וחסר צריך שינתן לו מאכליו מעט
ופעמים מעטים. וכן כשתהיה הכח חזקה והגוף בעניין החסרון או עניין מליחות נפסדים צריך   10
שיאכילו לחולה מאכל רב ופעמים רבות כי עניין גופו צריך אל מזון רב וכחו חזקה לעכל המזון.
ואם ימנעהו עתות הקדחת ולא נמצא עתות רבים להאכילו אז תן לו בפעמים מועטים.

וכן הוא ההוראה כפי כח החולי. ואמנם העת והשנה והמנהג ומה שינהג מנהג זה הוא על זה
המשקל: הקיץ ראוי להרבות הפעמים ולמעט מה שיגיעו לו בכל פעם והסתיו ראוי להרבות
המזון ולמעט הפעמים. ואמנם אמצע האביב בעבור שקרב אל הקיץ יצטרך אל מזון מעט בין   15
עתים רחוקים כי בעת הזאת מצוי שיהיו הגופים מלאים כי הכימוסים אשר נקפו בסתיו תזובנה
ותתחלחלו. ואמנם החורף מי שיחום יצטרך אל)י(ו תוספת מזון מעט ומשובח בעבור הפסד
הכימוסים בעת הזאת וכפי השנים והמנהגים זה מבואר.

(1.18)

[45] אמר אבוקרט: הקשה אשר יהיה מסבול המאכלים על הגופים הוא בקיץ ובחורף והנקל
מה שיהיה סובלו עליהם הוא בסתיו ואחריו באביב.   20

אמר המפרש: אמר ג'אלינו': דברו בזה הפרק הוא בחולה ודברו במה שקדם למעלה הוא
בבריאים.

(1.19)

[46] אמר אבוקרט: כאשר היתה עונת הקדחת כפי חיוב סבוביה לא יצטרך בזמנה שינתן
לחולה דבר שיזיקהו אבל ראוי שיחסרו לו מן התוספת בעבור עתות הפרקים.

_____

2 שישים מגמתו אל: أن يعطى ... حظّه a   6-5 וישים מגמתו גם כן אל: ويعطى أيضا ... حظّه a
10 חזקה: والكيموسات كثيرة. أمّا إذا كانت القوّة قويّة add. a   12 עתות: نوائب a   14 המשקל: المثال
a   15 בעבור שקרב: وإذا قرب a   16 מצוי שיהיו: يكاد أن تكون a   17 ונתחלחלו: وتحلّل a ‖ שיחום:
שיחוש MSS emendation editor ‖ אל)י(ו תוספת מזון מעט ומשובחה: إلى زيادة سابغة من غذاء
محمود a   18 וכפי)وأمّا B(: وأمر a   24 דבר שיזיקה: شيئا أو أن يضطرّ إلى شيء a ‖ הפרקים: الانفصال
a

אמר המפרש: אמר ג'אלינו': יראה באמרו בעבור עתות הפרקים עתות העונות. וכאשר
יהיה זה הזמן ראוי לו לחסר מן החומר שלא יגדל הקדחת והזהיר שלא תוסיף בו דבר
במזונותיו.

(1.20)

[47] אמר אבוקרט: הגופות אשר יבואנה או כבר בא לה הגבול על השלמות אין צריך שיטעון
ולא תחדש בהם חדוש לא בסם משלשל ולא בזולתו מן המעוררים אבל יונחו.   5

אמר המפרש: אמרו אשר יבואנה ירצה בו שכבר הוכנו סבותם ונראו אותותיהם ומזומן
שיהיה. ואמרו ולא בזולתו מן המעוררים כמו הקיא והזיעה והזלת השתן או הנידות. התנה
שיהיה הגבול שלם. אמנם הגבול החסר יתחייב שישלם חסרונו ויוציא מה שנשאר מן העובי
המחליא בצד הנקל שבו. ואמר ג'אלינו' כי הגבול השלם הוא מה שיתקבצו בו ששה ענינים:
הראשון שיקדמהו הבשול. השני שיהיה ביום מימי הגבול. השלישי שיהיה בהרקת דבר מבואר   10
שיוציא מן הגוף לא על יד מוציא בחוזק. הרביעי שיהיה הדבר המורק הוא הדבר המזיק אשר
היה עלת החולי. החמישי שיהיה הרקתו במצב בקומה מן הצד שיהיה בו החולי. הששי שיהיה
עם מנוחה וקלות הגוף.

אמר ג'אלינו': וכאשר חסר אחד מהם או יותר מאחד אין הגבול אמתי ולא שלם.

אמר המפרש: צריך לך שתשאל הנה תאמר איך ינוקה הליחה המחליאה בעצמה אחר הבשול   15
וביום הגבול ועל מצבו ולא יבא אחריו קלות ומנוחה הוא ראיה שכבר יגיעו התנאים החמשה
ולא יהיה עמו קלות ומנוחה כי ג'אלינו' יתנה תנאי שני והוא שיהיה עם קלות ומנוחה התשובה
שיתכן זה כשהפליג הנקיון ואף אם הוא מהמין שיצטרך יציאתו עם שאר התנאים מאחר
(כ)שהפליג לא יתחייב לו קלות ולא יהיה עמו מנוחה אבל חולשה ורכות מן הגוף וכבר יתכן
שיתעלף עלוף חזק ודע זה.   20

(1.21)

[48] אמר אבוקראט: הדברים הצריכים לנקותם ראוי שינוקו מן המקומות אשר הם נוטים
אליהם אבל האיברים הנאותים להנקות.

אמר המפרש: אמר ג'אלינו': הדברים הצריכים לנקותם הם הליחות המולידות לחליים אשר
יבוא בהם הגבול הבלתי שלם. והמקומות הנאותים לנקותם הם המעים והקיבה והשלפוחית
והרחם והעור ועם אלו גם כן החנכים והנחירים כשנרצה לנקות המוח. וצריך לרופא שיזכור   25

---

4 שיטעון: أَنْ تَحَرَّكَ a   7 הנידות: وَالدلك add. a   8 העובי: خلط a   11 על יד מוציא בחוזק:
بخراج a || המזיק: فقط add. a   12 במצב בקומה: على استقامة a   16 מצבו: استقامة a || ומנוחה:
لِأَنَّ جَالِينُوس يَشْتَرِطُ شَرْطًا سَادِسًا وَهُوَ أَنْ يَكُونَ مَعَ خِفٍّ وَرَاحَةٍ add. a   17 כי ג'אלינו' יתנה תנאי שני
והוא שיהיה עם קלות ומנוחה: om. a   22 אבל האיברים: بِالْأَعْضَاء a   25 החנכים: اللهوات a

בידיעת הטיית הטבע ואם מצא נטותה נגד הצד שיאות לנקיון ינקה בתקון מה שצריך אליה
יעזרנה. ואם ראה העניין בהפך זה וראה כי תנועתה תנועה מזקת)לא(ימנענה ויעתיקנה אל
הפך הצד אשר נטתה אליו. ואתן לזה משל: כשהיו בכבד כימוסים שחדשו חולי והצדדים
הנאותים שנטו אליהם שני צדדים: האחד לצד הקיבה וכאשר נטו אל זה הצד הנקותם בשלשול
יותר טוב משיהיה בקיא והצד השני)מ(צד הכליות והשלפוחית. ואמנם להטות הכימוסים
5 ההם אל צד החזה והריאה והלב אינו טוב.

(1.22)

[49] אמר אבוקרט: ראוי אמנם שתעשה הרפואה והתנועה אחר שתתבשל החולי ואמנם
מה שהתמיד נא בתחילת החולי אין צריך שיעשה זה אלא אם יהיה החולי מתעורר ואי אפשר
ברוב העניין שיהיה מתעורר.

אמר המפרש: אמר הרפואה ר״ל המשלשלת והחולי המתעורר הוא שיהיו הכימוסים עוקצים
10 לחולה והזיקוהו בחום שיהיה להם בחוזק ונזילתם מאבר לאבר בתחילת החולי ויכאיבוהו
ויחדשו לו עקיצה ולא יניחוהו לשקוט במקום אחד להיותם מתנועעים ונוזלים מאבר לאבר
וזה מעט מה שיהיה. ואמנם ברוב העניינים תהיינה הכימוסים נחות שוכנות באבר אחד ובאבר
ההוא יהיה בשולם באורך זמן החולי כלו עד שתחסור.

(1.23)

15 [50] אמר אבוקרט: לא יצטרך שיורה השיעור הראוי לנקותו מן הגוף מן רבויו. לכן צריך
להתמיד הנקיון בכל עת שהתמיד הדבר שצריך להריקו הוא אשר יריק ושהחולה יסבלנו בנקל
וקלות ובעת שיצטרך ויהיה הנקיון עד שיבואנו העלוף. ואמנם ראוי שיעשה זה כשיהיה החולה
סובלו.

אמר המפרש: (אמר) ג'אלינו: אם היה הדבר הגובר הוא שהורק אז גוף החולה יקל לו בהכרח
20 מפני זה. ואם הורק עם הדבר שיוצא מן הטבע דבר טבעי אז יבוא לחולה רפיון בהכרח ויחלש
כחו וירגיש צער וכובד. וצריך שיהיה הנקיון עד עת שיחדש עלוף בצמחים החדים אשר הם
בתכלית הגדול ובקדחות הדולקות מאד וכאבים החזקים בהפלגה. ותקדם על זה השיעור מן
הנקיון כשתהיה הכח חזקה. וכבר בחננו זה פעמים רבות אשר לא יסופר מרוב ומצאנוהו
מועיל תועלת חזקה ולא נדע בכאבים החזקים בהפלגה עזר גדול ומופלג מן ההרקה עד שיגיע
25 אל ההתעלפות אחר שיזהר וידע האם שיקיז עורק או הזיעה או אם יעשה השלשול
עד שיבא להתעלף.

---

1 ינקה בתקון מה שצריך אליה: أعدّ لها ما يحتاج إليه a   10 עוקצים: أقلقت a   12 עקיצה: قلقا a
14 בשולם: emendation editor: בשלום MSS   15 לכן: لكنّه a   16 להתמיד: أن يستغنم a   21 החדים:
الحارّة a   24 עזר: علاجا a   25 שיזהר (= أن تحذر): أن تحدّد a ‖ צריך לכן שיקיז עורק או הזיעה:
ينبغي أن يفصد عرق a

(1.24)

[51] אמר אבוקרט: כבר צריך בתחלואים החדים לפעמים שיעשה הרפואה המשלשלת
בתחלתה. וצריך שתעשה זה אחר שתקדם ותנהיג הענין על מה שיצטרך.

אמר המפרש: כבר נתבאר לנו שאין אנו רשאים לשלשל בתחלת החולי אלא בקצת החלאים
החדים והם החלאים המתבררים כמו שיבא לפנים. ועם זה צריך שיעשה בזהירות ובשמירה
גדולה ואחר תקנת הגוף מה שיתכן ואחר ידיעת דקות הליחות התערובויות. 5

אמר ג׳אלינו׳: הסכנה בנתינת הרפואות המשלשלות על זולת מה שראוי בתחלואים החדים
היא גדולה כי הסמנים המשלשלים כלם הם חמים ויבשים והקדחת מצד מה שהיא קדחת לא
יצטרך אל מה שיחמם וייבש אבל אמנם צריכה אל הפך זה ר״ל מה שיקרר וירטיב. ואמנם
יעשו זה כדי להסיר הכימוס הפועל לקדחת. וראוי שיהיו התועלות בהריק הכימוסים אשר
מהם נתחדש החולי יותר מן הנזקים אשר יבואו לגופים בזה הענין בסבת הסמנים המשלשלים. 10
ואמנם יהיו התועלות יותר כשיורק כל הכימוס בלי צער. וכבר צריך שתעיין החולה האם גוף
החולה מוכן מזומן לזה השלשול. כי אשר היה תחלת תחלואיהם מן עובי לחות רב או ממאכלים
דבקים עבים ואשר בהם מתחת הצלעות מתוח ונפוח או חום חזק מופלג או שיש לשם בקצת
המעים עם זה מורסא אין גוף אחד מאלו מזומנים לשלשול ויצטרך שלא יהיה זה דבר נמצא
ואם תהיינה הכימוסים בגוף החולה על הטוב שיתכן מקלות מרוצתם ר״ל שתהיינה רקיקות 15
ולא יהיה בהם דבר מן דביקות ושיהיו המעברים אשר יתפשט בהם מה שיצא בהשתלשלו
רחבים פתוחים שלא יהיה בהם דבר מן הסתומים. וכבר נעשה אנחנו זה הדבר ונכין הגוף בזה
הענין כשנרצה לשלשלו.

(1.25)

[52] אמר אבוקרט: כי הרקת הגוף מן המין שצריך שינקה יועיל זה ויקל סובלו ואם היה הענין
בהפך זה היה קשה. 20

אמר המפרש: זה הפרק נאמר כי אינו חזרת דברים למה שיכללהו הפרק ה׳ כי אותו הפרק
הוא במה שיורק מאליו וזה הפרק הוא במה שנריקנו אנחנו בסמים. וכאשר שם ג׳אלינו׳ הפרק
השני שיכלול שני העינים יחד נתחייב לתת סבה בהחזרת זה הפרק.

נשלם המאמר הראשון מפרקי אבוקרט.

---

1 לפעמים: في الندرة a 4 המתבררים: المتحاجة a 6 החדים: الحارّة a 9 כדי להסיר: لكان a 11 כל
הכימוס: الكيموس الضارّ a ‖ צער: أذى a ‖ החולה: أوّلا a 12 עובי לחות: تخم a 14 דבר זה: شيء
من هذا a 15 ואם: وأن a 16 אשר יתפשט בהם מה שיצא: التي تكون نفوذ ما يخرج a 17 הדבר:
وتقدّم add. a 21 ה׳: الثاني a 23 נתחייב: التجأ a

המאמר השני

(2.1)

[53] אמר אבוקרט: כשתהיה השינה בחלי מן החליים תחדש כאב זה מאותות מות.

אמר המפרש: ירצה באמרו כאב נזק ויש חליים ועתות מן החלי שתזיק בהם השינה ויצטרך
שיצוה החולה ביקיצה ואם ישן אז ינזק. ויש עתות שתועיל בהם השינה ואם ישן בהם החולה
וחידשה לו נזק זה אות מות כי תחת מה שקינו אל התועלת באתנו הנזק וזה אמנם יקרה
כאשר תהיינה ליחות הגוף רעות מאד וגוברות על החום היסודי. ואמנם החליים אשר תזיק
בהם השינה לעולם הוא בתחלת המורסות באיברים פנימיים או עם שפיכת החומר לקיבה או
בתחלת עונת הקדחת כ״ש כשיהיה עמו קור וסמור. והעתות אשר תועיל בהם השינה הוא
אחר סוף התחלת העונה והמורסא ובפרט בעת התכלית. והיותר מועילה שתהיה השינה הוא
עת הירידה ואם הזיקה בזו העת הוא אות מות. ואם הועילה לפי מה שהורה כבר על תועלת
השינה בזו העת לא יוסיף לנו בהוראה מאומה.

(2.2)

[54] אמר אבוקרט: כשהשקיט השינה ערבוב השכל זה אות יפה.

אמר המפרש: זה מורה על שהחום היסודי גבר על הכימוסים ונצחם.

(2.3)

[55] אמר אבוקרט: השינה והיקיצה כשעברה כל אחת מהם השיעור המכוון הוא אות רע.

אמר המפרש: זה מבואר.

(2.4)

[56] אמר אבוקרט: לא השובע ולא הרעב ולא זולתם מכלל הדברים משובח כשיעברו לשיעור
הטבעי.

אמר המפרש: זה מבואר.

(2.5)

[57] אמר אבוקרט: הליאות אשר לא יודע לו סבה יבִיט בחולי.

אמר המפרש: זה יורה על שהליחות כבר נתחדשו על בלתי המנהג הטבעי ולזה נזוקו מהם
האיברים או מרוע איכותם או מרוב כמותם ולזה יבִיט בחולי.

---

2 כשתהיה: النوم في مرض من الأمراض يحدث وجعا فذلك من علامات الموت وإذا كان a .add
19 יבִיט: يَنذرُ a 20 נתחדשו: تحرّكت a 21 יבִיט: يَنذرُ a

(2.6)

[58] אמר אבוקרט: מי שיכאיבהו דבר מגופו ולא ירגיש בכאבו מרוב עניניו ודאי שכלו מבולבל.

אמר המפרש: ירצה בכאב בכאן סבת הכאב כמו אם יהיה בחולה מורסא חמה או אדמדמת או מכה או פצע או חבורה והדומה לזה ולא ירגישנו ודאי שכלו מעורבב.

(2.7)

[59] אמר אבוקרט: הגופות אשר תכחשנה בזמן ארוך ראוי שיהיה החזרתם במזונות עד שישמנו בנחת והגופות אשר תכחשנה במעט זמן בזמן קצר. 5

אמר המפרש: וזה כי הגופות שכחשו בזמן מועט אמנם נתחדשה להם זאת הכחישות והרזות מהרקת הרטיבות לא מהתכת האיברים הנקפאים. ואמנם הגופים אשר כחשו וצמקו בזמן רב וכבר זב מהם הבשר ונתדקדק מהם וחלשו שאר האיברים אשר יהיה בהם ישול והתפשטות המזון בגוף והוליד הדם ולא יוכל שיבשל מן המזון השיעור שיצטרך אליו ולזה יצטרך שיוחזר 10 אל השמנות בזמן ארוך.

(2.8)

[60] אמר אבוקרט: הניצול מן החולי כשיקח מן המזון ולא יתחזק בו זה יורה על שעמס על גופו מן המזון יותר ממה שיסבול. וכאשר היה זה והוא לא יקח ממנו יורה על שגופו צריך אל ההרקה.

אמר המפרש: מבואר העלה בפרק אשר הודיענו כאשר הגוף הבלתי נקי כל מה שתזונהו 15 תוסיף בו רוע.

(2.9)

[61] אמר אבוקרט: כל גוף שתחפוץ לנקותו צריך שתשים מה שתחפוץ הוצאתו ממנו שיעבור בו בקלות.

אמר המפרש: יהיה זה כשירחיב ויפתח כל מעבריו ויחתוך וידקדק ויכין הרטיבות אשר בהם אם היה דבר מעובי וד(ב)קות. 20

(2.10)

[62] אמר אבוקרט: הגוף הבלתי נקי כל מה שתזוניהו תוסיף בו רוע.

---

4 או פצע: والفسخ a ‖ או חבורה: والشدخ a   15 מבואר: זה כי מבואר צ   19 ויכין: وتذيب a

אמר המפרש: מבואר העלה ורוב מה שיהיה זה הוא כשתהיה הקיבה מליאה מכימוסים
רעים ועם זה יקרה להם אשר זכר אבוקרט שיקרה לנמלטים מחולי והוא שלא יוכל ליקח
מן המאכלים.

(2.11)

[63] אמר אבוקרט: כשתמלא הגוף מן המשקים יותר נקל משתמלאנו מן מאכלים.

אמר המפרש: ר״ל הדברים הרטובים והמשקים אשר הם לגופינו מזון. וזה (כי) המזון הרטוב   5
וכ״ש אם היה חם בטבע יקל וימהר הזנתו לגוף.

(2.12)

[64] אמר אבוקרט: ההשארות אשר תשארנה מאחרי ימי הגבול מדרכן שתגברנה ותחזורנה
לחולי.

אמר המפרש: ברוב הענין תתעפש אותה ההשארות באורך הימים ותולד קדחת כי כל רטיבות
זרה מטבע הגשם אשר יקיף בה אי אפשר שתזונהא ולא יגיע ענינה אלא אל העפוש על הרוב.   10
וכאשר היה עם זה המקום אשר היא מקובצת בו חמימות יהיה שובב אל העפוש ביותר
מהירות ובחוזק.

(2.13)

[65] אמר אבוקרט: מי שיבואהו הגבול כבר יקשה עליו חליו בלילה שלפני בוא עונת הקדחת
שיבא בו הגבול ושוב בלילה שלאחריו יהיה יותר נקל.

אמר המפרש: עם הבדלת הטבע לדבר הרע מן הדבר הטוב והכין אותו אל הדחיה והיציאה   15
יחדש הפעמות שיצטער החולה ויכבד עליו חליו. וממנהג האנשים שישנו בלילה וכאשר מנע
ההצטערות ההוא מן השינה יתבאר סערת החולה)וראוי בהכרח עם אלי ההפעמות ההוא
בעבור השינה(וקושי חליו מבואר נגלה. וכבר זה יהיה ביום כשיהיה הגבול מוכן שיהיה בלילה
הבא אחריו. ואומרו יהיה יותר נקל מפני שרוב הגבולים יגיעו אל השלום.

(2.14)

[66] אמר אבוקרט: עם גרישת הבטן כבר יועיל התחלפות גווני הרעי כשלא יהיה שנויו אל   20
מינים המגונים ממנו.

אמר המפרש: כי רבוי גווניו מורה על הרקת מינים רבים מן הכימוסים והמינים המגונים הוא
שיהיה בו אותות התכת הגוף והוא הרעי השמן או מאותות העפוש והוא הריח המגונה.

---

7 תשארנה: מן الأمراض ‎.add. a‎   7–8 שתגברנה ותחזורנה לחולי: أن تجلب عودة من المرض ‎a‎
16 הפעמות: وواجب ضرورة عند هذا الاضطراب ‎.add. a‎

(2.15)

[67] אמר אבוקרט: כשנתמלא הגרון או שצמחו בגשמו שחין או אבעבועות צריך שתעיין
לרעי היוצא מן הגוף כי כשיהיה הגובר עליו המרה האדומה יהיה מזה חולאני ואם יהיה
מה שיצא מן הגוף כמו מה שיצא מגוף הבריא אז היה על השמירה מהתקדם על הזנת הגוף.

אמר המפרש: אמר ג׳אלינו׳: הגרון גם כן יקבל הכימוסים הבאים מהמוח. והשחין והאבעבועות
אמנם יתהוו בעבור התחמם הדם מפני המרה הכרכומית. וצריך שתתבקר ותעיין האם דחה
הטבע כל המותרות אל האיברים ההם אשר נכשלו ותדע זה כשהיה מה שיצא מן הגוף כמו
מה שיצא מגוף הבריא אין בהזנתו אז סכנה. ואם לא יהיה נקי מן הליחה עד תכליתו תמצא
הגובר על מה שיצא מן הגוף המרה וראוי אז שינוקה ויתרוקן קודם שיזון באשר הגוף כל מה
שתזונהו תוסיף בו רוע.

(2.16)

[68] אמר אבוקרט: כאשר יהיה באדם רעב אין ראוי שיתעמל.

אמר המפרש: עם מיעוט המזון יצטרך להרחיק ההתעמלות וסבת זה מבואר.

(2.17)

[69] אמר אבוקרט: כשירד על הגוף מזון יוצא מן הטבע הרבה זה יחדש חולי ויורה זה על
בריאותו.

אמר המפרש: יראה לי שכוונתו בזה הפרק שיספר בו כי כשיהיה המזון היורד על הגוף יוצא מן
הטבע יציאה רבה או יציאות האיכות יחדש אז חולי והגעת מה שיחדש מן החולי כפי שיעור
יציאתו אם יצא יציאה רבה חדש חולי גדול ואם היה יציאת המחליא יציאה מועטת יהיה החולי
מעט אמר ויורה שיעור על יציאתו במה שיורה מבריאותו כי כשהיתה היציאה מועטת יבריא
מהרה.

(2.18)

[70] אמר אבוקרט: מי שהיה מהדברים שיזונו מהרה בפתע גם יציאתו ימהר.

אמר המפרש: המופלג שבדברים כלם שיזונו מהרה בפתע גם יציאתו פתאום הוא היין ופי״
המהירות ר״ל אחר שתיתו בזמן מועט. ואמרו פתאום שיהיה תכף לירידתו בפעם אחת בגוף
יזונו לגוף כולו ולא ימשכוהו מעט מעט אבל פתאום.

---

1 כשנתמלא: اشتكى a ‖ בגשמו: في البدن a   3 על השמירה: على ثقة a   6 נכשלו: اعتلّت a   7 נקוי:
البدن a   8 הגוף: الذي ليس بالنقاء a. add.   15 יציאה רבה: الخروج في الكمية a   ‖ אז: emendation
editor או MSS ‖ והגעת: a ומבלغ ‖ מה: emendation editor מן MSS   20 גם יציאתו פתאום: a .om
22–21 תכף לירידתו בפעם אחת בגוף יזונו לגוף כולו: بعد أن يبتدى يغذو ويستوفي البدن غذاءها كلّه a

(2.19)

[71] אמר אבוקרט: ההקדמה לגזור בחליים החדים למות או לחיים לא תהיה בתכלית הדקדוק.

אמר המפרש: אמר ג'אלינו': הקדחת בחולי החד תהיה תמידית תכופה ברוב העיתים והמעט מן החליים חדים תהיינה בלתי קדחת כמו הפלג'.

(2.20)

[72] אמר אבוקרט: מי שהיה בבחרותו בטנו רך כשיזקין ייבש בטנו ומי שהיה בבחרותו יבש 5 הבטן כשיזקין ירך בטנו.

אמר המפרש: כשתבקש על האמת תדע כי זה הענין בלתי מחויב והוא דעת וגזירה כוזבת בלא ספק. והאמת אצלי כי אבוקרט ראה איש אחד או שנים קרה כך ושמהו גזירה מתמדת כמו שנהג מנהגו בספר הנכבד ספר אפידימיא אשר הסכימה ענין איש אחד או שנים תחזור אצלו הגזירה נשפטת על מין. זהו אצלי האמת. ואם לא תרצה זה ותרצה להשים לזה המאמר 10 הבלתי אמתי אופן אמתי ולהתנות לו תנאים ולרמוז לו רמיזות עליך זה כמו שזכר ג'אלינו' בזה הפרק.

(2.21)

[73] אמר אבוקרט: שתיית המשקה יכלה הרעב.

אמר המפרש: רוצה במשקה היין וירצה ברעב התאוה הכלביית כי שתיית היין אשר בו חום חזק יכלה זה הרעב ‹כי› התאוה הכלביית אמנם תהיה או מקור מזג הקיבה או מכימוס חמוץ 15 שוקה בגרמה והיין אשר זכרנוהו יכלה אלו השני ענינים יחד.

(2.22)

[74] אמר אבוקרט: ומי שהיה מן החליים שקרה מן המלוי תהיה רפואתו באשר יורק ומה שהיה מחודש מן ההרקה רפואתו יהיה בהמלאות.

אמר המפרש: זה מבואר.

(2.23)

[75] אמר אבוקרט: הגבול יבא בחליים החדים בארבע עשר יום.				20

---

2 הדקדוק (= الدقّة): الثقّة a 3 והמעט: فإنّ القليل a 9 אשר הסכימה: لأنّه باستقراء a 11 ולרמוז
לו רמיזות: وتفرض له فرضات ‖ זה כמו שזכר: بما ذكر a 13 יכלה: يشفي a 15 הקיבה: فقط add. a
18 בהמלאות: وشفاء سائر الأمراض يكون بالمضادّة add. a

אמר המפרש: אמר ג'אלינו': לא יעבור אחד מן החליים החדים אשר תנועתו תנועה אחת
ומהירה שיעבור י"ד יום. וכבר יבוא הגבול בהרבה מן החליים החדים באחד עשר יום ובתשיעי
ובשביעי ובחמישי. וכבר יבאו קצתם בששי אבל אינו משובח. והחליים אשר יבא בהם הגבול
השלם ביום הי"ד או קודם ומדרך אבוקרט שיקראם חלאים חדים במאמר משולח. ואמנם
החליים אשר יהיה בהם גבול חסר באחד מן הימים של הגבול הראשון ואחרי כן נשאר ממנו   5
השארות ישלם היות הגבול באחד מימי הגבול הנמנים עד יום הארבעים.

(2.24)

[76] אמר אבוקרט: הרביעי מביט בשביעי ותחלת השבוע השני הוא היום השמיני. והמביט
בי"ד הוא יום הי"א כי הוא הרביעי מן השבוע השני. והיום הי"ז גם כן הוא יום ההבטה כי הוא
הרביעי מן הי"ד והיום השביעי מן הי"א.

אמר המפרש: אמר ג'אלינו': היום הי"ז מביט בעשרים באשר יום העשרים הוא יום הגבול והוא   10
סוף השבוע השלישי.

(2.25)

[77] אמר אבוקרט: הקדחת הרביעית הקיציי ברוב העניין תהיה קצרה והחרפיי תארך וכ"ש
כשתגיע אל הסתיו.

אמר המפרש: לא הקדחת הרביעית לבד תהיה בקיץ קצרה אכן גם שאר החליים כי הכימוסים
יזובו ויתפשטו בכל הגוף ויתמוגגו ויתחייב מזה שלא יארך דבר מן החליים הקיציים. אבל   15
אבוקרט שם מאמרו בחולי יותר ארוך שבחליים כונתו להיות משל ויקרה בסתיו הפך זה
ר"ל שישכונו הכימוסים בעומק הגוף כמו אבן ותשארנה על חזקתן ואין החליים כלים כאשר
הכימוסים המולידים אותם נשארים ולא החליים ג"ב מתים באשר כחותם תשארנה ולא
תתמוגגנה.

(2.26)

[78] אמר אבוקרט: כשיהיה הקדחת אחר הקווץ יותר טוב מאשר יהיה הקווץ אחר הקדחת.   20

אמר המפרש: חולי הקיווץ יהיה ממילוי או מהרקה וכאשר יקרה הקווץ מן המלוי אמנם
יתמלאו העצבים מן הכימוס הנדבק הקר אשר ממנו הזנתו בהתחדש הקדחת אחר הקווץ.
הרבה פעמים תחמם הכימוס ותתיכהו ותדקדקהו ותמנעהו הקדחת ההיא. וכאשר קרה לאדם
קדחת שורפת ויבשה גופו כלו ועצביו ואחר כן קרה לו חולי הקווץ מפני היובש ודאי מכתו
אנושה.   25

1–2 תנועה אחת ומהירה: حركة حدّة وسرعة متصلة a   2 שיעבור י"ד יום: متّصلة هذا الحدّ a   6 הנמנים
(= الّتي تعدّ): الّتي بعد a   7 מביט: منذر a   8 ההבטה: إنذار a   16 כונתו להיות: فصيّره a
22 בהתחדש: وحدثت a   23 ותמנעהו: وتحلّله a   24–25 ודאי מכתו אנושה: فالآفة في ذلك عظيمة a

(2.27)

[79] אמר אבוקרט: אין ראוי לבטוח בקלות ימצאהו החולה בחלוף הדין ולא יבהילוך ענינים קשים יתחדשו על בלתי הקש כי רוב מה שיקרה מזה לא יעמד ולא יתקיים ולא יארך זמנו.

אמר המפרש: כאשר קרה חולי חזק ושוב הקל מעליו פתאום בלי קדימת בשול ולא הרקה לא תסמוך ולא תבטח על זה כי התערובות נתקררו ונקפאו וחסרו תנועותיהן לא זולת זה. וכן אם קדמה הבשול המבואר ושוב קרה אחריו השכל וכיוצא בזה לא יבהילוך כי הוא לא יתקיים 5 ורוב מה שיורה זה על פועל גבול משובח.

(2.28)

[80] אמר אבוקרט: מי שהיה בו הקדחת בלתי חלושה מאד אם ישאר גופו על ענינו לא יחסר ממנו כלום או יותך ביותר מן הראוי הוא רע כי הראשון יביט באורך חזלי והשני יורה על חלישות הכח.

אמר המפרש: צימוק הגוף לעולם הוא אות רע ומורה על חולשת הכח בין שהיה הקדחת בלתי 10 חלושה מאד או שהיתה הקדחת חזקה מאד.

(2.29)

[81] אמר אבוקרט: מי שהתמיד החולי בתחלתו ואם ראית שיתנועע דבר תניעהו. וכאשר היה החולי בתכליתו ראוי שיעמד החולה וינוח.

אמר המפרש: עוד יתן סבת זה בפרק שאחריו. ואמרו אם ראית שיתנועע דבר תניעהו ירצה בו ההקזה לבד ואיפשר גם כן על עשיית השלשול. ואין ראוי שיעשה אחד מאלו בעת 15 התכלית מהחולי כי בשול החולי יהיה בזו העת. והכחות הנפשיות תהיינה בזמן התכלית ברוב העינים רפויות. והטוב שבעזר על היות הבשול מהרה הוא לעשות ההקזה בהתחלת החולי כדי להקל מחמרו. ובעת התכלית הכחות החיוניות והכחות הטבעיות תשארנה על כחותיהן.

אמר המפרש: כבר קדם לך שלא יצטרך לשלשל בהתחלה אלא בחליים המתעוררים ומפני 20 זה אמר כך ואם ראית שיתנועע דבר תניעהו.

(2.30)

[82] אמר אבוקרט: כלל העינים בהתחלת החולי ובאחריתו הם יותר חלושים ובתכליתו יותר חזקים.

אמר המפרש: ירצה באמרו כלל הענינים המקריים כי הם בהתחלת החולי ובאחריתו יותר חלושים ר"ל עונות הקדחת והזיעה והכאב והמצוק והצמאון. ואמנם הענינים אשר יתחייבו מאלו המקרים והוא החולי יתחייב בהכרח שיהיה בעת התכלית יותר טוב כשיהיה החולי מן החליים אשר ימלטו.

(2.31)

5 [83] אמר אבוקרט: כאשר הקם מחליו יקח מהמאכלים ולא יתוסף גופו כלום זהו סימן רע.

אמר המפרש: זה מבואר וכבר קדם הענין.

(2.32)

[84] אמר אבוקרט: ברוב העתים כל מי שעניינו ברע ויקח מן המאכלים ולא יתוסף גופו כלל הנה באחריתו באשר לא (יקח) מן המאכלים. ואמנם מי שנמנע מתחלת ענינו הלקיחה מהמאכלים מניעה חזקה ואחר כך יקבל ממנו באחרונה ודאי ענינו יהיה יותר טוב.

10 אמר המפרש: המאמר הנה בקם מחליו ומבואר הוא כי מפני רוע מזג או השארות התערובות לא התחזקו איבריו ותאותו גדולה והוא אוכל ויתוספו התערובות או יתחזק רוע המזג ועדין תתבטל התאוה. וכאשר היה בתחלה לא יכסוף בעבור שהטבע מתעסק בבשול ומעת שמתחיל לכסוף תדע שכבר נתבשלו התערובות ודאי ענינו על הרוב לטוב.

(2.33)

[85] אמר אבוקרט: בריאות המחשבה בכל חולי אות טוב. וכן החריצה למאכל. והפך זה אות מגונה.

15

אמר המפרש: זה מבואר וכבר נתבאר זאת העלה בפרקים שחברתים.

(2.34)

[86] אמר אבוקרט: כאשר היה החולי נמשך אחר טבע החולי ושנותיו וגויתו והעת ההווה מעתות השנה אז סכנתו פחות מסכנת החולי אשר היה בלתי נמשך לאחד מאלו התנאים.

אמר המפרש: זה מבואר כי כשלא יהיה נמשך ונאות הוא אות על יציאה רבה משווי זה האיש.

2 يتحيّبو: تكون a ‖ 3–4 החולי מן החליים: المريض من المرضى a ‖ 8 באחריתו באשר: بآخره يؤول أمره إلى أن a ‖ (יקח): يحظى a ‖ 11 לא התחזקו: لم تغتذ a ‖ 11–12 ועדין תתבטל: فتستبطل a ‖ 13 ודאי ענינו: فتستمر حاله a ‖ 14 החריצה: الهشاشة a ‖ 17 נמשך אחר טבע החולי: ملائمًا لطبيعة المريض a ‖ וגויתו: وسحنته a ‖ 18 התנאים: الخصال

(2.35)

[87] אמר אבוקרט: היותר טוב בכל חולי שיהיה סביב הטבור ושפל הבטן יש בו עובי וכשהיה
דק מאד ודל הוא רע. וכשהיה כך והשלשול עמו הוא בסכנה.

אמר המפרש: שפל הבטן הוא מה שבין בית הערוה והטבור כי חלקי הבטן שלושה: המקום
אשר מתחת לצלעות ומה שאצל הטיבור ושפל הבטן. וכשהיו המקומות ההם עבים היה
העניין יותר טוב וכשהיו מצומקים היה העניין יותר רע וזה כי הוא אות וסבה רעה. אמנם רוע
האות בהיותו מורה על חולשת האיברים ההם אשר דקקן ונתכו. ואמנם רוע הסבה כי הזנת
המאכלים בקיבה והולדת הדם בכבד אי יהיו עם זה העניין כמו שצריך כי שני האיברים האלו
יתועלו בעובי מה שיכסה ושומנו כדי שיחמם.

(2.36)

[88] אמר אבוקרט: מי שהיה גופו בריא ונשתלשל או הקיא על ידי סם יקרב אליו העלוף. וכן
מי שנזון במזון רע,)עם עשיית הסם המשלשלת והמקיא.(

אמר המפרש: וכן מי שנזון במזון רע כשהקיא או השתלשל יקרב אליו העלוף כי בגופתם מותר
רע. וכשיפגשהו הסם פגישה כל שהוא תתבאר רעתו. זהו סבת ג׳אלינו׳. ואשר יראה לי בסבה
זו כי כי אשר יתמיד במזוונות הרעים והעלולים דמו דם מגונה מאד נפסד האיכות. והכשימשוך
הדם בכח המושכת הניע כל הדם שבו)ו(ירצה לסלק מעליו כל פסולותיו הרבה מאד מעורבים
אבל הם הרכבת חיי האיש הלזה להפסד ההנהגה שהנהיג. ויבא העלוף בהכרח לכח המושך
ורוב מה שישתדל למשכו והוא מעורב ומבולבל.

(2.37)

[89] אמר אבוקרט: מי שהיה גופו בריא עשיית הסם בו יקשה.

אמר המפרש: הבריאים כשיעשו הקיא או השלשול יקרה להם סבוב והמיה ויקשה צאת מה
שיצא מהם וימהר להם עם זה העלוף כי הסם תשתדל להמשכת הכימוס הניאות המחובר
לו וכשלוא מצאהו ימשוך הבשר)והדם(ויתעבום להסיר מהם מה שבם ממה שיאות
לו.

---

5 מצומקים: أهزل a   5–6 וסבה רעה. אמנם רוע האות בהיותו מורה על חולשת: צ .om   6 כי
הזנת: emendation editor כנתקן צ בותקין(?) ק   8 כדי שיחמם: بتسخينه لهما a   9 יקרב: أسرع
a   11 יקרב: أسرع a   12 וכשיפגשהו הסם פגישה כל שהוא: فإذا أثاره أدنى إثارة a ‖ סבת:
تعليل a   13 והעלולים: a .om   14 הדם: الدواء a ‖ מעורבים: ومتحدة a   15 הרכבת: مركب
a ‖ להפסד ההנהגה שהנהיג: الفاسد التدبير a   16 מעורב ומבולבל: متحد مختلط a   18 והמיה: ومغص
a   19–20 המחובר לו: a .om   20 הבשר)והדם(: الدم واللحم a

(2.38)

[90] אמר אבוקרט: מי שהיה מן המאכלים והמשקיות מגונה מעט אלא שהוא)יותר נמאס(
ינעם יותר ראוי שיובחר עליו מה שהוא מהם יותר משובח אלא שהוא יותר נמאס.

אמר המפרש: זה מבואר כי עכול הנעים הוא ייטב יותר.

(2.39)

[91] אמר אבוקרט: הזקנים הכהולים ברוב העניין יחלו פחות ממה שיחלו הבחורים אלא מה
5 שיקרה להם מן החליים הישנים ברוב העניין ימותו בעודם בהם.

אמר המפרש: הזקנים הכהולים הם יותר תופסים לעצמם הנהגה מן הבחורים והכחות בגופות
הזקנים חלושות לא יוכלו לבשל החליים מהרה והחליים הישנים כולם קרים ולזה יתחייב בם
המות.

(2.40)

[92] אמר אבוקרט: מי שיקרה מנזילה וירידת מים לישישים לא יתבשלו.

10 אמר המפרש: לא אלו התחלואים לבד אבל שאר מה שיקרה להם מן הליחות הקרות.

(2.41)

[93] אמר אבוקרט: מי שימצאהו פעמים רבות עלוף חזק מבלתי סבה נגלית הנה הוא ימות
פתאום.

אמר המפרש: מי שימצאהו עלוף באלו התנאים השלשה הוא שיהיה בלי סבה נראית וחזק
ופעמים רבות באמת ימצאהו זה מפני חולשת הכחות החיוניות.

(2.42)

15 [94] אמר אבוקרט: השתוק כשתהיה חזקה אי אפשר שיבריא בעליה ממנה וכשתהיה
חלושה לא יקל להבריא.

אמר המפרש: כל חולי השתוק אמנם תהיה כשלא יוכל הרוח הנפשיי לעבור אל מה שתחת
הראש מן הגוף או ממדוה מסוג המורסא נתחדש במוח או שבטני המוח נתמלאו מן רטיבות
הלבנה. ואם נעדר הנשתק מתנועת החזה זהו הגדול והיותר מסוכן שבהם. וכשיתנשם בתכלית
20 הרפיון זה השתוק חזק ג"כ. וכשיהיה נשימתו נשימה בלתי נעלמת ובלתי רפויה אלא שהיא

---

2 עליו מה: على ما a ‖ 4 הזקנים הכהולים: الكهول a ‖ 6 הם יותר תופסים לעצמם הנהגה: أضبط
لأنفسهم في التدبير a ‖ 9 שיקרה: من البحوحة a. add ‖ מנזילה וירידת מים: والنزل a ‖ לישישים: للشيخ
الفاني a ‖ 14 באמת: وإنّما a ‖ 18 שבטני: MSS emendation editor: שבטן ‖ 20 הרפיון: الاستكراه
a ‖ בלתי נעלמת ובלתי רפויה: من غير مجاهدة واستكراه a

מתחלפת בלתי מחוברת לסדר אחד אז שיתוקו ג״כ חזקה אלא שהיא חלושה יותר מן השניה. וכאשר בעליה ינשום נשימה מחוברת אז שיתוקו היא חלושה. ואם תשגיח בעניניו כל מה שראוי לעשותו אולי יבריא.

(2.43)

[95] אמר אבוקרט: אשר יחנקו ויבאו אל גדר העלוף ולא יגיע אל גדר המות לא יבריא מהם מי שנראה בפיו קצף. 5

אמר המפרש: זוכר ג׳אלינו׳ כי קצת ממי שנחנק ונראה קצף בפיהו הבריא אלא שזה לפעמים.

(2.44)

[96] אמר אבוקרט: מי שהיה גופו עב מאד בטבע ימהר אליו המות יותר ממי שגופו רזה.

אמר המפרש: עלת זה מבוארת לצרות העורקים ורוחבם כמו שנתבאר במזגים. אמר גאלינוס: כי שהיה הגוף טוב הבשר מיושר עד שלא יהיה עבה ולא רזה הוא המשובח ויותר יתכן שיחיה ויגיע מן הישישות בתכליתם. 10

(2.45)

[97] אמר אבוקרט: בעלי הכפייה כשהיה חדש בריאותו מעט יהיה בפרט בהעתקתו בשנים והאויר והעיר וההנהגה.

אמר המפרש: הכפיה והשתוק הכימוס הגורם לשניהם הוא הקור והעובי. וכשיעתק בעיר והשנים וההנהגה אל החום והיובש ויעתק ג״כ מן ההנהגה הרעה אשר הולידה הליחה הזאת אל הפך זאת ההנהגה אולי יבריא. 15

(2.46)

[98] אמר אבוקרט: כשהיו שני כאבים ביחד ואינם במקום אחד החזק שבהם יעלים האחר.

אמר המפרש: ההתעוררות הטבעי לצד האבר אשר בו הצער הגדול יותר יחסר הרגשת האבר האחר ולא ירגיש במה שבו מן הצער שיכאיבהו.

(2.47)

[99] אמר אבוקרט: בעת התילדות המוגלא יקרה הכאב והקדחת יותר ממה שיקרה אחר התילדה. 20

---

2 מחוברת: لازما لنظام a لنظام 6 שנחנק: خنق أو اختنق a שיחיה: emendation editor שיהיה MSS
11 מעט: om. a 12 והאויר: om. a 17 ההתעוררות הטבעי: إذا اتّجهت الطبيعة a ‖ הרגשת: الموضع
18 מן הצער: مّا add. a

אמר המפרש: כי אז ימתח מקום המורסא יותר ויחזק הכאב ויטה החום היסודי לצד הכימוס
לבשלו ויתפשט יותר ויתחזק הקדחת.

(2.48)

[100] אמר אבוקרט: אמנם בכל תנועה יניעה הגוף ותשכינהו עת שיתחיל בו הליאות תמנעהו
מהתחדש בו הליאות.

5   אמר המפרש: זה מבואר.

(2.49)

[101] אמר אבוקרט: מי שנהג בטורח אחד ואף אם הוא כחוש הגוף מאד או ישיש יותר סובל
לטורח ההוא אשר רגל בו ממי שלא רגל בו ואף כי היה כי איש גבור וחזק.

אמר המפרש: זה מובן.

(2.50)

[102] אמר אבוקרט: מי שכבר הנהיגו המזון מאורך הזמן ואף אם יזיק יותר ממי שלא הנהיגו
10   ודאי יקל עליו נזקו. וכבר ראוי שיעתק האדם אל מה שלא נהגו.

אמר המפרש: הקדים הקדמה צודקת והוליד בעבורה ואשר הוליד הוא שכל מי שירצה
להתמיד הבריאות בכל העתים ירגיל עצמו מהרגל להרגל בהדרגה. אמר ג'אלינו': היות הטוב
לכל אחד מבני אדם הוא שירגיל את עצמו לנסות כל דבר עד שלא יחסר לו בעת ההכרח דבר
שלא הרגילו ויבואהו נזק גדול. ואמנם יהיה זה כשלא ישאר האדם על מה שהרגילו תמיד אבל
15   יצא את עצמו בקצת העתים על הפכו.

(2.51)

[103] אמר אבוקרט: עשות ההרבה פתאום ממה שימלא הגוף או יריקהו או יחממו או יקררו
או יניעהו במין אחר מן התנועה אי זה מין שיהיה יסתכן. וכל מה שהוא הרבה הוא נגד הטבעי
וכל מה שיהיה מעט הוא בטוח כשתרצה להעתיק מדבר אל זולתו.

אמר המפר: זה מפורש.

1 היסודי: om. a   3 ותשכינהו: فإراحته a   6 כחוש: ضعيف a   7 איש גבור וחזק: كان قويّا شابّا
a   9 מי שכבר הנהיגו המזון: ما قد اعتاده الإنسان a   11–12 והוליד בעבורה ואשר הוליד הוא שכל
מי שירצה להתמיד הבריאות: وألزم عنها وعمّا يلزم من استدامة الصحّة a   12 עצמו: الانتقال add. a
13 שירגיל את עצמו: أن يحمل نفسه a ‖ יחסר לו: يصادفه a   15 יצא את עצמו: يحمل نفسه a   17 יסתכן:
خطر a   18 זולתו: ومتى أردت غير ذلك add. a

(2.52)

[104] אמר אבוקרט: אם עשית כל מה שראוי לעשותו לפי מה שצריך ולא יהיה מה שצריך
שיהיה לא תעתק אל זולת מה שאתה עליו כל שהתמיד מה שראיתיו מתחלת הענין קיים.

אמר המפרש: זה הפרק כולל דרך עצום מדרכי הרפואה ולא הפליג ג׳אלינו׳ בפירושו כל צרכו.
ופי׳ זה הוא כאשר הורוך האותות על דרך משל שהוא צריך שיתחמם והתמדת בחמום ולא
הבריא החולה אין ראוי לך שתעתק אל הסדור אבל תשתדל אל החמום כל עו׳ שראית העניינים   5
המורים על עשיית החמום קיימים. וזהו פירוש אמרו כל עוד שהתמיד מה שראית מתחלת
הענין קיים. זהו ענין אמרו כלום שלא תעתק ממין ההנהגה אבל צריך בהכרח שתעתק מסם
מחמם אל סם אחר מחמם ותהפך בסמנים הנפרדים והמרכבים אשר הם כולם מחממים כי
כשילמד הגשם סם אחד תמיד יקל רשומו עליו. ועו׳ כי בהתחלף מיני הסמנים שאכויותיהם
אחד נאותות למזג איש איש למזג אבר אבר ולמקרי חולי חולי. וזהו שרש גדול מסודות   10
הרפואות. וזהו הצד בעצמו יצדד במזונות ובמיני מה שינוקה בם הליחה ההיא המחלאיה או
בהתכה או בדיקוק או לבשל או לעבות החומר או להקפיא תמציד לעולם לצד ההנהגה אשר
הורו עליו ההוראות הקיימים ותהפך במיני המזונות והסמנים מצד אחד. והבן זה.

(2.53)

[105] אמר אבוקרט: מי שהיה בטנו רך בכל עוד שהוא בחור ייטב עניינו יותר ממי שבטנו יבש
ושוב יגיע עניינו בעת הישישות אל ענין יותר רע וזה כי בטנו ייבש כשיזקין על הרוב.   15

אמר המפרש: כבר קדם לנו זה הדעת ברכות הבטן ויבשותו בשנות הבחרות והישישות.
וג׳אלינו׳ ישתדל לתת סבת זה וכבר אמרתי מה שבדעתי ורך הטבע לעולם בכל השנים מסבות
התמדת הבריאות וכל יובש רע לבריאים ולחולים.

(2.54)

[106] אמר אבוקרט: גודל הגוף בבחורים אין למאסו אבל יאהב אבל שהיא יכבד עם הישישות
ויקשה סובלו ויהיה יותר רע מן הגוף אשר הוא חסר ממנו.   20

אמר המפרש: ג׳אלינו׳ יחשוב שרצה באמרו הנה גודל הגוף אורך הגוף עד שלא יהיה זה גזירה
שהיא שקר.

נשלם המאמר השני מפרקי אבוקרט.

3 הפליג: يَبلُغ a   5 אל הסדור: للتدبير a   6 שראית: emendation editor   שראיתיו MSS   7 כלום:
يعني a   9 כשילמד: متى ألف a   10 נאותות: عظيمة add. a   11 וזהו הצד בעצמו יצדד: وهذا النحو
بعينه يخص a יסדר צק add.   13 והסמנים מצד אחד: والأغذية التي هي كلّها من قبيل واحد a   18 יובש:
في الطبع a add.   20 סובלו: استعماله a   22 שקר: وهم محض a

המאמר השלישי

(3.1)

[107] אמר אבוקרט: התהפכות עתות השנה ממה שיעשה בהולדת החליים מיוחד ובעת האחד מהם השנוי החזק בקור או החום וכן בשאר העניינים על זה ההקש.

אמר המפרש: ר״ל שנוי טבעי הפרקים כמו שהיה פרק הסתיו חם או פרק הקיץ קר וכיוצא
בהם. וכן שנוי העת האחד ממזגו כשהיה חזק ואע״פ ששאר הפרקים לא נשתנו ודאי יוליד 5
תחלואים.

(3.2)

[108] אמר בקראט: כי מן הטבעים מה שיהיה בקיץ יותר טוב ובסתיו יותר רע ומהם מה שיהיה
עניינו בסתיו יותר טוב ובקיץ יותר רע.

אמר המפרש: ירצה באמרו מן הטבעים ממזגי האדם וזה מבואר כי בסתיו ייטב עניני החמים
ובקיץ ייטב עניני הקרים והקש על זה. 10

(3.3)

[109] אמר אבוקרט: כל אחד מן התחלואים עניינו עם דבר בלתי דבר ייטיב וירע. וקצת השנים
עם עתות מהשנה והעיירות ומינים מן המנהגות.

אמר המפרש: זה הפרק כשתסדר מילותיו יתבאר ביאור נכון וברור וכן סידורו כל אחד מן
התחלואים יהיה עניינו עם שנה בלתי שנה או עם עיר בלתי עיר או עם עת מהשנה בלתי עת
או עם הנהגה בלתי הנהגה למוטב או לרוע. דמיון זה כי בעל החולי הקר עם שנות הבחרות 15
ובעת הקיץ ובעיר החמה ובהנהגה חמה מוטב ובהפך זה הוא יותר רע. אמנם בעל השנים ישר
המזג ודאי הנהגת היושר והעת והעיר הישרים יאותו לו יותר. וכי בעל זה המזג לבדו הוא אשר
יתוקן עניינו במה שדומה לו. ואמנם בעלי המזג הנוטים מן היושר גם העיירות והעתות ומיני
ההנהגה ההפכיים להם הם יאותו להם יותר.

אמר אבוקרט: כי מן הטבעים מה שיהיה בקיץ יותר טוב ובסתיו יותר רע ומהם מה שיהיה 20
עניינו בסתיו יותר טוב ובקיץ יותר רע.

אמר המפרש: ירצה באמרו מן הטבעים ממזגי האדם וזה מבואר כי בסתיו ייטב עניני החמים
ובקיץ ייטב עניני הקרים והקש על זה.

---

16 ובהפך זה הוא יותר רע: والمثل الخارج عن الاعتدال عند المثل الخارج عن الاعتدال في تلك الجهة أردأ
a ‖ בעל emendation editor: עול MSS 20 אמר ... רע: a .om 23–22 אמר ... זה: a .om

(3.4)

[110] אמר אבוקרט: כשהיתה באי זה עת מעתות השנה פעם אחד חם ופעם קר יפלו מקרים
חוליים חורפיים.

אמר המפרש: זה מבואר.

(3.5)

[111] אמר אבוקרט: הרוח הדרומי יחדש כובד בשמיעה וסנויריות בראות וכובד בראש
ועצלות ורפיון. ועם כח זה הרוח ותגבורתו יקרה לחולים אלו המקרים. ואמנם הצפונים יחדשו   5
שעול וכאב הגרון ויובש הבטן וקושי ההשתנה והסמור וכאב הצלעות והחזה ועם תגבורת זה
הרוח וכחו ראוי שיפלו בחוליים חדשי אלו המקרים.

אמר המפרש: רוח דרומי חם ולח ולזה ירדים החושים וירטיב התחלת העצבים ויחדש העצלות
וקושי התנועה ורוח צפוני קר ויבש וישעיר הגרון והחזה ומגבת הבטן ויעבה המעברים ויחדש
כל מה שזכר.   10

(3.6)

[112] אמר אבוקרט: כשיהיה הקיץ דומה לאביב תפול בקדחות זיעה רבה.

אמר המפרש: ראוי כשהקיץ יבש חזק היובש אז יכין ויתיך הרטיבות. וכשיהיה דומה לאביב
ימשיך הרטיבות לרוב חמימותו אל מה שסמוך לעור ואי אפשר להתיכה בדרך קיטור בעבור
רטיבותו ומפני כי הרטיבות ההיא בעת הגבול והחלאים תורק בפתע יתהווה ממנה זיעה
רבה.   15

(3.7)

[113] אמר אבוקרט: בהעצר המטר יתחדשו חליים חדים ואם הגדיל העצירה בשנה ההיא
ואח״כ קרה באויר ענין יובש אז ראוי שיפלו ברוב אלו העניינים החליים האלו והדומה
להם.

אמר המפרש: מבואר הוא כי בהעצר המטר יתיבשו הליחות ויתחדשו הקדחות מעטי המניין
מחודדי האיכות.   20

(3.8)

[114] אמר אבוקרט: כשיהיו עתות השנה מחוברים לסדריהם והיה בכל עת מהם מה
שראוי שיהיה בו גם מה שיחודשו בהם מן התחלואים ייטב עמידתם וסדרם בגבול יפה.

_____

1 השנה: في يوم واحد a .add   8 ירדים: تكذّر a   9 וישעיר: فتخشّن a   10 כל: a .om   11 תפול: فتوقّع
a   12 ראוי: editor emendation ודאי MSS واجب a ‖ יכין: تهى a   16 חליים: حمّيات a   17 שיפלו:
أن يتوقّع a   22 גם: a .om

וכשהיו עתות השנה בלתי נאותים מחוברים לסדריהם יהיה מה שיתחדש בהם מן התחלואים
בלתי מסודרי הגבול.

אמר המפרש: זה מבואר.

(3.9)

[115] אמר אבוקרט: כי בחורף יהיו החליים יותר חדים ממה שיהיו ויותר ממיתים ברוב הענין
5   ואמנם האביב היותר בריא שבעתות החליים ומעטי המות.

אמר המפרש: האביב שוה וישר והחורף הוא בתכלית החלוף.

(3.10)

[116] אמר אבוקרט: החורף לבעלי הכליה רע.

אמר המפרש: להיותו קר ויבש מתחלף המזג ויזיק למושחתים מחולי הרבה.

(3.11)

[117] אמר אבוקרט: ואמנם בעתות השנה אספר בו: כשיהיה הסתיו במעט מטר
10   ורוח צפוני והיה האביב מגשים רוח דרומי ראוי בהכרח שיתחדש בקיץ קדחות חדות
ומורסות העין ושלשול הדם ורוב מה שיקרה שלשול הדם לנשים ולבעלי הטבעים
הרטובים.

אמר המפרש: זה מבואר אחר ידיעת שרשי המלאכה.

(3.12)

[118] אמר אבוקרט: וכשיהיה הסתיו דרומי ממטיר בצירוף והיה האביב מעט המטר
15   הצפוני דע כי הנשים ההרות כשיארך הריונם עד האביב מפילות מחמת סבה כל
שהוא. וההרות תלדנה מהם ילדים קטנים כחושי התנועה עטופים עד כי המה או
ימותו מיד או ישארו דלים צמוקים עטופים כל ימי חייהם. ואמנם שאר בני אדם יקרה
להם שלשול הדם ומורסת עין יבשה. והזקנים הכהולים יקרה להם מן הנזילה שיאבדו
מהר.

---

1 נאותים מחוברים: לازمة a   2 בלתי מסודרי הגבול: غير منتظم سمج البحران a   5 החליים: om. a
7 הכליה: السلّ a   8 למושחתים מחולי: للمسلولين a   11 ומורסות העין: ورمد a   14 בצירוף: دفعًا a
15 כשיארך הריונם: اللواتي تشقّ ولادتهنّ a   16 כחושי: ضعاف a ‖ עטופים: مسقامة a   17 עטופים:
مسقامة a

(3.13)

[119] אמר אבוקרט: וכשיהיה הקיץ מעט המטר צפוני ויהיה החורף ממטיר דרומי יקרה בסתיו מכאובי הראש חזקים ושעול ונמיכות קול וסתומי הנחירים ויקרה לקצת בני אדם הכליה.

(3.14)

[120] אמר אבוקרט: ואם יהיה צפוני ויבש יאות למי שטבעו רטוב ולנשים. ואמנם שאר האנשים יקרה להם מורסת עין יבשה וקדחות חדות וסתום הנחירים ישנה. ומהם מי שיקרה להם בלבול הדאגה השחורי שיארע מהמרה השחורה.

(3.15)

[121] אמר אבוקרט: כי מעניני האויר בשנה בכלל המיעוט המטר ביותר בריא מרבוי המטר ופחות ממית.

(3.16)

[122] אמר אבוקרט: ואמנם התחלואים המתחדשים בעבור רוב המטר ברוב העניינים הם קדחות ארוכות וגרישת הבטן ועפוש ומכאובי הראש ושתוק ואסכרה. ואמנם התחלואים המתחדשים בעבור מיעוט המטר הם הכליה ומורסת העין וכאב הפרקים וקושי השתן ושלשול הדם.

אמ' המפרש: כל מה שזכרו אבוקרט באלו החמשה פרקים מחמת החלופים הפלוניים יתחדש במין פלוני מבני אדם כשיהיה האויר כך אין זה תמיד בשום פנים ולזה אין צורך לתת סבה עליהם על פי חכמת עיון הפילוסופים אבן ג׳אלינו׳ רצה לתת סבה לכל אלה. ובכלל כי עם מה שתגיע מלאכת הרפואה מידיעת טבעי הפרקים והאנשים וסבות החליים באשר הרטיבות חומר העיפוש והחמימות תפעל בו נקל לתת סבות כל מה שזכר כאשר יקרה.

(3.17)

[123] אמר אבוקרט: ואמנם עניני האויר בכל יום יום מה שיהיה מהם צפוני הוא יקבץ הגויות ויקמץ ויחזקם וייטיב תנועותיהם וייפה מראיהם ויזכך השמע בהם וייבש הבטן ויחדש בעין עקיצה. ואם היה לעומת החזה כאב קדמוני יעוררהו ויוסיף עליו. ומה שהיה מהם דרומי הוא יתיך הגויות וירפם וירטיבם ויחדש כובד בראש וסתום בעינים ובכל הגוף קושי התנועה וירפה הבטן.

אמר המפרש: ידוע כי הצפוני קר ויבש והדרומי חם ולח וכל זה מבואר.

2 ונמיכות קול: وبحوحة a ‖ וסתומי הנחירים: وزكام a ‖ הכליה: السلّ a 4 וסתום הנחירים: وزكام a 5 בלבול הדאגה השחורי: الوسواس السوداوي a 9 ומכאובי הראש (= وصداع): وصرع a 10 הכליה: سلّ a 15 מה שתגיע מלאכת הרפואה: ما تأصّل في الصناعة الطبّية a 16 כאשר: مأشر צ 18 ויקמצם: وشّدها a 19 לעומת: في نواحي a 20 בראש: وثقلا في السمع a add. ‖ וסתום (= وسددا): وسددا a

(3.18)

[124] אמר אבוקרט: ואמנם בעתות השנה דע כי באביב ותחלת הקיץ יהיו הבחורים ואשר קרוב להם בשנים על מיטב ענייניהם ובהשלמת הבריאות. ובנשאר מן הקיץ ובקצה החורף יהיו הישישים ביופי ענינם. ובנשאר מן החורף ובסתיו יהיו הממוצעים ביניהם בשנים בענין טוב.

אמ' המפרש: כבר קדם לנו סבת זה בפרק אשר שנינו סדר מלותיו.

(3.19)

[125] אמר אבוקרט: והתחלואים כולם יתחדשו בעתות השנה כולם אלא שקצתם בקצת העתות יותר מן הדין שיתחדש בו ויתעורר.

אמר המפרש: זה מבואר.

(3.20)

[126] אמר אבוקרט: כבר יקרה באביב הדאגה השחורי והשטות וחולי הנופל והשתוק ונביעת הדם והאסכרה וסתום הנחירים ונמיכות הקול והשעול והחולי אשר יופשט בעבורו הגלד והילפת והבהק והכתמים גדולים אשר יתנגעו והאבעבועות וכאב הפרקים.

אמר המפרש: זה הפרק מבואר ממה שקדמו בפרק שלפניו וזה כי זכר בפרק הקודם לזה שכבר יתחדש כל מין ממיני החליים בכל פרק מפרקי השנה אכן קצת התחלואים בקצת הפרקים מהשנה יותר בדין כלומר שיתחדשו על הרוב באלו הפרקים. והשלים זה הענין בשאמר שכבר יתחדש באביב אשר הוא המיושר והשוה שבפרקים חוליים שחוריים כמו הדאגה השחורי והשטות וחליים לבנים והנכפה וסתום האף ונמיכות הקול והשעול וחליים מכורכמים ככתמים אשר יתנגע בהם הגלד והאבעבועות וחליים דמיים כהגרת הדם והאסכרה. ואמנם החליים המיוחדים באביב הם הנמשכים אחר זיבת הליחות ונביעתם לחוץ ותנועת הטבע לדחותם בכח. וכן הפרק שלאחר זה הוא נבנה על מה שביארתיו מהיות התחלואים כבר יתחדשו על חלוף טבע הפרק.

(3.21)

[127] אמר אבוקרט: ואמנם בקיץ יקרה להם קצת אלו התחלואים וקדחת תמידית ושורפת ושלישית הרבה וקיא ודפיקה ומורסת העין וכאב האזן ונגעים בפה ועפוש בנגעים ובשר מת.

8 השחורי: emendation editor השחרחורי MSS ‖ והשתוק (= والسكتة A:(A om. a 9 וסתום
הנחירים: والزكام a ‖ והחולי אשר יופשט בעבורו הגלד: والعلّة التي يتقشّر فيها الجلد a 10 והילפת:
والقوابي a ‖ והכתמים גדולים: والبثور الكثيرة a 15 והנכפה: الصرع a ‖ וסתום האף: والزكام a
16 ככתמים אשר יתנגע בהם הגלד: كالبثور التي يتقرّح فيها الجلد a 21 ודפיקה: وذرب a ‖ בנגעים
(= في القروح Arabic MSS): في الفروج emendation editor 22–21 ובשר מת: وحصف a

(3.22)

[128] אמר אבוקרט: ואמנם בחורף יקרה הרבה מתחלואי הקיץ וקדחת רביעית ארוכה
ומעורבת והטחול והשקוי והטפת השתן ושלשול הדם וחלקת המעים וכאב הירכים והאסכרה
ונזילה על הריאה וחולי מעים החזק אשר יקראוהו היונים איליאוש והכפיה והדאגה השחורי
והשטות.

5 אמר המפרש: כל זה מבואר ממה שקדמנו.

(3.23)

[129] אמר אבוקרט: ואמנם בסתיו יקרה חולי הצד והשטות וחולי הריאה וסיתום האף
ונמיכות הקול והשעול וכאב הצדדים והכסלים ומכאוב הראש והסתום והשתוק.

אמר המפרש: זה נבנה גם כן על מה שקדם שכבר יתחדש בסתיו חליים מיוחדים בו על הרוב
כסתום האף ונמיכות הקול והשתוק וחליים שאינם מטבעו כחולי הצד.

(3.24)

10 [130] אמר אבוקרט: ואמנם בשנים יקרו אלו המקרים: אמנם הילדים הקטנים עת יולדו יקרה
להם נגעי הפה והקיא והשעול והתעורה והפחד ומורסת הטיבור ורטיבות האזנים.

אמר המפרש: יקרה להם נגעי הפה מחמת רכות איבריהם ומה ש(ב)גופיהם מן רתיחת הדם
והקיא לרבוי ממה שיינקו וחולשת כח המחזיק בהם לחוזק הרטיבות. והשעול מחמת רטיבות
הריאה ורוב מה שיזוב ממוחם לרוב רטיבותם על הריאה והיא הסבה לרטיבות אזניהם כי
15 מותרי המוח ידחו אל האזנים. ומורסת הטיבור לקירוב זמן חתיכתו והפחד רובו בשינה בעבור
הפסד עיכול הקיבה יעשין המוח ויחדשו לו דמיונות מפחידות. ואמנם התעורה לא ידע לה
ג'אלינו' סבה אבל אמר כי הענין הנוהג בתינוקות הוא רבוי השינה וזהו אמת. אכן הרבה פעמים
יקרה להם התעורה והבכיה כל הלילה וסבת זה חזק הרגשתם מרכוז גשמיה וכחותיהם
כולם חלושות בלתי מוחזקים ומעט דבר מן הצער יקיצם. ואמר כי יבואם רוע העכול ומצוק
20 מפני הקיבה לרוב יניקותם יקיצום זה הצער ויעורו ובתוספת זה יבכו וזה נראה תמיד.

(3.25)

[131] אמר אבוקרט: כשיקרב הנער אל צמיחת השינים יקרה לו כאב בבשר השינים וקדחות
וקוץ ושלשול וכל שכן כשיצמחו לו השינים אשר כנגד העינים וירידת הריר מן התינוקות ולמי
מהם שבטנו רפה.

---

1 ארוכה: om. a 2 והשקוי: והשקוי emendation editor וחלקת: MSS וחלוקת add. a ‖ وسلّ 6 והשטות:
om. a 7 והסתום (= والسدد): والسدر a 12 ומה ש(ב)גופיהם מן רתיחת הדם: وما في اللبن من الجلاء
a 19 בלתי: emendation editor כלפי MSS ואמר: وقلّ a ‖ ומצוק: وقلق a 20 ובתוספת זה: وإن
زاد قليلا a 22 וירידת הריר (= واللعاب) מן התינוקות: وللعب من الصبيان a

אמר המפרש: זה כלו להיות השינים יבקעו וינקבו בבשר השינים וירחיבו הנקבים וימשך זה
הצער לקדחות והקוץ ולהיות המזון לא יתעכל יפה מפני הכאב והתעורה יחדש השלשול.
ורוב מה שיחדש הקיוץ וירידת הריר ורפיון הבטן הוא מרוב מותרות שבגופותיהם.

(3.26)

[132] אמר אבוקרט: כשיעבור הנער אלו השנים יקרה לו מורסת הגרון וכניסת חוליא
שבעורף ונזילה על הריאה והאבן והרימה ותולעים שבגוף והשומות התלויים והחזירים ושאר
האבעבועות.

אמ׳ המפרש: מאחרי צמיחת השינים עד קרוב לי״ג שנים יקחו הנערים המזונות הרבים ויוסיף
מכאובם וירבה רעתם ויכניסו מאכל אחר מאכל ותרבה תנועתם אחר אוכלם וכל זאת ההנהגה
מפסדת העכול ומרבה הליחות וגשמיהם עם זה רטוב ואיבריהם רכים ויתחייב מזה כל מה
שזכר כי כשיצמח העצל שבגרון ימשוך החוליא מן העורף לרכות קישוריהם.

(3.27)

[133] אמר אבוקרט: מי שעבר אלו השנים וקרוב שיצמח לו השיער בבית הערוה יקרה לו
הרבה מאלו התחלואים וקדחות יותר ארוכות ורעיפת דם הנחירים.

אמ׳ המפרש: באלו השנים ירבה החם ויעדיף בהם ולזה יתחדש בהם הרטיבות.

(3.28)

[134] אמר אבוקרט: ורוב מה שיקרה לנערים מן התחלואים יבא בקצתם הגבול בארבעים
יום ובקצתם בששה חדשים ובקצתם בשבעה שנים ובקצתם כשיתקשה צמיחת השיער בבית
הערוה. ואמנם מה שישאר מן החליים ולא ימס בעת הגדול ובנקבות בעת בא נדותן מדרכם
שיארך וישאר עם האדם כל ימי חייו.

אמר המפרש: ר״ל החליים הישנים.

(3.29)

[135] אמר אבוקרט: ואמנם הבחורים יקרה להם רקיקת דם וכליון וקדחות חדות וכפייה ושאר
החליים אלא שרוב מה שיקרה להם הוא מה שזכרנו.

אמר המפרש: כבר באר ג׳אלינו׳ כי אין פנים היות הכפיה מיוחדת לבחורים אלא הוא מתחלואי
הנערים.

1–2 וימשך זה הצער לקדחות: فيَتبع ذلك الألم الحمّى a   3 וירידת הריר: للعبل a ‖ ורפיון הבטן: والمعتقل
البطن a   5 והשומות התלויים: والثواليل المتعلّقة a   7–8 ויוסיף מכאובם וירבה רעתם: ويكثر شربهم
a   13 החם: الدم a ‖ הרטיבות: الرعاف في أمراضهم a   15 כשיתקשה: إذا شارفوا a   17 וישאר עם
האדם כל ימי חייו: .om a

(3.30)

[136] אמר אבוקרט: מי שעבר אלו השנים יקרה לו נזילה על הריאה וחולי הצד וחולי הריאה
ושכחה והקדחת אשר תהיה עמה התעורה והקדחת אשר יהיה עמה ערבוב השכל וקדחת
השורפת ושלשול היוצא הקיא ושלשול הארוך וגרידת המעים וחליקות המעים והתפתח פיות
העורקים ממטה.

אמר המפרש: ידוע כי השנים הם אלו שנות הכהול הליחה השחורית נראית בהם על הרוב
ולזה ייחדם ערבוב השכל ותעורה בקדחות והתפתח פיות העורקים. אמנם שאר מה שמנה
באלו השנים אינם מיוחדים לבעלי אלו השנים. וג׳אלינו׳ יחשוב לתת סבה מיוחדה באלו השנים
ואינו כד.

(3.31)

[137] אמר אבוקרט: ואמנם הישישים יקרה להם רוע הנשימה והנזילה אשר יקרה עמה
השעול והטפת השתן וקשיו וכאב הפרקים וכאב הכליות וסיבוב הראש והשתוק והנגעים
הרעים וחכוך הגוף ותעורה ורפיון הבטן ורטיבות העינים והנחירים וכהות הראות וכובד
השמע.

אמר המפרש: כל אלו הסבות מבוארות למי שידע מענין מזג הישישים.

נשלם המאמר השלישי מפ״א.

---

2 ושכחה: om. a ‖ 3 ושלשול היוצא הקיא: والهيضة a ‖ והתפתח (= وانفتاح MSS): وانتفاخ emendation editor 6 והתפתח (= وانفتاح CP): وانتفاخ a 7 באלו השנים: om. a ‖ יחשוב: يزعم a
11 הראות: والزرقة add. a

המאמר הרביעי

(4.1)

[138] אמר אבוקרט: ראוי שתשקה ההרה הסם המשלשל כשתהיינה התערובות מתעוררות
בגופה מעת שיעברו על העובר ארבעה חדשים ועד שיעבור עליו ז׳ חדשים ויהיה הקדמתך
לזה מעט. ואמנם מה שהיה העובר קטן מזה או גדול מזה ראוי שתזהר ותמנע.

5   אמר המפרש: זה מבואר כי העובר בתחלתו חלוש ויקל הפלתו ובאחריתו יכבד כי כבר גדל
ויעזור על הפלתו בכובדו.

(4.2)

[139] אמר אבוקרט: אמנם ראוי שאם יושקה מן הסם שיריק מן הגוף המין אשר אם נוקה
מאליו יועיל הרקתו. ואמנם מה שהיה הרקתו על חלוף זה ראוי שתפסיקנו.

אמר המפרש: זה מבואר.

(4.3)

10   [140] אמר אבוקרט: הרקת הגוף מן המין אשר צריך שיריק ממנו יועיל זה וסובלו בקלות ואם
היה הענין בהפך זה יהיה הענין קשה.

אמר המפרש: הודיענו בכאן שיהיה זה האות בידך שתדע אם הדרכת הדרך הישר או אם
חטאת ⟨ר״ל⟩ קלות סובלות ההרקה או קשיו.

(4.4)

[141] אמר אבוקרט: ראוי שיהיה מה שיעשה מן ההרקה בסם בקיץ למעלה יותר ובסתיו
15   למטה.

אמר המפרש: הגובר בקיץ היא המרה הכרכומית ובעבור חמימות התערובות ורתיחתם
יתנועעו לצד מעלה ולזה ישים ההרקה בקיץ ובסתיו בהפך זה.

(4.5)

[142] אמר אבוקרט: אחר עלית המזל הנקרא שערי העבור בערבי ובעת עלייתו ולפניו יקשה
ההרקה בסמנין.

---

3 ועד: emendation editor וְעם MSS   5 יכבד: emendation editor יכשר MSS   7 שאם יושקה ...
שיריק: أن تَسقي ... ما يستفرغ a   10 הרקת: إن استفرغ a   12 שתדע: emendation editor שתרעבו
MSS ‖ הדרכת הדרד הישר: أصبنا في الحدس a   16–17 המרה הכרכומית ובעבור חמימות התערובות
ורתיחתם יתנועעו: الصفراء والحرارة أجوّا الأخلاط متحرّكة a   17 ישים: يؤثّر a ‖ בקיץ: بالقيٴ a

אמר המפרש: זה הזמן הוא עיקר חזוק עת הקיץ והכחות חלושות מאד. וחום האויר מונע משיכת הסם ולא יגיע ממנו אלא חולשא.

(4.6)

[143] אמר אבוקרט: מי שהיה כחוש הגוף והקיא יקל לו שם הרקתך ברפואה מלמעלה והשמר שלא תעשה זה בסתיו.

(4.7)

[144] אמנם מי שיקשה עליו הקיא והיה ממוצע בבשר שים הרקתך בסם מלמטה והזהר שלא תעשה זה בקיץ. 5

אמר המפרש: זה מבואר.

(4.8)

[145] אמר אבוקרט: אמנם בעל הכליה כשתריקהו בסם הזהר מהריקו מלמעלה.

אמר המפרש: אמנם המזומנים לכליה והם צרי החזה והריאה שלהם גם כן צרי המעברים ולא יעבור בם החומר המורק. 10

(4.9)

[146] אמר אבוקרט: ואמנם מי שגובר עליו המרה השחורה יצטרך גם כן להריקו מלמטה בסם עבה כאשר נחבר שני הצדדים אל הקש אחד.

אמר המפרש: ירצה בסם עבה סם חזק והכרכומית תצוף)מ(למעלה והשחורה תצלול למטה וההקש האחד הוא אשר יעשה בזה בחירת אחד מן ההפכים לאחד מן הליחות כאשר נריק כל ליחה ממקומה הקרוב ליציאתה. 15

(4.10)

[147] אמר אבוקרט: ראוי שיעשה סם ההרקה בחליים החדים מאד כשתהיינה התערובות מעוררות מן היום הראשון כי איחורו בכמו אלו החליים רע.

אמר המפרש: זה מבואר וירא מהניח אלו התערובות הנשפכות ממקום למקום אחר בלתי מתקיים שמא יתקיימו באבר נכבד ויקדם להריקם קודם שתתחלש הכח או שיתקיימו באבר הנכבד. 20

---

1 עיקר חזוק עת הקיץ: أشدّ ما يكون من الصيف a   2 חולשא: واضطراب add. a   4 בסתיו: قال
المفسّر: حال القضيف دائمًا كحال أكثر الناس في الصيف وقد تقدّم النهي عن استعمال القيء في الشتاء add. a
5 אמנם מי: قال أبقراط: فأمّا من a   9 והריאה: a .om   10 המורק: a .om   13 תצלול: תצוף צ

(4.11)

[148] אמר אבוקרט: מי שהיה בו מצוק ומכאובים סביב לטבור וכאב הכסלים תמיד ולא יותר
לא בסם משלשל ולא בזולתו ודאי ענינו יגיע אל השקוי היבש.

אמר המפרש: כאשר לא יותר זה ברפואה הוא אות על)אלו האיברים מ(רוע מזג אשר המשיל
על אלו האיברים ומקויים בהם ויחדש השקוי התופיי אשר קרא אותו היבש בערך השקוי
5   הנודיי אשר בו המים והנודיי יתילד מקור גדול.

(4.12)

[149] אמר אבוקרט: מי שהיה בו חליקות המעים בסתיו הרקתו בסם מלמעלה הוא רע.

אמר המפרש: אע״פ שהמביא לחליקות המעים היא ליחה חמה ודקה תצוף אשר ראוי מן הדין
להריקם בקיא מאחר שהעת שהסתיו אין ראוי לעשות הקיא כמו שקדם.

(4.13)

[150] אמר אבוקרט: מי שצריך לשתות הכרבק והקיא לא יבואנו בקלות יצטרך ללחלח בטנו
10   לפני השקותו במאכל רב ובמנוחה.

אמר המפרש: זה מבואר.

(4.14)

[151] אמר אבוקרט: כשתשקה לאדם כרבק יהיה כונתך להניע גופו הרבה והשיכון יהיה מעט.
וכבר יורה על זה רכיבת הספינות שהתנועה תבלבל הגוף ותעורר הקיא.

אמר המפרש: ידוע כי הכרבק מקיא מאד והנעת הגוף בהעתקת המקומות הוא שיעור אל
15   הקיא והראיה רכיבת הספינות.

(4.15)

[152] אמר אבוקרט: כשתרצה שיהיה הרקת הכרבק הרבה מאד תניע הגוף וכשתרצה
להפסיקו אז תישן את השותה ולא תניעהו.

אמר המפרש: זה מבואר מוחזר.

(4.16)

[153] אמר אבוקרט: שתית הכרבק סכנה למי שבשרו בריא וזה כי הוא מחדש הקווץ.

20   אמר המפרש: זה מבואר.

---

4 ומקויים: وتمكّن a ‖ בערך: في مقابل a   7 חמה: حادّ a ‖ ראוי מן הדין: يوجب a   9 בטנו (= בטנה):
بدنه a   12 הרבה: ولتنويه add. a ‖ והשיכון: وتسكينه a   13 תבלבל הגוף ותעורר הקיא: ثوّر الأبدان a

(4.17)

[154] אמר אבוקרט: מי שאין לו קדחת ויש לו מניעה מהמאכל ונשיכה בפי האצטומכא וסבוב
ראש ומרירה בפה כל זה ראיה על צורך ההרקה בסם מלמעלה.

אמר המפרש: ר"ל במעים פי הקיבה והדקירה)ו(העקיצה והסבוב הוא שידמה האדם כי מה
שיראה כאלו הוא מסבב סביבו ויחסר חוש הראות פתאום עד שיחשוב שכבר כסה החשך
לכל מה שיראהו. ואלו המקרים יהיו כשתהיינה בפי הקיבה ליחות רעות עוקצות אותו ולזה
יצטרך כאשר יראו אלו המקרים שיתנקה על ידי קיא.

(4.18)

[155] אמר אבוקרט: הכאבים אשר למעלה מן הטרפשא יורו על נקוי בסם מלמעלה והכאבים
אשר למטה מן הטרפשא יורו על נקוי בסם מלמטה.

אמר המפרש: על אי זה צד אשר נטות הליחות ותשארנה שם מאותו הצד יתנקה בסם מקיא
מלמעלה או בסם משלשל מלמטה. ואמנם בעת שפיכת הליחות צריך למשכן אל הפך הצד.

(4.19)

[156] אמר אבוקרט: מי ששתה סם המריק והורק ולא יצמא ודאי לא פסקה ממנו ההרקה עד
שיצמא.

אמר המפרש: הצמאון אשר אחרי שתיית הסם כשלא יהיה מפני חום הקיבה או יבשותו או
מפני חדות הסם או מפני היות הליחה המתנקה חמה מורה על הנקות התערובות מאותה
הליחה שרצה להריקה.

(4.20)

[157] אמר אבוקרט: מי שהיתה בו קדחת ומצאתהו דאגה וכובד בארכובותיו וצער בכסליו
זה ראיה על צרכו להרקת הסם מלמטה.

אמר המפרש: זה מבואר.

(4.21)

[158] אמר אבוקרט: הרעי השחור הדומה לדם שיבא מעצמו היתה עם קדחת או עם בלתי
קדחת היא מן הרעות שבאותות. וכל מה שיהיו הגוונים בתוצאות יותר רעים היו האותות יותר
רעים. וכאשר היה זה עם שתיית סם היה האות יותר טוב. וכל מה שיהיו הגוונים ההם בתוצאות
יותר היה זה יותר רחוק מן הרעות.

---

1 ונשיכה בפי האצטומכא: נ"א דקירה במעים ק‎   3 במעים: الفؤاد a‎   11 פסקה: يَنقطع =‎
תפסק‎   14 התערובות: الأعضاء a‎   16 דאגה: مغص a‎   21 זה עם: emendation editor זה עם‎
MSS ‖ בתוצאות: om. a‎   22 הרעות: قال المفسّر: هذا بين add. a

(4.22)

[159] אמר אבוקרט: אי זה חולי שיצאה בהתחלתו המרה השחורה מלמטה או למעלה זו ראיה רעה מורה על מות.

אמר המפרש: כל מה שהתמיד החולי בהתחלתו אין ממה שיצא מן הגוף של החולה שיהיו תוצאותיו בתנועה מן הטבע אבל יהיה מקרה רע יציאתו הגוף יוצא כנגד הטבע. והמרה השחורה היא הליחה העבה הדומה לשמרים הנשרפים ויצאה שאי אפשר שישוב מרה שחורה טבעית. ותוצאות אלו התערובות הרעות לפני הבשול יורה על עקיצתו לאיברים לחזק רעתם ולא יוכלו האיברים להחזיק בהם עד שתתבשלנה.

(4.23)

[160] אמר אבוקרט: מי שכבר החלישו חולי חד או ישן או נפילה או זולת זה ואחר כך יצא ממנו מרה שחורה או כמו דם שחור מלמטה או מלמעלה זה ימות למחרת זה היום.

אמר המפרש: מי שזה עניינו טבעו חלוש כל כך שלא יוכל לבשל ולהבדיל ולהריק אלו התערובות אשר הנה רעות ככה. ולעוצם החולי וגדולתו ישפוך ויעבור כי אין דבר שיחזיקם. ואמרו או כמו דם שחור ר״ל הרעי השחור. וההפרש בין המרה השחורה ובין הרעי השחור שהמרה השחורה זב עמה דבר מפרק מעקיק בעקיצת החומץ ותרתיח בקרקע כשתפול עליה ואין דבר מזה ברעי השחורי.

(4.24)

[161] אמר אבוקרט: שלשול הדם כשהיתה התחלתו מן המרה השחורה זהו מאותות מות.

אמ׳ המפ׳: כאשר התחיל לצאת המרה הכרכומית וגרדה את המעים או נגעה אותם ובא הדם אחר זה יתכן שיבריא זו הגרידה או זה הנגע. ואמנם אם התערובת השחורי היא אשר גרדה ואחרי כן נגעה עד שבא הדם אי אפשר שלא תחדש במעים כמו סרטן המתחדש בשטח הגשם.

(4.25)

[162] אמר אבוקרט: יציאת הדם מלמעלה איך שיהיה הוא אות רע ויציאה מלמטה אות טוב וכל שכן כשיצא ממנו דבר שחור.

אמר המפרש: ירצה מלמעלה בקיא. ואמנם יהיה טוב מלמטה כאשר דחהו הטבע על צד קצת המותרות כמו שיקרה בטחורים ובתנאי שיהיה מעט.

4 רע: لازم a ‖ 5 ויצאה שאי אפשר שישוב: وخرج عن أن يكون a ‖ 9 מלמטה או מלמעלה (= من فوق أو من أسفل P): ולהריק a om. ‖ 10 ולהזיק MSS :emendation editor ‖ 13 מפרק: يريق a ‖ ותרתיח: وتقشر a ‖ 17 או זה הנגע: a om. ‖ 18 אי אפשר שלא תחדש: فلا برء له لأن يحدث a ‖ 21 וכל שכן: إذا a ‖ 22 קצת: نفض a

(4.26)

[163] אמר אבוקרט: מי שבו שלשול הדם ויוצא ממנו כמו חתיכות בשר זהו מאותות מות.

אמר המפרש: זה הראיה על חזקת הנגע במעים עד שיחתוך גרמיהם ולא יתכן לזה הבשר
מזור.

(4.27)

[164] אמר אבוקרט: מי שנשפך ממנו דם הרבה בקדחת מאי זה מקום שיהיה שפיכתו הוא
5   חסרונות המזון ירפה בטנו ביותר מהשיעור.

אמר המפרש: לחולשת החום היסודי מפני הרקת הדם ימעט משיכת האיברים למזון ויחלש
העכול וירפה הבטן.

(4.28)

[165] אמר אבוקרט: מי שהיה בו שלשול פעמים ומצאתהו צמח מתילד באזן כבר נפסק ממנו
השלשול ההוא. ומי שהיה חרש ונתחדש לו שלשול גדול נפסק מעליו החרשות.

10   אמר המפרש: סבת זה מבוארת להזלת החומר אל הפך הצד ומבואר הוא כי מאמרי הנה
בחרשות שיקרה פתאום בחליים ובפרט עם הקמת הגבול.

(4.29)

[166] אמר אבוקרט: מי שמצאו בקדחת ביום הששי מחוליו סמור בשר וראי גבולו יהיה
מגונה.

אמר המפרש: כאשר נתחדש הפלצות בקדחת וכש״(כ) בשורפת ממנהגו שיבא הנקיון אחריו
15   וכבר נודע רוע הנקיון בששי והוא ענין אמרו קשה.

(4.30)

[167] אמר אבוקרט: מי שהיה להתימות הקדחת וסת באי זו שעה שתניחנו וכן באי זו שעה
שתקחהו ויבא למחרתו באותה השעה בעצמה ודאי גבולו יקשה.

אמר המפרש: מבואר כי כשתהיינה וסתות הקדחת כולם יבאו על עת אחת בהתחלתה
ותכליתה זה ראיה על אורך. וזהו ענין אמרו גבולו יקשה כאלו אמר שיקשה שתכלה הקדחת
20   בגבול כי הגבול אמנם יהיה בחל(י)ים החדים אבל החל(י)ים הישנים הם יותכו על אורך זמן.

4-5 הוא חסרונות המזון: فإنّه عندما يبقه فيغذى a   8 פעמים: مرار a ‖ צמח מתילד באזן: صمم a
9 גדול: مرار a   11 הקמת: مقاربة emendation editor مفارقة a   13 מגונה: نكا a   16 שהיה
להתימות הקדחת: كانت لحاه a ‖ וסת: نوائب a ‖ וכן: إذا a   18 יבאו: ثابتة a   19 אורך: المرض add.
a

(4.31)

[168] אמר אבוקרט: בעל העייפות בקדחת רוב מה שיצאו בו צמחים בין פרקיו ולעומת לחייו.

אמר המפרש: בסבת חום הקדחת וחמימות האיברים מן בעל העייפות ידחו אל הפרקים ולעליון הגוף ויקבלם הבשר הרפה אשר בפרקי הלחיים.

(4.32)

[169] אמר אבוקרט: מי שנוצל מחוליו וחש מקום מגופו יתחדש במקום ההוא צמח.

אמר המפרש: יאמר כי הנמלט מחולי כשיסבול באבר מאבריו וימצאהו בו כאב ודאי שם יצא 5
צמח והסבה מבוארת. וכבר זכר ג'אלינו' כי חדוש הכאב גם כן יקרא חש.

(4.33)

[170] אמר אבוקרט: ואם יקרה לו סבל אבר מן האיברים קודם שיחלה בעליו ודאי באבר ההוא יהיה החזקת החולי.

אמר המפרש: זה מבואר סיפר בכאן מן הסבל הקודם לחולי עד שיהיה סבה לחולי. וזה הפרק שלפניו ספר בו מהסבל שיהיה אחר יציאת החולי. וזכר בפרק השלישי שלפניו זה הסבל 10
שיהיה בעצם החולי ואולם יפלו אלו הצמחים כולם בגבולים אשר יהיה בהם הרקה נגלית מבוארת.

(4.34)

[171] אמר אבוקרט: מי שהכשילו קדחת ואין בגרונו נפח וקרה לו חנוק בפתע פתאום זהו מאותות מות.

אמר המפרש: החנוק פתאום אמנם יקרה בעבור סתימת השפוי כובע הנקרא חנגרה 15
בערבי והמוקדח יצטרך אל שאיפת האויר הקר מאד. וכאשר נמנע האויר מלשאפו ימות בלא ספק. ואמנם התנה שלא יהיה שם נפח כי פעמים תהיה הקדחת נמשכת למורסת הגרון ויבא החנוק בו מעט מעט לתוספת המורסא ועם תכליתו יתכן שירד מעט וימלט החולה.

(4.35)

[172] אמר אבוקרט: מי שקרה לו קדחת ונתעוותה עמו צוארו ויכבד עליו הבליעה עד שלא 20
יוכל לבלוע אלא בקושי מבלתי שיראה בו נפח הנה זה מאותות מות.

2 ידחו: الفضل add. a ‏ 5 כשיסבול באבר: إن أتعب عضوه a ‏ 6 חש: كلال a ‏ 7 ואם יקרה לו סבל:
فإن كان أيضا قد تقدّم فتعب a ‏ 13 שהכשילו: اعتره a ‏ 16 מלשאפו: .om a

אמר המפרש: עוות הצואר וקושי הבליעה יהיה בעבור מורסא ופעמים יהיה לתגבורת היובש. ואשר רצה בו הנה הוא המתהוה מתגבורת היובש כי היא ראיה על שקיעת הפסד המזג באיברים מתגבורת היובש.

(4.36)

[173] אמר אבוקרט: הזיעה ישובח במחוממים אם התחילה ביום הג׳ או ביום הד׳ או בה׳ או בשביעי או בתשיעי או באחד עשר או בארבעה עשר או בעשרים או בארבע ועשרים או בשבע ועשרים או באחד ושלשים או בשלשה ושלשים או בשבע ושלשים. והזיעה אשר תהיה באלו הימים יהיה בה גבול התחלואים. ואמנם הזיעה אשר תהיה בזולת אלו ימים היא מורה על צער או על רקידה או על אורך חולי.

אמר המפרש: אין זה הדין בזיעה לבד אבל בכל הנקויים אשר יהיה בהם הגבול כי טבע אלו הימים הגבוליים כבר נודע בנסיון וכל גבול שיהיה בזיעה או בזולתה מן הנקויים כבר נמצאו בנסיון שהם על הרוב באלו הימים.

(4.37)

[174] אמר אבוקרט: הזיעה הקרה כשתהיה עם קדחת חדה תורה על מות. וכשתהיה עם קדחת רכה תורה על אריכות חולי.

אמר המפרש: תגבורת חום הקדחת תכבה את החום היסודי ולא תבשל התערוב(ו)ת הקרות מאד אשר בחיצון הגוף אשר מהם תצא הזיעה הקרה וראיית נאות אלו התערובות ותגבורת קרירותם מהיות חום הקדחת החזקה לא תוכל לחמם מה שיצא מהם.

(4.38)

[175] אמר אבוקרט: ועת שתהיה הזיעה באבר אחד מן הגוף הוא מורה על החולי נתחדש באבר ההוא.

אמר המפרש: ולזה היתה הזיעה מזה המקום לבדו אשר בו נעצרת הליחה.

(4.39)

[176] אמר אבוקרט: ואי זה מקום מן הגוף שיהיה קר או חם בו החולי.

אמר המפרש: זה מבואר.

1 يהיה: من زوال أحد الفقار وزواله قد يكون add. a   3 מתגבורת: واستيلاء a   4 או ביום הד׳: .om
a   5 עשר: أو في السابع عشر .om a   6 או בשלשה ושלשים או בשבע ושלשים: أو في الرابع والثلاثين a
8 או על רקידה: .om a   17 ועת: وحيث a

(4.40)

[177] אמר אבוקרט: וכשתתחדש שנוי בגוף כלו והיה הגוף פעמים יתקרר ואחר יתחמם פעם
אחרת או יצטבע בצבע ואחר ישתנה ממנו הוראה זה כלו על אריכות חולי.

אמר המפרש: החולי הבא ממינים רבים הוא לעולם יותר ארוך זמן מן החולי הבא ממין אחד.

(4.41)

[178] אמר אבוקרט: הזיעה המרובה שתהיה בעת השינה מבלתי סבה מבוארת תורה על
שבעליה סובל על גופו יותר ממה שיוכל שאתו. ואם היה כך שלא יוכל ליקח מן המאכלים דע
ש)ב(גופו צריך אל נקוי.

אמר המפרש: זה מבואר.

(4.42)

[179] אמר אבוקרט: הזיעה המרובה אשר תבא תדיר חמה היתה או קרה הקרה תורה על
שהחולי עצום והחמה תורה על שהחולי יותר קל.

אמר המפרש: הזיעה שתהיה בשאר ימות החולי לא על דרך הגבול מה שתהיה קרה יותר
תהיה יותר רע ⟨כי זה⟩ תורה על קרירות החומר.

(4.43)

[180] אמר אבוקרט: כשתהיה הקדחת בלתי מפסקת ואח״כ תתגבר ביום השלישי היא גדול
הסכנה. וכשתהיה הקדחת תפסיק על אי זה פנים שתהיה היא תורה על שאין בה סכנה.

אמר המפרש: זאת אשר היא תמידות ותדחוק בשלישי שיש בה סכנה היא נקראת שטר אלגב.

(4.44)

[181] אמר אבוקרט: מי שתמצאהו קדחת ארוכה וכאשר יקרהו או צמחים או רקונית חללים
הם בראשי פרקיו.

אמר המפרש: אריכות הקדחת הוא או לרוב החומר או לקרירות החומר או לעובי הליחות
והחומר אשר זה ענינו ברוב ידחה אמנם על אבר אחד ושם יחדש צמח או בראשי פרקיו
ויחדש כאב הפרקים.

_____

5 שלא יוכל ליקח: وهو لا يال a   10 מה: מה emendation editor בה MSS   14 ותדחוק: وتَشتَدّ a ‖ שטר:
ﭏﺞ‎ om.   15–16 רקונית חללים הם בראשי פרקיו: كلال في مفاصله a   18 בראשי פרקיו: لفضاء المفاصل

a

(4.45)

[182] אמר אבוקרט: מי שמצאו צמח או כאב בראשי פרקיו אמנם הקדחת הנה הוא מאשר לקח מן המאכלים יותר מכדי סובלו.

אמר המפרש: ר"ל אחר הקדחת אחר הסרת הקדחת לגמרי והוא עדין חלש.

(4.46)

[183] אמר אבוקרט: כשיקרה סמור בשר בקדחת בלתי מפסקת למי שכחו תש זה מאותות מות.

אמר המפרש: אמר ג'אלינו' כי אומרו זה הוא רומז על התמדת הסימור פעם אחר פעם ועדין הקדחת עומדת בלתי מפסקת הוא ראיה על היות הטבע משתדל לפלוט התערובת המחליאה ולהוציאה ולא יוכל בעבור קיומה והשארותה באיברים ויתוסף בכח תששות וחולשה וכליון להיותה בלתי סובלת רעידת הסמור וזעזוע הגוף.

(4.47)

[184] אמר אבוקרט: בקדחת אשר לא תפסק הרקיקה האדום והדומה לדם ומסרחת בשר אשר הם מסוג המרירות כלם רעים ואם תחסרנה חסרון טובה הנה משובחות. וכן הענין בתוצאות והשתן כי כאשר ייטב מה שיורק מהם היה משובח וכאשר יצא מה שאין תועלת ביציאתו מאחד מאלו המקומות זה רע.

אמר המפרש: המאמר הכולל כי הדברים הרעים אשר יורקו מורים על ענינים רעים שבגוף אשר יורקו ממנו אלא שהם אפשר שיהיה מה שיוציא כמו יציאת המוגלא מן הנגעים המעופשים ואין תועלת ביציאתם בחולי ההוא ואפשר שהיה יציאתם כמו יציאת המוגלא מן המורסא כשיפתח ויהיה בו נקי משובח לאבר אשר בו החולי. והאותות המורים על יציאת מה שיצא הוא טוב והוא בריאות הוא בשול בפרט וסבל הגוף למה שיצא בקלות והוקל בו עם זה טבע החולי. ואחריו העת ההווה מעתות השנה והארץ והשנים וטבע החולה.

(4.48)

[185] אמר אבוקרט: כשיהיה בקדחת הבלתי נפסקת חיצון הגוף קר ותוכה ניחר ו(ב)בעליו צמאון זה מאותות מות.

1 כאב חלל בראשי פרקיו: كلال في المفاصل a ‖ אמנם: بعد a   3 חלש: ناقه a   6 זה: إذا كانت تعرض
a   8 תששות וחולשה וכליון: نكاية وذبول a   10 האדום: الكَمِدة a ‖ ומסרחת: emendation editor
ורחיצת MSS ‖ ומסרחת בשר: والمَتِنة a   11 תחסרנה חסרון (= انتقصت انتقاصا): انتفضت انتفاضا
a   13-11 וכן ... רע: فإنّ خروج ما لا ينتفع بخروجه من أحد هذه المواضع فذلك ردي• a   14 רעים:
emendation editor רבים MSS   17 כשיפתח: ينفجر a

אמר המפרש: אמר ג׳אלינו׳ כי המקרים האלו לא ימצא תמיד אלא בקצת הקדחות אשר לא
יפסקו. וסבתו אמר כי תתחדש מורסא חמה בקצת האיברים הפנימיים וימשכו הדם והרוח
אל האבר העלול מן הגוף כלו ולזה יקל פנימי הגוף ויתחמם והעור קר כמו שיקרה בהתחלות
וסתות הקדחות. זהו למוד ג׳אלינוס והוא בלתי אמת כי אלו יתחייב זה היה מתחייב להיות אלו

5   המקרים לכל מורסא חמה שתתחדש באיברים פנימיים. ואנחנו רואים תמיד בעלי מדוה הצד
ומדוה הריאה ומדוה הכבד עורותם חמות מאד מפנימי גופותם. ואשר יראה לי כי סבת זה היות
החמרים אשר בחיצון הגוף עבים מאד הם קרים מאד לא ינצחם חום התערובות המעופשות
המהות הקדחת שנתעפשה בפנימי הגוף. וכל מה שנתלהב הדבר ההוא המעופש ועלה חומו
לצד חיצון הגוף יבקש נשימתו להתנשם ממנו ונתחדש מסך קר תחתיהם שימנע ויבדיל לחום
10   ההוא מהתפלש אל טבע הגוף וישוב ויחזור החום לאחור בחוזק מה שיתכן וישרוף פנימי
הגוף יותר ויתחזק הצמאון ויארע לחום כדמות מה שיעשו הנפחים מהזות המים על האש
כדי לחזק חום פנימי האש ותתיך את את הברזל וזאת היא סבה אמתית טבעית אין ספק
בה.

(4.49)

[186] אמר אבוקרט: כשיתעקם בקדחת בלתי מפסקת השפה או העין או האף או העפעפים
15   או שלא יראה החולה או לא ישמע אי זה מאלה שיהיה וכבר נחלש הגוף המיתה קרובה.

אמר המפרש: זה מבואר כשיראו אלה האותות עם חלשת הכח וכבר קדמה הקדחת בודאי
כי היובש כבר שלט על התחלת העצבים ולזה נתחדש העקום ההוא או זולתו מה שזכר.

(4.50)

[187] אמר אבוקרט: כשנתחדש בקדחת בלתי מפסקת רוע הנשימה וערבוב השכל זהו
מאותות מות.

20   אמר המפרש: זה מבואר כי החום כשהחזיק דבר באיברים עד שהוחלשו גם כן העצבים
המניעים לחזה ולטרפשה והריעה הנשימה.

(4.51)

[188] אמר אבוקרט כי הצמח המתחדש בקדחת ולא יותך בעת הגבולים הראשונים יביט
באריכות חולי.

אמר המפרש: זה מבואר.

1 הקדחות: emendation editor המקומות MSS 3 יקל ... ויתחמם: يَحترق ... حَرارة a 4 למוד:
تعليل a 6 מפנימי: مثل باطن a 8 המהות: المولّد a 9 נשימתו: منفسًا a 10 אל טבע הגוף (=
لطبع الجسد): لسطح الجسد a 11 מהות: emendation editor מהיות MSS ‖ האש: في الكور add. a
15 נחלש: emendation editor נכחש MSS 16 בודאי: علم a 20 כשהחזיק דבר: قد تمكّنت a

(4.52)

[189] אמר אבוקרט: הדמעות הנוזלות בקדחת או בזולתה מן החליים אם יהיה זה ברצון
החולה או למאסו ואם היה מבלי רצון הוא יותר רע.

אמר המפרש: (זה מבואר) להולשת הכח המחזיק ואמרו הוא יותר רע משמע על שהראשון
גם כן רע. וזה כי אע״פ שבכה ברצונו הוא ראיה על חולשת הכלי ולזה ימהר התפעלותו ויבואנו
הבכי.

(4.53)

[190] אמר אבוקרט: מי שנדבקו בשיניו בעת הקדחת ליחה דביקה חום קדחתו תהיה חזקה.

אמר המפרש: אלו הליחות הדבקות אמנם יתחדשו מחום חזק יפעל ברטיבות הליחה הלבנה
עד שייבשוה.

(4.54)

[191] אמר אבוקרט: מי שקרתהו בעת הקדחת השורפת שעול גדול יבש ואחר כן היתה
התעוררותו לו מעט אי אפשר לו שיצמא.

אמר המפרש: אי אפשר בשעול ואפילו לא ירוק מאומה שלא יתלחלח קנה הריאה ממה
שימשך אליו מחמת השעול ולזה לא יצמא.

(4.55)

[192] אמר אבוקרט: כל קדחת שתהיה עם מורסת הבשר הרך אשר בעגבות אלהאלבין בער״
וזולתם ממה שידומה לו הוא רע אלא אם כן יהיה קדחת יום.

אמר המפרש: כשהיתה סבת הקדחת מורסת ההאלבין והדומה לו מן הבשר הרך יהיה קדחת
יומית. אמנם כשהיתה לקדחת סבה אחרת ונתחבר עמה צמיחת ההאלבין והדומה לו אז הוא
אות רע כי סבת צמיחת ההאלבין והדומה לו אז הוא אות רע כי סבת הצמחת האלבין אז אמנם
יהיה נמשך לצמיחת אחד מבני מעיים וצמיחת הפנימי הזה הוא סבה לקדחת שקדמה ולזה
הוא סכנה.

(4.56)

[193] אמר אבוקרט: כשהיתה באדם קדחת ומצאו זיעה ולא יוסר ממנו הקדחת זה ודאי הוא
אות רע וזה כי הוא מביט באריכות מן חולי ומורה על רטיבות רבה.

אמר המפרש: זה מבואר.

---

2 או למאסו: فليس ذلك عندك a   3 משמע: دليل a   4 שבכה: emendation editor שהיה
MSS ‖ הכלי: قلبه a   11 המפרש: قال جالينوس add. a   13 בעגבות אלהאלבין בער׳: في الحالبين a
15 ההאלבין: الحالبين a   17 אות: om. a

(4.57)

[194] אמר אבוקרט: מי שארעו חולי הקווץ או המתוח ואחר כך אירע לו קדחת הותר בו
החולי.

אמר המפרש: חולי הקווץ הם שלשה מינים: הקווץ אשר לאחור והקווץ אשר לפנים והמתוח
(אשר לפנים בשוה המתוח בשוה(.)ו(לא יתראה באיברים כי מתחו לאחור ולפנים הוא
התמתחות שוה. ו)ל(כל מיני הקווץ אמנם הוא ממלוי האיברים העצביים ומן הרקתם. וכאשר
במשך הקווץ אחר הקדחת השורפת יתחייב שיהיה חדושו מן היבש. ומה שהיה מן הקווץ
מתחדש מתחלתו בפתע יתחייב חדושו מן המלוי. וכאשר קרה אחריו הקדחת הותרה קצת
הרטיבות המיותרת ותבשל קצת לחותם.

(4.58)

[195] אמר אבוקרט: כשהיה באדם קדחת שורפת וקרה לו סמור הותרה בו קדחתו.

אמר המפרש: כשיתנועע התערובת הכרכומית לצאת יחדש סמור וימשך אחריו קיא
הכרכומית וגרישת הבטן להוציא המותר ההוא המוליד בקדחת וכשיתנקו עורקיו הותרה
קדחתו.

(4.59)

[196] אמר אבוקרט: השלישית היותר ארוכה שתהיה תכלה בשבעה סבובים.

אמ׳ המפרש: אמר ג׳אלינוס: כבר חקרנו ובקרנו הגבול שברביעית והשלישית ומצאנוהו
שיהיה על חשבון מספר הסבובים לא כפי מספר מנין הימים.)מזה שהסבוב(השביעי בקדחת
השלישי יפול ביום השלשה עשר מתחלתה. וביום ההוא ברוב העניין יהיה גבול החולי ותכליתו
מבלתי שיעויין בו הארבעה עשר)ה( )ודברי אבוקרט בכאן בקדחת השלישית אמתית.

(4.60)

[197] אמר אבוקרט: מי שמצאתהו בקדחת החדה באזנו צמח הנקרא צמם בע׳ ויצא מנחיריו
דם או הותר בטנו בשלשול הותר בעבור זה חליו.

אמר המפרש: כבר קדם זכרון סבת זה.

(4.61)

[198] אמר אבוקרט: כשלא יהיה הסרת הקדחת מן המחומם ביום מן הימים הנפרדים מדרכה
שתחזור)והגבול אשר הוא בלתי שלם הוא קשה ויבא לידי חזרה מן החולי(.

---

1 קדחת: emendation editor האחת MSS   4)ו(לא יתראה באיברים: وليس ترى فيه الأعضاء تشنّج a
8 לחותם)= رطوبتها P(: رودتها a   11 וגרישת: وانطلاق a   17 שיעויין: أن ينتظر a   18 צמח הנקרא
צמם בע׳: صمم a

אמר המפרש: ג׳אלינו׳ יאמר כי זה טעות מן הנוסח ושמאמר אבוקרט הוא ביום מימי הגבול
או זוג היה או נפרד.

(4.62)

[199] אמר אבוקרט: כשקרה הירקרקות בקדחת לפני יום השביעי הוא סימן רע.

אמר המפרש: כבר יקרה זה הירקרקות על צד הגבול ולא יבוא הגבול בירקרקות לפני יום
השביעי אבל אמנם סבתו נגע מנגעי הכבד ולזה יהיה סימן רע.   5

(4.63)

[200] אמר אבוקרט: מי שמצאתהו בקדחתו סימור בשר בכל יום ודאי קדחתו תכלה בכל
יום.

אמר המפרש: רוצה באמרו תכלה בכל יום שהיא תוסר ממנו ותניחהו בכל יום עם הרקת
התערובת המביא לסמור עם התנועעו לחוץ וכן יקרה הענין בשלישית וברביעית.

(4.64)

[201] אמר אבוקרט: כשקרה הירקרקות בקדחת בשביעי או בתשיעי או באחד עשר או   10
בארבע עשר זה ישובח אלא אם כן שיהיה בצד הימני ממה שתחת הצלעות קושי. ואם היה
זה אין ענינו משובח.

אמר המפרש: סבת זה מבואר במה שקדם.

(4.65)

[202] אמר אבוקרט: כשהיתה בעת הקדחת התלהבות חזקה בקיבה ודפיקת הלב כל זה הוא
רע.   15

אמר המפרש: אם ירצה בתוך מעיו פי הקיב(ה) אז ענין אמרו דפיקת הלב עקיצת פי הקיבה
מפני שהושקתה בליחה הכרכומית. ואם ירצה באמרו בתוך מעיו הלב אז העלוף יזיק בו
להחזקת החום ממנו. אלו המקרים שניהם רעים מאד.

(4.66)

[203] אמר אבוקרט: הקווץ והכאבים הבאים בבני מעיו בקדחות החדות הוא אות רע.

---

4 יקרה: emendation editor יקשה MSS   9 לחוץ: emendation editor לחום MSS   11 בצד: emendation editor הצד MSS   14–15 כל זה הוא רע: فَتلكَ علامة رديئة a   16 בתוך מעיו: بِفؤاد a   אז:
באמרו: om. a   או MSS או emendation editor   17 בתוך מעיו: بالفؤاد a   אז: emendation editor או
MSS

אמר המפרש: הקדחת החזקה והגדולה תייבש העצבים כמו האש ותקווצם ועל אלו הפנים
יתחדש הקווץ הממית. ושמא יקרה בגוף כאב מאלו העניינים בעצמם מתגבורת ההתלהבות
והיובש.

(4.67)

[204] אמר אבוקרט: הבהלה והקווץ המתהוים בקדחת (מן) השינה מן האותות הרעות הם.

אמר המפרש: כשהיה הגוף מלא ליחות עם השינה ימלא ראשו ויכבד המוח. ואם תהיה הליחה
הגוברת נוטה אל השחרות יקרה ממנה הבהלה ואם אינו כן יקרה ממנה הכאב והקווץ. אמר   5
ג׳אלינוס שראה פעמים רבות בחליים הממיתים הבהלה והכאבים והקווץ יתחדשו מן השינה
והיה מדמה שקרה זה מהליכת הליחה המזיקה אל המוח בעת השינה.

(4.68)

[205] אמר אבוקרט: כשהאויר משתנה במעבריו שבגוף זה רע כי מורה על הקווץ.

אמר המפרש: ירצה באויר הנה אויר הנשימה כשיחבשהו שום דבר במעבריו עד שיפסוק   10
בעת כניסתו או ביציאתו או בשניהם יחד (לפי שיורה על העצבים המניעים החזה קרה להם
קצת קווץ).

(4.69)

[206] אמר אבוקרט: מי שהיה שתנו עבה דומה לטיט ומעט ואין גופו נקי מן הקדחת הוא
כשישתין שתן רב ורקיק יועיל בו ורוב מי שישתין זה השתן יצלול בזה בשתן מתחלת חליו או
אחריו בזמן מעט שמרים.   15

אמר המפרש: הענין ברוב במחוממים שיהיה השתן בתחלת החולי רקיק וכל מה שיקרב אל
תכליתו יתעבה עצמותו. והודיענו אבוקרט בזה הענין הבא לפעמים מעטים והוא שכבר יהיה
השתן דומה לטיט חוצות ומעט מתחלת החולי וסבת מעוטו שהוא לא יתפלש בכליות אלא
בקושי וכשהורק מזה רוב הליחה ההיא הרעה והתבשל מה שנשאר ממנה יורק אז מן השתן
מה שיהיה יותר רקיק והרבה.   20

(4.70)

[207] אמר אבוקרט: מי שהשתין בקדחת שתן מבולבל דומה לשתן עייר בן אתונות יש בו
כאב ראש עתה או יתחדש בו.

1 ותקווצם: فتعمّده وتجذبه a 5 הגוף: emendation editor בגוף MSS 10 הנה: om. a 13 לטיט:
بالعبيط a 16 השתן: emendation editor טוב MSS 17 עצמותו: emendation editor עצומו MSS
21 מבולבל: متثوّرا a ‖ עייר בן אתונות: الدوابّ a

אמר המפרש: אמנם יהיה השתן כן כשיעשה החום בחומר עבה ורב. ומה שהיה מן החמרים
על זה התואר ובפרט כשתעשה בו החום הנכרי יתילד ממנו הרוחות עד שיתבלבל כמי השעוה
או הזפת והראתינג׳. והרוחות העבות עם החום ימהרו לעלות אל הראש יראה הכאב ואפשר
שיהיה בלבול השתן לפני זה או איפשר שיהיה אחרי זה.

(4.71)

5   [208] אמר אבוקרט: מי שיבוא לו הגבול בשביעי כבר יראה בשתנו ברביעי ערפל אדומה
ושאר האותות תהיינה על זה ההקש.

אמר המפרש: הרביעי הוא יום ההבטה במה שיהיה בשביעי וכל אות בעל שעור יתראה בו
מורה על הבשול היא ראיה על הגבול המתהוה בשביעי. אכן הערפל הלבן יותר ראוי להורות
על זה והיותר ראוי ממנו הענן הלבן התלוי באמצע השתן. ואם יהיה החולי מהיר התנועה יהיה
10   שנוי הצבע לבדו ושנוי העצמות ראיה על הגבול שיבא בשביעי. ואמר ג׳אלינו׳ כי אבוקרט זכר
הערפל האדומה שהוא ראיה היותר חלושה להבין מזה עניני שאר הראיות שהם יותר חזקות
שהם מורות על הגבול מזומן. וכן האותות הנראות בימי ההבטה בתוצאות או ברוקין על זה
ההקש.

(4.72)

[209] אמר אבוקרט: כשיהיה השתן יבש ולבן הוא רע ובפרט (ב)בעלי הקדחת אשר עם
15   מורסת המוח.

אמר המפרש: זה השתן הוא בתכלית הרוחק מן הבשול ויורה על אריכות חולי ויורה גם על
שהמרה הירוקה תנועתה כלה למעלה לצד הראש.

(4.73)

[210] אמר אבוקרט: כשהיו המקומות אשר תחת הצלעות העליונים ממנו נפוחים ויהיה בהם
קרקור ואחר כן קרה לו כאב בשפל גבו דע כי בטנו ירפה אם לא יצאו ממנו רוחות רבות או
20   ישתין שתן רב וזהו בקדחת.

אמר המפרש: כשנתהוה הרוח עם הרטיבות המביאים קרקור ויתנועעו למטה וירד הנפח
לצד השפל השדרה וימתחו האיברים אשר לשם ויתחדש כאב. ואיפשר שתתפשט הרטיבות
ההיא אל העורקים ותצא בשתן והרוח יצא לבדו. וכבר יקרו שיצאו ביחד הרטיבות והרוחות
מן המעים וירפו הבטן. וכבר יקרה שינקבו שניהם אל העורקים ויעברו מהרה אל השלפוחית
25   ר״ל הרטיבות והרוחות. ו(ב)מי שיש לו קדחת בפרט ישען באלו האותות וידע כי הטבע כבר
הוכן ו(הו)זמן לדחות הדבר המזיק בשתן או ברעי.

─────────

2 הנכרי: الخارجة a   5 ערפל: غمامة a   10 ראיה: كافية a .add   12 ברוקין: في الرّزاق a   14 יבש:
مستشفّ a   17 כלה: emendation editor עלה MSS   18 העליונים: om. a   21 כשנתהוה: إذا
انحدرت a   22 שתתפשט: تأدّت a   24 שינקבו: ينفذان a   25 ר״ל: om. a   26 הוכן ו(הו)זמן:
عزمت a

(4.74)

‏[211] אמר אבוקרט: מי שיארע לו שיצאו לו צמחים באצילי פרקיו כבר נמלט מן אלו הצמחים‎
‏ברוב שתן עבה ולבן ישתין כשכבר התחיל ביום הרביעי בקצת מי שיש בו קדחת עייפות. ואם‎
‏הרעיף דם יהיה תכלית חליו עם זה במהרה לאלתר.‎

‏אמר המפרש: זה מבואר.‎

(4.75)

‏[212] אמר אבוקרט: מי שהיה משתין דם ומוגלא מורה זה על כי יש בו נגע בכליותיו או‎
‏בשלפוחיתו.‎

‏אמר המפרש: זה מבואר.‎

(4.76)

‏[213] אמר אבוקרט: מי שהשתין שתן עב ובו חתיכות בשר דקות או כמו השיער זה יוצא‎
‏מהכליות.‎

‏אמר המפרש: אמנם חתיכות הבשר הדקות הוא מעצם הכליות ואמנם מה שהוא כמו השיער‎
‏זה לא יהיה לא מעצם הכליות ולא מעצם השלפוחית. ואמר ג'אלינוס כי הוא ראה מי שקרה‎
‏להם שהשתינו אלו השערות וקצתם היה שיעור ארכם כמו חצי אמה מפני שהם התמידו‎
‏המאכלים המולידים ליחה עבה. וזאת הליחה העבה כשיפעול בו החום עד שישרפנה וייבשנה‎
‏בכליות יתילדו מזה השערות. ורפואות זה החולי יעיד על ההתאמתות זה ההקש בסבתו כי‎
‏אשר ימצאם החולי אמנם יבריאו בסמנים המדקדקים החותכים. ומאמר אבוקרט שאמר זה‎
‏יוצא מכליותיו הודענו במקום שיולדו השערות.‎

(4.77)

‏[214] אמר אבוקרט: מי שיצא בשתנו והוא עבה כמו סובין דע כי בשלפוחיתו גרב.‎

‏אמר המפרש: זה מבואר.‎

(4.78)

‏[215] אמר אבוקרט: מי שהשתין דם מבלתי דבר שקדם לו מורה על שהעורק שבכליות נסדק.‎

‏אמר המפרש: זה מבואר.‎

(4.79)

[216] אמר אבוקרט: מי שישקע בשתנו דבר דומה לחול אבן יתילד במקוה.

אמר המפרש: זה מבואר.

(4.80)

[217] אמר אבוקרט: מי שהשתין דם נקרש והיה בו קושי השתן ומצאתהו כאב בשפל בטנו
וסביב הערוה דע כי סביב לשלפוחיתו מכה.

5   אמר המפרש: זה מבואר.

(4.81)

[218] אמר אבוקרט: מי שהשתין דם ומוגלא וקליפות ושתנו יש בו ריח רע זה מורה על נגע
שבשלפוחית.

אמר המפרש: זה מבואר.

(4.82)

[219] אמר אבוקרט: מי שיצא לו שומא בטבעת החלוחלת(?) כשתתפתק ותשפוך דם תכלה
מעליו חליו.

10

אמר המפרש: זה מבואר.

(4.83)

[220] אמר אבוקרט: מי שהשתין בלילה שתן רב מורה על כי תוצאותיו מעטות.

אמר המפרש: זה מבואר.

נשלם המאמר הרביעי מפרקי אבוקרט.

---

4 וסביב הערוה: وعائه a ‖ מכה a ‖ מכה: وجع a   9 שומא: بُثرة a ‖ בטבעת החלוחלת(?): في إحليله
a ‖ כשתתפתק: انفتحت AC تقيّحت a ‖ ותשפוך דם: وانفجرت a

המאמר החמישי

(5.1)

[221] אמר אבוקרט: הקווץ אשר יהיה מן כרבק הוא מאותות מות.

אמר המפרש: יקרה הקווץ משתיית הכרבק הלבן והוא המכוון הנה כי הנה ההרקה או
לחזוק תנועת הקיא או לעקיצת הקיבה וזה כלו יתקשה רפואתו.

(5.2)

[222] אמר אבוקרט: הקווץ המתחדש מנגע הוא מאותות המות. 5

אמר המפרש: זה יהיה למורסות העצבים וינגע בהעלותו למוח. וכל מה שאמר אבוקרט בעבור
שהוא מאותות המות ירצה בזה גודל הסכנה ושהוא ימית ברוב.

(5.3)

[223] אמר אבוקרט: כשהלך מן הגוף דם רב וחדש פיהוק או קווץ זהו אות רע.

אמר המפרש: זה מבואר.

(5.4)

[224] אמר אבוקרט: כשיקרה קווץ או פיהוק אחר הרקה מרובה הנה הוא סימן רע. 10

אמר המפרש: זה מבואר.

(5.5)

[225] אמר אבוקרט: כשקרה לשכור חולי השתוק בפתע הוא יתקווץ וימות אלא אם כן
יתחדש בו קדחת או שידבר בעת שתסור מעליו שכרותו.

אמר המפרש: זה הקווץ יתהוה מפני מלוי העצבים ומשתיית היין בשימלא העצבים מהרה כי
היין יעבור לדקותו ולחמימותו. והיין כשירבה ממנו והוא לרוב עשנו ינצח לעצבים ויקוצם אלא 15
שהוא באיכותו יתרפא ויתוקן מה שנפסד לעצבים כשיחממם וייבשם. וכשלא יוכל לעשות
כבר יתחייב בהכרח שיבואנו הקווץ המתחדש ממנו המות. ובזה הכח אשר אמרנו כי היין יבא
בעבורו הקווץ כבר יבריאהו גם כן חולי הקדחת. והשכרות והוא ההזק שיקרה למי שהתמיד
בשתית היין.

---

3 כי: إمّا a ‖ 4 כלו: om. a ‖ 6 וינגע בהעלותו למוח: ويتراقى الألم للدماغ a ‖ בהעלותו: emendation editor בהפתו צ בהכותו(?) ק ‖ 15 יעבור: يغوص a ‖ עשנו: حمه a ‖ ינצח (يغلب): يجلب a
17–18 יבא בעבורו הקווץ: يرأ بها التشنّج a ‖ 18–19 למי שהתמיד בשתית: من شرب a

(5.6)

[226] אמר אבוקרט: מי שהכשילו המתוח הוא ימות בארבעה ימים. ואם יעבור הארבעה הוא
יבריא.

אמר המפרש: המתוח הוא חולי חד מאד באשר הטבע לא יוכל לסבול צער מתוחו מאחר
שהוא מורכב מן הקווץ אשר יהיה לאחור ומן הקווץ שיהיה לפנים ותכליתו יהיה ההבטה
הראשון מימי הגבול.   5

(5.7)

[227] אמר אבוקרט: מי שמצאתהו הכפייה קודם שיצמח לו השיער של בית הערוה הוא
יתחדש לו ההעתקה. ואמנם מי שקרה לו זה וכבר חלפו עליו מן השנים חמשה ועשרים הוא
ימות והוא בו.

אמר המפרש: אמר ג'אלינוס: רצה באמרו ההעתקה הכלות בחולי זה יהיה בתיקון התערובת
הקרה במזגה המולידה לכפייה והוא לבני רטוב בהעתקת השנים אל היובש ובהרגל ובהנהגה   10
המייבשת עם הסמנים הנאותים. ואבוקרט זכר בזה השנוי שיהיה בסבת השנים ומדת זמן
צמיחת שער הערוה)עד כלות זמן הגדול(הוא מה שבין תכלית השבוע השני עד)סוף זמן
הגדול והוא(חמשה ועשרים)יגיע לידי מוגלא(.

(5.8)

[228] אמר אבוקרט: מי שמצאו חולי הצד ולא ינקה בד' וה' הנה)ינקה((עינינו יגיע לעשות
מוגלא.   15

אמר המפרש: הרקת הליחה המולידה לחולי הצד על ידי רקיקה קורא אותו נקוי.

(5.9)

[229] אמר אבוקרט: דע מה שיהיה חולי הכלייה בשנות)הבחרות הוא(בין שמונה עשר
שנים ובין החמשה ושלשים שנה.

אמר המפרש: כבר קדם לנו כי הכלייה הוא מתחלואי הבחורים וכאשר זכר תחלואי החזה
והריאה זכר זה גם כן.   20

(5.10)

[230] אמר אבוקרט: מי שקרתהו שחיטה הנקרא אסכרה וימלט ממנו ונטה החומר אל ריאתו
הוא ימות בשבעה ימים. ואם יעברם יחזור להוצאת מוגלא.

אמר המפרש: מסופק אני אם הרבה לו הנסיון בזה החולי ודומיהם בזה המין מן ההעתקה ואין
ספק כי זה וההדומה לזה אמנם רוצה בו שהוא על הרוב.

(5.11)

[231] אמר אבוקרט: כשהיה באדם שדפון ויהיה מה שידחהו בשעול מן הרוק מאוסת הריח
כשישימנו על האש של גחלים ושער ראשו נושרות זה הוא מאותות מות.

אמר המפרש: מאיסות הריח מורה על הפסד הליחות וחוזק עפושם ונפילת שער הראש הוא
ממה שילקח ראיה על הפסד הליחה וגם כן יורה על העדר האיברים מן המזון.

(5.12)

[232] אמר אבוקרט: מי שנפל שיער ראשו מבעלי הכליה ואח״כ נתחדש לו שלשול הוא ימות.

אמר המפרש: שלשולם של אלו מורה על חולשת הכח ולזה יורה על קורבת המיתה.

(5.13)

[233] אמר אבוקרט: מי שירוק הדם בקצף הנה רקיקתו אמנם היא מריאתו.

אמר המפרש: הנה הוא מבואר כי הדם שיצא עם קצף הוא מגרם הריאה בעצמה.

(5.14)

[234] אמר אבוקרט: כשנתחדש שלשול במי שיש לו כליה יורה על מות ואם יהיה זה עם
סרחון ריח מה שירוקק ועם נשירת השערות יורה על קורבת מות כמו שקדם.

אמר המפרש: זה מבואר.

(5.15)

[235] אמר אבוקרט: מי שבאתהו העין במדוה הצד לידי פליטת מוגלא והוא אם נוקה
בארבעים יום למן היום אשר נשפך בו המוגלא אז חוליו יכלה. ואם לא ינוקה באלו הימים
יפול בחולי הכליון.

אמר המפרש: כשלא תצא המוגלה הנשפכה ונסגרה בתוך חדרי החזה היא תתעפש שם
ותצרב ותעפש את הריאה.

---

1 מסופק אני (= أَشُكّ): يوشك a   11 מות: قال المقسّر: إسهال أصحاب السلّ دليل الموت add. a   13 אמר
המפרש: זה מבואר :om. a   17 ונסגרה: وحصلت a ‖ חדרי: فضاء a ‖ שם :om. a   18 ותצרב: وتجمد
a ‖ ותעפש: وتقرّح a

(5.16)

[236] אמר אבוקרט: החום מזיק למי שירבה עשותו מדת זמן: ירפה הבשר ויפתח העצב
וירדים השכל ויגביר נזילת הדם ועלוף ויגיע בעליו אל המות.

אמר המפרש: יאמר כי מי שהפליג לנהוג בדברים החמים הוא ירפה בשרו ויפתח העצב עד
שירפהו בעבור התרת החום לעצמותו. ואמרו וירדים השכל אמר ג'אלינו': ירצה בו חולשת
השכל ויפסיד בכחו בהתרת עצם העצב ומבואר הוא שימשך אחר הזלת הדם העלוף וימשך   5
אחר העלוף המות.

(5.17)

[237] אמר אבוקרט: ואמנם הקור יחדש הקווץ והמתוח והסיתום והסימור שיהיה עמו קדחת.

אמר המפרש: זה מבואר.

(5.18)

[238] אמר אבוקרט: הקור מזיק לעצמות ולשינים ולעצב ולמוח ולחוט השדרה. ואמנם החום
הוא מועיל ונאות להם.   10

אמר המפרש: גם זה מבואר.

(5.19)

[239] אמר אבוקרט: כל מקום שנקרר כבר ראוי שיחומם אם לא תפחד על השפך הדם ממנו.

אמר המפרש: זה מבואר.

(5.20)

[240] אמר אבוקרט: הקור יעקוץ לנגעים ויקשה העור ויחדש)הסמור אשר עמה קדחת(
מהכאב מה שלא יהיה עמו מוגלא ויסתום ויחדש הסמור אשר עמה קדחת והקווץ   15
והמתוח.

אמר המפרש: זה מבואר.

---

1 מדת זמן: هذه المضار a ‖ ירפה: emendation editor ירפו MSS ‖ ויפתח (= ويفتح): ويفنخ a
2 נזילת: emendation editor עילת MSS   3 ירפה: emendation editor ירפא MSS ‖ ויפתח (=
ويفتح): ويفنخ a ‖ עד: يعني a   7 והסיתום: والاسوداد a   11 גם: om. a   15 ויסתום (= ويسد):
ويسود a

(5.21)

[241] אמר אבוקרט: אפשר אם ישפך על מי שיש בו מתוח בלי נגע והוא בחור טוב הבשר באמצע הקיץ מים קרים הרבה ונתחדש לו עטוף מן חום רב שיהיה המלטתו בחום ההוא.

אמר המפרש: זה מבואר.

(5.22)

[242] אמר אבוקרט: החום מוליד מוגלא אבל לא בכל נגע. וזה מגדולי האותות המורות על הבטחון והאמן)שיבשל המוגלא(וירטיב העור וידקדקהו וישקיט הכאב וישבר דקירת הסימור והקוץ והמתוח והמתוח ויתיר הכובד המתחדש בראש. והוא מן הנאותים שבעניינים לשברון העצמות וכ״ש לערומים מהם מן הבשר וכ״ש לעצמות הראש ולכל מי שאחזו הקור וניגעתהו. והנגעים המתרחבים והמתאכלים ולפי הטבעת והרחם והשלפוחית והחום לסובלי אלו החלאים מועיל ומרפא והקור מזיק להם וממית.

אמר המפרש: הוצאת המוגלא הוא אות טוב ומובטח בו בנגעים כי הוא מין ממיני הבשול כמו שידעת. ולא כל נגע מוציא מוגלא כי הנגעים הרעים כלם והקשים להרפא המתאכלות לא יתייל בהם מוגלא. ושאר מה שזכר מבואר כי כל אבר עצביי והעצמות גם כן יזיקם הקור.

(5.23)

[243] אמר אבוקרט: ואמנם הקור יצטרך שיעשה במקומות האלו ר״ל במקומות המגירות דם או שהוא מזומן להגרת דם. אין ראוי שיעשה במקום עצמו אשר יגר ממנו הדם כי אם סביבו ראוי שיעשה ובמה שהיה מן הצמחים החדים ובמקומות שיתחדש בם עקיצה סביב אל צמח אדמדם הנקרא אלחמרא בערבי וצבע הדם הלח)כי(כשיעשה הקור במה שכבר נתיישן בו הדם ישחירהו ובמורסא הנקרא האדומי אלחמרא בערבי כשלא יהיה עמו נגע כי מה שהיה עמו נגע הנה הוא יזיקהו.

אמר המפרש: זה מבואר.

(5.24)

[244] אמר אבוקרט: הדברים הקרים כמו השלג והברד מזיקים לחזה ומעוררים השעול ומביאים להגרת הדם והירידה.

אמר המפרש: זה מבואר.

---

2 עטוף: انعطاف a   5 דקירת: عادية a   7 שאחזו: أماته a   8 הטבעת: والفرج a   9 ומרפא: add. a ומרפא:
emendation editor ומרפק MSS   15 ראוי שיעשה: ومن حيث يجيء a   החדים: الحارّة a ‖ סביב:
مائل a   20–22 This aphorism features in the anonymous translation following aphorism 5.25

(5.25)

[245] אמר אבוקרט: המורסות שיתהוו בפרקי האיברים והכאבים שיהיו מבלתי נגע וכאבי
בעלי הנקרס וסובלי הקווץ המתחדשת במקומות העצביים ורוב מה שדומה לאלו אם ישפך
עליהם מים רבים קרים ישקיטם ויצמיקם וישקיט הכאב בהבאתו התרדמה כי מעט התרדמה
גם כן משקטת הכאבים.

אמר המפרש: ישקיט הכאב באלו המקומות שיחתוך הסבה המולידה אותו או בהרדים 5
לחושים.

(5.26)

[246] אמר אבוקרט: המים שיתחממו מהר או יתקררו מהר הם הקלים שבמימות.

אמר המפרש: מובן הוא שירצה באומרו הנה בכובד וקלות מהירות יציאתו מן הקיבה או
השארותו בה.

(5.27)

[247] אמר אבוקרט: מי שההביא אליו תאותו לשתות בלילה והיה צמאונו חזק ודאי אם ישן 10
אחריו זהו טוב.

אמר המפרש: כשישן אחר שתיית המים השינה תבשל התערובת המביאה לצמאון ולא יבא
לידי שתיית המים בלילה אלא מחוזק הצמאון.

(5.28)

[248] אמר אבוקרט: התחבושת בבושם הנקרא בערבי אפאיה מושך הדם הבא מן הנשים.
וכבר היה ראוי שיועיל במקומות אחרים הרבה לולי שיתחדש כובד בראש. 15

אמר המפרש: יאמר כי החבישה בבשמי האפויה ישלח דם הנדות או דם הלידה
כשנמנע כי זה ידקדק הדם אם היה עב או יפתח הסתום אם היה שם סתום או
ירחיב פיות העורקים אם נסתמו. וכבר היה ראוי להועיל בו גם כן לחמימות המקומות
הקרים או ליבש הרטיבות לולי היותו ממלא הראש כי כל חום יעלה לצד מעלה ויצער
הראש. 20

(5.29)

[249] אמר אבוקרט: ראוי שתשקה ההרה הסם המשלשל כשתהיינה הליחות בגופה
מתעוררות מעת שיעבור על העובר ארבעה חדשים עד שיעבור על העובר שבעה

---

2 וסובלי הקווץ: وأصحاب الفسخ a 3 ויצמיקם: emendation editor ויצמיתם MSS 12 יבא: يؤذن a
14 התחבושת בבושם הנקרא בערבי אפאיה: التكميد بالأفاوه a 16 החבישה בבשמי האפויה: التكميد
بالأفاوه a 17 סתום: om. a

חדשים ויהיה הקדמתך לזה מעט. ואמנם מי שהיה יותר קטן מזה או יותר גדול מזה ראוי שתזהר ותמנע.

אמר המפרש: אמנם אם יחזור חזרה בזה הפרק או החזירו בכוונה כדי להגיע הדבור בחליי הנשים.

(5.30)

5   [250] אמר אבוקרט: האשה ההרה כשתקיז דם תפיל וכל שכן אם עוברה כבר גדל.

אמר המפרש: זה מבואר.

(5.31)

[251] אמר אבוקרט: כשתהיה האשה הרה ויארע לה קצת התחלואים החדים זה מאותות מות.

אמר המפרש: אם היה מן החלאים החדים אשר עמהם קדחת אז ימית ברוע המזג המצריכה
10   לשאיפת אויר רב והאיברים עמוסים ובמיעוט המזון. אם היה כמו הפלאג' והקווץ אז היא לא תוכל לסבול חוזק הצער והמתוח באשר היא טעונה מהכובד.

(5.32)

[252] אמר אבוקרט: האשה כשתקיא דם ושוב נבע דם נדותה לה נפסק מעליה הקיא.

אמר המפרש: גם זה מבואר.

(5.33)

[253] אמר אבוקרט: האשה בנפסק נדותה אז רעיפת הדם טוב לה.

15   אמר המפרש: זה מבואר גם כן.

(5.34)

[254] אמר אבוקרט: האשה ההרה אם בא לה גרישת הבטן לא יאמן עליה שלא תפיל.

אמר המפרש: כשתניע הכח הדוחה באלו האיברים השכנים לרחם בכח תירא פחד גם כן שתניע הכח הדוחה שברחם.

---

3 אמנם אם:إمّا أنّه a   9 ימית:emendation editor ימות MSS   10 עמוסים:مضغوطة a   13 גם:.om
a   16 גרישת הבטן:استطلاق البطن a || הבטן:emendation editor הבדן MSS   17 פחד:-emenda
tion editor פרק צ תורה ק

(5.35)

[255] אמר אבוקרט: כשהיתה באשה חולי הרחם או קושי הלידה ומצאתה עטוש זה טוב.

אמר המפרש: כי האשה כשתתבטל נשימתה בחולי הרחם הנקרא התחנקות הרחם.
והעטוש מורה על התעוררות הטבע לפעול פעולתו והוא גם כן סבה להתפלטות האיברים
ולפלוט מה שנדבק בהם ונסתבך בהם מן התערובות המזיקות ובזה הצד יבריא העטוש
5 לפיהוק.

(5.36)

[256] אמר אבוקרט: כשהיתה דם הנדות מהאשה משונה המראה ולא תהיה בעת וסתה
תמיד מורה זה על שגופה צריך אל נקוי.

אמר המפרש: זה מבואר.

(5.37)

[257] אמר אבוקרט: כשהיתה האשה הרה וצמקו שדיה בפתע היא תפיל.

10 אמר המפרש: ידוע הוא השתתפות השדים לרחם וכאשר צומקה זה ראיה על מיעוט המזון
המגיע אליהם וכאשר ימעט המזון המגיע לרחם גם כן תפיל העובר.

(5.38)

[258] אמר אבוקרט: כשהיתה האשה הרה וצמק אחד משדיה פתאום והרתה תאומים אז
תפיל אחד מעובריה. אם הצמוק הוא מצד הימני תפיל הזכר ואם הצמוק בצד השמאלי תפיל
הנקבה.

15 אמר המפרש: הזכר הוא בצד הימני על הרוב.

(5.39)

[259] אמר אבוקרט: כשהאשה לא תתעבר ולא תלד ואחר היה לה חלב נדותה נפסקה.

אמר המפרש: לפעמים עם פסיקת הנדות ימלאו העורקים המגיעים אל השדים מלוי רב ויחדש
החלב לרוב הדם המגיע אל השדים. ויראה לי כי זה אינו אמת אלא אם כן היתה האשה בתכלית
הנקיון ושהיו מזונותיה בתכלית הטובה.

---

2 כי האשה כשתתבטל נשימתה בחולי הרחם הנקרא התחנקות הרחם: يريد بعلّة الأرحام اختناق الرحم
a 4–3 להתפלטות האיברים ולפלוט: لتنفض الأعضاء a 10 צומקה: emendation editor צומתה
a האשה: بدن المرأة 18 a לפעמים: في الندرة MSS 17 היא emendation editor: הוא MSS 15

(5.40)

[260] אמר אבוקרט: כשיקפיא הדם בשדי האשה יורה מעניניה על השטות.

אמר המפרש: הקרוב אצלי שראה זה פעם או פעמים וגזר אומר כמו שנהג מנהגו בספר אפידימיא. וכבר זכר ג'אלינוס כי לא ראה זה מעולם וזהו האמת ר"ל שאין זה סבה מסבות השטות. ואמנם קרה זה במקרה פעם או פעמים וראהו אבוקרט וחשבהו לסבה.

(5.41)

[261] אמר אבוקרט: כשתרצה לדעת האם האשה הרה אם לא תשקנה כשרוצה לישן מי הדבש. ואם מצא אותה המיה במעיה היא הרה ואם לא ימצאנה המיה אינה הרה.

אמר המפרש: ירצה באמרו כשרוצה לישן עם המנוחה והמלוי מן המאכלים ומי הדבש הם מולידים רוחות ויעזור לזה מלוי הבטן. וכשלא ימצא הרוח מקום מנוס לצאת בעבור דחיקת הרחם דרך יציאת הרוח יתחדש עלוף.

(5.42)

[262] אמר אבוקרט: כשהיתה האשה הרה בזכר תהיה יפת מראה וכשתהיה הרה בנקבה תהיה רעת המראה.

אמר המפרש: כל זה מבואר והוא על הרוב.

(5.43)

[263] אמר אבוקרט: כשתתחדש באשה הרה המורסא הנקראת האדום ברחמה ודאי זה הוא מאותות מות.

אמר המפרש: יראה לי מדברי ג'אלינוס שירצה לומר מות העובר וכן שאר המורסות החדות.

(5.44)

[264] אמר אבוקרט: כשתהר האשה והיא מן הכחישות על ענין יוצא מן הטבע היא תפיל קודם שתשמין.

אמר המפרש: כשתהר האשה והיא מן הכחישות המזון המגיע לאיברים יקחוהו האיברים בכללם ולא יותר עמה דבר שיזון בו העובר כשיגדל ולזה תפיל קודם שתגיע בענין השמנות לא לחזירתה לטבעה בעובי גופה.

---

5 מי: emendation editor מן MSS   6 המיה: مغص a   9 עלוף: المغص a   13 האדום: الحمرة a
15 החדות: الحارّة a   18 כשתהר: يقول إنّها إذا حبلت a ‖ מן הכחישות: في غاية الهزال a   19 בענין:
حيز a

(5.45)

[265] אמר אבוקרט: כשתהיה האשה הרה וגופה מיושר ותפיל בחדש השני)ת(או השלישי
מבלי סבה מבוארת ודאי נשתנה הרחם שלה ונתמלא ליחה דומה לליחה יוצאת מהנחירים
ולא תוכל לתפוש העובר לכובדו אבל ישמט ממנה.

אמר המפרש: זה מבואר.

(5.46)

[266] אמר אבוקרט: כשתהיה האשה על ענין יוצא מהטבע מן השמנות ודאי לא תתעבר כי   5
הקרום הפנימי מקרומי הבטן הנקרא החלב ידחוק ברחמה ולא תתעבר עד שתכחש.

אמר המפרש: יש לרחם לו צואר ארוך וקצה זה הלול הוא מחובר או פנימי הירכים מחושק(?)
הטבעת (ו)הנקרא פי הרחם על דרך האמת והוא התחלת הלול ממה שהוא לצד הרחם והוא
אשר ידחוק בו החלב מן האשה השמנה המופלגת בשמנות.

(5.47)

[267] אמר אבוקרט: כשתתפתח הרחם עד שיגיע אל הירך ראוי בהכרח אל צורך המעשה   10
לפתילות.

אמר המפרש: ירצה באמרו המעשה מלאכת היד כלומר הכנסת הפתילות וכשיבוא לידי
טרומה אז כבר צריכה אל הפתילות.

(5.48)

[268] אמר אבוקרט: כשיהיה העובר זכר ראוי שיהיה הריונו מן הצד הימין וכשיהיה נקבה מן
הצד השמאלי.   15

אמר המפרש: זה מבואר כי הצד הימין הוא יותר חם. וכבר זכר ג'אלינו' כי הזרע הבא מן
האשה מהצד הימין מאחת מהביצים שלה יש בה חום ועובי ומה שבא מן הצד השמאלי הוא
רקיק ומימי יותר קר מן האחר. ומי יתן ידעתי האם בא לו זה בנבואה או הראה לו זה ההקש
והסברא. ואפילו אם היה לפניו וארג זאת האריגה בסברא ודאי זה ההקש וסברא הם מאד.

---

2 ודאי נשתנה: فتقعير a   6 עד: دون أنْ a   7 הלול: الرقبة a   8–7 הוא מחובר או פנימי הירכים
מחושק(?) הטבעת: الذي يلي الفرج وفي داخله يلج الإحليل a يسمّى فم رقبة الرحم وقد يسمّى فم الرحم
add. a   8 הלול: الرقبة a ‖ לצד: يلي a   10 כשתתפתח: تفتح a (= تفتح): تقيح a   11–10 המעשה לפתילות
الفتل A العمل a   13–12 וכשיבוא לّدי טרומה: وإذا تقيّح ممّا يلي منه خارج a   13 טרומה (?):(= trauma?)
emendation editor טרימה MSS   18 הראה לו: وداه a   19 ואפילו אם היה לפניו וארג זאת האריגה
בסברא: فإنْ كان حدّد وحرّر هذا التحرير بقياس a ‖ ודאי זה ההקש וסברא הם מאד: فهذا قياس عجيب
غريب a ‖ מאד: عجيب غريب a غريب BP

(5.49)

[269] אמר אבוקרט: כשתרצה להפיל השליא תכניס באפה סם מעטיש וסתום נחיר(י)ה וגם
פיה.

אמר המפרש: כי יתחדש לבטן בעבור זה מתוח וקושי ויעזור על נפילת השליא.

(5.50)

[270] אמר אבוקרט: כשתרצה להפסיק דם נדות אשה תשים על כל אחד משדיה כלי המציצה
5   מהגדול שאיפשר להמצא.

אמר המפרש: זה מבואר כי הוא מושך אל הפך הצד.

(5.51)

[271] אמר אבוקרט: פי הרחם של אשה הרה יהיה סתום.

אמר המפרש: זה מבואר.

(5.52)

[272] אמר אבוקרט: כשיצא החלב משדי המעוברת יורה זה על חולשת העובר וכאשר יהיו
10   עצורים יורה זה על שהעובר יותר בריא.

אמר המפרש: אמנם יצא החלב ויגר מן האשה המעוברת למלוי העורקים אשר בין הרחם
והשדים לרבויו ואמנם ירבה שם להמצא הדם כשיהיה העובר מעט המזון ולא ימשוך
מהעורקים ההם כי אם מעט דבר.

(5.53)

[273] אמר אבוקרט: כשיהיה ענין האשה הולך אל ההפלה הנה שדיה יצמקו. ואם הענין בהפך
15   זה ר"ל שיהיו שדיה קשים הנה ימצאנה כאב בשדים או בירכים או בעינים או בשני ארכובותיה
(ו)לא תפיל.

אמר המפרש: צמיקות השדים ראיה על מעוט הדם כמו שזכרנו וגדלם ראיה על שווי שעורו
וקשים ראיה על רבוי הדם ועביו. ולכן ישתדל הטבע לדחות המותר ההוא הנוסף לאבר אחר
(...) כאב. ובכלל אלו הראיות ענין כולן בלתי אמתיות ולא שיהיו ברוב. וכל אלו הפרקים
20   והדומה להם נמשך אחר מה שקרה פעם או שתי פעמים וראה אותו כי החכם אבוקרט התחיל
במלאכה.

---

3 וקושי: وَتوتّر a   10 עצורים: مكتنزين a   12 ימשוך: يمتار a   17 שזכרנו: ذكّ a ‖ וגדלם (=
واكتبارهما): واكتنازهما a   18 ישתדל: يمكن أنْ a   19 (...): قريب من الرحم أو من الثدي فيحدث
في ذلك العضو a ‖ ענין: om. a   20 להם: عندي add. a

(5.54)

[274] אמר אבוקרט: כשיהיה פי הרחם קשה הנה יתחייב בהכרח שיהיה סתום.

אמר המפרש: זה מבואר.

(5.55)

[275] אמר אבוקרט: כשיקרה הקדחת לאשה הרה ונבערה בחום מופלג בלי סבה נראת תקשה בלידתה ותסתכן או תפיל בסכנה.

5   אמר המפרש: צריך לקלות הלידה שיהיו שתי הגופים חזקים גוף האם וגוף העובר.

(5.56)

[276] אמר אבוקרט: כשיקרה אחר זיבת הנדות קווץ ועלוף זה רע.

אמר המפרש: זה מבואר.

(5.57)

[277] אמר אבוקרט: כשיבוא הנדות ביותר שעור מחוקה יקרה מזה חליים מן הרחם.

אמר המפרש: זה מבואר.

(5.58)

10   [278] אמר אבוקרט: כשיקרה בפי הטבעת או תוך הרחם מורסא יבוא מזה טפטוף השתן וכן כשיגלו הכליות ימשך לזה טפת השתן וכשנתחדש בכבד מורסא יבוא מזה פיהוק.

אמר המפרש: טפטוף השתן יבוא לחולשת הכח המחזיק בשלפוחית או לחדות השתן.)אמר אבוקרט(חולשת הכח יהיה מרוע מזג או מצמח יתחדש שם וחדוד השתן ממה שיתערב בו מן הליחות העוקצות.)אמר המפרש(כשתהיה המורסא באחד מאלו שני האיברים תזיק לשלפוחית לשכנות המקום ותחלשנה כחותיה. וכשתהיה המדוה בכליות ויחדש עקיצה בשתן ולא יבוא מן מורסא בכבד הפיהוק אלא כשהיא גדולה.

(5.59)

[279] אמר אבוקרט: כשהאשה לא תהר ורצונך שתדע אם תהר אם לא תכסנה בשמלה והקטר מתחתיה. אם תראה כי רוח הקטורת יעבור בגופה עד שיגיע אל נחיר)י(ה ואל פיה דע כי אין סבת העדר ההריון ממנה.

20   אמר המפרש: הקטורת יהיה בעניינים טובי הריח כמו מר ולבונה ומיעה ואשטורק.

(5.60)

[280] אמר אבוקרט: כשהאשה ההרה יבוא נדותה בעתה לא יתכן שיהיה העובר בריא.

אמר המפרש: יאמר ג'אלינו': כמדומה שיהיה הנדות הנגר מן ההרות מן העורקים אשר בצואר הרחם כי השליא תלויה בפיות של כל העורקים אשר מבפנים בחלל הרחם ולא יתכן יצא ממנו מאומה לחדרי הרחם.

(5.61)

[281] אמר אבוקרט: כשלא נגרה דם נדות האשה בעתה ולא נתחדש בה סמור ולא קדחת אבל קרה לה מצוק ועלוף ורוע נפש דע כי היא הרה.

אמר המפרש: זה מבואר.

(5.62)

[282] אמר אבוקרט: כשתהיה פי הרחם מן האשה קר ומקשיי לא תתעבר וכשתהיה גם כן רטובה מאד לא תהר כי רטיבותה תקפיא הזרע ותכבנו וכשתהיה יבשה יותר מדאי או חמה שורפת לא תהר כי הזרע יעדר מן המזון ויפסד וכשתהיה מזג הרחם שוה בין שני אלו העניינים תהיה האשה רבת בנים.

אמר המפרש: זה מבואר.)אמר אבוקרט: כשתהיה האשה הרה ומצאתה קושי זה מורה על ההפלה. אמר המפרש: זה מבואר(

(5.63)

[283]

(5.64)

[284] אמר אבוקרט: החלב לסובלי כאב הראש רע והוא גם כן רע למחוממים ולמי שהיה לו המקומות אשר מתחת צלעותיו שטוחות ובו קרקור ולמי שיש לו צמא ולמי שגובר המרה על תוצאותיו)ו(למי שהוא בקדחת חדה ולמי שיש לו שלשול דם הרבה. ויועיל לסובלי השדפון כשלא יהיה בהם חום חזק מאד ולבעלי הקדחת הארוכה והחלושה כשלא יהיה עמה דבר ממה שזכרנו ותהיינה גופותם נתכים על זולת מה שיחייבהו החולי.

אמר המפרש: החלב הוא מן הדברים הממהרים להשתנות אמנם בקיבה אשר היא קרה יתחמץ אמנם בקיבה אשר היא חמה יותד אל העשניות ואמנם הנזונים ממנו לפי הדין יוליד

---

6 ועלוף (= وغشي P): وغشّي a ‖ ומקשיי: متكاثفا a ‖ om. a 8 פי: a 9 מאד: emendation editor بزولت(؟) MSS ‖ רטיבותה: emendation editor رطيبوتها MSS ‖ תקפיא הזרע ותכבנו: تغمر
المني وتجمده وتطفئه a 14 This aphorism is missing in the Arabic and Hebrew translations
16 שטוחות: مشرفة a 20 אמנם: إمّا a 21 אמנם: وإمّا a ‖ ואמנם: وإمّا a

מזון דק ומשובח אלא שהוא בעת הזנתו יחדש נפח במה שתחת הצלעות ויכאיב הראש. זהו
פעולתו בבריאים ואמנם בחולים הוא כל מה שזכר.

(5.65)

[285] אמר אבוקרט: מי שנתחדש בו מכה ונתנפח בעבורה אי איפשר שיבואנו חולי הקווץ
ולא חולי השגעון. ואם נעלם זה ההתנפחות פתאום ושוב היתה המכה מגבי יקרה לו הקווץ או
המתוח. ואם היתה המכה מלפניו יקרה לו שגעונות או כאב חד בצדדים או בלוי או שלשול
דם אם היה זה ההתנפחות אדומה.

אמר המפרש: איני צריך להשיב לך פעמים באלו הגזרות אשר אמרם אבוקרט קצתם הם על
הרוב או על הנכון והיושר וימצאו קצת גזרותיו על המעט ואולי ראה זה הוא פעם אחת וייחס
הענין בזה לסבה אחת אשר אינה סבה אמתית.

וביאור זה הפירוש לג'אלינוס שהוא רוצה באמרו ההתנפחות המורסא וכל תערובת יוצא מן
הטבע. ומה שהוא ממנו מגבו של הגוף הוא עצביי ומה שהוא ממנו מלפניו יהיה הגובר עליו
הגידים הדופקים. וכשתעלה התערובת המולידה למורסא מן העצבים אל המוח יהיה חולי
הקווץ וכשעלה בעורקים אל המוח אז יהיה השגעון. ואם באה זאת התערובת אל החזה יהיה
הכאב בצדדים. ורוב מה שימצא לסובלי מדוה הצד עשיית המוגלא.

(5.66)

[286] אמר אבוקרט: כשנתחדשו צמחים גדולים ורעים ושוב לא יתראה עמהם שום נפח הנזק
עצום.

אמר המפרש: ר״ל הצמחים הרעים אשר יהיו בראשי העצלים או בסופם או מה שיהיה מן
העצלים שגובר עליהם העצב. וכשלא תתחדש מורסא במי שזה ענינו מן הצמחים לא יאמן
שלא תהיינה התערובות הנשפכות אל הצמחים נעתקות מהם אל מקומות אשר הם יותר
נכבדות ממקומות הצמחים.

(5.67)

[287] אמר אבוקרט: הרכות משובח והרפיון מגונה.

---

1 דק: غزيرا a ‖ הזנתו: استقرائه a   3 מכה: قرحة a   4 המכה: القرحة a ‖ מגבו: مכהו צ من خلف a
5 בלוי: تقيح a   7 איני צריך להשיב לך פעמים באלו הגזרות: لا أحتاج أنْ أكرّر أنّ أكثر هذه القضايا a
8 וימצאו: وعند التحقيق فتوجد a   10 הפירוש: الفصل a ‖ תערובת (= خلط) a   13 יהיה: ولَد
a   15 צמחים (= خراجات A): جراحات a ‖ ושוב: ثمّ a   17 הצמחים (= بالجراحات AP): بالجراحات a
18 במ: في ما a ‖ הצמחים (= الجراحات AP): الجراحات a   19 הצמחים (= الجراحات AP): الجراحات
a   20 הצמחים (= الجراحات AP): الجراحات a   21 והרפיון: والبيئة a

אמר המפרש: אמר ג'אלינוס: ירצה ברפיון בכאן קושי דחוי התוצאות והוא הפך הרכות כי כל קושי ודאי הוא מתערובת בלתי מבושלת.

(5.68)

[288] אמר אבוקרט: מי שמצאתהו כאב במאוחר ראשו ונחתך העורק הנצב אשר במצח יעזר בחתוך ההוא.

אמר המפרש: המשיכה אשר בחלוף הצד בצואר הוא למשוך מן המאוחר אל המוקדם ומן   5
המוקדם אל המאוחר.

(5.69)

[289] אמר אבוקרט: עקיצת הסמור ברוב מה שיתחיל בנשים הוא משפל השדרה ושוב יעלה בשדרה אל הראש. והוא גם כן באנשים יתחיל מגביהם יותר ממה שיתחיל מלפניהם כמו מה שיתחיל מן השוקים ומן הירכים. וזה כי העור גם כן בפני הגוף ספוגיי ויורה לך על זה
השער.   10

אמר המפרש: הקור ימהר אל הגב יותר להיותו קר לרוב העצמות שיש לשם ומעוט הבשר. והנשים יותר קרים מן האנשים והראיה על ספיגות העור מלפנים מצמיחת השערות.

(5.70)

[290] אמר אבוקרט: מי שקרה לו קדחת רביעית אי איפשר לו הקווץ ואם קרה לו הקווץ לפני הרביעית ואחר כן נתחדש לו קדחת רביעית תשקיט הקווץ.

אמר המפרש: ביאור ג'אלינו' אמר כי זה המין מן הקווץ הוא המתהוה מן המלוי ורפואתו יהיה   15
בחסר התערובת הוצאה מן הטבע או לבשלה. ובקדחת רביעית תצא בחזוק ותתבשל בחום הקדחת.

(5.71)

[291] אמר אבוקרט: מי שעורו נמתח ושחור וקשה ימות בלא זיעה ומי שעורו רפה ספוגי ימות בזיעה.

אמר המפרש: ר"ל בזיעה של מות ממי שהיה עורו כן.   20

---

1 ברפיון: بالتيع a ‖ דחוי: المدافع a ‖ התוצאות ‖ om. a הרכות: ‖ emendation editor הרקות MSS
7 עקיצת הסמור: النافض a ‖ ושוב: ثمّ a   9 השוקים: الساعدين a   11 לרוב: emendation editor
לחבור MSS   12 השערות: هناك add. a   16 בחסר (= بنقاص): باتفاض a ‖ הוצאה מן הטבע:
خارج a ‖ בחזוק: النافض add. a   18 ושחור: قلا a   20 בזיעה של מות: من أشرف على الموت a

(5.72)

[292] אמר אבוקרט: מי שבו ירקון אי אפשר שיולדו בו רוחות.

אמר המפרש: מן הסבות המולידות רוחות הוא מציאות הליחה הלבנה אשר במקומות התילדותם וזה לא יהיה עם חולי הירקות לתגברות המרה האדומה.

נשלם המאמר החמשי.

המאמר הששי

(6.1)

[293] אמר אבוקרט: כשנתחדש הגיהוק החמוץ במדוה הנקרא חלקות המעים אחרי
שנתארך ולא היה זה לו מקודם זה אות משובח.

אמר המפרש: כשהיה חולי חלקות המעים מפני חולשת כח המחזיק ויצא המאכל קודם
שנתעכל ואחרי כן חודש לו הגיהוק החמוץ זהו ראיה על שהמאכל כבר חזר להשאר בקיבה
שיעור מה שיתכן שיתחיל המאכל להשתנות קצת שנוי שיעור כדי שיתחמץ ושהטבע התחיל
לחזור לפעולתו.

5

(6.2)

[294] אמר אבוקרט: מי שהיה בנחיריו בטבע רטיבות יתירה והיתה שכבת זרע רקיק ודאי
בענין הבריאות הוא חלוש וקרוב להיות חולאני. ומי שענינו בהפך זה הוא יותר בריא הגוף.

אמר המפרש: אלו הדברים מורים על רטיבות המוח ויובש שאר האיברים ולזה הורקק שכבת
זרעו.

10

(6.3)

[295] אמר אבוקרט: מניעת האכילה בשלשול דם המיושן הוא אות רע ועם קדחת הוא יותר
רע.

אמר המפרש: שלשול הדם כשהיה מגרידת המעים הדקים ואורך רעתו ושרפתו יוסיף לחפור
בעומק האיברים ושב מכה ונגע עם עפוש ונתזנק הקיבה בהשתתפותה להם ויגיע לעכולה
הנזק. וכשעלתה המכה על פי הקיבה תפול התאוה והיה זה ראיה על תפישה והחזקת החולי
ואריכות הזיקו.

15

(6.4)

[296] אמר אבוקרט: מי שהיה מן הנגעים ינשרו ויפלו מה שיש בסבובה הוא רע.

אמר המפרש: נשירת השיער שבסביב הנגע ופשיטת העור היא ראיה על חדוד מה שישפך
אליה ולזה תאכל מה שבסביב מקומו.

20

---

5 חזר: صار a   9–8 ודאי בענין הבריאות הוא חלוש וקרוב להיות חולאני: فإنّ صحّته أقرب إلى السقم a
14 ואורך רעתו ושרפתו: وطال لبثه a   15 מכה ונגע: قرحة a   16 על פי הקיבה: لفم المعدة a ‖ תפישה
והחזקת החולי: تمكّن المرض a   17 ואריכות: وامتداد a   18 ינשרו: ينتثر a   19 ופשיטת: emendation
editor ופשיתת MSS   20 מה שבסביב מקומו: ما حوله أخيرا a

(6.5)

[297] אמר אבוקרט: ראוי שתבקר מן הכאבים ההווים בצלעות ופני החזה וזולת זה משאר האיברים גודל התחלפותם.

אמר המפרש: ר״ל שלא יכוין על בקור מקום הנזק בלבד מבלתי שיעויין בגודל החולי או חולשתו. והראיה על זה מחוזק הכאב ומה שיתחבר עמו מן הדקירה והעקיצה והמתוח והדומה בזה מהתחלפות המקרים וחוזקם הנמשכים אל נזק האבר ההוא.

(6.6)

[298] אמר אבוקרט: המדוים שיהיו בשלפוחית (ו)בכליות יקשה רפואתם בישישים.

אמר המפרש: זה מבואר.

(6.7)

[299] אמר אבוקרט: מי שהיה מן הכאבים אשר יקרה בבטן העליון הוא יותר נקל ומה שהיה מהם בלתי כך הוא יותר חזק.

אמר המפרש: אמר ג׳אלינו: רוצה לומר בעליון הוא מקום מה שסמוך אל השדרה העליונה למעלה מן הטרפש השטוח על המעים והקיבה ואמרו ומה שהיה מהם בלתי כך ר״ל מה שהיה מהם במעים ובקיבה.

(6.8)

[300] אמר אבוקרט: מה שיקרה מן הנגעים בגופות סובלי השקוי לא יקל להתרפ(א)ות.

אמר המפרש: הנגעים לא יתרפאו עד שיקל יובשם בשלמות ואין זה נקל במשוקים.

(6.9)

[301] אמר אבוקרט: הכתמים הרחבים לא יתכן היות עמם חכוך.

אמר המפרש: היות הכתמים והנגעים יומתחו ברוחב ולא יהיה להם עובי הוא ראיה על היות החמר יותר קר. ולזה לא יתחדש החכוך לקרירות החומר.

---

3 יכוין על: يقتصر على a ‖ הנזק: الألم a ‖ 4 שיתחבר: يوجد a 6-7 צק This aphorism features in
10 השדרה העליונה: ظاهر البطن a after aphorism 6.8 14 שיקל יובשם (= تخفّ جفافا): تجفّ
جفافا a ‖ במשוקים: في مزاج المستسقين a 15 הכתמים: البثور a ‖ לא יתכן היות: لا يكاد تكون a
16 הכתמים: البثور a ‖ עובי: تخصوص a 17 החכוך: emendation editor החתוך MSS

(6.10)

[302] אמר אבוקרט: מי שהיה לו צער וכאב חזק בראשו ויצא באפיו או באזנו או בפיו נגע או מים ודאי הותר זה.

אמר המפרש: זה מבואר.

(6.11)

[303] אמר אבוקרט: סובלי הדאגה השחוריי וסובלי צמר המוח הנקרא ברסם בערבי כשנתחדש להם הטחורים היה זה להם סימן טוב.

אמר המפרש: הדאגה השחוריית הוא ערבוב השכל ההווה מן השחורה והוא הנקרא בלשון יון מלכוניא והברסם הוא צמר בקרומי המוח. ומבואר הוא כשיפנה החמר אל ⟨חלוף⟩ הצד ובא לידי התפתחות פיות העורקים זהו תקונו.

(6.12)

[304] אמר אבוקרט: מי שנתרפא מן הטחורים המיושנים עד שהבריא ושוב לא הניח מהם אחד לא יאמן עליו שלא יתחדש בו השקוי או הכליה.

אמר המפרש: כי הוא כשלא יניח מהם אחד שיורק ממנו הדם ⟨שב⟩ זה הדם ונתרבה על הכבד ויכבה חומו ברבויו ויחדש השקוי או ימשך בעורקים אחרים וישקה העורק שבריאה ויחדש הכליה ר״ל שהוא כבר יחדש אלו שני החליים וכבר יתחדש מזה זולתם מהתחלואים.

(6.13)

[305] אמר אבוקרט: כשקרה לאדם הפיהוק ונתחדש לו עטוש שקט פיהוקו.

אמר המפרש: רוב מה שיקרה הפיהוק מן המלוי וזהו אשר יבריאהו העטוש להתחסר הרטיבות ההוא בתנועת העטוש הדוחה ברעישה.

(6.14)

[306] אמר אבוקרט: כשיהיה באדם השקוי ונגר המים ממנו בעורקים אל בטנו היה זה כלות חוליו.

אמר המפרש: זה מבואר שכבר יפעל הטבע באלו המים מה שיפעל בגבולי החלאים החדים בחמר המחליא.

---

1 או בפיו נגע: قيح a‏ 2 ודאי הותר זה: فإنّ مرضه يحَلّ بذلك a‏ 4 וסובלי: emendation editor כסובלי צ ⟨...⟩ ק ‖ צמר המוח הנקרא ברסם בערבי: البرسام a‏ 7 והברסם הוא צמר: والبرسام ورم حارّ a‏ 11 הדם: العكر a‏ 12 ברבויו: emendation editor ורבויו MSS ‖ ימשך: تبعّته a ‖ וישקה: فينفتق a‏ 16 הדוחה ברעישה: المزعجة a

(6.15)

[307] אמר אבטקרט: כשיהיה לאדם שלשול ארוך ונתחדש לו הקיא מעצמו נפסק ממנו שלשולו.

אמר המפרש: זה מבואר כי הטבע משך החמר בחלוף הצד.

(6.16)

[308] אמר אבוקרט: מי שפגעו חולי הצד או מדוה הריאה ונתחדש לו שלשול זה בו סימן
רע.   5

אמר המפרש: אמנם יהיה השלשול אות רע באלו שני החליים כשהיה החולי גדול מאד עד
שירפה (הטבע) מחולשת הכח.

(6.17)

[309] אמר אבוקרט: כשהיה באדם צמח העין הנקרא רמד בער' ובאתהו שלשול זהו משובה.

אמר המפרש: זה מבואר.

(6.18)

[310] אמר אבקרט: כשנתחדש בשלפוחית השריפה הנקרא בערבי אלחרק או במוח או בלב   10
או בכוליא או בטרפשא או בקץ)ו(ת המעים הדקים או בקיבה או בכבד זהו הריגה.

אמר המפרש: אמר ג'אלינו': אבוקרט יגזור הריגה במה שיהרג בהכרח ובמה שיהרג על
הרוב. וכבר ראיתי איש אחד שמצאו במוחו פציעה גדולה בתכלית ונתרפא אלא שזה לעתים
רחוקים.

(6.19)

[311] אמר אבוקרט: כשנחתך עצם או חלל או עצב או מקום הרקיק מן הלחי או קצה הערלה   15
לא יצמח ולא יתאחד.

אמר המפרש: לא יצמח ר"ל לא יתחדש כמוהו בנגע עמוק ואם היה בקיעה לא יתחבר כי הם
איברים יבשים ויתרחבו גם בסדיקה ובכריתה רוחב גדול.

---

10 השריפה הנקרא בערבי אלחרק (= حرق): خرق a (حرق): om. a   11 בטרפשא a   הריגה: قتّال || יגזור:
يستعمل a || הריגה: قتّال a   13 שמצאו: emendation editor   יצא צ (...) ק || בתכלית: غائرة a
15 חלל: غضروف a || קצה הערלה: القلفة a

(6.20)

[312] אמר אבוקרט: כשנשפך הדם אל חדרי הבטן על חלוף הצד הטבעי אי אפשר שלא יבלה.

אמר המפרש: רצה באמרו יבלה כי ישתנה ויפסד הדם בהכרח.

(6.21)

[313] אמר אבוקרט: מי שנשתנה ונתחדש בו רוחב העורקים הנקראים דליות או הטחורים
הותר בזה שטותו.

אמר המפרש: זה מבואר כשנפנה החמר אל חלוף הפך הצד ובתנאי שתהיה זאת התערובת   5
המולידה לשטות היא אשר נטתה אל השוקים. וכבר ידעת כי גזרותיו אינם כללים.

(6.22)

[314] אמר אבוקרט: הכאבים הבאים מן השדרה אל המפרקים יתיכם הקזת העורקים.

אמר המפרש: זה כשתהיינה ⟨תערובות⟩ סבה אל אלו הכאבים ונטו לצד המפרק על ידי
הרקתם מן המקום שנטו אליו יועיל בו בלי ספק.

(6.23)

[315] אמר אבוקרט: מי שהתמיד בו הפחד ורוע הנפש זמן ארוך ודאי חליו מן המרה השחורה.   10

אמר המפרש: כשקרה לאדם הבהלה ורוע הנפש מבלי סבה נגלית אז סבתו מדרך הדאגה
שחורית ואע"פ שלא יהיו אלו המקרים מתמידים. וכשהיו אלו המקרים מסבה ידועה כמו
כעס ויגון או אבל ואח"כ ארך שהייתו והתמיד יורה ג"כ על הדאגה השחורית.

(6.24)

[316] אמר אבוקרט: אם נחתכו קצת מן המעים הדקים לא יתאח⟨ד⟩ו.

אמר המפרש: זה מבואר.   15

(6.25)

[317] אמר אבוקרט: העתקת הצמח הנקרא אדום מחוץ לצד פנים אינו משובח. ואמנם
העתקתו מפנים לצד חוץ הוא משובח.

_____

1 חדרי הבטן: فضاء a ‖ הצד: الأمّ a ‖ יבלה: يَقيح a   2 יבלה: يَقيح a ‖ הדם: صورته الدمية
a ‖ בהכרח: om. a   3 שנשתנה: أصابه جنون a   7 המפרקים: المرفقين a (= המרפקים)   8 ונטו:
emendation editor וכמו MSS ‖ המפרק: المرفق a (= המרפק)   13 ויגון: أو غيظ a ‖ שהייתו: emendation editor ⟨...⟩ צ (?)שלהתו ק   15 אמר המפרש: זה מבואר: om. a.

אמר המפרש: זכר המורסא האדומה למשל והוא הדין בכל מורסא ובכל חומר הנפלשים
מפנים לחוץ הם אות טוב. וכשהענין בהפך זה הוא אות רע כי זה יורה על חולשת הטבע.

(6.26)

[318] אמר אבוקרט: מי שקרה לו בקדחת השורפת רעישה אז ערבוב השכל יתירנה ממנו.

אמר המפרש: כבר ביאר ג'אליני' בלבול)זה(המאמר שבזה הפרק. וזה כי חומר הקדחת
השורפת הוא בעורקים וכשנעתק החומר לעצבים חדש הרעש וכשתפשה בחוזק במוח   5
יתערבב השכל והוא יותר מסוכן מן הקדחת השורפת. ולא בכמו זה יאמר כי הותרה הקדחת
אחר כי הענין אשר נתחדש בו יותר מסוכן ויותר רע.

(6.27)

[319] אמר אבוקרט: מי שנכוה או נכרת מן הבלויים או מן המשוקים ונגר ממנו מוגלא או מים
הרבה מאד בפתע הוא יאבד בלי ספק.

אמר המפרש: הבלויים יקראו כל מי שהיה בו מוגלא ברוחב החדר אשר בין החזה והריאה.   10
ויצטרך שיכוה סובל זה החולי ליבש זה הרטיבות כשנלאו לצאת ברקיקה. וכן סובל השקוי
המימיי יוכרתו. וזכר כי זאת ההרקה הפתאומית מאבדת. וכבר יראה גם כן בשאר האיברים
כשנתחדש באחד מהם מורסא גדולה ובלתה והורק הבלוי ממנה בפתע מסתכן כי יקרה
לבעליו ממנו העלוף לאלתר ונפילת הכח ואחר כן כשישאר בחלישותו קשה להשיבו.

(6.28)

[320] אמר אבוקרט: הסריסים לא יקרה להם חולי הנקרס והוא חולי ברגל ולא יקרחו.   15

אמר המפרש: כי הם כמו הנשים וכמו שלא יקרה לנשים הקרחות בעבור רטיבות מזגיהם כן
לא יקרה לאלו. ומיעוט נפילת הנקרס בהם כמו שיתבאר.

(6.29)

[321] אמר אבוקרט: האשה לא יבואנה הנקרס בהם אלא בהפסק נדותן.

אמר המפרש: כבר נתן הסבה במיעוט נפילת הנקרס בנשים וזה להתרוקנות מותריהן בדם
נדותן.   20

(6.30)

[322] אמר אבוקרט: הנער לא יבואנו הנקרס טרם שיתחיל בעשיית המשגל.

---

8 הבלויים: المتقيّحين a ‏ 10 ברוחב החדר: في الفضاء a ‏ 12 יוכרתו: emendation editor: יכרותו צ ‹...›

ובלתה: فتقيّح a ‏ 13 ק

אמר המפרש: (אמר) ג'אלינו' כי לעשיית המשגל יש לו בהולדת הנקרס כח גדול מאד ולא
ביאר סבת זה. והקרוב לפי דעתי כי סבת זה היות הרגלים מעטי הבשר רבי העצבים והמיתרים
והם בולטים אל האויר. וכשהחזיק המשגל לעצבים על הכלל להתרוקנות רוחו והתקררו אותו
תהיה החלישות בעצבי הרגלים יותר חזק. ואנחנו רואים תמיד כשיתקררו הרגלים תבטל קושי
האבר. וזה ראיה על ההשתתפות שבין המשגל והעצבים.

(6.31)

[323] אמר אבוקרט: מכאובי העינים יתירם שתיית היין החי או המרחץ או החבוש או הקזת
העורקים או שתיית המשלשל.

אמר המפרש: כבר ביאר ג'אלינו' אופני בלבול זה הפרק אשר לא יבא על דרך הלמוד המועיל
במלאכת הרפואה. וזכר כי כשהיה החומר חד והיה הגוף נקי מועיל המרחץ להשקיט הכאב.
וכשפסק גם כן פליטת החומר עם נקוי הגוף מועילה התחבושת במים חמים. וכשיהיו עורקי
העין מלאים ונשקע בהם דם עב מבלתי שיהיה שאר הגוף כלו מלא והיתה העין יבשה אז שתיית
היין יתיך המורסא ההיא ויפליט מהעורקים הדבר הנשקע בהם.

וזכר ג'אלינו' (כי) אלו המינים השלשה מן הרפואה הם מסוכנים מאד כי לא ימצא בם מקום
לאמתות. אמנם הקזת העורקים אם נתמלאו דם או הרקת התערובת הגוברת על ידי שלשול
הוא ענין מבואר האמת והוא הנעשה תמיד.

(6.32)

[324] אמר אבוקרט: העלגים הנקרא אלתאג' בע' יקרה להם שלשול הארוך.

אמר המפרש: רוב מה שיהיה סבת הלתאג' הוא מפני רוב רטיבות או רכות ולזה ילתג'ז הנערים
לרוב רטיבותם ורכותם ועם זה המזג ירפה הטבע לרוב.

(6.33)

[325] אמר אבוקרט: בעל הגיהוק החמוץ אי אפשר שימצאנו מדוה הצד.

אמר המפרש: רוב התילדות חולי הצד אמנם הוא מליחה חדה ודקה וקלה (נגרה) אל הקרום
שבפנים לצלעות ותשתקע בו. ובעלי הגיהוק החמוץ רחוק שיתילד בהם זאת הליחה.

(6.34)

[326] אמר אבוקרט: הקרח(ות) לא יקרה לו שיתרחבו העורקים הנקראים דליות ברוב העניין
ומי שנתחדש בו מבעלי הקרחות רוחב הדליות יחזירו שער ראשו.

---

4 החלישות: نكاية ذلك a   12 המורסא ההיא: ذلك الدم a ‖ ויפליט: ويستفرغه ويزعجه من a
16 העלגים הנקרא אלתאג' בע': اللثغ a   17 ילתג'ז: يلثغ a   19 אי אפשר: لا يكاد a   20 ודקה וקלה:
رقيق a   21 רחוק: قلّ a

אמר המפרש: אמר ג'אלינו' כי ר"ל הקרחות בכאן בעלי הנתק. כשנעתק החומר הרע למטה
נתחדש הדליות ויצמח השער.

(6.35)

[327] אמר אבוקרט: כשנתחדש בסובל השקוי השעול (הוא) אות רע.

אמר המפרש: ר"ל כשהיתה סבת השעול השקוי וזה כאשר רבתה רטיב(ו)תו המימית עד
5 שתגיע אל קנה הריאה אז גבה המשקה בשיעור שתחנקהו הרטיבות ההיא.

(6.36)

[328] אמר אבוקרט: הקזת העורקים מתיר קושי השתן (ו)ראוי שיחתכו העורקים הפנימיים.

אמר המפרש: תקן ג'אלינו' זה הפרק בשאמר: כבר יתיר לקושי השתן כשהיתה סבתו מורסא
דמית עם רוב דם. ושאר הפרק אמר שהוא נוסף במאמר אבוקרט והראוי שיהיה ההקזה אז
בעורק הארכובה.)בכל מקום יאמר אבוקרט כי החליים שהם למעלה מהכבד שיקח מעורק
10 הזרועות והחליים שהם למטה מהכבד מן העורקים שהם תחת הארכובות(.

(6.37)

[329] אמר אבוקרט: כשנראית מורסת הגרון מחוץ במי שמצאתהו האסכרה היא אות
משובח כי החולי הותר לחוץ.

אמר המפרש: מבואר הוא כי היותר טוב הוא העתק החולי מן האיברים הפנימיים לצד חוץ.

(6.38)

[330] אמר אבוקרט: כשנתחדש חולי הסרטן הארוך הנסתר היותר טוב הוא שלא יתרפא.
15 ואם יעשה רפואה ימות. ואם לא יעשה רפואה ישאר)כד(זמן ארוך.

אמר המפרש: רצה באמרו הנסתר אשר יהיה בעומק הגוף ולא יראה או שיהיה נגלה ואין עמו
נגע ור"ל בהנחת הרפואה ממין הכריתה או הכויה או החמום.

(6.39)

[331] אמר אבוקרט: חולי הקווץ הוא מן המלוי ומן ההרקה וכן הפיהוק.

אמר המפרש: זה מבואר העלה.

---

1 ר"ל הקרחות בכאן בעלי הנתק: يريد هنا القرع 4 רבתה: emendation editor עَرفة MSS 5 או
גבה המשקה בשיעור: فيكون قد أشفى على a 8 נוסף: دخيل a 9 בעורק הארכובה: في مأبض الركبة
a 11 במי: emendation editor כמו צ)...(ק 12 כי החולי הותר לחוץ: om. a 14 הארוך: om. a
17 או החמום (= أو التسكين): لا التسكين

(6.40)

[332] אמר אבוקרט: מי שקרה לו כאב תחת הצלעות מבלתי צמח ואחר כן נתחדש לו קדחת
הותר זה הכאב מעליו.

אמר המפרש: כשהיה זה הכאב בסבת הרוח או הסתום אז תתיכהו הקדחת וכאלו אמר כבר
התיכהו הקדחת מעליו. וכבר שניתי לך משפטי האיש הלזה באשר גזירותיו רובם והגדולים
שבהם חסירי התנאים או הם באים לפעמים וקצתם הם שגגות באשר נפלו במקרה וחשב הוא
כי שני דברים שנתדבקו במקרה שאחד מהם הוא סבת האחר. כן יאמר מי שאינו עקש ואמנם
המתעקש יאמר מה שירצה.

(6.41)

[333] אמר אבוקרט: כשהיה מקום מן הגוף כבר עשה מוגלא ולא יובן בלותו אמנם לא יובן
מפני עובי החומר או המקום.

אמר המפרש: מבואר כי מפני עובי החומר או עובי המקום יורע ידיעת המוגלא.

(6.42)

[334] אמר אבוקרט: כשהיה הכבד של בעל הירקון קשה הוא אות רע.

אמר המפרש: זה מבואר.

(6.43)

[335] אמר אבוקרט: כשנתחדש בבעל הטחול שלשול מדם ואחר בו יבואהו השקוי או
חליקות המעים וימות בו.

אמר המפרש: בעל הטחול הוא אשר יש בטחול קושי ישן וכשנתחדש שלשול הדם על דרך
העתקת הליחה ההיא העבה השחורית אשר נשתקעה בתוך הטחול הועיל בזה כמו שאמר
אחר כן. ואם ארך השלשול ועבר השיעור יחדש כחות המעים בהסתבכות אלו הליחות הרעות
בהם וחדש חליקות המעים ויכבה החום הטבעי. ומפני השתתפות המעים אל הכבד יחלש
הכבד ויחדש השקוי.

(6.44)

[336] אמר אבוקרט: מי שבא לו הטפת השתן בחולי המעים הנקרא איליאוש ונפסד ממנו
הרגלו בהוצאות הוא ימות בתוך שבעת ימים אלא אם כן יתחדש בו קדחת ונגר ממנו שתן רב.

---

4 שניתי לך: اطّردت a   5 לפעמים: نادرة a ‖ שגגות: وهم a   6 עקש: يتعصّب a   9 החומר: المدّة
a   10 יורע: يعسر a   17 יחדש: (...) ק هلّ a ‖ בהסתבכות: بمرور a   20 בחולי המעים: القولنج a
20–21 ונפסד ממנו הרגלו בהוצאות: وتفسيره المستعاذ منه a

אמר המפרש: כבר נסתפק ג'אלינו' בזה הפרק ולפרש פירושים רחוקים לאמת דברים שהם
גלויים חולשה הוא מפעולת הבטל.

(6.45)

[337] אמר אבוקרט: כשעבר על הנגע שנה או זמן ארוך מזה יתחייב מזה שיוציאו ממנו עצמות
אם יהיה מקום הנגע אחר התרפאו עמוק.

אמר המפרש: רוב מה שיארך זמני הנגעים הוא מפני מכה באה לעצם וכ(ש)יצא העצם יפסד   5
הצורה ונשאר המקום משונה.

(6.46)

[338] אמר אבוקרט: מי שמצאתהו חטוטרת מנזילת ליחה על הריאה אלרבו בערבי ושעול
קודם שצמחו לו שערות שלבית הערוה הוא ימות בקל.

אמר המפרש: כשנתחדשה החטוטרת מבלי סבה מתחלת הוא ממורסא קשה וכשנמשך אחר
זה צרות על הריאה או מפני חזק המורסא ובזמן הגדול תתוסף הריאה ולכן לא יתכן שיתרחבו   10
חדרי החזה ולא יוכל גופו להתגדל מפני החטוטרת ויובשה ולזה יחנק וימות.

(6.47)

[339] אמר אבוקרט: מי שצריך להקיז או לשתות סם משלשל ראוי שישתה הסם או שיקיז
בזמן האביב.

אמר המפרש: זה מבואר למי שצריך אליו על השמירה כמו שיעשו הבריאים תמיד.

(6.48)

[340] אמר אבוקרט: כשיתחדש בבעלי הטחול)תמיד(שלשול הדם הוא אות טוב.   15

אמר המפרש: כבר קדם פירוש זה.

(6.49)

[341] אמר אבוקרט: מי שהיה מתחלואי הנקרס ועמו מורסא חמה אז מורסתו תשקוט
בארבעים יום.

אמר המפרש: כבר קדם לך על איזה צד יתן אלו הגבולים.

---

1 ולפרש פירושים: وتكلّف تأويلات a   2 מפעולת הבטל: من فعل البطّالين a   3 שיוציאו: أنْ يتبيّن
a || עצמות: emendation editor עש(.)תות צ (...) ק   4 הנגע: الأُرَ a   6-5 וכ(ש)יצא העצם יפסד
הצורה: وإذا خرج العظم الفاسد برأت a   7 אלרבו: emendation editor אלרבי   6 משונה: غائِرا a   6 משונה: غائِرا a
8 בקל. MSS   om. a   10 או מפני חזק המורסא: لأجل التقوس a   11 חדרי: فضاء a || גופו: كلّه
a || ויובשה: وسببها a   17 מי: ما a

(6.50)

[342] אמר אבוקרט: מי שנתחדש במוחו כריתה אי אפשר שלא יבא לו קדחת וקיא המרה.

אמר המפרש: כשיצמח במוח מפני החתוך בהכרח ימשך אחריו קדחת וקיא המרה מפני
השתתפות המוח אל הקיבה.

(6.51)

[343] אמר אבוקרט: מי שנתחדש בו בעת בריאותו כאב פתאום בראשו ונשתתק מיד וקרה
5   לו מהומה יאבד בשבעה ימים אם לא יבואנו הקדחת.

אמר המפרש: המהומה הוא אות על חזק השתוק. וכבר ידעת שהיא תמית אם לא שיתחדש
קדחת ואז יתכן שתותר זאת הליחה העבה או הרוח העבה.

(6.52)

[344] אמר אבוקרט: כבר ראוי שתבקר פנימי העין בעת התנומה בחליים החדים. ואם נגלה
מאומה מלובן העין והעפעף אינו סגור בטוב ואין זה מפני שלשול שקדם ולא שתית משקה
10   סם אז הוא אות ממית מאד.

אמר המפרש: אמנם נגלה לובן העין כשלא יסגרו העפעפים ופתיחת העפעפים אמנם הוא מפני
היובש וימהר לאדם כשהוא יבש בטבע או מפני חולשת הכח כמו שיחלוש בחליים החלושים
שאינם יכולים לסתום פיהם.

(6.53)

[345] אמר אבוקרט: מי שהיה מבולבל השכל עם שחוק הוא יותר בטוח. ומי שהיה ממנו עם
15   אבל ויגון הוא יותר מסוכן.

אמר המפרש: אין שום מין מבלבול השכל שהוא בטוח והיותר מזיק שבו מה שהיה עם אבל
ויגון והוא השטות. והפחות מזיק מה שיהיה עם שחוק ושמחה מבלתי שהוא נהוג כסבאות יין
ואשר הוא עם דאגה ופחד ומחשבה הוא ממוצע. וכלם הם מן חולי במוח עצמו או בשכנותו אל
אבר אחר)נזוק(. ואשר הוא מחום לבד מבלתי ליחה הוא דומה לבלבול הדעת שיצא משתית
20   היין ואשר יבא מן המרה הכרכומית יהיה עמו דאגה ומחשבה ופחד. וכשנתוסף אחד מהם
ונטה אל המרה השחורה נטה הבלבול אל השטות.

---

4 פתאום: emendation editor פתאות צ ⟨...⟩ ק   5 מהומה: غطيط a   6 המהומה: الغطيط a
8 בחליים החדים: في وقت النوم a   9 אינו סגור בטוב: مطبق a   10 אות: رديئة a   add. a   12 בחליים:
في المرضى a   16–17 אבל ויגון: إقدام وتهجّم a   17 כסבאות: كشارب a   18 בשכנותו: من أجل
المشاركة a   20 דאגה ומחשבה ופחד: هم وحرص a ‖ אחד מהם: احتراقا a

(6.54)

[346] אמר אבוקרט: נשימה של בכי בחליים החדים אשר עם קדחת הוא אות רע.

אמר המפרש: ר"ל שתהיה נשימ(ה)(ת) החולה נפסקה ותחזור כנשימת מי שחנקו הבכי וזה
יהיה מפני חולשת הכח מחזרת הנשימה או מפני יובש כלי הנשימה וקושיו עד שאין לו כח
להתפשט הנשימה או מפני ענין קרוב אל חולי הקווץ וכל זה בחליים החדים רע מאד.

(6.55)

5   [347] אמר אבוקרט: חולי הנקרס יתעורר באביב ובחורף על הרוב.

אמר המפרש: באביב מפני מרוצת הליחות ותוסיף להתוך קפיאתם מהסתיו ובחורף מפני
(מה) שקדם מאכילת הפירות בקיץ.

(6.56)

[348] אמר אבוקרט: התחלואים השחוריים יפחד מהם שיבוא לידי חולי השתוק או הפלג' או
הקווץ או השטות או אל הדאגה.

10   אמר המפרש: השתוק והפלג' והקווץ והדאגה כבר יבאו מליחה לבנה ומליחה שחורה. ואמנם
חולי השטות לא יבא אלא משרפת הכרכומית עד שתשוב שחורה.

(6.57)

[349] אמר אבוקרט: השתוק והפלג' תתחדשנה בפרט למי שיהיה מן השנים ב(י)ן הארבעים
והששים.

אמר המפרש: באר ג'אלינו' זה הפרק כדי שישוב מאמר אמתי. ר"ל השתוק והפלג'
15   המתחדשות מהמרה השחורה כי המרה השחורה תגבר על בעלי אלו השנים. ואמנם
לפי ביאור האמת חדושיהן תהיינה מן השחורה הקרה מאד והוא בדרך זרות גדול וברוב
תתחדשנה מהלבנה. ומזמן הששים שנה עד סוף החיים.

(6.58)

[350] אמר אבוקרט: כשיצא לחוץ החלב הנה הוא בלא ספק יתעפש.

אמר המפרש: זה מבואר.

---

3 מחזרת הנשימה: عن استيفاء التنفّس a‏ 3–4 עד שאין לו כח להתפשט הנשימה: حتّى لا تقدر القوّة أنْ
تبسطه a‏ 4 מאד a‏ 9 הדאגה (= الغمّ): om. a‏ 10 המפרש: قال جالينوس add. a‏ ‖ והדאגה
(= والغمّ): والعمى a‏ 16 חדושיהן תהיינה מן השחורה הקרה מאד והוא בדרך זרות גדול: حدوث هذين
من السوداء نادر جدًّا a

(6.59)

[351] אמר אבוקרט: מי שהיה בו כאב גיד הנשה ונשמטה ירכו ושוב חזרה ודאי כבר נולד בו
רטיבות רירי דומה לליחה היוצאת מהנחירים.

אמר המפרש: מפני רטיבות הרירי המדובק יתבטלו המיתרים וימהר השמטת עצם הקולית
מהירך.

(6.60)

[352] אמר אבוקרט: מי שבאתהו כאב מיושן בירכיו ונשמטה ירכו ודאי יצטמק רגלו מכל וכל   5
ואם לא יכוה יהיה צולע.

אמר המפרש: נגוב זה הרטיבות הרירי הוא בכויה וכשלא יתנגב זה הרטיבות בכויה יתחדש
הצליעה ולא יזונו הרגלים על מנהגיהם ויצטמקו.

נשלם המאמר הששי מפרקי אבוקרט.

---

1 נולד בו: נולד ⟨...⟩ **צק** حدثت به a   2 דומה לליחה היוצאת מהנחירים: a .om   3 המדובק: .om
a ׀׀ יתבטלו: (= تبطّل): تبطّل a

המאמר השביעי

(7.1)

[353] אמר אבוקרט: קור הקצוות בתחלואים החדים אות רע.

אמר המפרש: זהו אצלי ראיה על חולשת החום היסודי והיותה לא תתפשט אל הקצוות
עם היות החולי חד ר״ל חם כי אבוקרט כבר יקרא חוליים חדים לתחלואים אשר
תהיה בהם הקדחת ארוכה מתמדת. והקצוות הם קצה האף וקצה האזנים והידים 5
והרגלים.

(7.2)

[354] אמר אבוקרט: כשהיה חולי בעצם והיה מראה הבשר עליו כהה זה הוא אות רע.

אמר המפרש: זה המראה נמשך אחר הכבות החום הטבעי.

(7.3)

[355] אמר אבוקרט: התחדשות הפיהוק ואודם העינים אחרי הקיא אות רע.

אמר המפרש: כשלא יוסר הקווץ אחר הקיא הוא אות שסבתו הוא או מצמח בראש העצבים 10
ר״ל המוח או מצמח בקיבה ואודם העינים הוא נמשך אחר אלו שני הצמחים.

(7.4)

[356] אמר אבוקרט: כשנתחדש אחר הזיעה סימור אינו אות יפה.

אמר המפרש: כבר אמר אבוקרט שמקרה הגבול כשלא יבא אחריהם נקיון מורה על מות או
על קושי הגבול כי הטבע נכשל.

(7.5)

[357] אמר אבוקרט: כשנתחדש בעבור חולי השטות שלשול הדם או שקוי או גרה הוא אכול 15
העינים הוא אות יפה.

אמר המפרש: אמנם השקוי והשלשול יבריאנו מפני העתק החומר. ואמנם הגרה כי המקרים
כשנתוספו ונתחזקו ידחו את הטבע ויעוררהו לדחות כל מה שיזיק על דרך הגבול כן פירשו
ג׳אלינו׳.

15–16 גרה הוא אכול העינים: حيرة‎ a   17 הגרה: الحيرة‎ a

(7.6)

[358] אמר אבוקרט: הפסד תאות המאכל בחלי הישן והרעי הזך שלא יתערב בו מן הרטיבות המיימית ואמנם יצא החולי אשר בגוף לבדו ולמיני המרה הכרכומית או ממיני השחורה. וכל זה ראיה על שהרטיבות היסודיית כלה נשרפה מפני חום הקדחת.

(7.7)

[359] אמר אבוקרט: כשתתחדש מרוב שתיית היין הסמור והרתת וערבוב שכל הוא אות רע.

אמר המפרש: התקבץ הסמור עם בלבול השכל יקרה מעט אלא בקצת סובאי יין המשתכרים   5
ויכבה החום היסודי ויתחדש הסמור וימלא המוח דם חם ועשן חם ויתבלבל השכל.

(7.8)

[360] אמר אבוקרט: כשנתפתח הצמח ונשפך לצד פנימי הגוף יבא מזה נפילת הכח וקיא ומריכות נפש.

אמר המפרש: זה מבואר ור״ל בצמח הנקרא דבילה בער׳ ור״ל פנימי הגוף הקיבה.

(7.9)

[361] אמר אבוקרט: כשנתחדש מפני נזילת הדם בלבול השכל או קווץ הוא אות רע.   10

אמר המפרש: בלבול השכל אחר ההרקה יהיה להפעמות המוח בתנועתו והוא לעולם בחולשא ואבוקרט (קורא) לבלבול השכל החלוש הזיה.

(7.10)

[362] אמר אבוקרט: כשיתחדש עם חולי מעים (הנקרא) קולנג׳ שינהג אחריו הקיא או הפיהוק או ערבוב שכל וקווץ זה הוא אות רע.

אמר המפרש: זה מבואר.   15

(7.11)

[363] אמר אבוקרט: כשיתחדש ממדוה הצד מדוה הריאה זהו אות רע.

אמר המפרש: כשלא יספוק הליחה המתחדש לחולי הצד מקומה יעדיף ממנה דבר אל הריאה. ואמנם מדוה הריאה אי אפשר שימשך אחריו חולי הצד.

---

1 הזך: دليل ردي‌ء. قال المفسّر: يريد بالبراز الصرف add. a   3 נשרפה: emendation editor: ושרפה MSS
5 סובאי יין המשתכרים: مكثري السكر a   8 ומריכות: (...) ק وذبول a   11 להפעמות: لاضطراب a
13 עם: عن a ‖ שינהג אחריו: المستعاذ منه a

(7.12)

[364] אמר אבוקרט: ומן מדוה הריאה מדוה השרסם הוא צמח במות.

(7.13)

[365] אמר אבוקרט: ומן השריפה החזקה חולי הקווץ והמתוח.

(7.14)

[366] אמר אבוקרט: ומן מכת הראש הבהלה ובלבול השכל.

(7.15)

[367] אמר אבוקרט: ומרקיקת הדם רקיקת המוגלא.

(7.16)

5   [368] אמר אבוקרט: ומרקיקת המוגלא הכליון והנזילה. וכשנפסק הרוק ימות בעל החולי.

(7.17)

[369] אמר אבוקרט: ו(מ)מורסות הכבד הפיהוק.

(7.18)

[370] אמר אבוקרט: ומן התעורה הקווץ ובלבול השכל.

אמר המפרש: זה מבואר ופירושו כאשר גדלו הכאבים ונושנו פעמים יתחדש ממנו כך וכך כמו
כי צמח הכבד כשהגדיל והזיק פי הקיבה חדש הפיהוק. וכבר ידעת כי הקווץ ובלבול השכל
10   כבר ימצא מיובש. והיובש ימשך אחרי רוב ההרקה והתנועה הנפשיית והתעורה.

(7.19)

[371] אמר אבוקרט: ומהתגלות העצם המורסא הנקרא אדום אלחמרה בער׳.

אמר המפרש: ביאר ג׳אלינו׳ כי התגלות העצם לא תתחדש בעבור(ו) זאת המורסא אלא
לפעמים מועטים אבל הוא זכר כל מה שאפשר שימשך אחר דבר ואפילו על המעט.

(7.20)

[372] אמר אבוקרט: ומן המורסא הנקרא חומרה העפוש והבלוי.

15   אמר המפרש: זה מבואר לפי מה שקדם כמה פעמים שר״ל כבר תתחדש כך וכך.

---

3 השכל: ردي، a add. a   8 זה: كلّ هذا a ‖ הכאבים: هذه العلل a ‖ ונושנו: وفاقت a   10 והתעורה:
אמר אבוקרט: ومحولي השכחה הרעש צק. add. a   14 והבלוי: والتقيّح a   15 שקדם: emendation editor
שקרה צ ⟨...⟩ ק

(7.21)

[373] אמר אבוקרט: ומן ההכאה החזקה בנגע השפך הדם.

אמר המפרש: זה מבואר כי לחוזק הצער יתנועעו העורקים תנועה מופלגת לדחות המזיק.

(7.22)

[374] אמר אבוקרט: ומן הכאב הישן לעומת הקיבה מוגלא.

אמר המפרש: הכאב הישן אמנם יהיה בעבורו המורסא. וזאת המורסא עתיד להגלות.

(7.23)

[375] אמר אבוקרט: ומן הרעי הזך שלשול הדם.   5

אמר המפרש: ר״ל שיהיה הרעי ליחה מהליחות בלבד שכבר חדש אכול ונגע במעים.

(7.24)

[376] אמר אבוקרט: ומכריתות העצם הבהלה ובלבול השכל אם הגיע בחלל.

אמר המפרש: כשיחתך העצם של הראש עד שיגיע החתך למקום החלול המקיף למוח יחדש
ערבוב השכל.

(7.25)

[377] אמר אבוקרט: הקווץ הבא משתיית הסם המשלשל ממית.   10

(7.26)

[378] אמר אבוקרט: קרירות הקצוות מכאב חזק ההוה שלעומת הקיבה הוא רע.

(7.27)

[379] אמר אבוקרט: כשנתחדש בהרה שלשול של זחיר עצור יהיה סבה שתפיל.

אמר המפרש: זה מבואר.

---

4 עתיד להגלות: سيتقيّح a   6 שיהיה ... שכבר חדש: إنْ يكون ... فقط قد يحدث a   7 הבהלה: om.
a   8 המפרש: يقول إنَّ add. a   10 ממית: قال المفسّر: هذا بيّن add. a   11 רע: قال المفسّر: هذا بيّن add.
a   12 שלשול של זחיר עצור: زحير a

(7.28)

[380] אמר אבוקרט: כשנחתך דבר מן העצם או מן החלל או מן העצבים לא יתאחה.

אמר המפרש: כבר הודה ג'אלינו' שזה חזרת המאמר.

(7.29)

[381] אמר אבוקרט: אם חודש במי שגבר עליו הליחה הלבנה שלשול חזק הותר חליו מעליו.

אמר המפרש: הלבנה הוא השקוי הבשריי. אמר המחבר: וכבר ראיתי זה פעמים.

(7.30)

[382] אמר אבוקרט: מי שהיה בו שלשול והיה מה שישלשל הדבר מקוצף כבר היה סבת   5
שלשולו דבר שיצא מן הראש.

אמר המפרש: סבת הדבר המקוצף הוא התערב האויר לו התערבות חזקה. כבר יהיה זה
הרטיבות הבא מן הראש או מן האיברים האחרים או שיתילד בקיבה והמעים.

(7.31)

[383] אמר אבוקרט: מי שהיה לו קדחת ויצלול בשתנו שמרים דומים לשחיקת הגריסים יורה
על אורך החולי.   10

אמר המפרש: התערובת אשר יהיה זה ממנו הוא רחוק מהתבשל ולזה זכר אבוקרט כי אלו
ימותו על הרוב. ומי שינצל מהם יארך חליו כמו שזכר הנה.

(7.32)

[384] אמר אבוקרט: כשגבר על השמרים שבשתן המרירה והיה עליונו דק מורה על שחליו
חד.

אמר המפרש: זה מובן וירצה באמרו דק שיהיה עליון השמרים דק ויהיה תמונתו כמו הלב   15
הפיניא.

(7.33)

[385] אמר אבוקרט: מי ששתנו מתפזר זה יורה על שיש בגופו התפעמות חזק.

אמר המפרש: ר"ל מחולף החלקים וזה מורה על התחלפות פעולת הטבע בליחות.

---

1 החלל: الغضروف a ‖ או מן העצבים- :om. a, but cf. Galen, *In Hippocratis Aphorismos commenta*-
rius 7.28, ed. Kühn, vol. 18a, p. 126: ἢ νεῦρον ‖   6 שיצא: يخدر a   15 וירצה: emendation editor
ויראה MSS

(7.34)

[386] אמר אבוקרט: מי שהיה על שתנו רב אבעבועות יורה על שהחולי בכליות וההבטה ממנו באריכות.

אמר המפרש: שהוא מורה על רוח עבה בתוך תערובת מדובקת ולזה מביט באריכות חולי.

(7.35)

[387] אמר אבוקרט: מי שנראה בעליון שתנו שומן הרבה מורה על שבכליותיו חולי חד.

אמר המפרש: כשהשומן בא פתאום באחת הוא מורה על התכת חלב הכליות וזה הוא פירוש   5
אמרו הרבה שאם יבא מהתכת חלב של שאר האיברים היה בא מעט מעט.

(7.36)

[388] אמר אבוקרט: מי שהיה בו חולי הכליות וקרה לו המקרים שזכרנו למעלה
(ו)מתחדש (בו) כאב כבד)או(אם היה הכאב במקומות החיצונים יפלו בו צמחים
שיצאו ממנו לחוץ. ואם היה זה הכאב במקומות הפנימיים הדין שיהיה צמח דבילה בער'
מבפנים.   10

אמר המפרש: זה מובן.

(7.37)

[389] אמר אבוקרט: אשר יקיא הדם מבלתי הקדחת ינצל וראוי שיעזור בעליו בדברים
הקובצים והדם שיוציא בקיא עם קדחת הוא רע.

אמר המפרש: ר"ל כשלא יהיה עמו מורסא בקיבה אשר נמשכה אחריה קדחת בהכרח.
או הדם היה מפני עורק שנתק או נגע נתחדש עתה ואיפשר שיבריא מהרה בדברים   15
הקובצים.

(7.38)

[390] אמר אבוקרט: הנזילה הבאה אל הגוף העליון יעשה מוגלא בעשרים יום.

אמר המפרש: הגוף העליון הוא חדר החזה אשר בו הריאה ויום העשרים הוא יום הגבול להיותו
סוף השבוע השלישי. ונאמר שזה הרחוק מה שיתכן שיתבשל בו הנזילה.

1 רב (= עב?) אבעבועות: عنب a   4 הרבה: جملة a   6 הרבה: جملة a ‖ שאם: أمّا الذي a   8 כבד:
في عضل صلبه a   12 שיעזור: أنْ يعالج a   15 או הדם היה: وكان قيء هذا الدم a   17 הבאה: التي تنحدر
a ‖ הגוף: الجوف a

(7.39)

[391] אמר אבוקרט: מי שהשתין דם הקרוש והיה בו הטפת השתן וקושיו ומצאתהו כאב אצל
הטבור ובית הערוה זה אות על שיש בשלפוחיתו הכאב.

אמר המפרש: השיב דבריו פעמים.

(7.40)

[392] אמר אבוקרט: כשנעדר האדם מלשונו פתאום או רפיון אבר מאבריו אז החולי מן
השחורה.

אמר המפרש: כבר הודה ג׳אלינו׳ שלא יתחייב שיהיה זה מן השחורה בהכרח.

(7.41)

[393] אמר אבוקרט: כשבא לזקן בסבת הרקת שלשול או קיא הפיהוק אינו סימן יפה.

אמר המפרש: הפיהוק אחר ההרקה רע כי הוא נמשך אחר יובש ובזקנים הוא יותר רע ליובש
מזגם מכל השנים.

(7.42)

[394] אמר אבוקרט: מי שמצאתהו קדחת לא ממרה ונשפך על ראשו מים חמים לרוב יחסר
מזה חמימותו.

אמר המפרש: ג׳אלינו׳ ישתדל לפרש זה הפרק בשאמר כי כונתו באמרו קדחת לא ממרה
שאינה קדחת מעפוש אבל קצת מפני קדחת יומיית ואין ספק כי המרחץ בו מועיל ובו תותר
הקדחת.

(7.43)

[395] אמר אבוקרט: האשה לא תהיה בעלת שני ימינים. אמר גאלינוס: עלת זה חולשת עצבים
ועצלים כי בעלת שני ימינים אמנם סבתו הוא מכח העצבים.

(7.44)

[396] אמר אבוקרט: מי שנכוה מהבלוייס ויצא ממנו מוגלא נקיה לבנה פתאום ינצל. ומי שיצא
ממנו מוגלא כמו טיט וירוקה מוסרחת ימות.

---

2 הטבור (= السِّرَّة ACP): الشَّرج (= السِّرَّة ACP)   Pᴵᵗ S, fol. 148ª   3 השיב דבריו פעמים: تَكَرَّر معناه a   4 מלשונו:
قوّه add. a ‖ رפיון (= اسْترْخاء): اسْترْخى a ‖ אז: אז emendation editor: MSS או   10 יחסר (= نَقَصت):
انقَضت a   13 קצת מפני קדחת יומיית: بعض أنواع حمّى يوم a   17 שנכוה: أوبطّ add. a (except for
BCP)   18 כמו טיט וירוקה: كَرة a

אמר המפרש: הבלויים הם אשר יתקבצו חמר הרבה בין חזיהם והריאה שלהם ולאותם
החליים היה מנהג הקדמונים לכוותם להוציא החומר הנעצר.

(7.45)

[397] אמר אבוקרט: מי שהיה לו בכבדו מוגלא ונכוה ויצא ממנו מוגלא נקיה לבנה הוא ינצל.
וזה אם היתה זאת המוגלא בו בקרום הכבד ואם יצא ממנו כדמות שמרי השמן ימות.

5   אמר המפרש: כשהיתה המוגלא בקרום ובגוף הכבד ינצל והוא אפשר ההתנצלות.

(7.46)

[398] אמר אבוקרט: כאב העינים טוב לו שישתה בעליו יין חי ואחרי כן יכנס במרחץ וישפוך
עליו מים חמים לרוב ואחרי כן יקיז)ובזה יותר ממנו מכאוביו(.

אמר המפרש: ג'אלינו')אמר(כי זה הפרק נחשד אל אבוקרט אחר ובכלל הוא טעות גמור
אמרו מי שאמרו.

(7.47)

[399] אמר אבוקרט: כשנתחדש בבעל השקוי שעול לא יבריא.
10

אמר המפרש: זכרנו פירוש זה.

(7.48)

[400] אמר אבוקרט: קושי השתן והטפתו יתירנו שתיית היין וההקזה ויצטרך שיקיז העורק
הפנימי.

אמר המפרש: זה המאמר הוא נגלה הפסדו אבל ג'אלינו' כבר הציל להוציא לתחלת זה הפרק
15   אופן האמתת. ואמר כשהיתה סבת זה קור או סתום מחודשת מדם עב מבלתי מלוי שאר הגוף
אז היה שתיית היין הרב מועיל לזה. ואמנם אמרו בזה הפרק ויצטרך להקיז העורק הפנימי וכן
מאמר שאמר בפרק שלפני זה כבר פירש ג'אלינו' כי זה בלתי אמת ואין זה דעת אבוקרט.

(7.49)

[401] אמר אבוקרט: כשנראית המורסא האדומה אלחמרה בער' במי שבא לו האסכרה הנה
זה אות יפה כי החולי כבר נטה לצאת לצד חוץ.

20   אמר המפרש: זה מבואר.

1–2 ولאותם החליים: وهم الذين a   2 הנעצר: om. a   5 ובגוף הכבד ינצל: وجرم الكبد سالم a
8 נחשד אל אבוקרט אחר: دلّس على أبقراط a   10 יבריא: يرجا a   14 הציל: قد تكلّف a ‖ להוציא:
emendation editor לנמצא צ למצא ק   15 שאר: om. a   18 המורסא האדומה אלחמרה בער': الورم
والحمرة a

(7.50)

[402] אמר אבוקרט: מי שמצאהו במוחו החולי הנקרא סקקלינוס כליון ימות בשלשה ימים
ואם יעברם ינצל.

אמר המפרש: זה החולי הוא הפסד המות עצמו ואין לו בריאות כשגבר. אמנם כשהתחיל זה
החולי ועבר שלשה ימים הנה הוא ראיה על שלא גבר בו ושהטבע גבר והצליח.

(7.51)

5 [403] אמר אבוקרט: העטוש)ש(יהיה בראש כשנתחמם המוח ונרטב המקום החלל אשר
בראש ונלכד שמה הרוח ונשמע לו קול רעם כי התפלשותו ויציאתו יהיה במקום צר.

אמר המפרש: כבר יהיה העטוש כשנתחמם המוח ונרטב המקום החלול אשר בו והותרה
זאת הרטיבות לעשן. וכבר ידחה עם השעול רוח מלמטה וכשבא במעברות הנחירים היה סבה
להתחדשות העטוש. ומעברות האף יעברו אל שני מקומות אל הפה ואל המות. ונקב המפולש
10 אל הפה ינוקה ברוח ונדחה מלמטה. ואמנם המעברות אשר יתפלשו אל המוח יתנקו ברוח
אשר רועם ממנו. ואמרו המקום החלל רוצה לומר בטן המוח.

(7.52)

[404] אמר אבוקרט: מי שהיה בו כאב חזק בכבדו ובא לו קדחת הותר זה הכאב מעליו.

אמר המפרש: כאב חזק בכבד בלתי קדחת אמנם יהיה מרוח עב ולכן כשנתחדשה הקדחת
הותר זה הרוח.

(7.53)

15 [405] אמר אבוקרט: מי שצריך להוצאת דם מן העורקים ראוי שיקטע העורק בזמן האביב.

אמר המפרש: זה הפרק הוחזר פעמים.

(7.54)

[406] אמר אבוקרט: מי שהרגיש בו ליחה לבנה במה שבין הקיבה והטרפש ובא לו כאב
מאשר אין לה מקום מנוס לצאת אל אחד החדרים אז זאת הליחה כשנגרה בעורקים אל
השלפוחית הותר מעליו חליו.

20 אמר המפרש: כבר נאמר כי זה הפרק אינו דברי אבוקרט ואמר ג'אלינו' כי לא ימנע עבור אלו
הליחות לעורקים באידיות כי הטבע מתעסק לדקק הליחות ולהוציאם בכל דרך שיוכל ואפילו

_____
1 החולי הנקרא סקקלינוס: سفاقلوس a ‖ עצמו: .om a   3 כשגבר: إذا استحكم a ‖ אמנם: يريد أنه
a   4 ימים: ولم يهلك add. a   6 ונלכד: فانحدر a ‖ גבר: يستحكم a ‖ add. a   רעם: فانحدر a   8 ידחה =)
يدفع): يرتفع a   10 ונדחה: التي ترتفع a   11 רועם: تنحدر a   17 שהרגיש: تحيّز a

מאחרי הקרומים כמו שידחה המוגלא המתקבצת במה שבין החזה והריאה. ובכלל הוא מאמר
שנופל על המעט ומעט התועלת בו מאד.

(7.55)

[407] אמר אבוקרט: מי שנמלא כבדו מים ואחרי כן נשפכו אלו המים אל הקרום הפנימי לבטן
יתמלא בטנו מים וימות.

אמר המפרש: כבר יתחדש זה הנפח הרבה פעמים בכבד ואמרו מי שנתמלא בטנו מים שימות   5
הוא על הרוב.

(7.56)

[408] אמר אבוקרט: המצוק והעלוף והסמור ירפאם כשנמזג היין בשוה עם המים.

אמר המפרש: רוב המצוק יבא מרטיבות מזקת אשר בפי הקיבה ושתיית היין המזוג מעט כמו
שזכר ירפאנו מכל זה להכבסו העורקים ותקונו לתערובות.

(7.57)

[409] אמר אבוקרט: מי שיצא בו שחין דק בטבעתו כשיבלה ויצא יתחסר מעליו כאבו.   10

אמר המפרש: זה מוחזר פעמים.

(7.58)

[410] אמר אבוקרט: מי שיזעזע וינוע מוחו ימצאנו מיד השתוק.

אמר המפרש: כשיהיה זעזוע המוח בחוט השדרה בעבור הכאה או כיוצא בו.

(7.59a–b)

[411]

(7.60)

[412] אמר אבוקרט: מי שבשרו רטוב ראוי שירעיב עצמו כי הרעב מיבש הגויות.   15

אמר המפרש: זה מבואר.

---

1 מאחרי הקרומים: بعد ودقّ a   2 שנופל על המעט: قليل الوقوع a   5 הנפח: النفّاخات a   7 והעלוף:
والثاؤب a   9 להכבסו העורקים: להכנסו בעורקים MSS لغسله a emendation editor   10 בטבעתו:
في إحليله a   כשיבלה: إذا تقيّحت a ‖ יתחסר (= نقص): انقضى a   13 כשיהיה: إنّما يكون a ‖ בעבור
הכאה: بسقطة a   14 This aphorism is missing in the Arabic and Hebrew MSS, as it is a repetition
of aphorisms 4.34–35

(7.61)

[413] אמר אבוקרט: כשתתחדש בגוף כלו שינויים ויתקרר קור גדול ושוב יתחמם ויצטבע מגוונים ושוב ישתנה ויתהפך לגוון אחר זה מביט באריכות חולי.

אמר המפרש: זה מבואר.

(7.62)

[414] אמר אבוקרט: הזיעה הרבה הנגרת תמיד חמה תהיה או קרה יורה על שצריך להוציא

5 מגופו רטיבות אמנם מלמעלה לחזק אמנם מלמטה למי שהוא חלוש.

אמר המפרש: אמרו כי הרטיבות ינוקה מן החזק בקיא ומן החלוש בשלשול לא ינהג זה תמיד. וכבר ידעת דרכי האיש הלזה וכבר נסתפק ג׳אלינו׳ בזה הפרק האם הוא מאמר אבוקרט או זולתו.

נשלמו פרקי אבוקרט.